COMPLETE GUIDE TO

SPORTS INJURIES

HOW TO TREAT —
Fractures, Bruises, Sprains, Strains, Dislocations, Head Injuries

---

By H. Winter Griffith, M.D.

Illustrations by Mark Pederson

THE BODY PRESS/PERIGEE

Withdrawn

A Perigee Book
Published by The Berkley Publishing Group
A division of Penguin Group (USA) Inc.
375 Hudson Street
New York, New York 10014

Perigee edition: March 2004

ISBN 978-0-399-52954-2

Visit our website at
www.penguin.com

Printed in the United States of America
10 9 8 7 6 5 4 3 2

Contents

About the Author

H. Winter Griffith, M.D., a Fellow of the American Academy of Family Physicians, has had a lifelong participation and interest in athletics and exercise. A high school and college athlete, Dr. Griffith was team physician for several years for Florida State University athletic teams. Dr. Griffith has authored several medical books, including the best-selling *Complete Guide to Prescription & Nonprescription Drugs* and *Complete Guide to Symptoms, Illness & Surgery*. Dr. Griffith received his medical degree from Emory University in 1953, and spent more than 20 years in private practice. He established a basic medical science program at Florida Slate University and was director of the family practice residency program at Tallahassee Memorial Hospital. Dr. Griffith then became associate professor of Family & Community Medicine at the University of Arizona College of Medicine. Until his death in 1993, Dr. Griffith lived in Tucson, Arizona.

Mark Pederson is a certified medical illustrator (CMI) and has been published in more than 100 journal articles and books. He has been director of the Visual Communications Department, Annenberg Center for Health Sciences, in Rancho Mirage, California, since 1991. Mr. Pederson was head of the Medical Illustration Section, Division of Biomedical Communications, College of Medicine, University of Arizona, in Tucson for more than 17 years. He taught in the Department of Anatomy at the University of Michigan while earning a master of science degree in medical and biological illustration. He is a member of the Association of Medical Illustrators. Mr. Pederson is a sports enthusiast and remains active in a number of sports activities.

Technical Consultants

David A. Friscia, M.D.
Orthopedic surgeon, Rancho Mirage, CA.

Karen Friscia P.T.
Rancho Mirage, CA

Ruth Schaller
Nurse practitioner, Tucson, AZ

Preface

The recent increase in organized and recreational sports participation for all ages and both sexes has been accompanied by a significant increase in the number of injuries sustained by these athletes. Most of these injuries are minor sprains, strains and bruises, and many are due to overuse rather than to external force. Other injuries are more serious and usually require the attention of a physician or other members of the medical team. Some of these injuries require hospitalization and surgery. Rarely, athletic participation may result in a catastrophic injury with prolonged disability, paralysis or even death.

This book will be extremely beneficial in the recognition and care of minor injuries, helping the reader to know not only what is wrong, but also how to administer first aid and determine when to be seen by a physician. Even in the case of more serious injuries, the injured person and his or her family will be able to better understand the condition and what might be expected before full recovery is reached.

This book is recommended reading for all coaches, parents and athletes-regardless of age or sex.

SPORTS, EXERCISE & YOUR HEALTH

We are living at a time when interest in sports and fitness has never been higher. Correspondingly, our knowledge about injury and illness as a result of physical activity has also increased. The purpose of this book is to share this knowledge with you, giving you some guidelines about prudent physical activity and athletic participation. But first we must examine the relationship between physical activity and good health.

THE BENEFITS OF EXERCISE

Regular exercise or athletic activity plays a key role in staying healthy. Not only is exercise an important part of treating medical problems such as hypertension, depression and high blood fat levels (especially high levels of low-density cholesterol)—it can also be important in *preventing* many of these same medical problems.

Regular exercise also improves your body image and increases your energy level. It helps control weight and reduces stress.

If you are an athlete engaged in a competitive sport or if you are a fitness enthusiast participating in a regular exercise program, you are familiar with the many benefits of regular physical activity. If you do not participate in a sport or fitness program, the following suggestions will help you choose and begin the right program for you. Exercise comes in many forms— everyone should be able to find some activity enjoyable.

7 STEPS TO CHOOSING A SPORT OR EXERCISE PROGRAM

(1) Obtain a physical examination from your doctor so you will know if you have any limitations that affect your choice of activity.

(2) Choose an activity you enjoy. Some people prefer an exercise they can do alone so they don't have to coordinate plans with others. Other people enjoy the company and extra incentive provided by workout partners. The best sport or exercise for you is one you *do*. So look around, join a club, find others to join you or set out on your own—but begin!

(3) Set aside time to work out. It's best to start at three sessions per week, then increase gradually to four, five or more. Some people schedule a session every day. When interruptions occur, they still get the recommended minimum of three exercise sessions a week.

Most people find that setting aside a consistent time each day helps them get into the habit of working out. The time of day is not important as long as you don't try to exercise or play on a full stomach. On the other hand, exercising on an empty stomach first thing in the morning is not always a good idea either. A light meal 30 minutes to one hour before your workout should not interfere with your performance. Common-sense measures, such as avoiding the heat of the day and not exercising when sick, are important.

(4) Be prudent as to the amount of time you exercise each day. The ideal duration is 30 minutes of continuous activity. Some people find it necessary

to begin with 10 to 15 minutes and build up. Except for those who train for athletic competition, it is not necessary to spend many hours a day exercising. (5) Choose the proper intensity of exercise. Appropriate intensity varies greatly depending on your age, sex and medical condition. Many doctors recommend aerobic exercise as beneficial for most persons. It can be geared to an individual's fitness level and increased as one's ability allows.

Exercise is aerobic if it accelerates the heart rate to a prescribed level, sustains the physical activity for at least 20 minutes, uses major muscle groups of the body and is regulated in intensity and duration. Aerobic exercise should be done at least three times a week to achieve cardiopulmonary-vascular fitness—a strong and healthy heart, lungs and blood vessels.

The best forms of aerobic exercise include brisk walking, swimming, bike riding, jogging, rope jumping, rowing or aerobic dance. Sports such as tennis and golf have good recreational effects, but they do not require enough sustained effort to reach and maintain aerobic levels for a sufficient period of time.

Although we have defined aerobic exercise here, we strongly recommend that you read one of the many books on this subject to get a broader view of the benefits and techniques of this important category of exercise. Check your library or bookstore.
(6) Incorporate additional exercise into your day whenever you can. Park your car far enough from your destination to allow a good walk. Use the stairs instead of taking the elevator. Use manual rather than power tools.
(7) Vary your activity, alternating sports and forms of exercise to avoid boredom. It takes about a month of good, regular exercise before you will begin to see and feel the benefits. Meanwhile, use whatever tricks you can think of to keep yourself going.

THE RISKS OF EXERCISE

Despite the many healthy benefits obtained through sports and exercise, injuries and illnesses can occur as a result of physical activity. Anyone participating in a contact sport such as football can expect some of the contact to be hard on the body. Bruises, sprains, broken bones, concussions—even deaths—have been known to occur. We are now aware of many factors that can help prevent injuries, and prevention is the best cure. For example, protective equipment kept in good repair, a well-conditioned body and adequate warm-up go a long way toward preventing serious injuries in athletics. But accidents do happen.

In addition, certain preexisting conditions can increase the danger or difficulty of participation in physical activity. For example, if a person has an infection, his performance will not be up to par—he may make himself sicker or be more prone to injury. Some pre-existing conditions are permanent, such as diabetes mellitus, and these have a bearing on how a person can participate. The whole body is involved in any kind of exercise program, and its state must be taken into account. The presence of such preexisting medical illnesses requires consultation with your doctor prior to beginning any exercise program.

THE GOALS OF THIS BOOK

This book is designed to help you maintain or achieve a satisfactory level of good health. Good physical and mental health is essential to winning in competitive sports and achieving an optimal level of fitness. This book is *your* resource—it has been written for you with the following objectives:

• To present a concise, comprehensive, clear guide to sports injuries and illnesses.

• To address the benefits and risks of competitive athletics and to minimize the frequency of the only major risk: injury.

• To provide parents with information about the physical requirements for competing and the various aspects of injuries to athletes of all ages, including youngsters and adolescents. This will help parents make informed decisions regarding sports activities for their children.

• To equip young people with enough information to make wise decisions about their participation in sports.

• To encourage safe participation in sports among all age groups by providing information on how to prevent and treat illness and injury.

• To provide coaches and trainers with a guide to technical concepts they need to know so they can instruct and supervise the athletes they direct. Trainers and coaches can be effective teachers—they have great influence over impressionable young people, and they attract great devotion.

• To make it possible for athletes or parents to render self-care when it is appropriate.

• To call attention to situations when parents or athletes need to obtain professional help.

• To provide information and understanding when surgery or other drastic measures have been recommended.

The information in this book comes from experienced, authoritative experts in the field of sports injuries and sports medicine, and it represents a consensus among professionals when such a consensus exists.

To organize and present information as clearly as possible, this book has been divided into two major sections, Sports Injuries and Sports Medicine. Each of these sections is made up of easy-to-use charts. A chart format was chosen to make it easy to find the information you need quickly. Other smaller sections—entitled Rehabilitation, Appendix, Glossary, Index and Emergency First Aid— follow the first two sections. The smaller sections do not include charts.

Each sports injury chart addresses one specific injury, including text and an illustration that allows you to compare normal and injured anatomy. It includes information about how to identify the injury, how to prevent the injury and what first aid to administer if you find someone injured. It can serve as an informal second opinion for the treatment of each injury. It also covers what to expect as you are treated and during recovery, what activity level you can expect to be allowed, what rehabilitation you might need and any diet restrictions needed.

Each sports medicine chart addresses a common noninjury medical problem that might occur among athletes and others engaged in vigorous physical activity. Some problems are caused by conditions such as crowded locker rooms or the use of athletic equipment. Others are not unique to athletes, but can affect athletic performance either temporarily or permanently. Still others can be caused or made worse by athletic activity. Information on how to recognize the medical problem, how to prevent it, how it is usually treated and how you can expect it to affect your performance is included.

The Guide to Sports Injury Charts, page 14, and Guide to Sports Medicine Charts, page 21, explain in detail what is included on each chart.

Following is a brief explanation of the other book sections.

The Rehabilitation section is an important adjunct to the sports injury charts. This section provides programs of exercise and conditioning that can be followed after injury to the major areas of the body. Most of the injury charts contain a reference to this section.

The exercises are simple and generally don't require special equipment. However, consult your doctor before attempting the exercises following any moderate to severe injury

The Appendix deals with sports medicine topics of a more general nature that apply to most charts, such as Aging & Exercise, Safe Use of Crutches or Nutrition for Athletes.

The Glossary gives brief definitions of medical terms and concepts associated with sports medicine, especially if they are referred to in the book.

The Index is your key to finding the information you need. Every topic is cross referenced by its most common names. Refer to the index to find your topic before trying to find it by leafing through the charts.

An Emergency First Aid section completes the major areas covered in this book. Most emergencies are covered under the individual injury entries, but life-threatening emergencies are dealt with separately in this section. *In case of emergency, refer to the last four pages of this book.* Emergencies are listed alphabetically in this section.

YOUR DOCTOR'S ROLE

Condensing the mass of information available about sports medicine and injuries into one volume has required some shortening and simplification. We have made every effort to include all major facts and concepts.

However, this book does not promise that you will always be able to diagnose and treat your own injuries or illnesses. Printed words cannot replace the knowledge and expertise that your doctor provides.

It is impossible to include in a book all the factors and circumstances that affect each *individual's* health. Your team physician or health care provider may take into account other factors not included here when he or she makes a precise diagnosis and recommends treatment for you. Most athletes are basically healthy people to begin with. More important, the athlete has great motivation to get well quickly so he or she can resume competition. All these factors make diagnosis, treatment and rehabilitation different—and usually quicker—for athletes than for the general population.

Your active participation in your medical program is a key element in winning, not only in athletic pursuits and sports competition, but also in life. We hope this book will be an important reference and guide to help you take care of your body so you can achieve your maximum athletic potential.

NORMAL ANATOMY

These illustrations are for general orientation to anatomy and provide brief explanations of function. They are frequently repeated throughout the book without further explanation. This section is by no means a complete explanation of anatomy or body parts. However, it concerns those body parts that are usually most affected by sports and exercise. These include the musculoskeletal system, the brain and central nervous system, the cardiovascular system and the respiratory tract. Most sports injuries affect these areas—especially the musculoskeletal system.

SKELETON

See Figure 1, front view of the female skeleton, and Figure 2, rear view of the male skeleton.

Both males and females have 206 bones: 29 in the skull, 26 in the spine, 25 in the chest, 64 in the arms and 62 in the legs.

Female bones are slightly smaller and lighter than corresponding male bones, and female limbs are shorter in proportion to total body length. Females have an increased shoulder slope and an increased angle at the elbows and knees.

The hip joint is smaller and more delicate. The female pelvic cavity, surrounded by the hip bones and sacrum, is wider than the male pelvis to allow for childbirth.

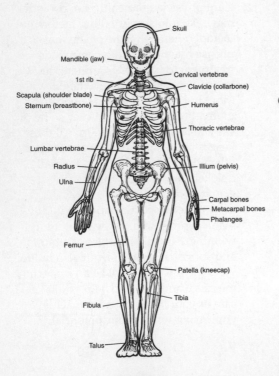

FIGURE 1

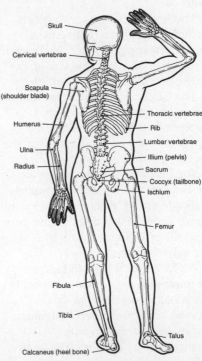

FIGURE 2

BRAIN, SPINAL CORD & NERVES

See Figure 3.

Billions of nerve cells in the brain control body movement and other functions associated with speech, learning, emotions and memory. The spinal cord and nerves branching from it are an extension of the same complicated nerve cells that form the brain. They provide the path by which messages are transmitted from the brain to all parts of the body.

The brain is protected by the rigid bones of the skull; the spinal cord is protected by the bones of the spine (vertebral column). The nerves outside the brain and spine are less well protected and more subject to injury during competitive sports and other vigorous activity.

HEART & MAJOR BLOOD VESSELS

See Figure 4.

The heart is a thick, strong muscle about the size of a clenched fist. The blood vessels are of two types: arteries and veins. To avoid confusion, the illustration shows only arteries. Veins and arteries usually run parallel. Arteries carry blood from the heart through narrower and narrower branches to capillaries that provide oxygen and nourishment to every body cell. In the capillaries, the blood absorbs waste materials from the cells.

Beyond the capillaries, veins begin. Veins carry the blood back to the heart to be pumped to the lungs. There carbon dioxide is eliminated and oxygen from the inhaled air is

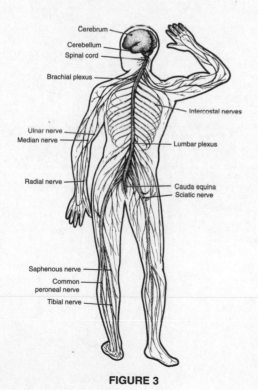

Cerebrum
Cerebellum
Spinal cord
Brachial plexus
Intercostal nerves
Ulnar nerve
Median nerve
Lumbar plexus
Radial nerve
Cauda equina
Sciatic nerve
Saphenous nerve
Common peroneal nerve
Tibial nerve

FIGURE 3

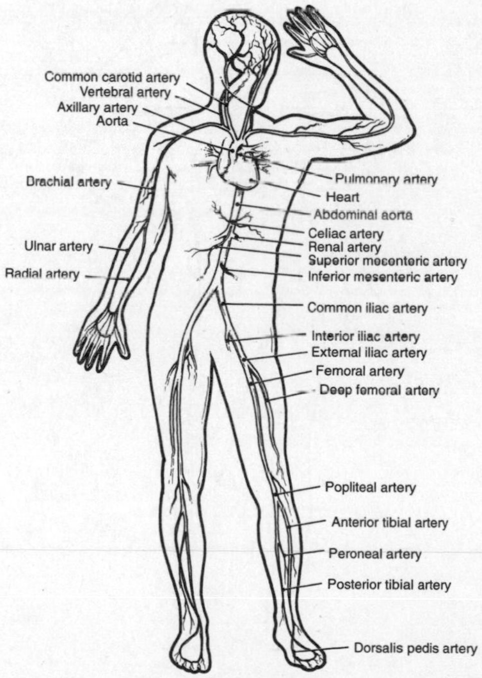

Common carotid artery
Vertebral artery
Axillary artery
Aorta
Drachial artery
Pulmonary artery
Heart
Abdominal aorta
Celiac artery
Ulnar artery
Renal artery
Superior mesenteric artery
Radial artery
Inferior mesenteric artery
Common iliac artery
Interior iliac artery
External iliac artery
Femoral artery
Deep femoral artery
Popliteal artery
Anterior tibial artery
Peroneal artery
Posterior tibial artery
Dorsalis pedis artery

FIGURE 4

absorbed. The oxygenated blood then returns to the heart to be pumped once again through arteries to the body cells.

Nourishment enters the blood stream by absorption through the capillaries of the intestinal tract. Waste materials (other than carbon dioxide) pass through the kidneys to be eliminated. Gases pass into the lung capillaries to be eliminated along with carbon dioxide.

RESPIRATORY SYSTEM

See Figure 5.

The major parts of the respiratory system include the nose and mouth, trachea, bronchial tubes and lungs. The lungs contain about 300 million tiny air sacs where absorption of oxygen from inhaled air takes place. Carbon dioxide and other waste gases are eliminated by exhaling.

The respiratory rate is closely related to the intensity of exercise. Exercise immediately increases the respiratory rate to provide more oxygen to sustain increased body needs.

GASTROINTESTINAL SYSTEM & URINARY TRACT

See Figure 6.

During the process of digestion, food passes through the esophagus to the stomach, then into the small and large intestines. The liver and pancreas (among other functions) manufacture enzymes that pass into the intestinal tract to aid in the digestion of the nutrients and their absorption into the bloodstream.

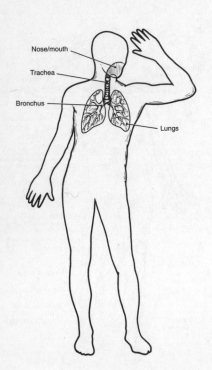

FIGURE 5

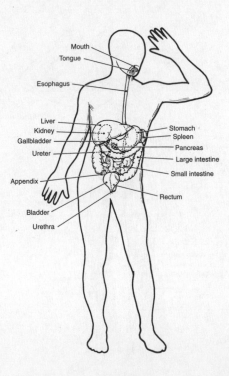

FIGURE 6

The urinary tract is composed of the kidneys, ureters, bladder and urethra. Blood brought to the functioning part of the kidneys is filtered, and waste materials are extracted and become urine. Urine passes through the ureters to the bladder, where it is stored until it is eliminated through the urethra.

MAJOR MUSCLE GROUPS

See Figure 7, front view, and Figure 8, rear view, of major muscle groups.

There are over 600 named muscles in the body that attach to bone to allow our bodies to move. Females and males have the same muscles, with the exception of those associated with the sexual organs. The muscles shown here (skeletal muscles) are all under voluntary control. That is, we can command the movement of these muscles. Chemical and electrical activity generated in our brains is transmitted through nerves to the muscles we wish to contract or relax. Another set of muscles in the body, mainly those in the heart, blood vessels, intestines and other body organs, functions automatically or involuntarily—completely out of conscious control.

Muscles receive nutrition through the bloodstream via the circulatory system. Extra nutrition and oxygen are needed by muscles during exercise. These needs are met in three ways: (1) increased respiratory rate, (2) increased cardiac output (the amount of blood pumped per minute by the heart) and (3) redistribution of blood flow from inactive organs, such as the gastrointestinal tract, to active skeletal muscles.

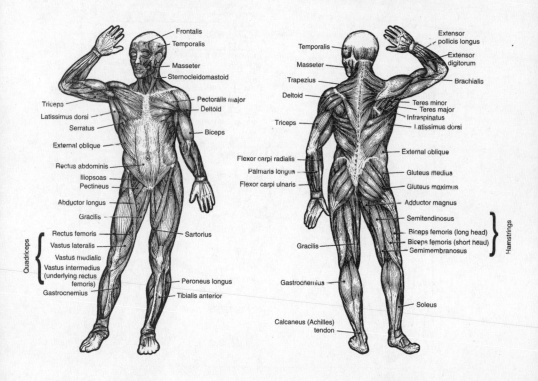

FIGURE 7

FIGURE 8

GUIDE TO SPORTS INJURY CHARTS

In this guide, the information about injuries associated with sports and vigorous physical exercise is organized in easy-to-read, illustrated charts.

The injuries described in this section are the most common ones that occur during vigorous physical activity or in competitive sports. Some injuries, such as those of the ankle, are quite common. Others are relatively rare, but

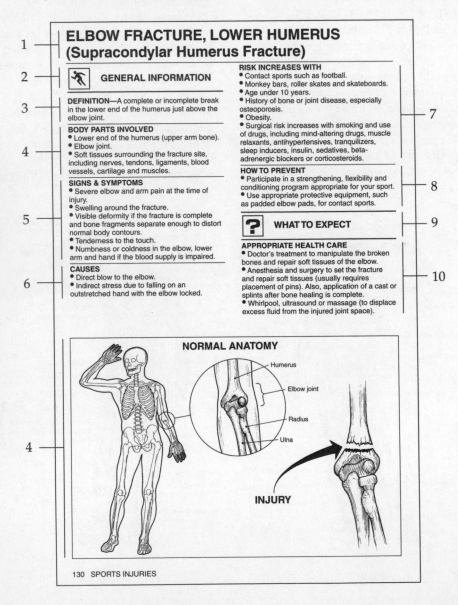

1 — ## ELBOW FRACTURE, LOWER HUMERUS (Supracondylar Humerus Fracture)

2 — ### GENERAL INFORMATION

3 — **DEFINITION**—A complete or incomplete break in the lower end of the humerus just above the elbow joint.

4 — **BODY PARTS INVOLVED**
- Lower end of the humerus (upper arm bone).
- Elbow joint.
- Soft tissues surrounding the fracture site, including nerves, tendons, ligaments, blood vessels, cartilage and muscles.

5 — **SIGNS & SYMPTOMS**
- Severe elbow and arm pain at the time of injury.
- Swelling around the fracture.
- Visible deformity if the fracture is complete and bone fragments separate enough to distort normal body contours.
- Tenderness to the touch.
- Numbness or coldness in the elbow, lower arm and hand if the blood supply is impaired.

6 — **CAUSES**
- Direct blow to the elbow.
- Indirect stress due to falling on an outstretched hand with the elbow locked.

RISK INCREASES WITH
- Contact sports such as football.
- Monkey bars, roller skates and skateboards.
- Age under 10 years.
- History of bone or joint disease, especially osteoporosis.
- Obesity.
- Surgical risk increases with smoking and use of drugs, including mind-altering drugs, muscle relaxants, antihypertensives, tranquilizers, sleep inducers, insulin, sedatives, beta-adrenergic blockers or corticosteroids. — 7

HOW TO PREVENT
- Participate in a strengthening, flexibility and conditioning program appropriate for your sport.
- Use appropriate protective equipment, such as padded elbow pads, for contact sports. — 8

? WHAT TO EXPECT — 9

APPROPRIATE HEALTH CARE
- Doctor's treatment to manipulate the broken bones and repair soft tissues of the elbow.
- Anesthesia and surgery to set the fracture and repair soft tissues (usually requires placement of pins). Also, application of a cast or splints after bone healing is complete.
- Whirlpool, ultrasound or massage (to displace excess fluid from the injured joint space). — 10

NORMAL ANATOMY

- Humerus
- Elbow joint
- Radius
- Ulna

4 —

INJURY

130   SPORTS INJURIES

still possible. Each injury is presented in a two-page format, including text and detailed illustrations. A sample chart, *ELBOW FRACTURE, LOWER HUMERUS*, is used here as an example. The major sections of this chart are explained on the following pages to help you become familiar with the chart format.

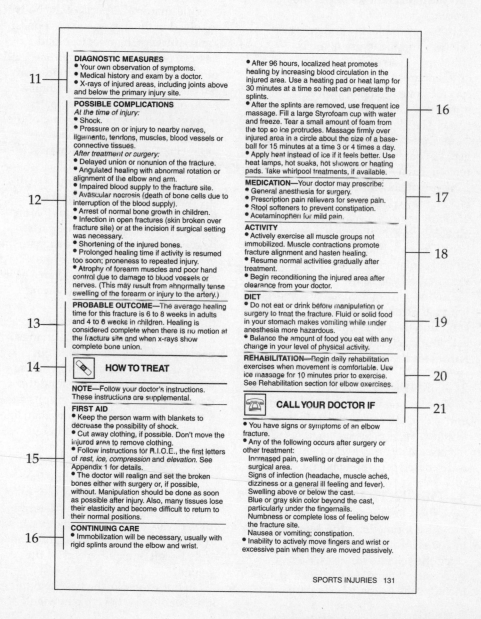

11

DIAGNOSTIC MEASURES
- Your own observation of symptoms.
- Medical history and exam by a doctor.
- X-rays of injured areas, including joints above and below the primary injury site.

POSSIBLE COMPLICATIONS
At the time of injury:
- Shock.
- Pressure on or injury to nearby nerves, ligaments, tendons, muscles, blood vessels or connective tissues.

After treatment or surgery:

12
- Delayed union or nonunion of the fracture.
- Angulated healing with abnormal rotation or alignment of the elbow and arm.
- Impaired blood supply to the fracture site.
- Avascular necrosis (death of bone cells due to interruption of the blood supply).
- Arrest of normal bone growth in children.
- Infection in open fractures (skin broken over fracture site) or at the incision if surgical setting was necessary.
- Shortening of the injured bones.
- Prolonged healing time if activity is resumed too soon; proneness to repeated injury.
- Atrophy of forearm muscles and poor hand control due to damage to blood vessels or nerves. (This may result from abnormally tense swelling of the forearm or injury to the artery.)

13

PROBABLE OUTCOME—The average healing time for this fracture is 6 to 8 weeks in adults and 4 to 6 weeks in children. Healing is considered complete when there is no motion at the fracture site and when x-rays show complete bone union.

14

🩹 **HOW TO TREAT**

NOTE—Follow your doctor's instructions. These instructions are supplemental.

FIRST AID
- Keep the person warm with blankets to decrease the possibility of shock.
- Cut away clothing, if possible. Don't move the injured area to remove clothing.

15
- Follow instructions for R.I.C.E., the first letters of *rest, ice, compression* and *elevation.* See Appendix 1 for details.
- The doctor will realign and set the broken bones either with surgery or, if possible, without. Manipulation should be done as soon as possible after injury. Also, many tissues lose their elasticity and become difficult to return to their normal positions.

16

CONTINUING CARE
- Immobilization will be necessary, usually with rigid splints around the elbow and wrist.

- After 96 hours, localized heat promotes healing by increasing blood circulation in the injured area. Use a heating pad or heat lamp for 30 minutes at a time so heat can penetrate the splints.

16
- After the splints are removed, use frequent ice massage. Fill a large Styrofoam cup with water and freeze. Tear a small amount of foam from the top so ice protrudes. Massage firmly over injured area in a circle about the size of a baseball for 15 minutes at a time 3 or 4 times a day.
- Apply heat instead of ice if it feels better. Use heat lamps, hot soaks, hot showers or heating pads. Take whirlpool treatments, if available.

17

MEDICATION—Your doctor may prescribe:
- General anesthesia for surgery.
- Prescription pain relievers for severe pain.
- Stool softeners to prevent constipation.
- Acetaminophen for mild pain.

18

ACTIVITY
- Actively exercise all muscle groups not immobilized. Muscle contractions promote fracture alignment and hasten healing.
- Resume normal activities gradually after treatment.
- Begin reconditioning the injured area after clearance from your doctor.

19

DIET
- Do not eat or drink before manipulation or surgery to treat the fracture. Fluid or solid food in your stomach makes vomiting while under anesthesia more hazardous.
- Balance the amount of food you eat with any change in your level of physical activity.

20

REHABILITATION—Begin daily rehabilitation exercises when movement is comfortable. Use ice massage for 10 minutes prior to exercise. See Rehabilitation section for elbow exercises.

21

☎ **CALL YOUR DOCTOR IF**

- You have signs or symptoms of an elbow fracture.
- Any of the following occurs after surgery or other treatment:
  Increased pain, swelling or drainage in the surgical area.
  Signs of infection (headache, muscle aches, dizziness or a general ill feeling and fever).
  Swelling above or below the cast.
  Blue or gray skin color beyond the cast, particularly under the fingernails.
  Numbness or complete loss of feeling below the fracture site.
  Nausea or vomiting; constipation.
- Inability to actively move fingers and wrist or excessive pain when they are moved passively.

1—CHART NAME

The charts are arranged alphabetically by body part, followed by the most common name for the injury. Other names (usually medical terms or sports medicine jargon) appear in parentheses under the main heading.

In our example, the body part is "elbow" and the injury name is "fracture." Fractures can occur in different areas of the elbow, so the specific bone segment, "lower humerus," is included after the injury name. The alternate name, "supracondylar humerus fracture," is listed in parentheses and cross referenced in the index.

If you are not sure what your injury is, you may compare the different types of elbow injuries, because they appear alphabetically in the same part of the book. Yet each injury has its own chart so you can quickly obtain the specific information you need.

To find information about a sports injury, check first in the index. If you can't find the injury chart you need, ask your doctor or trainer for alternate names for the injury.

2—GENERAL INFORMATION

This section includes the illustration and six topics: *Definition, Body Parts Involved, Signs & Symptoms, Causes, Risk Increases With* and *How to Prevent*. Each is discussed separately below.

3—DEFINITION

A short definition of the injury is provided. Sometimes the definition includes information from other categories, such as Causes, Risk Increases With or How to Treat. It also includes the primary body parts (bones, muscles, ligaments, nerves and other tissues) involved in the injury at the time the injury occurs.

4—BODY PARTS INVOLVED & ILLUSTRATION

This is a list and illustration of specific anatomical parts of the body involved in the injury, such as bones, joints, muscles, ligaments, blood vessels, nerves, lining membranes and others. The list usually includes body parts involved at the time of injury.

In our example, the body parts involved include the lower end of the humerus, or upper arm bone, the elbow joint and many soft tissues surrounding the injury area.

The illustration helps you visualize the nature of the injury and the detailed anatomy of the body parts involved. It consists of three parts: (l) A whole-body view to designate the general area of the injury occurs. (2) An enlarged view of the injured area as it appears before the injury (normal anatomy).
(3) A close-up illustration of the area after the injury showing the change in normal anatomy due to the injury.

By using the illustration with the text, the reader can understand the nature of the injury. Photographs and x-rays are harder to interpret than line drawings and are not used here.

5—SIGNS & SYMPTOMS

A *sign* may be observed by the patient or by someone else, or it may represent physical findings determined by x-ray examinations and other diagnostic measures. A *symptom* can only be felt or experienced by the patient.

In our example, the first item under this heading is "Severe elbow and arm pain at the time of injury." This is a symptom that can be experienced only by the patient. The next two items, "swelling" and "deformity," are signs. They can be observed by others around the patient.

6—CAUSES

The causes of most athletic injuries are usually obvious, because the symptoms begin immediately after injury. However, some injuries produce delayed symptoms, and their causes are not readily apparent. Other injuries may occur simultaneously as a complication of a primary injury. For example, indirect elbow injuries frequently accompany direct trauma to the wrist. Both types of causes are mentioned for our sample injury.

7—RISK INCREASES WITH

Risk factors are usually preexisting medical disorders. For example, an athlete with arthritis may be at increased risk of joint and bone injuries because these body parts are already weakened or misshapen.

The type of sport in which a person participates can also be a risk factor. For example, boxing is a sport particularly likely to lead to fractures of bones in the hand.

Our example includes risk factors in both categories. A person with osteoporosis has a greater risk of suffering an elbow fracture, and elbow fractures of the lower humerus are most likely in contact sports.

8—HOW TO PREVENT

Prevention may be of two kinds, prevention of the initial injury or prevention of a reinjury after healing. Prevention of any injury is the best of all possible treatments.

In general, the most important way to prevent injury is to follow a supervised conditioning program before beginning competition. Protective equipment designed for individual sports, such as elbow pads in our example, can also prevent or lessen the severity of injuries.

9—WHAT TO EXPECT

This section includes four topics: *Appropriate Health Care, Diagnostic Measures, Possible Complications* and *Probable Outcome*. Each is discussed separately below.

10—APPROPRIATE HEALTH CARE

A doctor's diagnosis and prescription of treatment are usually the most appropriate forms of health care for all moderate or serious injuries. In a few cases, total self-care is sufficient, especially if the patient has had previous experience in treating a specific sports injury. Then he can use this book to verify his approach and as a source of additional information concerning treatment and rehabilitation. In no case should this book replace a doctor's instructions.

Even the simplest injuries sometimes result in the development of complications. These usually require professional care. To cover such cases, a doctor's treatment is listed on some charts as appropriate even though it may apply to only a small fraction of cases.

One of the most important aspects of appropriate health care—but one that is not listed on the charts—is a positive mental attitude about getting well. Having a positive outlook, being determined to heal quickly and maintaining a sense of humor can be powerful assets in helping you regain strength, flexibility and skill so you can return quickly to your athletic activities.

If you have a particularly serious athletic injury, you may benefit from seeking care from a sports medicine specialist. But beware! Sports medicine is a fairly new medical specialty. While there are several certifying boards for sports medicine providers, their requirements vary dramatically. Some people who designate themselves as sports medicine specialists may not have any relevant special training and may use the term "sports medicine" merely as a marketing tool.

Check out the credentials of any physician you choose. Your family doctor or a nearby medical school can usually provide referrals to qualified sports medicine specialists. Be certain that the doctor you select communicates well with you. The best doctor-patient relationship is one of mutual respect.

11—DIAGNOSTIC MEASURES

Your own observation of signs and symptoms is usually the first—and often, the most important—diagnostic measure. It is the first step toward appropriate medical treatment. For this reason, it is listed under this heading on almost all injury charts. Exceptions are made for a few injuries, such as those involving unconsciousness, when self-observation is impossible.

A medical history and physical examination by a doctor, trainer or physical therapist are almost universal requirements before treatment of any serious injury. Additional studies include x-rays, laboratory studies or

other specialized tests. See the Glossary for an explanation of any diagnostic test you don't understand.

You may not require all the diagnostic tests listed on the chart; conversely, you may undergo tests not listed. Some tests are performed only if previous tests have not provided enough information. Others are performed only when complications develop.

12—POSSIBLE COMPLICATIONS

Complications are additional medical problems triggered by or resulting from the original injury. Complications can sometimes occur despite accurate diagnosis and competent treatment. In our example, possible complications of an elbow fracture range from shock at the time of injury to long-term problems, such as arrested bone growth in children. As a rule, serious complications occur in only a small percentage of cases.

13—PROBABLE OUTCOME

The outcome of an injury or illness is generally the area of greatest concern to the patient. Athletes are keenly concerned with how the injury will affect future performance. Unfortunately, doctors can't always provide definite answers. No one can predict how long an injury will require to heal—or even how completely it will heal—with absolute accuracy.

The predictions in this section are educated guesses based on the average expected outcome. For instance, an elbow fracture of the lower humerus requires an *average* healing time of 6 to 8 weeks in adults and 4 to 6 weeks in children. Responses to treatment vary greatly from person to person. They are affected by such variables as age, sex, general state of health before the injury, specific preexisting medical conditions and fitness level.

14—HOW TO TREAT

This section provides a summary and reminder of instructions you may have been given by your trainer or doctor. It is not intended to replace your doctor's instructions. If the instructions don't seem to fit your problem, ask your doctor or trainer for answers that apply uniquely to you.

The six major headings in this section include *First Aid, Continuing Care, Medication, Activity, Diet* and *Rehabilitation.*

15—FIRST AID

The instructions here are intended for people who have not had previous training in first aid.

Our example gives simple instructions for treating someone with a fracture at the elbow. The victim should be covered to prevent shock, the arm should not be moved and the steps for R.I.C.E. (rest, ice, compression and elevation) should be followed.

16—CONTINUING CARE

The instructions under this heading apply to home treatment, including treatment following surgery when that has been necessary. They cover common matters, such as applications of heat or cold, postoperative care of surgical wounds, appropriate clothing, bandages and bathing. These continuing care instruction cannot be complete or apply to everybody, but they provide a good review of general measures that are helpful for most injured athletes.

17—MEDICATION

Information listed under this heading is generally of two types: drugs your doctor may prescribe or administer and nonprescription medicines you can safely administer yourself.

Prescription drugs are usually named by generic name or drug class. A brief description of a drug's purpose and effect is given.

You may obtain complete information regarding drugs and medications by referring to the book *Complete Guide To Prescription & Non-Prescription Drugs,* published by Berkley Publishing Group. It is available in most bookstores, or you can order direct from the publisher at 1-800-788-6262, ext. 1.

18—ACTIVITY

This section is of vital interest to an injured person accustomed to vigorous exercise. It tells you whether to stay in bed, when to rest the injured part and when you may resume activity.

As a rule, you should keep the uninjured parts of the body active while the injured part rests. Rest is essential for recovery. For example, someone with an elbow fracture of the lower humerus should begin exercising the uninjured arm, legs, shoulders and other muscle groups—as well as engaging in cardiovascular (aerobic) training—as soon as possible. See your doctor for specific instructions.

19—DIET

A diet for an injured person usually does not vary from a normal diet. In some cases, if surgery is anticipated, food and liquids are restricted. Nutrition plays an important part in healing. The body requires certain nutritional building blocks to repair tissue. Opinions vary about the best diet for competitive athletes, but the general rules of good nutrition are the same for athletes as for others.

20—REHABILITATION

Rehabilitation is a crucial part of treating any injury, particularly injuries to competitive athletes. Its importance cannot be overemphasized. Details of rehabilitation for specific regions of the body may be found in the Rehabilitation & Conditioning section of this book.

21—CALL YOUR DOCTOR IF

The person with no previous medical experience should be able to determine from the chart whether he or she needs to see a doctor. For example, our sample chart leaves no doubt that a doctor should be seen immediately following a possible elbow fracture.

In addition, instructions are given for signs of complications that may arise after the initial injury. These instructions are especially important for injuries that are more serious than they first appear.

After your doctor has made a diagnosis, the course of recovery may differ from what is expected. If so, your doctor wants to be the first to know. Many developing complications can be averted with prompt medical treatment. Specific symptoms are listed that indicate the most common complications.

For example, a person with an elbow fracture would almost certainly have a cast. Our example lists telltale signs of problems due to a cast, including swelling and color changes in the hand.

Of course, if you have my symptoms other than those listed in this section that you believe are related to the injury or the medicines you take, call your doctor about them, too.

GUIDE TO SPORTS MEDICINE CHARTS

The sports medicine charts cover topics that affect or result from your participation in sports, physical exercise or athletic competition.

Any illness or disorder that affects health has some effect on physical activity. This book deals only with those most applicable to sports and exercise.

Each of the medical problems is described in a one-page format as shown in the sample chart, DEHYDRATION, on page 23. The format is similar to but slightly different from the one used in the Sports Injuries section.

Major sections of the chart format are numbered and explained in the next few pages.

1—CHART NAME

Charts are arranged alphabetically by the most common name for the illness, disorder or medical problem. Other names for these appear in parentheses below the main heading. DEHYDRATION does not have another name, so it appears alone. However, a disease such as ATHLETE'S FOOT is also known as "Ringworm of the Foot," so this second name appears as a subheading. All names in this book, including alternate names, are cross referenced in the index.

To find information about a medical problem, check the index. If you can't find the illness chart that you need, it may not be included in this reference.

2—GENERAL INFORMATION

This section includes four topics: Definition, Signs & Symptoms, Causes & Risk Factors and How to Prevent. Each is discussed separately below.

3—DEFINITION

Here you will find a short definition of the problem or disease. In the DEHYDRATION chart, the definition is short and simple. Charts for other ailments may be more detailed. Sometimes an illness or disorder cannot be defined without including information about causes, risks or general treatment—even if this information is covered in greater detail elsewhere on the chart.

4—SIGNS & SYMPTOMS

The distinction between signs and symptoms is important. A sign is observed. A symptom is felt or experienced.

In our sample chart, the first item mentioned under this heading is "dry mouth." This is a symptom that only the patient can experience. The next three items ("decreased or absent urination, sunken eyes, wrinkled skin") are signs. They can be observed by the patient or by others.

Signs and symptoms are listed together in this book. No attempt has been made to separate the two. A wide range of possible signs and symptoms is listed on most charts. It is unlikely that any patient will have all, or even most, of the possible signs and symptoms.

The presence or absence of signs and symptoms may vary according to:
• The age and sex of the patient.
• The patient's general state of health at the onset of the disorder.
• The extent and stage of the illness.
The charts in this book are written from the perspective of the effect of disease on an athlete. For more general information, including a separate

section devoted to symptoms, please refer to the book *Complete Guide to Symptoms, Illness & Surgery*, published by Berkley Publishing Group.

5—CAUSES & RISK FACTORS

Many times the cause of a disorder is unknown. At the same time, many disorders have factors that are known to increase the risk of succumbing to them. These include factors that may trigger the problem, make it more likely to occur or cause it to increase in duration or intensity. Because it is sometimes hard to know when risks end and causes begin, these two factors are listed together on the illness charts.

Common causes of illness in athletes include:
• Inherited (congenital) defects.
• Infections from bacteria, viruses, parasites, yeast or fungi. All of these are sometimes referred to as "germs," but most people associate "germs" with bacteria only.
• Allergies.
• Physical injury, including that caused by cold or heat.
• Toxins (poisons) from a wide range of sources, including environmental pollution.

Risk factors affecting how a person reacts to the causes above include:
• Age.
• Stress, either physical or emotional.
• Fatigue or overwork.
• Poor nutrition due to improper diet, disease or the special demands of strenuous physical activity.
• Obesity.
• Recent or chronic illness that can lower resistance to other disorders.
• Recent surgery or injury.
• Use of drugs, such as alcohol, tobacco, caffeine, narcotics, psychedelics, hallucinogens, marijuana, sedatives, hypnotics or cocaine.
• Use of prescription or nonprescription medications. Even necessary drugs may cause adverse reactions and side effects that can complicate the treatment and outcomes of medical problems and affect athletic performance.
• Crowded or unsanitary conditions, including locker rooms.
• Poor personal hygiene.
• Mental or emotional disorders, such as anxiety and depression.
• Defects in the body's immune system.

6—HOW TO PREVENT

Prevention can be of two types— prevention of the initial disease or prevention of a relapse or recurrence after recovery.

Prevention of any medical problem is the best treatment. Many diseases cannot be prevented because we cannot control all of their causes. However, we *can* control many risk factors. In our example, an athlete can decrease the risk of becoming severely dehydrated by remembering to drink adequate water, especially during hot weather and when sweating heavily.

7—WHAT TO EXPECT

This section includes four topics: *Diagnostic Measures, Surgery, Normal Course of Illness* and *Possible Complications*. Each is discussed separately below.

8—DIAGNOSTIC MEASURES

As with injuries, your own observation of symptoms is usually the first diagnostic measure of an illness. The next logical step is often a medical

DEHYDRATION

🏃 GENERAL INFORMATION

DEFINITION—Loss of water and essential body salts (electrolytes) needed for normal body function. Necessary salts contain sodium, potassium, calcium, bicarbonate and phosphate. Water accounts for about 60% of a man's weight and 50% of a woman's weight and needs to be kept within fairly narrow limits to maintain cells and body tissue.

SIGNS & SYMPTOMS
* Dry mouth and swollen tongue.
* Decreased or absent urination; urine color may be deep yellow.
* Sunken eyes and wrinkled skin.
* Inability to sweat.
* Fatigue.
* Dizziness; confusion; coma.
* Low blood pressure.
* Severe thirst.
* Increase in heart rate and breathing.

CAUSES & RISK FACTORS
* Heavy sweating; too much exercise.
* Persistent vomiting or diarrhea from any cause.
* Persistent high fever.
* Use of drugs that deplete fluids and electrolytes, such as diuretics ("water pills").
* Overexposure to sun or heat.
* Not taking in a sufficient amount of water.
* Diabetes mellitus, chronic lung disease, chronic kidney disease or adrenal disease.
* Injuries to the skin, such as burns, can cause fluid loss through the damaged skin.

HOW TO PREVENT
* Obtain medical treatment for underlying causes of dehydration.
* If you are vomiting or have diarrhea, drink enough water to keep urine consistently pale (you may not feel thirsty, but fluid intake is essential).
* If you use diuretics, weigh daily.
* Carry water with you to outdoor activities; drink plenty of water while exercising and avoid exercising outdoors in very hot weather.
* Avoid drinking alcohol in hot weather..

❓ WHAT TO EXPECT

DIAGNOSTIC MEASURES
* Your own observation of symptoms.
* Medical history and physical exam by a doctor if needed.
* Laboratory blood studies, including blood counts and electrolyte measurement (see Glossary).

SURGERY—Not necessary or useful for this disorder.

NORMAL COURSE OF DISORDER—Curable with control of the underlying cause and replacement of necessary fluids.

POSSIBLE COMPLICATIONS
* Depends on seriousness of underlying cause. Usually with mild to moderate symptoms, no complications are expected.
* Severe dehydration or electrolyte imbalance may lead to heartbeat irregularities, cardiac arrest and death.

✏️ HOW TO TREAT

NOTE—Follow your doctor's instructions if provided. These instructions are supplemental.

MEDICAL TREATMENT—Hospitalization to be sure you get enough fluids (with a severe or prolonged illness only).

HOME TREATMENT
* For minor dehydration, take frequent small amounts of clear liquids. Sip through a straw or suck on ice chips .Large amounts may trigger vomiting.
* Take off excess clothing and loosen any other clothes. Place a wet towel around the person. Don't use ice packs on the skin; they can actually raise a person's temperature.
* Get the person to an air conditioned area, or near a fan. If outside, get the person to a shady area.

MEDICATION—Your doctor may prescribe fluids given through a vein (IV) to replace lost water, anti-emetic drug if vomiting is severe, drugs for diarrhea if it is persistent or to lower fever.

ACTIVITY—Rest in bed until you recover.

DIET—Drink carbohydrate/electrolyte solutions. For adults, diluting commercial solutions such as Gatorade or Recharge with an equal amount of water may be adequate. Suck on popsicles made from juices or sports drinks. For children, use special commercial products (Pedialyte or Ricelyte). Instructions are on the labels.

☎️ CALL YOUR DOCTOR IF

* If symptoms are severe, seek emergency care
* You have mild to moderate symptoms of dehydration that are not relieved by self-treatment.
* Fever is over 101°F (38.3°C).
* Diarrhea or vomiting continues for over 2 days.

422 SPORTS MEDICINE

history and physical exam by a doctor. Even if a problem can be treated at home, a doctor's history and exam will be necessary if complications develop that require medical treatment.

Additional diagnostic measures include laboratory studies and other medical tests. The most common are listed in this section by name and are described in the Glossary. The list of diagnostic tests is only a guide. Your doctor may not need every one listed, or additional ones may be required if diagnosis is difficult or if complications develop.

9—SURGERY

When surgery is necessary or useful to cure the illness, it is indicated here. Sometimes the name or description of the procedure is given. If you are uncertain what the name means, refer to the Glossary. As is the case with most ailments, our sample shows that dehydration does not require surgery.

10—NORMAL COURSE OF DISORDER

A very important concern in any illness is how the illness will affect the patient's life. Most illnesses last a short time, but some may continue to hinder performance permanently. These issues are discussed in this section. For dehydration, we see that as soon as the underlying cause is removed, the patient should have no lasting difficulties.

Illnesses and injuries are similar in that no one can completely predict the course of either. This section describes the average patient's experience, but individuals will vary. Medicine is an inexact science. Response to treatment depends on many variables, and there remain many questions about health and disease.

11—POSSIBLE COMPLICATIONS

Complications are additional medical problems triggered by the original illness. Some complications are preventable, a few are inevitable—but most are rare. With dehydration, life-threatening shock can occur as a complication. However, this is a rare occurrence, resulting only when dehydration is ignored and untreated in its earlier stages.

12—HOW TO TREAT

This section provides a general list of instructions for treating your illness. Your doctor may have given you instructions, and this information should not replace your doctor's instructions. Treatments vary a great deal from individual to individual.

The five major headings in this section include *Medical Treatment, Home Treatment, Medication, Activity* and *Diet*. They are explained in detail below.

13—MEDICAL TREATMENT

Some ailments can be treated successfully at home. This section covers those cases for which medical treatment is essential. It explains the type of treatment generally used for a particular disorder. Many times medical treatment is necessary only if home treatment has not proven successful. For instance, in the case of dehydration a person may need to be hospitalized for intravenous fluids.

Rehabilitation is sometimes mentioned here. It can be useful for illnesses that cause temporary or permanent disability. Rehabilitation may be provided by trained physical therapists or by physiatrists (medical doctors who specialize in physical therapy).

14—HOME TREATMENT

This section covers the various things a patient can do at home to help himself or herself get better. Some of the instructions elaborate on what your doctor may have told you to do. Others give you suggestions for treating yourself. The measures mentioned here are not complete and may not apply to everyone, but they provide a good review of home treatment that is helpful for many patients. For example, our sample chart for dehydration explains the importance of weighing daily and recording rapid fluid loss.

15—MEDICATION

Medication is often an important part of treatment. This chart section tells you which nonprescription drugs you can take safely, and it lists the prescription drugs your doctor is most likely to recommend. Drugs are usually named by generic name or drug class.

16—ACTIVITY

Patients are often confused about whether they must stay in bed during an illness. They are often concerned about returning to their favorite sport or physical activity, and they want to know if activity will be restricted after recovery. These questions are answered under this heading.

Exercise references are often included, and when they do not specify otherwise, references to regular physical exercise mean aerobic exercise.

In the case of dehydration, it is necessary to rest in bed only until you recover. No permanent reduction in activity is necessary, nor is it useful.

17—DIET

Diet information can vary from "No special diet" to references to the diets that hasten healing or recovery time. Nutrition plays a big part in health and disease.

In the case of dehydration, the diet prescribed depends on the underlying cause of the disorder. For additional specialized diet instructions, consult your doctor or a dietitian.

18—CALL YOUR DOCTOR IF

For most medical problems, a phone call or visit to your doctor is recommended to establish a diagnosis.

After diagnosis, when the course of an illness differs from what is expected, your doctor wants to know. Many developing complications can be averted with prompt medical treatment. The symptoms listed usually indicate complications.

Of course, if any other symptoms begin that you believe are related to your illness or the drugs you take, call your doctor about them, too.

Sports Injuries

ABDOMINAL WALL STRAIN

GENERAL INFORMATION

DEFINITION—Injury to the muscles or tendons of the abdominal wall, or injury to the places where muscles or tendons attach to pelvic bones. Tendons, muscles and their attached bones comprise contractile units. These units stabilize the pelvis and rib cage and allow their motion. A strain occurs at the weakest part of a unit. Strains are of 3 types:
- Mild (Grade I)—Slightly pulled muscle without tearing of muscle or tendon fibers. There is no loss of strength.
- Moderate (Grade II)—Tearing of fibers in a muscle or tendon or at the attachment to bone. Strength is diminished.
- Severe (Grade III)—Rupture of the muscle-tendon-bone attachment, with separation of fibers. Severe strains may require surgical repair. Chronic strains are caused by overuse. Acute strains are caused by direct injury or overstress.

BODY PARTS INVOLVED
- Abdominal muscles and tendons.
- Bones in the abdominal area (ribs, pubic bone and iliac crest bone).
- Soft tissues surrounding the strain, including nerves, periosteum (covering of bone), blood vessels and lymph vessels.

SIGNS & SYMPTOMS
- Pain when moving or stretching abdominal muscles.
- Muscle spasm, especially with hard breathing or twisting.
- Swelling in the abdominal area. Loss of strength (moderate or severe strain).
- Crepitation ("crackling" feeling and sound when the injured area is pressed with fingers).
- Calcification of the muscle or its tendon (visible with x-ray).
- Inflammation of the tendon sheath.

CAUSES
- Prolonged overuse of muscle-tendon units in the abdominal wall.
- Single violent injury or force applied to the muscle-tendon units in the abdominal wall.

RISK INCREASES WITH
- Stretching exercises.
- Pole vaulting, high jumping and hurdling.
- Contact sports.
- Any cardiovascular medical problem that results in decreased circulation.
- Medical history of any bleeding disorder.
- Obesity.
- Poor nutrition.
- Previous abdominal wall strain.
- Poor muscle conditioning.

HOW TO PREVENT
- Participate in a strengthening, flexibility and conditioning program appropriate for your sport.
- Warm up before practice or competition.

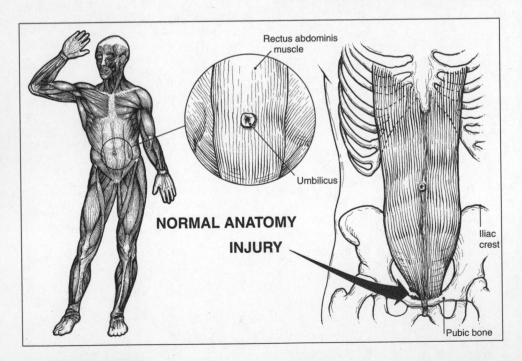

Rectus abdominis muscle

Umbilicus

Iliac crest

Pubic bone

NORMAL ANATOMY

INJURY

WHAT TO EXPECT

APPROPRIATE HEALTH CARE
- Doctor's diagnosis.
- Self-care during rehabilitation.
- Physical therapy (moderate or severe strain).
- Surgery (severe strain).

DIAGNOSTIC MEASURES
- Your own observation of symptoms.
- Medical history and exam by a doctor.
- X-rays of injured areas to rule out fractures.

POSSIBLE COMPLICATIONS
- Prolonged healing time, if activity is resumed too soon.
- Proneness to repeated injury.
- Inflammation at attachment to bone (periostitis).
- Abdominal hernia.
- Prolonged disability (sometimes).

PROBABLE OUTCOME—If this is a first-time injury, proper care and sufficient healing time before resuming activity should prevent permanent disability. Torn ligaments and tendons require as long to heal as fractured bones. Average healing times are:
- Mild strain—2 to 10 days.
- Moderate strain—10 days to 6 weeks.
- Severe strain—6 to 10 weeks.
If this is a repeat injury, complications listed above are more likely to occur.

 HOW TO TREAT

NOTE—Follow your doctor's instructions. These instructions are supplemental.

FIRST AID—Follow instructions for R.I.C.E., the first letters of *rest, ice, compression* and *elevation* (if possible). See Appendix 1 for details.

CONTINUING CARE
- Use ice massage 3 or 4 times a day for 15 minutes at a time. Fill a large styrofoam cup with water and freeze. Tear a small amount of foam from the top so ice protrudes. Massage firmly over the injured area in a circle about the size of a softball.
- After the first 24 hours, apply heat instead of ice if it feels better. Use heat lamps, hot soaks, hot showers, heating pads or heat liniments and ointments.
- Take whirlpool treatments, if available.
- Wrap the injured abdominal wall muscles loosely with an elasticized bandage, or wear a corset between treatments.
- Massage gently and often to provide comfort and decrease swelling.

MEDICATION
- For minor discomfort, you may use:
  aspirin, acetaminophen or ibuprofen.
  topical liniments and ointments.
- Your doctor may prescribe:
  Stronger pain reliever.
  Injection of a long-acting local anesthetic to reduce pain.
  Injection of a corticosteroid, such as triamcinolone, to reduce inflammation.

ACTIVITY—Resume your normal activities gradually after pain subsides.

DIET—During recovery, balance the amount of food you eat with any change in your level of physical activity. Eat a variety of foods to get the energy, protein, vitamins, minerals and fiber you need for good health and healing.

REHABILITATION—Begin a supervised weightlifting program when supportive wrapping is no longer needed. Use ice massage for 10 minutes prior to exercise.

 CALL YOUR DOCTOR IF

- You have symptoms of a moderate or severe abdominal wall strain or a mild strain persists longer than 10 days.
- Pain or swelling worsens despite treatment.
- Symptoms of a hernia develop:
  A lump in the groin or umbilical area that usually returns to its normal position with gentle pressure or after lying down.
  Scrotal swelling, with or without pain.

ACHILLES TENDINITIS

GENERAL INFORMATION

DEFINITION—Inflammation of the Achilles tendon.

BODY PARTS INVOLVED
- Achilles tendon, which attaches the lower leg muscles to the heel.
- Soft tissues in the surrounding area, including blood vessels, nerves, ligaments, periosteum (covering of bone) and connective tissues.

SIGNS & SYMPTOMS
- Constant pain or pain with motion.
- Limited motion of the ankle.
- Crepitation (a "crackling" sound when the tendon moves or is touched).
- Heat and redness over the inflamed Achilles tendon.
- Tenderness directly over the Achilles tendon.

CAUSES
- Strain from unusual use or overuse of the lower leg muscles and Achilles tendon.
- Partial tearing of the tendon.
- Direct blow or injury to the lower leg, foot or ankle. Tendinitis becomes more likely with repeated injury.
- Infection introduced through broken skin at the time of injury.

RISK INCREASES WITH—Contact sports, especially those involving kicking, jumping and quick starts.

HOW TO PREVENT
- Engage in a program of physical conditioning and flexibility before beginning regular sports participation.
- Achilles stretching exercises before any sports activity.
- Warm up adequately before practice or competition.
- Learn proper moves and techniques for your sport.

WHAT TO EXPECT

APPROPRIATE HEALTH CARE
- Doctor's examination and diagnosis.
- Self-care during recovery.

DIAGNOSTIC MEASURES
- Your own observation of symptoms and signs.
- Medical history and physical examination by your doctor.
- X-rays of the area to rule out other abnormalities (insertional spurs).

POSSIBLE COMPLICATIONS
- Prolonged healing time if activity is resumed too soon.
- Proneness to repeated injury.
- Achilles tendon rupture.

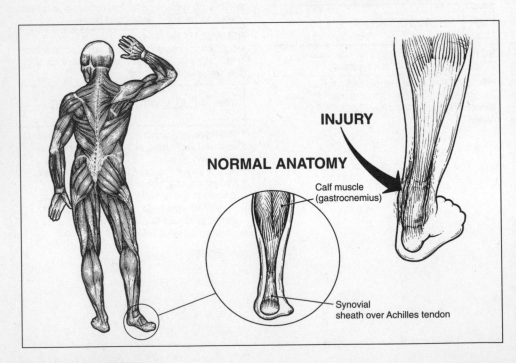

INJURY

NORMAL ANATOMY

Calf muscle (gastrocnemius)

Synovial sheath over Achilles tendon

PROBABLE OUTCOME
● Achilles tendinitis is usually curable in about 6 weeks with anti-inflammatory medications, stretching exercises, physical therapy and rest of the inflamed area.
● Recovery is usually quicker if the inflammation is caused by a direct blow rather than by a strain or sprain.

 ## HOW TO TREAT

NOTE—Follow your doctor's instructions. These instructions are supplemental.

FIRST AID—None. This problem develops slowly.

CONTINUING CARE
● You may need a walking boot cast for 10 to 14 days. See Appendix 2 (Care of Casts). Then wrap the ankle area with an elasticized bandage until healing is complete.
● Heel lifts in shoes may be helpful.
● Apply heat frequently. Use heat lamps, hot soaks, hot showers, heating pads or heat liniments and ointments.
● Take whirlpool treatments, if available.
● To prevent a recurrence, wear protective strapping or an adhesive bandage for several weeks after healing is complete.

MEDICATION
● You may use nonprescription drugs such as acetaminophen for minor pain.
● Your doctor may prescribe:
Stronger pain relievers.
Nonsteroidal anti-inflammatory medication (either prescription or nonprescription) for 7 to 14 days.

ACTIVITY—Resume normal activities gradually.

DIET—During recovery, balance the amount of food you eat with any change in your level of physical activity. Eat a variety of foods to get the energy, protein, vitamins, minerals and fiber you need for good health and healing. Your doctor may suggest vitamin and mineral supplements to promote healing.

REHABILITATION
● Begin daily rehabilitation exercises when supportive wrapping is no longer needed and you can walk without pain.
● Use ice massage for 10 minutes before and after exercise. Fill a large styrofoam cup with water and freeze. Tear a small amount of foam from the top so ice protrudes. Massage firmly over the injured area in a circle about the size of a softball.
● See Rehabilitation section for ankle and foot exercises.

 ## CALL YOUR DOCTOR IF

● You have symptoms of Achilles tendinitis.
● Significant weakness occurs or a wound or indentation is evident over the Achilles tendon (see Achilles Tendon Strain).
● New, unexplained symptoms develop. Drugs used in treatment may produce side effects.

ACHILLES TENDON STRAIN
(Partial or Complete Heel Cord Rupture)

GENERAL INFORMATION

DEFINITION—Injury to the Achilles tendon or its adjoining muscle or bone. These 3 parts comprise a contractile unit. The strain occurs at the weakest part of the unit. Strains are of 3 types:
Mild (Grade I)—Slightly pulled muscle without tearing of muscle or tendon fibers. There is no loss of strength.
Moderate (Grade II)— Partial tearing of fibers in a muscle or tendon or at the attachment to bone. Strength is diminished.
Severe (Grade III)—Rupture of the muscle-tendon-bone attachment, with separation of fibers. Ruptures usually require surgical repair. Chronic strains are caused by overuse. Acute strains are caused by direct injury or overstress.

BODY PARTS INVOLVED
- Achilles tendon; heel bone (calcaneus).
- Muscle attached to the Achilles tendon.
- Soft tissues surrounding the strain, including nerves, periosteum (bone covering), blood vessels and lymph vessels.

SIGNS & SYMPTOMS
- Pain when flexing or extending the foot.
- Muscle spasm at the rear of the calf.
- Tenderness directly over the Achilles tendon.
- Swelling around the Achilles tendon.
- Loss of strength (moderate or severe strain).
- Crepitation ("crackling" feeling and sound when the injured area is pressed with fingers).
- Calcification of the muscle or its tendon (visible with x-ray).
- Inflammation of the sheath covering the Achilles tendon.
- Abnormal Thompson test—foot does not flex when squeezing calf.

CAUSES
- Prolonged overuse of muscle-tendon units in the ankle.
- Single episode of stressful overactivity, as in hurdling, long jumping, high jumping or starting a sprint.
- Degeneration of tendon (classic in weekend athlete between age 30 and 50).

RISK INCREASES WITH
- Contact sports.
- Running.
- Sports that require quick starts, such as long jumping, hurdling or running races.
- Any cardiovascular medical problem that results in decreased circulation.
- Medical history of any bleeding disorder.
- Obesity.
- Poor nutrition.
- Previous Achilles tendon injury.
- Poor muscle conditioning.

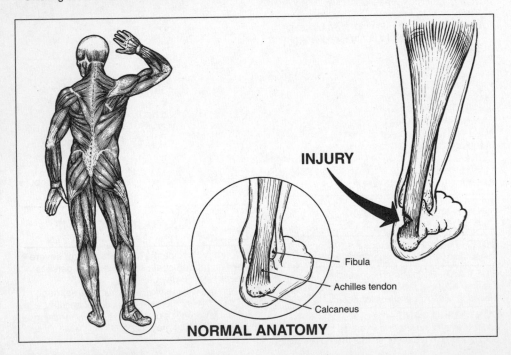

INJURY

Fibula

Achilles tendon

Calcaneus

NORMAL ANATOMY

HOW TO PREVENT
- Participate in a strengthening, flexibility and conditioning program appropriate for your sport.
- Achilles stretching exercises before athletic activities.
- Warm up before practice or competition.
- Tape the Achilles tendon area before practice or competition.
- Wear proper protective shoes.

 WHAT TO EXPECT

APPROPRIATE HEALTH CARE
- Doctor's diagnosis.
- Application of tape, plaster splints or casts (sometimes).
- Self-care during rehabilitation.
- Physical therapy (moderate or severe strain).
- Surgery (severe strain).

DIAGNOSTIC MEASURES
- Your own observation of symptoms.
- Medical history and exam by a doctor.
- X-rays of injured areas to rule out fractures.
- Diagnostic ultrasound to identify severe strain (complete tear).

POSSIBLE COMPLICATIONS
- Prolonged healing time if activity is resumed too soon.
- Proneness to repeated injury.
- Limp and weakness of push-off with repeated injury.
- Inflammation at the attachment to bone (periostitis).
- Prolonged disability (sometimes), especially if complete tear is missed. Early examination by doctor is necessary.

PROBABLE OUTCOME—If this is a first-time injury, proper care and sufficient healing time before resuming activity should prevent permanent disability. Torn ligaments and tendons require as long to heal as bone fractures. Average healing times are:
- Mild strain—2 to 10 days.
- Moderate strain—10 days to 6 weeks.
- Severe strain—6 to 10 weeks.

If this is a repeat injury, complications listed above are more likely to occur.

 HOW TO TREAT

NOTE—Follow your doctor's instructions. These instructions are supplemental.

FIRST AID—Follow instructions for R.I.C.E., the first letters of *rest, ice, compression* and *elevation. See* Appendix 1 for details.

CONTINUING CARE—If a cast or splints are used, leave toes free and exercise them occasionally. If a cast or splints are not used:

- Use ice massage 3 or 4 times a day for 15 minutes at a time. Fill a large styrofoam cup with water and freeze. Tear a small amount of foam from the top so ice protrudes. Massage firmly over the injured area in a circle about the size of a softball.
- After the first 24 hours, apply heat instead of ice if it feels better. Use heat lamps, hot soaks, hot showers, heating pads or heat liniments and ointments.
- Take whirlpool treatments, if available. Wrap the injured ankle with an elasticized bandage between treatments. Insert a heel lift in your shoe.
- Massage gently and often to provide comfort and decrease swelling.
- The most important aspect of treatment of a severe tear is immobilization, with or without surgery. Continued movement in this situation makes long-term or permanent disability likely.

MEDICATION
- For minor discomfort, you may use:
  Aspirin, acetaminophen or ibuprofen.
  Topical liniments and ointments.
- Your doctor may prescribe:
  Stronger pain relievers.
  Injection of a long-acting local anesthetic to reduce pain (rare).
  Nonsteroidal anti-inflammatory medication (either prescription or nonprescription) for 7 to 14 days.

ACTIVITY
- For a moderate or severe strain, walk with crutches for at least 72 hours—longer with a cast or splints. See Appendix 3 (Safe Use of Crutches).
- Resume normal activities gradually after pain has subsided.

DIET—During recovery, balance the amount of food you eat with any change in your level of physical activity. Eat a variety of foods to get the energy, protein, vitamins, minerals and fiber you need for good health and healing.

REHABILITATION
- Begin daily rehabilitation exercises and stretching when supportive wrapping is no longer needed.
- See Rehabilitation section for ankle and foot exercises.

 CALL YOUR DOCTOR IF

- You have symptoms of a moderate or severe Achilles tendon strain or a mild strain persists longer than 10 days.
- Pain or swelling worsens despite treatment.
- The following occur with a cast or splints:
  Pain, numbness or coldness below the injury.
  Dusky, blue or gray toenails.

ANKLE CONTUSION

GENERAL INFORMATION

DEFINITION—Bruising of skin and underlying tissues of the ankle due to a direct blow. Contusions cause bleeding from ruptured small capillaries that allow blood to infiltrate muscles, tendons or other soft tissues. Ankle contusions are common, but they are not serious injuries.

BODY PARTS INVOLVED—Ankle tissues, including blood vessels, muscles, tendons, nerves, covering of bone (periosteum) and connective tissues.

SIGNS & SYMPTOMS
- Local swelling—either superficial or deep.
- Pain and tenderness over the bruise.
- Feeling of firmness when pressure is exerted at the injury site.
- Discoloration under the skin, beginning with redness and progressing to the characteristic "black-and-blue" bruise.

CAUSES—Direct blow to the ankle, usually from a blunt object or collision in sports.

RISK INCREASES WITH
- Violent contact sports such as field hockey, football, ice hockey and soccer, especially when ankles are not adequately protected.
- Medical history of any bleeding disorder, such as hemophilia.
- Poor nutrition, including vitamin deficiency.
- Use of anticoagulants or aspirin.

HOW TO PREVENT—Wear appropriate protective gear and equipment, such as high-ankle shoes and shin guards, during competition or other athletic activity if there is risk of an ankle contusion.

WHAT TO EXPECT

APPROPRIATE HEALTH CARE
- Doctor's care unless the contusion is quite small.
- Self-care for minor contusions and for serious contusions during rehabilitation.
- Physical therapy for serious contusions.

DIAGNOSTIC MEASURES
- Your own observation of symptoms.
- Medical history and physical exam by a doctor for all except minor injuries.
- X-rays of the injured area to assess total injury to soft tissues and to rule out the possibility of underlying fracture. The total extent of injury may not be apparent for 48 to 72 hours.

POSSIBLE COMPLICATIONS
- Excessive bleeding, leading to disability. Infiltrative-type bleeding can sometimes lead to calcification and impaired function of the injured muscle.
- Infection if skin over the contusion is broken.
- Fracture of bone not recognized on initial x-rays.

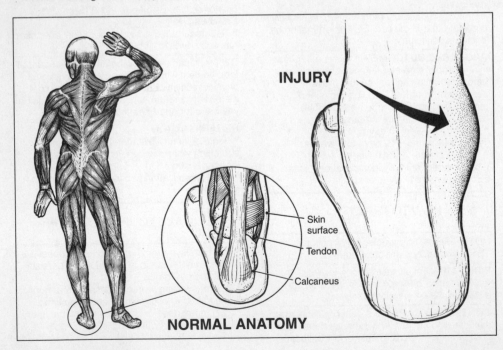

INJURY

Skin surface

Tendon

Calcaneus

NORMAL ANATOMY

PROBABLE OUTCOME—Healing time varies with the extent of injury, but uncomplicated ankle contusions will heal within 2 to 4 days.

HOW TO TREAT

NOTE—Follow your doctor's instructions These instructions are supplemental.

FIRST AID—Use instructions for R.I.C.E., the first letters of *rest, ice, compression* and *elevation.* See Appendix 1 for details.

CONTINUING CARE
• Wrap an elasticized bandage over a piece of sponge rubber on the injured area. Keep the area compressed for about 72 hours.
• Continue ice massage. Fill a large styrofoam cup with water and freeze. Tear a small amount of foam from the top so ice protrudes. Massage gently over the injured area in a circle about the size of a softball. Do this for 15 minutes at a time 3 or 4 times a day, and also before workouts or competition.
• After 72 hours, apply heat instead of ice If it feels better. Use heat lamps, hot soaks, hot showers, heating pads, heat liniments and ointments or whirlpool treatments.
• Massage gently and often to provide comfort and decrease swelling. Stroke toward the heart from the toes.

MEDICATION
• For minor discomfort, you may use:
  Acetaminophen or ibuprofen or other anti-inflammatory medications.
  Topical liniments and ointments.
• Your doctor may prescribe stronger medicine for pain.

ACTIVITY—As soon as underlying damage can be ruled out, normal activity can begin within a day or two.

DIET—Balance the amount of food you eat with any change in your level of physical activity. Eat a variety of foods to get the energy, protein, vitamins, minerals and fiber you need for good health and healing.

REHABILITATION
• For serious contusions, begin daily rehabilitation exercises when supportive wrapping is no longer needed.
• See Rehabilitation section for ankle and foot exercises.

CALL YOUR DOCTOR IF

• You have a contusion that doesn't improve in 1 or 2 days.
• Skin is broken and signs of infection (drainage, increasing pain, fever, headache, muscle aches, dizziness or a general ill feeling) occur.

ANKLE DISLOCATION

GENERAL INFORMATION

DEFINITION—An injury to the ankle so that the talus bone is displaced out of the socket formed by the tibia and fibula. Ankle dislocations are almost always associated with sprains (damage to ligaments) and fractures.

BODY PARTS INVOLVED
- Bones of the ankle, including the tibia, fibula and talus; ligaments that hold the bones of the ankle together.
- Soft tissues surrounding the dislocated bones, including nerves, tendons, muscles and blood vessels.

SIGNS & SYMPTOMS
- Excruciating pain at the time of injury.
- Loss of ankle function and severe pain when attempting to move the ankle.
- Locking of the dislocated bones in the abnormal position or spontaneous reposition, leaving no apparent deformity.
- Tenderness over the site of the dislocation, fracture and sprain.
- Ankle swelling and bruising.
- Numbness or paralysis of the foot from pressure or pinching of blood vessels or nerves.

CAUSES
- Serious injury with stress on the side of the ankle, forcing the ankle through a motion for which it is not designed.
- End result of a severe ankle sprain (injury to ligaments, fibers or attachment due to overstress).
- Recurrent sprains and strains that leave weakened ligaments.
- Powerful muscle contractions.

RISK INCREASES WITH
- Running, jumping or fast walking, especially on uneven terrain.
- Severe trauma such as fall from a height.
- Participation in contact sports.
- Repeated ankle injuries of any sort, especially dislocations or sprains.
- Poor muscle conditioning.

HOW TO PREVENT
- Protect ankle joints with protective devices (e.g., wrapped elastic bandages or tape wraps).
- Develop a high level of lower leg and ankle strength and conditioning.
- Warm up adequately before physical activity.
- Avoid irregular surfaces for running or track events.

? WHAT TO EXPECT

APPROPRIATE HEALTH CARE
- Doctor's care.
- Surgery to reduce ankle and fix fractures with screws and plates, and to repair ruptured tendons or ligaments.
- Physical therapy after the cast is removed.
- Self-care during rehabilitation.

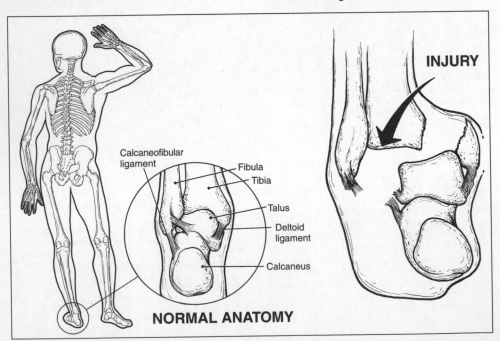

Calcaneofibular ligament
Fibula
Tibia
Talus
Deltoid ligament
Calcaneus

NORMAL ANATOMY

INJURY

DIAGNOSTIC MEASURES
- Your own observation of symptoms.
- Medical history and exam by a doctor.
- X-rays of injured areas to assess total injury. Dislocations of the ankle bones are frequently associated with fractures and sprains (torn ligaments) of the ankle.

POSSIBLE COMPLICATIONS
- Excessive bleeding or postoperative infection.
- Prolonged healing time if usual activities are resumed too soon.
- Avascular necrosis (bone cell death), with resultant bone collapse and arthritis.
- Proneness to repeated ankle injury.
- Unstable or permanently arthritic ankle joint.

PROBABLE OUTCOME
- A dislocated ankle with a fracture and/or sprain requires an average of 15 to 20 weeks to heal completely. Surgical pins or screws are usually removed after full healing if symptomatic. If this is a first-time injury, proper care, surgery and sufficient healing time before resuming activity should prevent permanent disability.
- If nonsurgical treatment is chosen, as much as 20 weeks healing time may be required before returning to sports activity. The period of crutch use and non-weight-bearing will be prolonged.

 ## HOW TO TREAT

NOTE—Follow your doctor's instructions. These instructions are supplemental.

FIRST AID—Use instructions for R.I.C.E., the first letters of *rest, ice, compression* and *elevation.* See Appendix 1 for details.

CONTINUING CARE
- The doctor will reduce (realign) the dislocated bones with surgery or, if possible, without. The setting will line up the dislocated bones as close to their normal positions as possible. Setting should be done as soon as possible after injury. Also, many tissues lose their elasticity and become difficult to return to a normal position.
- Following surgery, the physician may apply a stirrup splint from below the knee to the toes. A stirrup splint is less likely to cause problems with swelling at this time than a cast may cause. This will support the ankle enough to allow you to walk with crutches, but you should not put weight on the injured ankle.
- When the swelling subsides several days later, sutures may be removed and the splint replaced by a walking boot or cast. depending on the injury, weight-bearing may be allowed. This cast may need to stay in place for 10 to 21 days.

- After the cast is removed, strapping may be necessary for a minimum of 6 weeks.
- Bathe and shower as usual after the cast is removed.
- Use ice massage. Fill a large styrofoam cup with water and freeze. Tear a small amount of foam from the top so ice protrudes. Massage firmly over the injured area in a circle about the size of a baseball. Do this for 15 minutes at a time 3 or 4 times a day, and also before workouts or competition.
- Apply heat instead of ice if it feels better. Use heat lamps, hot soaks, hot showers, heating pads or heat liniments and ointments.
- Take whirlpool treatments, if available.
- Gentle massage will frequently provide comfort and decrease swelling.

MEDICATION
- For minor discomfort, you may use:
  Nonprescription medicines such as aspirin, acetaminophen or ibuprofen.
  Topical liniments and ointments.
- Your doctor may prescribe stronger medicine for pain.

ACTIVITY
- Walk with crutches until your doctor applies the walking cast. See Appendix 3 (Safe Use of Crutches).
- Resume your normal activities gradually.

DIET—During recovery, balance the amount of food you eat with any change in your level of physical activity. Eat a variety of foods to get the energy, protein, vitamins, minerals and fiber you need for good health and healing. Your doctor may suggest vitamin and mineral supplements to promote healing.

REHABILITATION
- Begin daily rehabilitation exercises when supportive wrapping is no longer needed. Use ice massage for 10 minutes prior to exercise.
- See Rehabilitation section for ankle and foot exercises.

 ## CALL YOUR DOCTOR IF

- You have symptoms of any severe ankle injury.
- Pain, swelling or bruising increases despite treatment.
- You notice numbness or discoloration of the toes when the walking cast is in place.
- Signs of postoperative infection occur, such as fever, drainage from the surgical wound or increasing pain at the operative site.

ANKLE EXOSTOSIS
(Bone Spurs; Calcium Deposits)

GENERAL INFORMATION

DEFINITION—A piling up of bone at the site of a new or repeat injury, usually caused by direct trauma.

BODY PARTS INVOLVED
• Lower part of the tibia and fibula(lower leg bone).
• Top of ankle bone (talus).
• Blood vessels, nerves, periosteum (covering of bone), and other soft tissues close to the exostosis.

SIGNS & SYMPTOMS
• Loss of "push" or "drive" (the ability to push off rapidly and forcefully in running).
• Inability to run, cut or jump at full speed.
• Low level of ankle pain with activity. Sometimes no pain exists.
• No tenderness or pressure with a physical examination. Sometimes pain and tenderness in the ankle and top of the heel bone can be detected only by special examination of a trained medical professional.
• Change in ankle bone contours. This begins as a small irregular bump that progresses to a large calcified spur (1 cm or more in length). In the worst cases, the exostosis may break away and appear on the x-ray as a calcified loose body.

• "Locking" if the tendon catches on the exostosis during exercise.

CAUSES
• Repeated ankle or foot injury, even mild injury.
• Participation in sports that require "pushing off" or "springing" from a position with the foot bent upward.
• Early arthritic changes.

RISK INCREASES WITH
• Medical history of repeated ankle injury.
• Vitamin and mineral deficiency, which makes complications following injury more likely.
• Poor muscle strength or conditioning, which fosters improper movement and allows undue stress on the ankle and foot bones.
• Improper or inadequate strapping prior to participation in contact sports (recurrent sprains).

HOW TO PREVENT
• Participate in a strengthening, flexibility and conditioning program appropriate for your sport.
• Allow full healing time after an ankle or foot injury before resuming any sport that requires you to push off and run.
• Warm up adequately before competition or workouts.

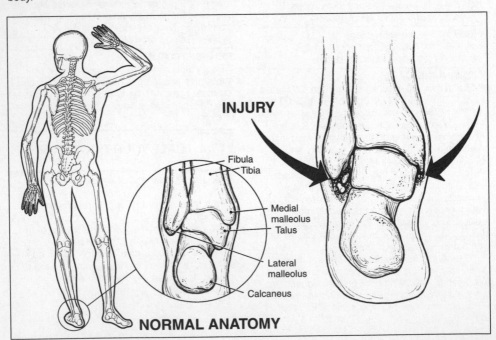

INJURY

Fibula
Tibia

Medial malleolus
Talus

Lateral malleolus

Calcaneus

NORMAL ANATOMY

? WHAT TO EXPECT

APPROPRIATE HEALTH CARE
- Doctor's diagnosis and care.
- Surgery to remove the exostosis (sometimes).
- Self-care during recovery.

DIAGNOSTIC MEASURES
- Your own observation of symptoms.
- Medical history and physical exam by a doctor.
- X-rays of the foot, ankle and knee.

POSSIBLE COMPLICATIONS
- Disability severe enough to diminish an athlete's competitive ability if the exostosis is untreated. Because mild exostosis is not readily apparent, coaches and other athletes often attribute the decline in performance to emotional causes or a loss of competitive drive in the athlete rather than understanding that it is caused by a physical disability (exostosis).
- Proneness to repeated injury.
- Degenerative arthritic changes in the ankle joint and cartilage in later life.
- Pressure on or injury to nearby nerves, ligaments, tendons, blood vessels or connective tissues.
- Tendinitis from direct irritation.

PROBABLE OUTCOME—Exostosis usually causes no disability with proper treatment, including rest of the injured ankle, heat treatments, corticosteroid injections and protection against additional injury. In a few cases, surgery is necessary. No surgical treatment is required for mild conditions that do not interfere with performance.

HOW TO TREAT

NOTE—Follow your doctor's instructions. These instructions are supplemental.

FIRST AID—None. The problem develops gradually.

CONTINUING CARE
- Apply heat frequently. Use heat lamps, hot soaks, hot showers, heating pads or heat liniments and ointments.
- Take whirlpool treatments, if available.
- Gentle massage will frequently provide comfort and decrease swelling.

MEDICATION
- Medicine usually is not necessary for this disorder. For minor discomfort, you may use nonprescription drugs such as aspirin or ibuprofen.
- If surgery is necessary, your doctor may prescribe:
  Nonsteroidal anti-inflammatory drugs to help control swelling.
  Stronger pain relievers.
  Antibiotics to fight infection.

ACTIVITY—Rest the affected ankle for 2 to 4 weeks. Use splints or crutches, if necessary, to prevent weight-bearing. Elevate the foot when sitting or lying down. Resume your normal activities gradually.

DIET—During recovery, balance the amount of food you eat with any change in your level of physical activity. Eat a variety of foods to get the energy, protein, vitamins, minerals and fiber you need for good health and healing. Your doctor may suggest vitamin and mineral supplements to promote healing.

REHABILITATION
- Begin daily rehabilitation exercises when pain subsides and you have clearance from your doctor.
- Use ice massage for 10 minutes before and 10 minutes after exercise. Fill a large styrofoam cup with water and freeze. Tear a small amount of foam from the top so ice protrudes. Massage firmly over the injured area in a circle about the size of a baseball.
- See Rehabilitation section for ankle and foot exercises.

CALL YOUR DOCTOR IF

- Your ability to push off with the foot and ankle diminishes for no apparent reason.
- Any of the following occurs after surgery:
  Numbness or discoloration of the toes when the walking cast is in place.
  Signs of infection (headache, muscle aches, dizziness or a general ill feeling and fever).
  Increased pain, swelling, redness, drainage or bleeding in the surgical area.

ANKLE FRACTURE, BIMALLEOLAR

GENERAL INFORMATION

DEFINITION—A break in the bones of both sides of the ankle. A temporary dislocation of the talus and rupture of ligaments of the ankle joint may also accompany this injury. The fracture sites include the lower ends of both the tibia and the fibula. The full extent of injury may not be recognized immediately.

BODY PARTS INVOLVED
• Three main bones of the ankle joint—the talus, tibia and fibula.
• Ligaments that support the ankle joint.
• Blood vessels, nerves, periosteum (covering of bone), and other soft tissues close to the injury site.

SIGNS & SYMPTOMS
• Severe, immediate ankle pain.
• A feeling of popping or tearing in the outer or inner part of the ankle. Sometimes it will feel as if the ankle joint was temporarily dislocated and popped back into joint. A sound may be heard at the time of fracture.
• Severe tenderness at the injury site.
• The injured person usually falls at the time of injury and has great difficulty walking.
• General swelling and bruising immediately throughout the ankle and foot.
• Visible deformity of the ankle.

CAUSES—Direct blow or stress imposed from either side of the ankle joint. The ligament or ligaments that normally hold the joint in place are stretched and sometimes torn.

RISK INCREASES WITH
• Sports that demand quick changes in direction, such as football and skiing.
• Activities involving jumping, such as basketball, soccer, volleyball, distance jumping and high jumping. Participants often accidentally land on the side of the foot or someone else lands on their foot.
• Walking or running on rough surfaces, such as roads with potholes.
• Shoes with inadequate support to prevent the foot from rolling over when stress occurs.
• Poor nutrition.
• Poor muscle strength or conditioning.
• Inadequate strapping prior to contact or collision sports.
• Previous ankle injury.

HOW TO PREVENT
• Build your strength with a conditioning program appropriate for your sport.
• Warm up before practice or competition.
• Tape the ankle from midfoot to midcalf before practice or competition. If you cannot use tape, wrap the ankle with elastic bandages.
• Wear proper protective shoes.
• Provide the ankle with substantial support during sports activities for 12 months following any significant ankle injury.

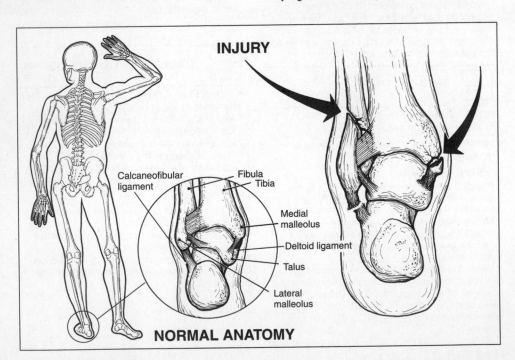

INJURY

Calcaneofibular ligament
Fibula
Tibia
Medial malleolus
Deltoid ligament
Talus
Lateral malleolus

NORMAL ANATOMY

WHAT TO EXPECT

APPROPRIATE HEALTH CARE
• Surgery to pin broken bones.
• Doctor's care.
• Physical therapy after the cast is removed.
• Self-care during rehabilitation.

DIAGNOSTIC MEASURES
• Your own observation of symptoms.
• Medical history and exam by a doctor.
• X-rays of injured areas to assess total injury. Fractures of the ankle bones are often associated with torn ligaments (sprains).

POSSIBLE COMPLICATIONS
• Excessive postoperative bleeding or infection.
• Prolonged healing time if usual activities are resumed too soon.
• Proneness to repeated ankle injury.
• Unstable or permanently arthritic ankle joint. Arthritic changes may also occur in the knee joint, because an ankle fracture sometimes causes added stress on the knee due to changes in weight-bearing.

PROBABLE OUTCOME
• Ankle fractures require an average of 12 to 16 weeks to heal completely. If this is a first-time injury, proper care, surgery and sufficient healing time before resuming activity should prevent permanent disability.
• If nonsurgical treatment is chosen, as much as 20 weeks' healing time may be required before returning to sports activity. The period of crutch use and non-weight-bearing will be prolonged.

 HOW TO TREAT

NOTE—Follow your doctor's instructions. These instructions are supplemental.

FIRST AID—Use instructions for R.I.C.E., the first letters of *rest, ice, compression* and *elevation*. See Appendix 1 for details.

CONTINUING CARE
• Following surgery, the physician may apply a stirrup splint from below the knee to the toes. A stirrup splint is less likely to cause problems with swelling than a cast may cause. This will support the joint effectively enough to walk on crutches, but you should not bear weight on the injured ankle.
• When the swelling subsides in several days, sutures are usually removed and the splint is replaced by a walking boot cast. This cast may need to stay in place for 14 to 28 days. You may walk on the walking cast as your doctor directs.

• After the cast is removed, strapping may be necessary for a minimum of 6 weeks.
• Bathe and shower as usual after the cast is removed.
• Use an ice pack 3 or 4 times a day. Wrap ice chips or cubes in a plastic bag. Wrap the bag in a moist towel, and place it over the injured ankle. Use for 20 minutes at a time.
• Apply heat instead of ice if it feels better. Use heat lamps, hot soaks, hot showers, heating pads or heat liniments and ointments.
• Take whirlpool treatments, if available.
• Massage the ankle gently and often to provide comfort and decrease swelling.

MEDICATIONS
• For minor discomfort, you may use:
 Nonprescription medicines such as aspirin, acetaminophen or ibuprofen.
 Topical liniments and ointments.
• Your doctor may prescribe stronger medicine for pain, if needed.

ACTIVITY
• Walk with crutches until your doctor applies the walking cast or boot. See Appendix 3 (Safe Use of Crutches).
• Assume your normal activities gradually, but don't drive until healing is complete.

DIET—During recovery, balance the amount of food you eat with any change in your level of physical activity. Eat a variety of foods to get the energy, protein, vitamins, minerals and fiber you need for good health and healing.

REHABILITATION
• Begin daily rehabilitation exercises when movement is comfortable.
• Use ice massage for 10 minutes before and 10 minutes after exercise. Fill a large styrofoam cup with water and freeze. Tear a small amount of foam from the top so ice protrudes. Massage firmly over the injured area in a circle.
• See Rehabilitation section for ankle and foot exercises.

 CALL YOUR DOCTOR IF

• You have symptoms of any severe ankle injury.
• Pain, swelling or bruising increases during treatment or rehabilitation.
• You notice numbness or discoloration of the toes when the walking cast is in place.
• You develop signs of postoperative infection (fever or increasing pain or drainage from the surgical wound).

ANKLE FRACTURE, SINGLE BONE
(Medial or Lateral Malleolar Ankle Fracture)

 GENERAL INFORMATION

DEFINITION—A fracture, usually in either side of the ankle, often including a total tear of one or more ankle ligaments. A temporary dislocation of the ankle joint may also occur.

BODY PARTS INVOLVED
- Lowest part of the lower leg bones (tibia and fibula).
- Ligaments on either side of the ankle that support the ankle joint.
- Three main bones of the ankle joint (talus, tibia, and fibula) involved with the dislocation or sprain.
- Blood vessels, nerves, periosteum (covering of bone), and other soft tissues close to the injury site.

SIGNS & SYMPTOMS
- Severe ankle pain immediately after injury.
- Popping or feeling of tearing in the outer or inner part of the ankle. Sometimes there will be a sensation that the ankle joint is dislocated or has popped back into joint.
- Severe tenderness at the injury site.
- The injured person usually falls at the time of injury and has difficulty walking.
- Forcing the ankle in the direction of pain may reveal some looseness in the joint.
- General swelling throughout ankle and foot.
- Bruising immediately or soon after injury.
- Visible deformity if fractured bone is displaced.

CAUSES—Stress imposed from either side of the ankle joint that temporarily forces or pries the ankle or heel bone (talus) out of its socket. The ligament or ligaments that normally hold the joint in place are stretched and torn.

RISK INCREASES WITH
- Previous ankle injury.
- Contact sports.
- Running, walking and jumping in such sports as basketball, soccer, volleyball, skiing or distance and high jumping. Persons in these often accidentally land on the side of the foot.
- Shoes with inadequate support to prevent lateral displacement when stress occurs.
- Osteoporosis or other bone disease.
- Poor nutrition, especially calcium deficiency.
- Poor muscle strength or conditioning.
- Inadequate strapping prior to participation in contact sports.
- Walking or running on rough surfaces, such as roads with potholes.

HOW TO PREVENT
- Participate in a strengthening, flexibility and conditioning program appropriate for your sport.
- Wear high-top athletic shoes for contact sports.
- Apply adequate taping or bracing (midfoot to midcalf) before participation in risky activities.

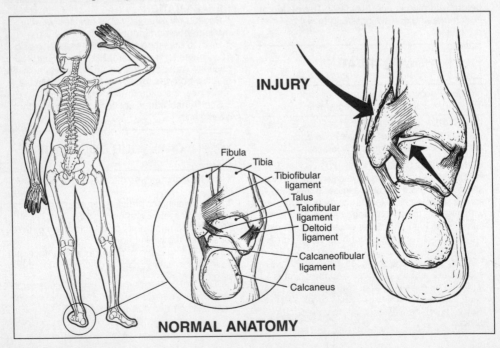

INJURY

Fibula
Tibia
Tibiofibular ligament
Talus
Talofibular ligament
Deltoid ligament
Calcaneofibular ligament
Calcaneus

NORMAL ANATOMY

- Wear supportive elastic ankle wraps (not as good as tape, but better than nothing).
- Support the ankle well during sports activities for 12 months after any significant ankle injury.

 ## WHAT TO EXPECT

APPROPRIATE HEALTH CARE
- Surgery to pin broken bones together and to repair ruptured tendons.
- Doctor's care.
- Physical therapy after the cast is removed.

DIAGNOSTIC MEASURES
- Your own observation of symptoms.
- Medical history and exam by a doctor.
- X-rays of injured areas to assess total injury.

POSSIBLE COMPLICATIONS
- Full extent of the injury may not be recognized immediately, delaying treatment.
- Excessive postoperative bleeding or infection.
- Prolonged healing time if usual activities are resumed too soon.
- Proneness to repeated ankle injury.
- Unstable or permanently arthritic ankle joint, if many repeat injuries occur or if bones are not set adequately.

PROBABLE OUTCOME
- After surgery, an ankle fracture and/or sprain requires an average of 10 to 12 weeks to heal completely. If this is a first-time injury, proper care, surgery and sufficient healing time before resuming activity should prevent permanent disability. Torn ligaments require as much healing time as fractured bones.
- If nonsurgical treatment is chosen, as much as 20 weeks' healing time may be required before returning to sports activity. The period of crutch use and non-weight-bearing will be prolonged.

 ## HOW TO TREAT

NOTE—Follow your doctor's instructions. These instructions are supplemental.

FIRST AID—Use instructions for R.I.C.E., the first letters of *rest, ice, compression* and *elevation*. See Appendix 1 for details.

CONTINUING CARE
- Following surgery, the doctor may apply a stirrup splint from below the knee to the toes. A stirrup splint is less likely to cause problems with swelling than cast may cause. This will support the ankle effectively enough to walk on crutches, but you should not bear weight on the injured ankle.
- When the swelling subsides several days later, sutures may be removed. The splint is replaced by a removable boot or cast for 14 to 28 days. See Appendix 2 (Care of Casts). Your doctor will allow weight-bearing between 4-6 weeks.
- After the cast has been removed, strapping or a brace will be necessary for at least 6 weeks.
- Bathe and shower as usual after cast is removed.
- After cast removal, use frequent ice massage. Fill a large styrofoam cup with water and freeze. Tear a small amount of foam from the top so ice protrudes. Massage firmly over the injured area in a circle about the size of a baseball. Do this for 15 minutes at a time 3 or 4 times a day.
- Apply heat instead of ice if it feels better. Use heat lamps, hot soaks, hot showers or heating pads; take whirlpool treatments, if available.
- Gentle massage will frequently provide comfort and decrease swelling.

MEDICATION
- For minor discomfort, you may use aspirin, acetaminophen or topical liniments and ointments.
- Your doctor may prescribe stronger medicine for pain, if needed.

ACTIVITY—Walk with crutches until you have a walking cast. See Appendix 3 (Safe Use of Crutches). Resume your normal activities gradually. Don't drive until cast is removed and mobility has returned.

DIET
- Do not eat or drink before manipulation or surgery to treat the fracture. Fluid or solid food in your stomach makes vomiting while under anesthesia more hazardous.
- During recovery, balance the amount of food you eat with any change in your level of physical activity. Eat a variety of foods to get the energy, protein, vitamins, minerals and fiber you need for good health and healing.

REHABILITATION—Begin daily rehabilitation exercises when supportive wrapping is no longer needed. Use ice massage for 10 minutes prior to exercise. See Rehabilitation section for ankle and foot exercises.

 ## CALL YOUR DOCTOR IF

- You have signs or symptoms of any severe ankle injury.
- Pain, swelling or bruising increases during treatment or rehabilitation.
- You notice numbness or discoloration of the toes when the walking cast is in place.
- Signs of postoperative infection occur, such as fever, drainage from the surgical wound or increasing pain at the surgical site.

ANKLE FRACTURE, TALUS
(Osteochondral Fracture)

 GENERAL INFORMATION

DEFINITION—A fracture of the ankle involving both bone and cartilage of the talus, accompanied by a total tear (or sprain) of one or more ligaments. A temporary dislocation of the ankle joint may also occur. A two-ligament sprain with a chondral fracture of the ankle will cause more disability than a single-ligament sprain.

BODY PARTS INVOLVED
• Bones and cartilage of the ankle joint.
• Ligaments that support the ankle joint.

SIGNS & SYMPTOMS
• Severe pain in the ankle, appearing at the time of the injury.
• Popping or a feeling of tearing in the outer or inner part of the ankle. Sometimes there will be a sensation that the ankle joint is dislocated or was temporarily dislocated and popped back into joint.
• Severe tenderness at the injury site.
• Loss of function. The injured person usually falls at the time of injury and has great difficulty when attempting to walk.
• Looseness in the joint if the foot is forced in the direction of pain.
• Generalized swelling immediately throughout the ankle and foot.
• Bruising immediately or soon after injury.

• Continuing signs and symptoms with little improvement, indicating an injury more severe than a simple sprain.

CAUSES—Stress imposed from either side of the ankle joint that temporarily forces or pries the ankle bone (talus) out of its socket. The ligaments that normally hold the joint in place are stretched and torn, and a piece breaks off the surface of the wedged talus bone.

RISK INCREASES WITH
• Previous ankle injury and ankle instability.
• Activities in which the foot may land sideways, such as running, walking, and jumping in such sports as basketball, soccer, volleyball, skiing, distance jumping and high jumping.
• Shoes with inadequate support to prevent sideways displacement when stress occurs.
• Poor nutrition, especially calcium deficiency.
• Poor muscle strength or conditioning.
• Inadequate ankle strapping prior to participation in contact sports.
• Walking or running on rough surfaces, such as roads with potholes.

HOW TO PREVENT
• Participate in a strengthening, flexibility and conditioning program appropriate for your sport.
• Tape ankle adequately (midfoot to midcalf) before participation in contact sports. Otherwise, wear supportive elastic ankle wraps or braces.

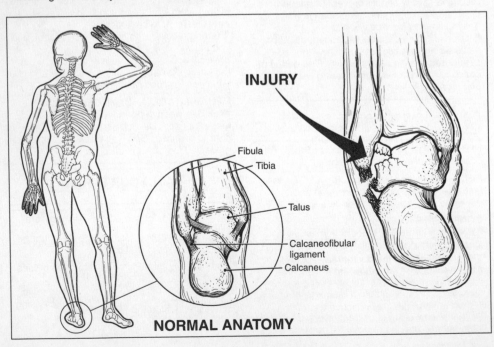

INJURY

Fibula
Tibia
Talus
Calcaneofibular ligament
Calcaneus

NORMAL ANATOMY

• Provide the ankle with substantial support during sports activities for 12 months following any significant ankle injury.

 ## WHAT TO EXPECT

APPROPRIATE HEALTH CARE
• Surgery to insert metal pins or screws to hold broken bits of bone together and to repair the ruptured ligaments.
• Doctor's care for application of a walking cast after surgery and ankle taping when the cast is no longer needed.
• Physical therapy after the cast is removed.

DIAGNOSTIC MEASURES
• Your own observation of symptoms.
• Medical history and exam by a doctor.
• X-rays of injured areas to assess total injury. Chondral fractures of ankle bones are often associated with torn ligaments (sprains).

POSSIBLE COMPLICATIONS
• Full extent of the injury is sometimes not recognized immediately, delaying treatment.
• Prolonged healing time if activity is resumed too soon.
• Proneness to repeated ankle injury.
• Unstable or arthritic ankle joint following repeated injury.
• If unrecognized, the ankle may have chronic pain or giving way periodically due to loose pieces of bone or cartilage.

PROBABLE OUTCOME—Healing time after surgery averages 12 to 16 weeks. If this is a first-time injury, proper care (including surgery) and sufficient time for healing before resuming activity should prevent permanent disability. Torn ligaments require as much time to heal as fractured bones.

 ## HOW TO TREAT

NOTE—Follow your doctor's instructions. These instructions are supplemental.

FIRST AID
• Use instructions for R.I.C.E., the first letters of *rest, ice, compression* and *elevation*. See Appendix 1 for details.
• To prevent further injury to the ankle, avoid any weight-bearing. Go to your doctor's office or hospital emergency room right away.

CONTINUING CARE
• Following surgery, the doctor may apply a stirrup boot splint from below the knee to the toes. Stirrup boots are less likely to cause problems with swelling than a cast may cause. This will support the joint effectively enough to walk on crutches, but you should not bear weight on the injured ankle.

• When the swelling subsides several days later, sutures may be removed and the splint will be replaced by a removable boot or cast. See Appendix 2 (Care of Casts). This cast may need to stay in place for 10 to 21 days. Start walking on the cast as your doctor directs.
• After the cast has been removed, strapping may be necessary for a minimum of 6 weeks.
• After cast removal, use frequent ice massage. Fill a large styrofoam cup with water and freeze. Tear a small amount of foam from the top so ice protrudes. Massage firmly over the injured area in a circle about the size of a baseball. Do this for 15 minutes at a time 3 or 4 times a day.
• Apply heat instead of ice if it feels better. Use heat lamps, hot soaks, hot showers, heating pads or heat liniments and ointments.
• Gentle, frequent massage will provide comfort and decrease swelling.

MEDICATION
• For minor discomfort, you may use:
Nonprescription medicines such as aspirin, acetaminophen or ibuprofen.
Topical liniments and ointments.
• Your doctor may prescribe stronger medicine for pain, if needed.

ACTIVITY—Walk with crutches until your doctor applies the walking cast. See Appendix 3 (Safe Use of Crutches). Resume normal activities gradually. Don't drive until healing is complete.

DIET
• Do not drink or eat before manipulation or surgery to treat the fracture. Fluid or solid food in your stomach makes vomiting while under anesthesia more hazardous.
• During recovery, balance the amount of food you eat with any change in your level of physical activity. Eat a variety of foods to get the energy, protein, vitamins, minerals and fiber you need for good health and healing.

REHABILITATION—Begin daily rehabilitation exercises after clearance from your doctor. Use ice massage for 10 minutes prior to exercise. See Rehabilitation section for ankle and foot exercises.

 ## CALL YOUR DOCTOR IF

• You have signs or symptoms of any severe ankle injury.
• Pain, swelling or bruising increases during treatment or rehabilitation.
• You notice numbness or discoloration of toes when the walking cast is in place.
• Signs of postoperative infection occur: fever, drainage from the surgical wound or increasing pain at the surgical site.

ANKLE SPRAIN, GRADE 1
(Mild or 1st-Degree Ankle Sprain)

 GENERAL INFORMATION

DEFINITION—Stretching and slight or partial tearing of one or more ligaments in the ankle. A two-ligament sprain causes more disability than a single-ligament sprain.

BODY PARTS INVOLVED
• Ligaments that support the ankle joint.
• Three main bones of the ankle joint—the talus (ankle bone) and the tibia and fibula (lower leg bones).
• Blood vessels, nerves, periosteum (covering of bone) and other soft tissues close to the injury.

SIGNS & SYMPTOMS
• Ankle pain at the time of injury.
• A feeling of popping or tearing in the outer part of the ankle.
• Mild tenderness at the injury site.
• Little loss of function. The injured person can bear weight and walk without help for 30 minutes or so following injury. Then, depending on the extent of injury, the joint may seem to lose some of its capacity for weight-bearing as swelling occurs.
• Swelling in the ankle.
• Little or no visible bruising for several hours after injury. Then some bruising may appear.

CAUSES—Stress imposed from either side of the ankle joint, temporarily forcing or prying the ankle or heel bone out of its normal socket. The ligaments that normally hold the joint in place are stretched without tearing.

RISK INCREASES WITH
• Previous ankle injury.
• Any sport in which sideways displacement of the ankle is likely. Runners, walkers, and participants in such sports as basketball, soccer, volleyball, skiing, distance jumping and high jumping are prone to ankle sprains. When jumping, they often accidentally land on the side of the foot.
• Use of shoes with insufficient support to prevent sideways displacement when stress occurs.
• Poor muscle strength or conditioning.
• Inadequate strapping prior to participation in contact sports.
• Walking or running on rough surfaces, such as roads with potholes.

HOW TO PREVENT
• Participate in a strengthening, flexibility and conditioning program appropriate for your sport.
• Warm up before practice or competition.
• Tape the ankle from midfoot to midcalf before practice or competition. If you cannot use tape, wrap the ankle with elastic bandages or use an elastic brace.

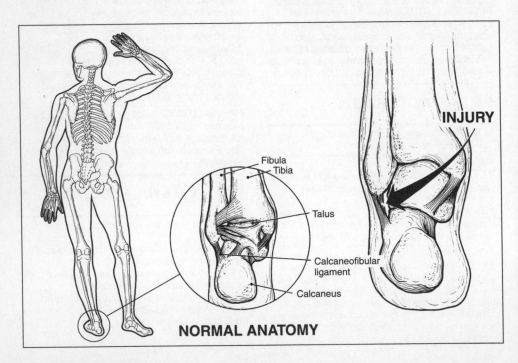

NORMAL ANATOMY

Fibula
Tibia
Talus
Calcaneofibular ligament
Calcaneus

INJURY

- Wear proper protective shoes.
- Provide the ankle with substantial support during sports activities for 12 months following any significant ankle injury.

 ## WHAT TO EXPECT

APPROPRIATE HEALTH CARE
- Doctor's care only if discomfort is great or doesn't improve in 24 hours.
- Self-care after diagnosis.
- Whirlpool, ultrasound or massage (to displace fluid from the injured joint space).

DIAGNOSTIC MEASURES
- Your own observation of symptoms.
- Medical history and exam by a doctor.
- X-rays of the ankle, foot and knee to rule out fractures.

POSSIBLE COMPLICATIONS
- Prolonged healing time or more severe ligament injury if activity is resumed too soon.
- Proneness to repeated injury.
- Unstable or arthritic ankle joint following repeated injury.

PROBABLE OUTCOME—The full extent of the injury cannot be determined for 12 to 24 hours. A first-degree ankle sprain usually heals enough in 5 to 7 days to allow modified activity. Complete healing requires an average of 6 weeks.

 ## HOW TO TREAT

NOTE—Follow your doctor's instructions. These instructions are supplemental.

FIRST AID—The goal is to prevent further injury to the torn ligaments. Follow instructions for R.I.C.E., the first letters of *rest, ice, compression* and *elevation*. See Appendix 1 for details.

CONTINUING CARE
- Continue using an ice pack 3 or 4 times a day. Wrap ice chips or cubes in a plastic bag. Wrap the bag in a moist towel, and place it over the injured area. Use for 20 minutes at a time.
- After 96 hours, apply heat instead of ice if it feels better. Use heat lamps, hot soaks, hot showers, heating pads, or heat liniments and ointments.
- Take whirlpool treatments, if available.
- Keep the foot elevated whenever possible to decrease swelling.
- Massage the ankle gently and often to provide comfort and decrease swelling.

MEDICATION
- For minor discomfort, you may use:
  Nonprescription medicines such as aspirin, acetaminophen or ibuprofen.
  Topical liniments or ointments.
- Your doctor may prescribe:
  Nonsteroidal anti-inflammatory drugs.
  Stronger medicine for pain, if needed.

ACTIVITY—Except for very minor injuries, walk with crutches for about 72 hours. See Appendix 3 (Safe Use of Crutches). Resume your normal activities gradually.

DIET—During recovery, balance the amount of food you eat with any change in your level of physical activity. Eat a variety of foods to get the energy, protein, vitamins, minerals and fiber you need for good health and healing. Your doctor may suggest vitamin and mineral supplements to promote healing.

REHABILITATION
- Begin daily rehabilitation exercises when supportive wrapping is no longer needed.
- Use ice massage for 10 minutes before and 10 minutes after exercise. Fill a large styrofoam cup with water and freeze. Tear a small amount of foam from the top so ice protrudes. Massage firmly over the injured area in a circle about the size of a baseball.
- See Rehabilitation section for ankle and foot exercises.

 ## CALL YOUR DOCTOR IF

- You have symptoms of an ankle sprain that does not improve within 1 week.
- Ankle pain, swelling or bruising increases despite treatment.

ANKLE SPRAIN, GRADE 2
(Moderate or 2nd-Degree Ankle Sprain)

 GENERAL INFORMATION

DEFINITION—Partial tearing of the lateral ligaments of the ankle, resulting in weakening and some loss of ankle function. A two-ligament sprain causes more disability than a single-ligament sprain.

BODY PARTS INVOLVED
• Ligaments that support the ankle joint.
• Three main bones of the ankle joint—the talus (ankle bone), and the tibia and fibula (lower leg bones).
• Blood vessels, nerves, periosteum (covering of bone) and other soft tissues close to the injury.

SIGNS & SYMPTOMS
• Severe ankle pain at the time of injury.
• A feeling of popping or tearing in the outer part of the ankle.
• Moderate tenderness at the injury site.
• Loss of function. The injured person usually falls, but can walk a little, since direct weight-bearing does not place stress on the injured ankle. Then, depending on the extent of the injury, the joint may seem to lose some of its capability to weight bear as swelling occurs.
• Mild looseness in the joint if the foot is forced in the direction of the pain.

• Generalized moderate swelling immediately throughout the ankle and foot.
• Bruising that appears soon after injury.

CAUSES—Stress imposed from either side of the ankle joint, temporarily forcing or prying the ankle or heel bone out of its socket. The ligaments that normally hold the joint in place are stretched and partially torn.

RISK INCREASES WITH
• Previous ankle injury.
• Any sport in which sideways displacement of the ankle is likely. Runners, walkers, and participants in sports such as basketball, soccer, volleyball, skiing, distance jumping and high jumping are prone to ankle sprains. They often accidentally land on the side of the foot.
• Use of shoes with inadequate support to prevent sideways displacement when stress occurs.
• Poor muscle strength or conditioning.
• Inadequate strapping prior to participation in contact sports.
• Walking or running on rough surfaces, such as roads with potholes

HOW TO PREVENT
• Build your strength with a conditioning program appropriate for your sport.
• Warm up before practice or competition.

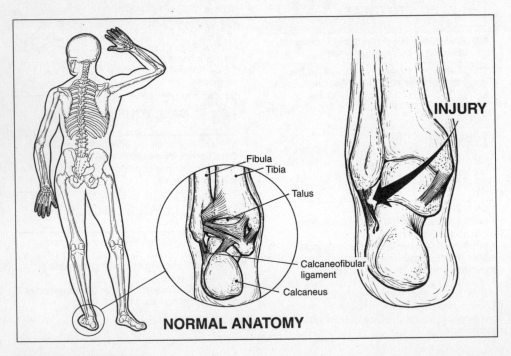

Fibula
Tibia
Talus
Calcaneofibular ligament
Calcaneus

NORMAL ANATOMY

INJURY

- Tape the ankle from midfoot to midcalf before practice or competition. If you cannot use tape, wrap the ankle with elastic bandages or use an elastic brace.
- Wear proper protective shoes.
- Provide the ankle with substantial support during sports activities for 12 months following any significant ankle injury.

 ## WHAT TO EXPECT

APPROPRIATE HEALTH CARE
- Doctor's care to apply a walking cast or brace and to apply tape after cast removal.
- Whirlpool, ultrasound and massage (to displace accumulated fluid in injured joint spaces).

DIAGNOSTIC MEASURES
- Your own observation of symptoms.
- Medical history and exam by a doctor.
- X-rays of the injured areas to rule out fractures.

POSSIBLE COMPLICATIONS
- Prolonged healing time if activity is resumed too soon.
- Proneness to repeated injury.
- Unstable or arthritic ankle joint following repeated injury.

PROBABLE OUTCOME—The full extent of injury cannot be determined for 12 to 24 hours. Complete healing requires an average of 6 to 10 weeks. However, a return to modified, supported activity may begin in 10 to 21 days. If this is a first-time injury, proper treatment and sufficient healing time before resuming activity should prevent permanent disability. Ligaments have a poor blood supply, and torn ligaments require as much healing time as fractures.

 ## HOW TO TREAT

NOTE—Follow your doctor's instructions. These instructions are supplemental.

FIRST AID—The goal is to prevent further injury to the torn ligaments. Follow instructions for R.I.C.E., the first letters of *rest, ice, compression* and *elevation.* See Appendix 1 for details.

CONTINUING CARE
- Keep ice packs on the injured area almost continuously for 24 hours.
- Wrap an elastic bandage over a sponge-rubber donut placed over the sprained area to compress the area for about 72 hours.
- After the first 24 hours, your doctor may apply a stirrup splint from below the knee to the toes. This will support the ankle enough to walk on crutches, but you should not bear weight on the injured ankle yet.

- When the swelling subsides in several days, the splint is replaced by a walking boot cast for 10 to 21 days. You may walk on the walking cast when your doctor directs.
- After the cast has been removed, strapping may be necessary for a minimum of 6 weeks.
- After cast removal (or if a cast was not used), continue using an ice pack 3 or 4 times a day. Wrap ice chips or cubes in a plastic bag. Wrap the bag in a moist towel, and place it over the injured area. Use for 20 minutes at a time.
- Apply heat instead of ice if it feels better. Use heat lamps, hot soaks, hot showers, heating pads or heat liniments and ointments.
- Take whirlpool treatments, if available.
- Keep the foot elevated whenever possible to decrease swelling.
- Gentle massage will frequently provide comfort and decrease swelling.

MEDICATION
- For minor discomfort, you may use:
  Nonprescription medicines such as aspirin, acetaminophen or ibuprofen.
  Topical liniments and ointments.
- Your doctor may prescribe:
  Stronger medicine for pain, if needed.
  Nonsteroidal anti-inflammatory drugs.

ACTIVITY—Use a splint and crutches or a walking boot or walking cast as prescribed by your doctor. After the cast is removed, resume your normal activities gradually. Don't drive until the ankle is completely healed.

DIET—During recovery, balance the amount of food you eat with any change in your level of physical activity. Eat a variety of foods to get the energy, protein, vitamins, minerals and fiber you need for good health and healing.

REHABILITATION
- Begin daily rehabilitation exercises when supportive wrapping is no longer needed.
- Use ice massage for 10 minutes before and 10 minutes after exercise. Fill a large styrofoam cup with water and freeze. Tear small amount of foam from the top so ice protrudes. Massage firmly in a circle over the injured area.
- See Rehabilitation section for ankle and foot exercises.

 ## CALL YOUR DOCTOR IF

- You have symptoms of a second-degree ankle sprain.
- Ankle pain, swelling or bruising increases despite treatment.
- You experience numbness or discoloration of toes when the walking cast is in place.

ANKLE SPRAIN, GRADE 3
(Severe or 3rd-Degree Ankle Sprain)

GENERAL INFORMATION

DEFINITION—A severe injury to the ankle in which the lateral ligaments are stretched and totally torn (ruptured). A severe sprain may include a temporary or fixed dislocation (the joint slips out of place, and may move back in).

BODY PARTS INVOLVED
* Usually, the three lateral ligaments that support the ankle joint and connect the bones to each other.
* Three main bones of the ankle joint—the talus (ankle bone) and the tibia and fibula (lower leg bones).
* Blood vessels, nerves, periosteum (covering of bone) and other soft tissues close to the injury.

SIGNS & SYMPTOMS
* Severe ankle pain at the time of injury.
* A feeling of popping or tearing in the outer or inner part of the ankle. Sometimes there will be a sensation that the ankle joint is dislocated or was temporarily dislocated and popped back into joint.
* Severe tenderness at the injury site.
* Loss of function. The injured person usually falls and has great difficulty walking. The joint loses its stability.
* Looseness in the joint if the foot is forced in the direction of pain.
* Immediate, marked, generalized swelling throughout the ankle and foot.

* Bruising that appears immediately or soon after injury.

CAUSES—Stress imposed from either side of the ankle joint, temporarily forcing or prying the ankle or heel bone out of its socket. The ligament or ligaments that normally hold the joint in place are stretched and torn.

RISK INCREASES WITH
* Previous ankle injury.
* Any sport in which sideways displacement of the ankle is likely. Runners, walkers and participants in such sports as basketball, soccer, volleyball, skiing, distance jumping and high jumping are prone to ankle sprains. They often accidentally land on the side of the foot.
* Use of shoes with inadequate support to prevent sideways displacement when stress occurs.
* Poor muscle strength or conditioning.
* Inadequate strapping prior to participation in contact sports.
* Walking or running on rough surfaces, such as roads with potholes.

HOW TO PREVENT
* Build your strength with a conditioning program appropriate for your sport.
* Warm up before practice or competition.
* Tape the ankle from midfoot to midcalf before practice or competition. If you cannot use tape, wrap the ankle with elastic bandages or use an elastic brace.

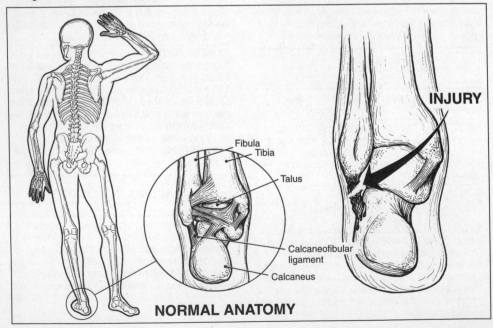

Fibula
Tibia
Talus
Calcaneofibular ligament
Calcaneus

NORMAL ANATOMY

INJURY

- Wear proper protective shoes.
- Provide the ankle with substantial support during sports activities for 12 months following any significant ankle injury.

 # WHAT TO EXPECT

APPROPRIATE HEALTH CARE
- Doctor's care.
- Application of a walking cast or brace and taping of the ankle when the cast is no longer needed.
- Physical therapy after the cast is removed.
- Surgery (sometimes) to repair the torn ligaments, especially in repeated injury (usually for chronic instability).

DIAGNOSTIC MEASURES
- Your own observation of symptoms.
- Medical history and exam by a doctor.
- X-rays of injured areas to assess total injury. Grade-3 sprains are often accompanied by fractures of the ankle bones.

POSSIBLE COMPLICATIONS
- Prolonged healing time or further, more extensive injury if activity is resumed too soon.
- Proneness to repeated injury.
- Unstable or arthritic ankle joint following repeated injury.

PROBABLE OUTCOME—The full extent of injury cannot be determined for 12 to 24 hours. A third-degree ankle sprain usually requires 21 to 42 days to return to supported, modified activity. Complete healing requires 12 to 16 weeks. If this is a first-time injury, proper care, surgery and sufficient healing time before resuming activity should prevent permanent disability. Ligaments have a poor blood supply, and torn ligaments require as much healing time as fractures.

 # HOW TO TREAT

NOTE—Follow your doctor's instructions. These instructions are supplemental.

FIRST AID—The goal is to prevent further injury to the torn ligaments. See a doctor immediately for proper diagnosis and care. Follow instructions for R.I.C.E., the first letters of *rest, ice, compression* and *elevation*. See Appendix 1 for details.

CONTINUED CARE
- The doctor may apply a stirrup splint from below the knee to the toes. A stirrup splint is less likely to cause problems with swelling than a cast may cause. This will support the joint effectively enough to walk on crutches, but you should not bear weight on the injured ankle.

- When the swelling subsides in several days, the splint is replaced by a walking cast for 10 to 21 days. You may walk on the walking cast as your doctor directs.
- After the cast has been removed, ankle taping will be necessary for a minimum of 6 weeks.
- After cast removal, use an ice pack 3 or 4 times a day. Wrap ice chips or cubes in a plastic bag. Wrap bag in a moist towel, and place over the injured area. Use for 20 minutes at a time.
- After 96 hours, apply heat instead of ice if it feels better. Use heat lamps, hot soaks, hot showers, heating pads or heat liniments and ointments.
- Take whirlpool treatments, if available.
- Keep the foot elevated whenever possible to decrease swelling.
- Massage the ankle gently and often to provide comfort and decrease swelling.

MEDICATION
- For minor discomfort, you may use: Nonprescription medicines such as aspirin, acetaminophen or ibuprofen. Topical liniments and ointments.
- Your doctor may prescribe: Nonsteroidal anti-inflammatory drugs. Stronger medicine for pain if needed.

ACTIVITY—Walk with crutches until your doctor applies the walking cast. See Appendix 3 (Safe Use of Crutches). Resume normal activities gradually. Don't drive until healing is complete.

DIET—During recovery, balance the amount of food you eat with any change in your level of physical activity. Eat a variety of foods to get the energy, protein, vitamins, minerals and fiber you need for good health and healing.

REHABILITATION
- Begin daily rehabilitation exercises when supportive wrapping is no longer needed.
- Use ice massage for 10 minutes before and 10 minutes after exercise. Fill a large styrofoam cup with water and freeze. Tear a small amount of foam from the top so ice protrudes. Massage firmly in a circle over the injured area.
- See Rehabilitation section for ankle and foot exercises.

 # CALL YOUR DOCTOR IF

- You have symptoms of a third-degree ankle sprain.
- Ankle pain, swelling or bruising increases despite treatment.
- You notice numbness or discoloration at the toes when the walking cast is in place.
- You develop signs of postoperative infection (increased pain or drainage from surgical site).

ANKLE STRAIN

GENERAL INFORMATION

DEFINITION—A stretch or tear (partial or complete) of any muscles or tendons that surround the ankle. Muscles, tendons and their attached bones comprise contractile units. These units stabilize the ankle and allow its motion. A strain occurs at the weakest part of a unit. Strains are of 3 types:
- Mild (Grade I)—Slightly pulled muscle without tearing of muscle or tendon fibers. There is no loss of strength.
- Moderate (Grade II)—Tearing of fibers in a muscle-tendon unit in the ankle muscle or tendon or at the attachment to bone. Strength is diminished.
- Severe (Grade III)—Rupture of the muscle-tendon-bone attachment, with separation of fibers. Severe strain may require surgical repair. Chronic strains are caused by overuse. Acute strains are caused by direct injury or overstress.

BODY PARTS INVOLVED
- Tendons and muscles surrounding the ankle.
- Lower leg bones (tibia and fibula) and foot bones.
- Soft tissues surrounding the strained muscle and attached tendon, including nerves, periosteum (covering of bone), blood vessels and lymph vessels.

SIGNS & SYMPTOMS
- Pain when moving or stretching the ankle.
- Muscle spasm in the calf.
- Tenderness to the touch; swelling in the ankle.
- Loss of strength (moderate or severe strain).
- Crepitation ("crackling" feeling and sound when the ankle is pressed and actively moved with fingers).
- Calcification of the muscle or its tendon (visible with x-ray).
- Inflammation of the sheath covering the tendon.

CAUSES
- Prolonged overuse of muscle-tendon units in the ankle.
- Single violent injury or force applied to the muscle-tendon unit in the ankle.

RISK INCREASES WITH
- Sports that require quick starts, such as starting a race.
- Contact sports.
- Medical history of any bleeding disorder.
- Obesity.
- Poor nutrition.
- Previous ankle injury.
- Poor muscle condition.

HOW TO PREVENT
- Participate in a strength, flexibility and conditioning program appropriate for your sport.
- Warm up before practice or completion.
- Tape the ankle area before practice or competition.
- Wear proper shoes and protective equipment.

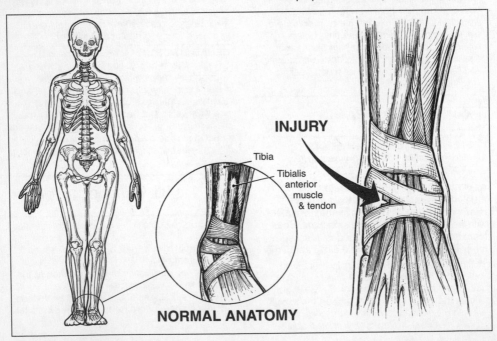

INJURY

Tibia

Tibialis anterior muscle & tendon

NORMAL ANATOMY

WHAT TO EXPECT

APPROPRIATE HEALTH CARE
- Doctor's diagnosis.
- Application of tape, splints or walking casts (sometimes).
- Self-care during rehabilitation.
- Physical therapy (moderate or severe strain).
- Surgery (severe strain).

DIAGNOSTIC MEASURES
- Your own observation of symptoms.
- Medical history and exam by a doctor.
- X-rays of the leg, foot and ankle to rule out fractures.
- MRI scan to rule out tendon rupture.

POSSIBLE COMPLICATIONS
- Prolonged healing time if activity is resumed too soon.
- Proneness to repeated injury.
- Unstable or arthritic ankle following repeated injury.
- Inflammation at the attachment to bone (periostitis).
- Prolonged disability (sometimes), especially weakness.

PROBABLE OUTCOME—If this is a first-time injury, proper care and sufficient healing time before resuming activity should prevent permanent disability. Torn ligaments and tendons require as long to heal as fractured bones. Average healing times are:
- Mild strain—2 to 10 days.
- Moderate strain—10 days to 6 weeks.
- Severe strain—6 to 10 weeks.

If this is a repeat injury, complications listed above are more likely to occur.

HOW TO TREAT

NOTE—Follow your doctor's instructions. These instructions are supplemental.

FIRST AID—Use instructions for R.I.C.E., the first letters of *rest, ice, compression* and *elevation*. See Appendix 1 for details.

CONTINUING CARE
- Use ice massage 3 or 4 times a day for 15 minutes at a time. Fill a large styrofoam cup with water and freeze. Tear a small amount of foam from the top so ice protrudes. Massage firmly over the injured area in a circle about the size of a softball.
- After the first 72 hours, apply heat instead of ice if it feels better. Use heat lamps, hot soaks, hot showers, heating pads or heat liniments and ointments.
- Take whirlpool treatments, if available.
- If a cast was used, wrap the injured ankle with an elasticized bandage between treatments after cast is removed.
- Massage gently and often to provide comfort and decrease swelling.

MEDICATION
- For minor discomfort, you may use:
  Aspirin, acetaminophen or ibuprofen.
  Topical liniments and ointments.
- Your doctor may prescribe:
  Stronger pain relievers,
  Injection of a long-acting local anesthetic to reduce pain (rare).
  Injection of a corticosteroid, such as triamcinolone, to reduce inflammation (rare).

ACTIVITY
- For a moderate or severe strain, walk with crutches for at least 72 hours—longer with a cast or splints. See Appendix 3 (Safe Use of Crutches).
- Resume your normal activities gradually.

DIET—During recovery, balance the amount of food you eat with any change in your level of physical activity. Eat a variety of foods to get the energy, protein, vitamins, minerals and fiber you need for good health and healing.

REHABILITATION—Begin daily rehabilitation exercises when supportive wrapping is no longer needed. Use ice massage for 10 minutes prior to exercise. See Rehabilitation section for ankle and foot exercises.

CALL YOUR DOCTOR IF

- You have symptoms of moderate or severe ankle strain or a mild strain persists longer than 10 days.
- Pain or swelling worsens despite treatment.
- The following occur with a cast or splints:
  Pain, numbness or coldness below the injury.
  Dusky, blue or gray toenails.

ANKLE SYNOVITIS

GENERAL INFORMATION

DEFINITION—Inflammation of the synovium, the smooth, lubricated lining of the ankle joint. The synovium's lubricating fluid helps the ankle move freely and prevents bone surfaces from rubbing against each other. Synovitis is often a complication of an injury, such as a fracture, or of rheumatological diseases, such as gout or rheumatoid arthritis, or of infection.

BODY PARTS INVOLVED
• Ankle joint.
• Synovial membrane surrounding the entire joint.
• Space between the joint and the synovial membrane.

SIGNS & SYMPTOMS
• Pain and heat in the ankle.
• No visible ankle swelling. Swelling and fluid accumulation is deep within the joint.

CAUSES
• Any injury to the ankle and ankle joint.
• Bacterial infection.
• Metabolic disturbance, such as an acute attack of gout or rheumatoid arthritis.

RISK INCREASES WITH
• Repeated ankle injury.
• Poor muscle strength or conditioning, which makes ankle injury more likely.
• Inadequate ankle strapping prior to participation in contact sports.
• Medical history of gout, rheumatoid arthritis or other inflammatory joint diseases.
• Infection in another joint or tissues.
• Vitamin or mineral deficiency, which makes complications following injury more likely.

HOW TO PREVENT
• Tape the ankle securely from midfoot to midcalf before participation in contact sports. If taping is not possible, wear supportive elastic ankle wraps.
• Protect the ankle with substantial support during sports activities for 12 months after a significant ankle injury.

WHAT TO EXPECT

APPROPRIATE HEALTH CARE
• Doctor's diagnosis and application of a walking cast and tape.
• Self-care during rehabilitation.
• Whirlpool, ultrasound or massage to displace excess fluid from the injured joint space.
• Occasionally, surgery or arthroscopy necessary to remove inflamed synovium.

DIAGNOSTIC MEASURES
• Your own observation of symptoms.
• Medical history and exam by a doctor.
• X-rays of the ankle, foot and knee to rule out fractures or developing arthritis.

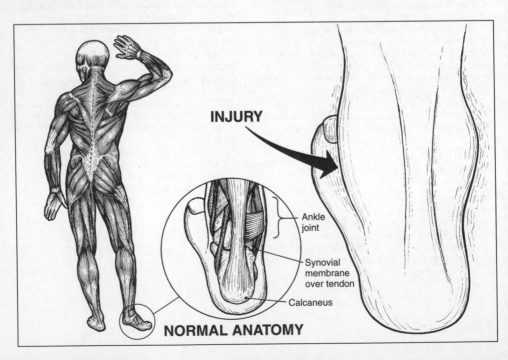

INJURY

Ankle joint

Synovial membrane over tendon

Calcaneus

NORMAL ANATOMY

POSSIBLE COMPLICATIONS
- Prolonged healing time if activity is resumed too soon.
- Proneness to repeated ankle injury.
- An arthritic ankle or permanent stiffness of the joint following repeated bouts of synovitis.
- Chronic synovitis that may prevent athletic participation.

PROBABLE OUTCOME—Healing is possible in 3 to 5 weeks with heat treatments, corticosteroid injections (sometimes) and rest (of the ankle). In many cases, ankle synovitis does not heal completely and becomes chronic. This is because the ankle joint is subjected to continual stress.

 HOW TO TREAT

NOTE—Follow your doctor's instructions. These instructions are supplemental.

FIRST AID—No first aid. This condition develops gradually

CONTINUING CARE
- Obtain treatment for any underlying medical condition, such as gout or infection.
- For greater comfort, keep the foot elevated whenever possible.
- You may need a walking plaster boot cast for 10 to 14 days. See Appendix 2, Care of Casts.
- After the cast is removed, apply heat frequently. Use heat lamps, hot soaks, hot showers, heating pads or heat liniments and ointments.
- Take whirlpool treatments, if available.
- Massage gently and often to provide comfort and decrease swelling.
- Chronic synovitis may require ankle strapping before any workout or competition.
- Chronic synovitis may require surgery. In an arthroscopy synovectomy, a tiny cut is made in the skin over the joint and a thin tube is inserted into the joint to remove the lining.

MEDICATION
- Your doctor may prescribe:
  Antibiotics if infection is present.
  Nonsteroidal anti-inflammatory drugs or antigout medicine.
  Injection of a long-acting local anesthetic mixed with a corticosteroid to help reduce pain and inflammation.
- You may take aspirin or ibuprofen for minor discomfort.

ACTIVITY—Resume normal activities slowly as swelling, pain, redness and disability diminish.

DIET—During recovery, balance the amount of food you eat with any change in your level of physical activity. Eat a variety of foods to get the energy, protein, vitamins, minerals and fiber you need for good health and healing. Your doctor may suggest vitamin and mineral supplements to promote healing.

REHABILITATION
- Rest the ankle for 3 to 5 weeks. Elevate it whenever possible.
- Begin daily rehabilitation exercises when a walking cast is no longer needed.
- Use ice massage for 10 minutes before and 10 minutes after exercise. Fill a large styrofoam cup with water and freeze. Tear a small amount of foam from the top so ice protrudes. Massage firmly over the injured area in a circle about the size of a baseball.
- See Rehabilitation section for ankle and foot exercises.

 CALL YOUR DOCTOR IF

- You have symptoms of ankle synovitis
- Symptoms worsen or persist longer than 5 weeks despite treatment outlined above.

ANKLE TENOSYNOVITIS

GENERAL INFORMATION

DEFINITION—Inflammation of a tendon or the lining of a tendon sheath in the ankle. This lining secretes a fluid that lubricates the tendon. When the lining becomes inflamed, the tendon cannot glide smoothly in its covering.

BODY PARTS INVOLVED
● Any ankle tendon and its lining (tendon sheath).
● Soft tissues in the surrounding area, including blood vessels, nerves, ligaments, periosteum (covering of bone) and connective tissues.

SIGNS & SYMPTOMS
● Constant pain or pain with motion.
● Limited motion of the ankle.
● Crepitation (a "crackling" sound when the tendon moves or is touched).
● Heat and redness over the inflamed tendon.

CAUSES
● Strain from unusual use or overuse of muscles and tendons in the ankle.
● Direct blow or injury to the ankle. Tenosynovitis becomes more likely with repeated ankle injury.
● Ill-fitting boots or shoes, creating excess pressure on tendon pathway.
● Infection introduced through broken skin at the time of injury or through a surgical incision after injury. .

RISK INCREASES WITH
● Contact sports, especially kicking sports such as football or soccer.
● Skiing.
● If surgery is needed to remove inflamed synovium, surgical risk increases with smoking, poor nutrition, alcoholism or drug abuse and recent or chronic illness.

HOW TO PREVENT
● Participate in a strength, flexibility and conditioning program appropriate for your sport.
● Warm up adequately before practice or competition.
● Wear protective footgear appropriate for your sport.
● Learn proper moves and techniques for your sport.

WHAT TO EXPECT

APPROPRIATE HEALTH CARE
● Doctor's examination and diagnosis.
● Surgery (sometimes) to enlarge the tendon's covering, remove inflamed synovium and restore a smooth gliding motion.

DIAGNOSTIC MEASURES
● Your own observations of symptoms and signs.
● Medical history and physical examination by your doctor.

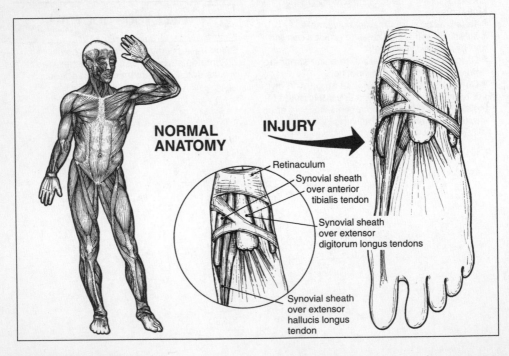

NORMAL ANATOMY

INJURY

Retinaculum

Synovial sheath over anterior tibialis tendon

Synovial sheath over extensor digitorum longus tendons

Synovial sheath over extensor hallucis longus tendon

- X-rays of the area to rule out other abnormalities.
- MRI to evaluate integrity of tendon and soft tissues,
- Laboratory studies: Blood and urine studies before surgery. Tissue examination after surgery.

POSSIBLE COMPLICATIONS
- Prolonged healing time if activity is resumed too soon.
- Proneness to repeated injury.
- Adhesive tenosynovitis: The tendon and its covering become bound together. Restriction of motion may be complete or partial. Surgery may be necessary to remove the covering or transfer the tendon to a less constrictive area.
- Constrictive tenosynovitis: The walls of the covering thicken and narrow, preventing the tendon from sliding through. Surgery is necessary to cut away part of the covering.

PROBABLE OUTCOME—Tenosynovitis of the ankle is usually curable in about 2 to 4 weeks with heat treatments, corticosteroid injections and rest of the inflamed area. Recovery is usually quicker if the inflammation is caused by a direct below rather than by a sprain or strain.

 HOW TO TREAT

NOTE—Follow your doctor's instructions. These instructions are supplemental.

FIRST AID—None. This problem develops slowly.

CONTINUING CARE
- If surgery is not necessary, you may need a walking boot cast for 10 to 14 days. See Appendix 2 (Care of Casts). Then wrap the ankle with an elasticized bandage until healing is complete.
- Apply heat frequently. Use heat lamps, hot soaks, hot showers, heating pads or heat liniments and ointments.
- Take whirlpool treatments, if available.

MEDICATION—You may use nonprescription drugs such as acetaminophen for minor pain. Your doctor may prescribe:
- Nonsteroidal anti-inflammatory drugs.
- Stronger pain relievers, if needed.
- Injection of the tendon covering with a long-acting local anesthetic and a nonabsorbable corticosteroid to relieve pain and inflammation.

ACTIVITY—Resume normal actively slowly and stretch before activities.

DIET—During recovery, balance the amount of food you eat with any change in your level of physical activity. Eat a variety of foods to get the energy, protein, vitamins, minerals and fiber you need for good health and healing. Your doctor may suggest vitamin and mineral supplements to promote healing.

REHABILITATION
- Begin daily rehabilitation exercises when supportive wrapping is no longer needed.
- Use ice massage for 10 minutes before and after exercise. Fill a large styrofoam cup with water and freeze. Tear a small amount of foam from the top so ice protrudes. Massage firmly over the injured area in a circle about the size of a softball.
- See Rehabilitation section for ankle and foot exercises.

 CALL YOUR DOCTOR IF

- You have symptoms of ankle tenosynovitis.
- Any of the following occurs after surgery:
  Increased pain, swelling, redness, drainage or bleeding in the surgical area.
  Signs of infection (headache, muscle aches, dizziness or a general ill feeling and fever).
  New, unexplained symptoms. Drugs used in treatment may produce side effects.

ARM & SHOULDER TENOSYNOVITIS, BICEPS TENDON SHEATH (Biceps Tendinitis)

 GENERAL INFORMATION

DEFINITION—Inflammation of the lining of the biceps tendon sheath in the upper arm and shoulder. This lining secretes a fluid that lubricates the tendon. When the lining becomes inflamed, the tendon cannot glide smoothly in its covering.

BODY PARTS INVOLVED
- Biceps tendon, which attaches the biceps muscle to the shoulder.
- Lining and covering of the biceps tendon.
- Soft tissues in the surrounding area, including blood vessels, nerves, ligaments, periosteum (covering of bone) and connective tissues.

SIGNS & SYMPTOMS
- Constant pain or pain with motion.
- Limited motion of the shoulder and elbow.
- Crepitation (a "crackling" sound when the tendon moves or is touched).
- Heat and redness over the inflamed tendon.
- Restriction of movement, followed by a sudden painful snap if the tendon breaks away from its attachment to bone.

CAUSES
- Strain from unusual use or overuse at the biceps muscle.
- Direct blow or injury to the shoulder. Tenosynovitis becomes more likely with repeated injury to the biceps muscle-tendon unit.
- Infection introduced through broken skin at the time of injury or through a surgical incision after injury.

RISK INCREASES WITH
- Contact sports.
- Throwing sports.
- Gymnastics.
- Weightlifting.
- If surgery is needed, surgical risk increases with smoking, poor nutrition, alcoholism or drug abuse and recent or chronic illness.

HOW TO PREVENT
- Engage in a conditioning program before beginning regular sports participation.
- Warm up adequately before practice or competition.
- Wear protective gear appropriate for your sport.
- Learn proper moves and techniques for your sport.

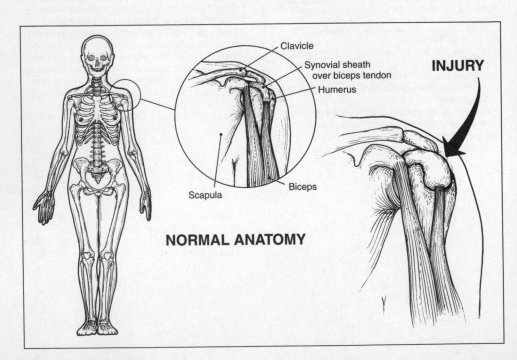

Clavicle
Synovial sheath over biceps tendon
Humerus
INJURY
Biceps
Scapula

NORMAL ANATOMY

WHAT TO EXPECT

APPROPRIATE HEALTH CARE
- Doctor's examination and diagnosis.
- Surgery (sometimes) to enlarge the tunnel of the tendon covering and restore a smooth, gliding motion. The surgical procedure is performed under general anesthesia in an outpatient surgical facility or hospital operating room.

DIAGNOSTIC MEASURES
- Your own observation of symptoms and signs.
- Medical history and physical examination by your doctor.
- X-rays of the area to rule out other abnormalities, especially fractures.
- Diagnostic ultrasound or MRI (see Glossary for both) to confirm diagnosis and to rule out rotator cuff tear.

POSSIBLE COMPLICATIONS
- Prolonged healing time if activity is resumed too soon.
- Proneness to repeated injury of the biceps tendon.
- Adhesive tenosynovitis: The tendon and its covering become bound together. Loss of motion may be complete or partial. Surgery is necessary to remove the covering or transfer the tendon to a new area.
- Constrictive tenosynovitis: The walls of the covering thicken and narrow the opening, preventing the tendon from sliding through. Surgery is necessary to cut away part of the covering.
- Rupture of the tendon if motion is forced when the tendon and its covering are bound together.

PROBABLE OUTCOME—Tenosynovitis is usually curable in about 6 weeks with heat treatments, corticosteroid injections and rest of the inflamed area. Recovery is usually quicker if the inflammation is caused by a direct blow rather than by a strain or sprain.

 # HOW TO TREAT

NOTE—Follow your doctor's instructions. These instructions are supplemental.

FIRST AID—None. This problem develops slowly.

CONTINUING CARE
- Wrap the shoulder with an elasticized bandage, or use a sling until healing is complete.
- Apply heat frequently. Use heat lamps, hot soaks, hot showers, heating pads or heat liniments and ointments.

MEDICATION—You may use nonprescription drugs such as acetaminophen for minor pain. Your doctor may prescribe:
- Stronger pain relievers.
- Injection of the unruptured tendon covering with a combination of a long-acting local anesthetic and a nonabsorbable corticosteroid such as triamcinolone.

ACTIVITY—Resume normal activities slowly.

DIET—During recovery, balance the amount of food you eat with any change in your level of physical activity. Eat a variety of foods to get the energy, protein, vitamins, minerals and fiber you need for good health and healing.

REHABILITATION
- Begin daily rehabilitation exercises when supportive wrapping is no longer needed.
- Use ice massage for 10 minutes before and after exercise. Fill a large styrofoam cup with water and freeze. Tear a small amount of foam from the top so ice protrudes. Massage firmly over the injured area in a circle about the size of a softball.
- See Rehabilitation section for elbow exercises and shoulder exercises.

 # CALL YOUR DOCTOR IF

- You have symptoms of biceps tenosynovitis.
- Any of the following occurs after surgery:
  Increased pain, swelling, redness, drainage or bleeding in the surgical area.
  Headache, muscle aches, dizziness or a general ill feeling and fever.
- New, unexplained symptoms develop. Drugs used in treatment may produce side effects.

ARM CONTUSION, FOREARM

GENERAL INFORMATION

DEFINITION—Bruising of skin and underlying tissues of the forearm caused by a direct blow. Contusions cause bleeding from ruptured small capillaries, allowing blood to infiltrate muscles, tendons or other soft tissues.

BODY PARTS INVOLVED—Tissues of the forearm, including blood vessels, muscles, tendons, nerves, covering of bone (periosteum) and connective tissues.

SIGNS & SYMPTOMS
- Forearm swelling—either superficial or deep.
- Pain and tenderness in the forearm.
- Feeling of firmness when pressure is exerted on the injured area.
- Discoloration under the skin, beginning with redness and progressing to the characteristic "black-and-blue" bruise.
- Restricted forearm mobility proportional to the extent of injury.

CAUSES—Direct blow to the forearm, usually from a blunt object.

RISK INCREASES WITH
- Violent contact sports, especially when the forearm is not adequately protected.
- Medical history of any bleeding disorder.
- Poor nutrition, including vitamin deficiency.
- Use of anticoagulants or aspirin.

HOW TO PREVENT—Wear appropriate protective gear and equipment during competition or other athletic activity if you have had a recent contusion or the activity makes a contusion likely.

WHAT TO EXPECT

APPROPRIATE HEALTH CARE
- Doctor's care, unless the contusion is quite small.
- Self-care for minor contusions and for serious contusions during rehabilitation.
- Physical therapy for serious contusions.

DIAGNOSTIC MEASURES
- Your own observation of symptoms.
- Medical history and physical exam by a doctor for all except minor injuries.
- X-rays of the injured area to assess total injury to soft tissues and to rule out the possibility of underlying fracture. Total extent of injury may not be apparent for 48 to 72 hours.

POSSIBLE COMPLICATIONS
- Excessive bleeding, leading to disability. Infiltrative-type bleeding can sometimes lead to calcification and impaired function of injured muscles and tendons.
- Decreased blood supply to forearm muscles, causing tissue death, loss of function and contraction of affected muscles (known as acute compartment syndrome).

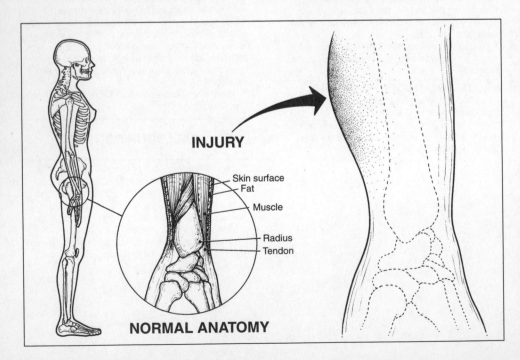

INJURY

Skin surface
Fat
Muscle
Radius
Tendon

NORMAL ANATOMY

- Prolonged healing time if usual activities are resumed too soon.
- Possible infection if skin is broken over the contusion.

PROBABLE OUTCOME—Healing time varies with the extent of injury, but average healing time for forearm contusions is 1 to 2 weeks. Expect a return to activity when mobility and protective strength return.

 ## HOW TO TREAT

NOTE—Follow your doctor's instructions. These instructions are supplemental.

FIRST AID—Use instructions for R.I.C.E., the first letters of *rest, ice, compression* and *elevation*. See Appendix 1 for details.

CONTINUING CARE
- Use a sling to immobilize the arm.
- Wrap an elasticized bandage over a felt pad on the injured area. Keep the area compressed for about 72 hours.
- Continue ice massage. Fill a large styrofoam cup with water and freeze. Tear a small amount of foam from the top so ice protrudes. Massage gently over the injured area in a circle about the size of a softball. Do this for 15 minutes at a time 3 or 4 times a day, and also before workouts or competition.
- After 72 hours, apply heat instead of ice if it feels better. Use heat lamps, hot soaks, hot showers, heating pads, heat liniments and ointments or whirlpool treatments.
- Massage gently and often to provide comfort and decrease swelling.

MEDICATION
- For minor discomfort, you may use: Acetaminophen or ibuprofen. Topical liniments and ointments.
- Your doctor may prescribe stronger medicine for pain.

ACTIVITY—Begin activities slowly, and stop exercise as soon as pain begins. Increase activity as healing progresses.

DIET—During recovery, balance the amount of food you eat with any change in your level of physical activity. Eat a variety of foods to get the energy, protein, vitamins, minerals and fiber you need for good health and healing.

REHABILITATION
- Begin daily rehabilitation exercises when supportive wrapping is no longer needed.
- See Rehabilitation section for wrist and hand exercises.

 ## CALL YOUR DOCTOR IF

- You have symptoms of a forearm contusion that doesn't improve within a day or two.
- Skin is broken and signs of infection (drainage, increasing pain, fever, headache, muscle aches, dizziness or a general ill feeling) occur.

ARM CONTUSION, RADIAL NERVE

GENERAL INFORMATION

DEFINITION—Injury from a direct blow to the area over the radial nerve in the upper arm, close to the elbow. Contusions cause bleeding from ruptured small capillaries that allow blood to infiltrate nerves, muscles, tendons or other soft tissues.

BODY PARTS INVOLVED
• Radial nerve.
• Blood vessels, muscles, tendons, covering of bone (periosteum) and connective tissues.

SIGNS & SYMPTOMS
• Swelling at the contusion site—either superficial or deep.
• Pain and tenderness at the elbow.
• Shocking, tingling sensation, with numbness in the wrist and hand.
• Dropped wrist and loss of some movement in the fingers and thumb.
• Feeling of firmness when pressure is exerted at the injury site.
• Discoloration under the skin, beginning with redness and progressing to the characteristic "black-and-blue" bruise.
• Restricted elbow activity proportional to the extent of injury.

CAUSES
• Direct blow to the elbow and radial nerve from a blunt object.
• Falling on an elbow.

RISK INCREASES WITH
• Contact sports such as football, hockey or baseball, especially when elbows and arms are not adequately protected.
• Medical history of any bleeding disorder.
• Poor nutrition, including vitamin deficiency.

HOW TO PREVENT—Wear appropriate protective gear and equipment, such as elbow pads, during competition or other athletic activity if there is risk of an elbow or radial nerve contusion.

? WHAT TO EXPECT

APPROPRIATE HEALTH CARE
• Doctor's care unless the contusion is quite small.
• Surgery is very rarely needed and is reserved for those with extended periods of numbness and weakness.
• Self-care for minor contusions or for serious nerve contusions during rehabilitation after surgery.
• Physical therapy to demonstrate and teach stretching and use of positioning splints.

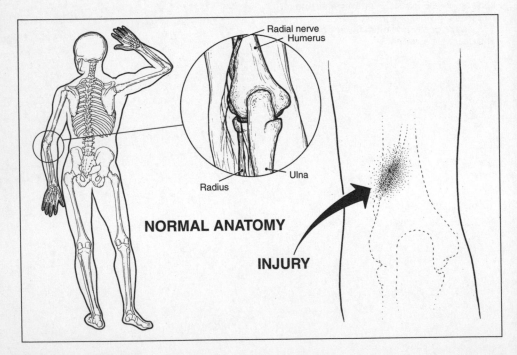

Radial nerve
Humerus
Radius
Ulna

NORMAL ANATOMY

INJURY

DIAGNOSTIC MEASURES
- Your own observation of symptoms.
- Medical history and physical exam by a doctor for all except minor injuries.
- X-rays of the elbow to assess total injury to soft tissues and to rule out the possibility of underlying fractures. The total extent of injury may not be apparent for 48 to 72 hours.

POSSIBLE COMPLICATIONS
- Permanent damage to the radial nerve, leading to disability in the forearm and hand.
- Prolonged healing time if usual activities are resumed too soon.
- Infection if skin over the contusion is broken.

PROBABLE OUTCOME—Healing time for contusion to tissues around the nerve averages 1 to 2 weeks. However, healing time for the radial nerve itself may be considerably longer, averaging at least 6 to 8 weeks. In some cases, symptoms never disappear and surgery may be necessary.

 HOW TO TREAT

NOTE—Follow your doctor's instructions. These instructions are supplemental.

FIRST AID—Use instructions for R.I.C.E., the first letters of *rest, ice, compression* and *elevation*. See Appendix 1 for details.

CONTINUING CARE
- Support the arm in a sling.
- Wrap an elasticized bandage over a sponge-rubber donut placed on the injured area. Keep the area compressed for about 72 hours.
- Continue ice massage. Fill a large styrofoam cup with water and freeze. Tear a small amount of foam from the top so ice protrudes. Massage gently over the injured area in a circle about the size of a softball. Do this for 15 minutes at a time 3 or 4 times a day, and also before workouts or competition.

- Apply heat instead of ice when skin warmth over the injury becomes the same as for the noninjured areas. Use heat lamps, hot soaks, hot showers, heating pads, heat liniments and ointments or whirlpool treatments
- Massage gently and often to provide comfort and decrease swelling.

MEDICATION
- For minor discomfort, you may use:
  Acetaminophen or ibuprofen
  Topical liniments and ointments.
- Your doctor may prescribe stronger medicine for pain.

ACTIVITY—Begin activities slowly, and stop exercise as soon as any pain begins. Increase activity as healing progresses.

DIET—During recovery, balance the amount of food you eat with any change in your level of physical activity. Eat a variety of foods to get the energy, protein, vitamins, minerals and fiber you need for good health and healing.

REHABILITATION
- Begin daily rehabilitation exercises when supportive wrapping is no longer needed.
- See Rehabilitation section for elbow exercises.

 CALL YOUR DOCTOR IF

- You have symptoms of a radial nerve contusion.
- Any of the following occurs after surgery:
  Increased pain, swelling, redness, drainage or bleeding in the surgical area.
  Signs of infection: headache, muscle aches, dizziness, fever or a general ill feeling.
  Nausea or vomiting.
  Constipation.
- New, unexplained symptoms develop. Drugs used in treatment may produce side effect.

ARM CONTUSION, UPPER ARM

GENERAL INFORMATION

DEFINITION—Bruising of the skin, muscle and underlying tissues of the upper arm due to a direct blow. Contusions cause bleeding from ruptured small capillaries, allowing blood to infiltrate muscles, tendons or other soft tissues. Muscle tissues is damaged most by a contusion in this area.

BODY PARTS INVOLVED
• Upper arm, particularly the biceps or triceps muscle.
• Other soft tissues, including blood vessels, tendons, nerves, covering of bone (periosteum) and connective tissues.

SIGNS & SYMPTOMS
• Local swelling—either superficial or deep.
• Pain and tenderness over the bruised area.
• Feeling of firmness when pressure is exerted on the injured area.
• Discoloration under the skin, beginning with redness and progressing to the characteristic "black-and-blue" bruise.
• Restricted arm mobility proportional to the extent of injury.

CAUSES—Direct blow to the upper arm, usually from a blunt object.

RISK INCREASES WITH
• Violent contact sports such as football or hockey, especially when the upper arm is not protected adequately.
• Medical history of any bleeding disorder.
• Poor nutrition, including vitamin deficiency.
• Use of anticoagulants or aspirin.

HOW TO PREVENT—Wear appropriate protective gear and equipment, such as foam rubber or felt pads, during competition or other athletic activity if there is risk of an upper arm contusion.

WHAT TO EXPECT

APPROPRIATE HEALTH CARE
• Doctor's care unless the injury is quite small.
• Self-care for minor contusions or for serious contusions during rehabilitation.
• Physical therapy for serious contusions.

DIAGNOSTIC MEASURES
• Your own observation of symptoms.
• Medical history and physical exam by a doctor for all except minor injuries.
• X-rays of the arm, shoulder and elbow to assess total injury to soft tissues and to rule out the possibility of underlying fracture. The total extent of injury may not be apparent for 48 to 72 hours.

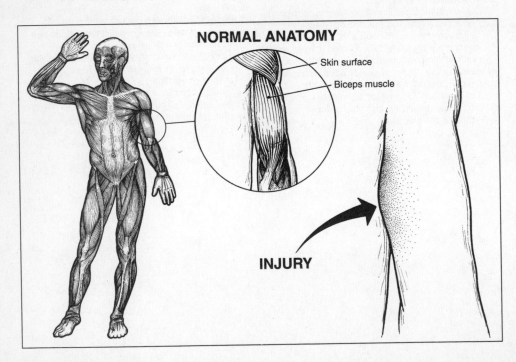

NORMAL ANATOMY

Skin surface

Biceps muscle

INJURY

POSSIBLE COMPLICATIONS
- Excessive bleeding, leading to disability. Infiltrative-type bleeding can occasionally lead to calcification and impaired function of injured muscle with stiffness.
- Prolonged healing time if usual activity is resumed too soon.
- Infection if skin over the contusion is broken.

PROBABLE OUTCOME—Healing time varies with the extent of injury, but all except the most serious upper arm contusions should heal in 1 to 2 weeks. Return to activity when mobility and protective strength return.

 ## HOW TO TREAT

NOTE—Follow your doctor's instructions. These instructions are supplemental.

FIRST AID—Use instructions for R.I.C.E., the first letters of *rest, ice, compression and elevation*. See Appendix 1 for details.

CONTINUING CARE
- Wrap felt or sheet wadding over the injured area. Then wrap the arm with an elasticized bandage from fingertips to armpit. Keep area compressed for about 72 hours.
- Continue ice massage. Fill a large styrofoam cup with water and freeze. Tear a small amount of foam from the top so ice protrudes. Massage gently over the injured area in a circle about the size of a softball. Do this for 15 minutes at a time 3 or 4 times a day, and also before workouts or competition.

- After 72 hours, apply heat instead of ice if it feels better. Use heat lamps, hot soaks, hot showers, heating pads, heat liniments and ointments or whirlpool treatments.
- Massage gently and often to provide comfort and decrease swelling.

MEDICATION
- For minor discomfort, you may use: Acetaminophen or ibuprofen. Topical liniments and ointments.
- Your doctor may prescribe stronger medicine for pain.

ACTIVITY—Begin activities slowly, and stop exercise as soon as pain begins. Increase activity as healing progresses.

DIET—During recovery, balance the amount of food you eat with any change in your level of physical activity. Eat a variety of foods to get the energy, protein, vitamins, minerals and fiber you need for good health and healing.

REHABILITATION
- Begin daily rehabilitation exercises when supportive wrapping is no longer needed.
- See Rehabilitation section for Shoulder Exercises.

 ## CALL YOUR DOCTOR IF

- You have an upper arm contusion that doesn't improve in 1 or 2 days.
- Skin is broken and signs of infection (drainage, increasing pain, fever, headache, muscle aches, dizziness or a general ill feeling) occur.

ARM EXOSTOSIS
(Blocker's Exostosis)

GENERAL INFORMATION

DEFINITION—An overgrowth of bone in the upper arm. An exostosis occurs at the site of repeated injury, usually from direct blows. This benign overgrowth of bone can be mistaken for a bone tumor.

BODY PARTS INVOLVED
• Middle third (usually) of the humerus, the upper arm bone.
• Soft tissues surrounding the exostosis, including muscles, nerves, lymph vessels, blood vessels and periosteum (covering of bone).

SIGNS & SYMPTOMS
• No symptoms for mild cases.
• Pain and tenderness in the upper arm at the site of the exostosis.
• Extreme sensitivity in the upper arm to pressure or minor injury.
• Change in the contour of the bone, ranging from a slight lump to a large calcified spur (1 cm or more in length) on the humerus. In the worst cases, the exostosis may break away and feel like a distinct foreign body in the arm. An x-ray will show it to be loose in the tissues of the upper arm.

CAUSES
• Repeated injury (contusions, sprains or strains) that involve the upper arm bone.
• Chronic irritation to an already damaged bone area.

RISK INCREASES WITH
• Contact sports, particularly football or other sports that require blocking with the arms.
• Other direct blows to the arms.
• History of bone or joint disease, such as osteomyelitis, osteomalacia or osteoporosis.
• Vitamin or mineral deficiency.
• Poor muscle strength or conditioning, making injury more likely.
• If surgery or anesthesia is needed, surgical risk increases with smoking, use of mind-altering drugs, muscle relaxants, tranquilizers, sleep inducers, insulin, sedatives, beta-adrenergic blockers or corticosteroids.

HOW TO PREVENT
• Allow adequate time for recovery from any arm injury.
• During participation in contact sports, wear fiberboard pads over the upper arms and shoulder pads to prevent injuries.
• Learn proper moves and techniques for the sports activities you pursue to decrease the risk of injury.

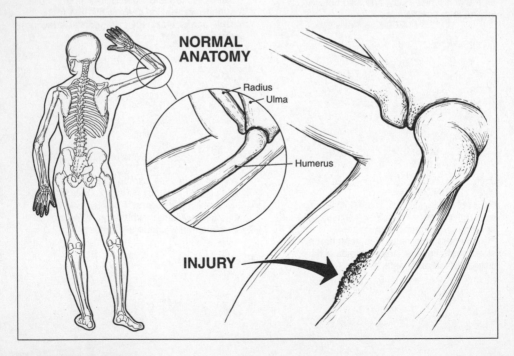

NORMAL ANATOMY

Radius
Ulma
Humerus

INJURY

WHAT TO EXPECT

APPROPRIATE HEALTH CARE
- Doctor's care.
- Surgery (sometimes) to remove the exostosis.
- Self-care during rehabilitation.
- Physical therapy.

DIAGNOSTIC MEASURES
- Your own observation of signs and symptoms.
- Medical history and physical exam by a doctor.
- X-rays of the elbow, arm and shoulder.

POSSIBLE COMPLICATIONS
- Overlooking a mild exostosis that produces no symptoms, despite signs of diminished performance. Athletes and coaches frequently assume that decreased performance results from loss of competitive drive or emotional causes rather than from the physical disability that actually exists.
- Prolonged healing time if activity is resumed too soon.
- Proneness to repeated arm injury.
- Unstable or arthritic shoulder or elbow following repeated injury.
- Pressure on or injury to nearby muscles, nerves, ligaments, tendons, blood vessels or connective tissues.
- Impaired blood supply to the injured area.
- Tendinitis from direct irritation.

PROBABLE OUTCOME—Upper arm exostosis usually causes no disability if it is treated properly. Treatment usually involves resting the injured arm for 2 to 4 weeks, heat treatments, corticosteroid injections and protection against additional injury. In a few cases, surgery is necessary to remove the exostosis.

HOW TO TREAT

NOTE—Follow your doctor's instructions. These instructions are supplemental.

FIRST AID—None. This condition develops gradually.

CONTINUING CARE
- Rest the injured arm. Use a sling if needed to prevent weight-bearing. Don't subject yourself to reinjury until completely healed.
- Apply heat frequently. Use heat lamps, hot soaks, hot showers, heating pads or heat liniments and ointments.
- Take whirlpool treatments, if available.
- Follow instructions under How to Prevent to avoid a recurrence of the injury. Use proper protection during competition and workouts.

MEDICATION
- Medicine usually is not necessary for this disorder. For minor pain, you may use non-prescription drugs such as aspirin or other anti-inflammatories.
- If surgery is necessary, your doctor may prescribe:
  Nonsteroidal anti-inflammatory drugs to help control swelling or adjacent tendinitis.
  Stronger pain relievers.
  Antibiotics to fight infection.

ACTIVITY—Decrease activity for 2 to 4 weeks. If surgery is necessary, resume normal activity gradually.

DIET—During recovery, balance the amount of food you eat with any change in your level of physical activity. Eat a variety of foods to get the energy, protein, vitamins, minerals and fiber you need for good health and healing. Your doctor may suggest vitamin and mineral supplements to promote healing.

REHABILITATION
- Begin daily rehabilitation exercises when movement is comfortable. Weightlifting done under supervision can help provide a quick return of strength and flexibility.
- Use ice massage for 10 minutes prior to exercise. Fill a large styrofoam cup with water and freeze. Tear a small amount of foam from the top so ice protrudes. Massage firmly over the injured area in a circle about the size of a softball.
- See Rehabilitation section for shoulder exercises.

CALL YOUR DOCTOR IF

- You have symptoms of upper arm exostosis.
- You notice no improvement despite treatment.
- Any of the following occurs after surgery:
  Increased pain, swelling, redness, drainage, or bleeding in the surgical area.
  Signs of infection (headache, muscle aches, dizziness or a general ill feeling and fever).
  New, unexplained symptoms. (Drugs used in treatment may cause side effects).

ARM FRACTURE, FOREARM

GENERAL INFORMATION

DEFINITION—A complete or incomplete break in one or both bones of the forearm (the radius and the ulna).

BODY PARTS INVOLVED
- Ulna and radius bones; elbow and wrist joints.
- Soft tissues around the fracture site, including nerves, tendons, ligaments and blood vessels.

SIGNS & SYMPTOMS
- Severe arm pain at the time of injury.
- Swelling of soft tissues around the fracture.
- Visible deformity if the fracture is complete and the bone fragments separate enough to distort normal arm contours.
- Tenderness to the touch.
- Numbness and coldness in the lower arm and hand if the blood supply is impaired.

CAUSES—Direct blow or indirect stress to the bone. Indirect stress may be caused by twisting, violent muscle contraction or falling on the outstretched arm.

RISK INCREASES WITH
- Contact sports, especially football, soccer or hockey.
- History of bone or joint disease, especially osteoporosis.
- Poor nutrition, especially calcium deficiency.
- If surgery or anesthesia is needed, surgical risk increases with smoking and use of drugs, including mind-altering drugs, muscle relaxants, antihypertensives, tranquilizers, sleep inducers, insulin, sedatives, beta-adrenergic blockers or cortisone.

HOW TO PREVENT
- Build your strength with a good conditioning program before beginning regular athletic practice or competition. Increased muscle mass helps protect bones and underlying tissues.
- If you have had a previous arm injury, use padded arm splints when competing in contact sports.

WHAT TO EXPECT

APPROPRIATE HEALTH CARE
- Doctor's treatment.
- Anesthesia and surgery to set the fracture or to insert a metal plate that immobilizes broken bones until they heal.
- Adults usually require surgery to place plate(s) and screws. Children may heal satisfactorily with closed reduction and casting.
- Whirlpool, ultrasound or massage (to displace excess fluid from the elbow and wrist).

DIAGNOSTIC MEASURES
- Your own observation of symptoms.
- Medical history and exam by a doctor.
- X-rays of injured areas, including the elbow above and the wrist below the primary injury site. In young people, x-rays of the normal side should be made for comparison.

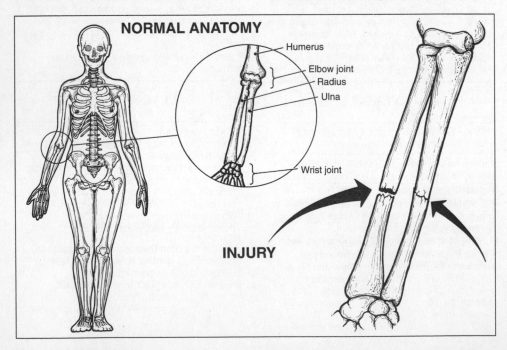

NORMAL ANATOMY

Humerus
Elbow joint
Radius
Ulna
Wrist joint

INJURY

POSSIBLE COMPLICATIONS

At the time of injury:
• Shock.
• Pressure on or injury to nearby nerves, ligaments, tendons, muscles, blood vessels or connective tissues.
After treatment or surgery:
• Delayed union or nonunion of the fracture.
• Impaired blood supply to the fracture site.
• Avascular necrosis (death of bone cells) due to interruption of the blood supply.
• Death of muscle cells if the arm swells inside the cast.
• Arrest of normal bone growth in children.
• Infection in open fractures (skin broken over fracture site) or at the incision if surgical setting was necessary.
• Shortening of the injured bones.
• Proneness to repeated injury.
• Unstable or arthritic wrist or elbow following repeated injury.
• Prolonged healing time if activity is resumed too soon.
• Stiffness, with limitation of forearm rotation.

PROBABLE OUTCOME—The average healing time (after surgery) for this fracture is 6 to 8 weeks in adults and 5 to 6 weeks in children (usually casted). Healing is complete when there is no motion at the fracture site and when x-rays show complete bone union.

HOW TO TREAT

NOTE—Follow your doctor's instructions. These instructions are supplemental.

FIRST AID
• Keep the person warm with blankets to decrease the possibility of shock.
• Cut away clothing, if possible, but don't move the injured arm to do so.
• Splint the broken arm for comfort and travel.
• Follow instructions for R.I.C.E., the first letters at *rest, ice, compression* and *elevation*. See Appendix 1 for details.
• The doctor will manipulate and set the broken bones with surgery or, if possible in children, without. Manipulation should be done as soon as possible after injury. Also, many tissues lose their elasticity and become difficult to return to a normal position.

CONTINUING CARE
• Immobilization will be necessary. A rigid cast or plaster splints will be placed around the injured arm to immobilize the elbow and wrist.
• After 96 hours, localized heat promotes healing by increasing blood circulation in the injured area. Use a heat lamp or heating pads so heat can penetrate the cast.
• After the cast is removed, use frequent ice massage. Fill a large styrofoam cup with water and freeze. Tear a small amount of foam from the top so ice protrudes. Massage firmly over the injured area in a circle about the size of a baseball. Do this for 15 minutes at a time 3 or 4 times a day.
• Apply heat instead of ice if it feels better. Use heat lamps, hot soaks, hot showers, heating pads or heat liniments and ointments.
• Take whirlpool treatments, if available.

MEDICATION—Your doctor may prescribe:
• General anesthesia, local anesthesia or muscle relaxants to make bone manipulation and fixation of bone fragments possible.
• Prescription pain relievers for severe pain.
• Stool softeners to prevent constipation due to inactivity.
• Acetaminophen (available without prescription) for mild pain after initial treatment.

ACTIVITY
• Actively exercise all muscle groups not immobilized. Muscle contractions promote fracture alignment and hasten healing.
• Begin reconditioning the injured arm after clearance from your doctor.
• Resume normal activities gradually after treatment.

DIET
• Do not eat or drink before manipulation or surgery to treat the fracture. Fluid or solid food in your stomach makes vomiting while under anesthesia more hazardous.
• During recovery, balance the amount of food you eat with any change in your level of physical activity. Eat a variety of foods to get the energy, protein, vitamins, minerals and fiber you need for good health and healing.

REHABILITATION—Begin daily rehabilitation exercises when movement is comfortable. Use ice massage for 10 minutes prior to exercise. See Rehabilitation section for elbow exercises and for wrist and for hand exercises.

CALL YOUR DOCTOR IF

• You have signs or symptoms of a forearm fracture.
• Any of the following occurs after surgery or other treatment:
  Increased pain, swelling or drainage in the surgical area.
  Signs of infection (headache, muscle aches, dizziness or a general ill feeling and fever).
  Swelling above or below the cast.
  Blue or gray skin color beyond the cast, particularly under the fingernails.
  Numbness or complete loss of feeling below the fracture site.
  Nausea or vomiting; constipation.

ARM FRACTURE, HUMERUS

GENERAL INFORMATION

DEFINITION—A complete or incomplete break in the humerus, the large bone in the upper arm extending from the elbow to the shoulder. The most common fractures of the humerus occur at the tubercles (top part of the humerus that fits into the shoulder joint) or in the neck or shaft of the humerus.

BODY PARTS INVOLVED
- Humerus.
- Elbow and shoulder joints.
- Soft tissues around the fracture site, including nerves tendons ligaments and blood vessels.

SIGNS & SYMPTOMS
- Severe arm pain at the time of injury.
- Swelling of soft tissues around the fracture.
- Visible deformity if the fracture is complete and the bone fragments separate enough to distort normal arm contours.
- Tenderness to the touch.
- Numbness and coldness in the arm and hand if the blood supply is impaired.

CAUSES—Direct blow or indirect stress to the bone. Indirect stress may be caused by twisting, violent muscle contraction or falling on the outstretched arm.

RISK INCREASES WITH
- Contact sports such as football or hockey.
- History of bone or joint disease, especially osteoporosis.
- Age under 12 or over 60.
- Obesity.
- If surgery or anesthesia is needed, surgical risk increases with smoking or use of drugs, including mind-altering drugs, muscle relaxants, antihypertensives, tranquilizers, sleep inducers, insulin, sedatives, beta-adrenergic blockers or corticosteroids.

HOW TO PREVENT
- Build your strength with a good conditioning program before beginning regular athletic practice or competition. Increased muscle mass helps protect bones and underlying tissues.
- If you have had an arm injury, use padded arm splints when participating in contact sports.

WHAT TO EXPECT

APPROPRIATE HEALTH CARE
- Doctor's treatment.
- Anesthesia and surgery to set the fracture.
- Whirlpool, ultrasound, or massage to displace excess fluid from the injury area.

DIAGNOSTIC MEASURES
- Your own observation of symptoms.
- Medical history and exam by a doctor.
- X-rays of injured areas, including joints above and below the primary injury site.

POSSIBLE COMPLICATIONS
At the time of injury:
- Shock.

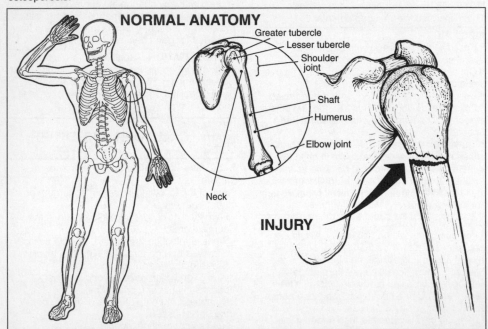

NORMAL ANATOMY

Greater tubercle
Lesser tubercle
Shoulder joint
Shaft
Humerus
Elbow joint
Neck

INJURY

• Pressure on or injury to nearby nerves, ligaments, tendons, muscles, blood vessels or connective tissues.

After treatment or surgery:
• Delayed union or nonunion of the fracture.
• Impaired blood supply to the fracture cells.
• Avascular necrosis (death of bone cells) due to interruption of the blood supply.
• Arrest of normal bone growth in children.
• infection in open fractures (skin broken over the fracture) or at the incision following surgery.
• Shortening of the injured humerus.
• Unstable or arthritic shoulder or elbow joint following repeated injury.
• Prolonged healing time if activity is resumed too soon.

PROBABLE OUTCOME—The average healing time for this fracture is 6 to 8 weeks. Healing is considered complete when there is no motion at the fracture site and when x-rays show complete bone union.

 ## HOW TO TREAT

NOTE—Follow your doctor's instructions. These instructions are supplemental.

FIRST AID
• Keep the person warm with blankets to decrease the possibility of shock.
• Cut away clothing, if possible, but don't move the injured arm to do so.
• Splint the shoulder by wrapping the arm to the trunk.
• Follow instructions for R.I.C.E., the first letters of *rest, ice, compression* and *elevation*. See Appendix 1 for details.
• If necessary, the doctor will realign the broken bones with surgery or, if possible, without. This manipulation should be done as soon as possible after injury. Also, many tissues lose their elasticity and become difficult to return to a normal position.

CONTINUING CARE
• Immobilization will be necessary. It can take several forms, depending on the fracture:
  Placement of surgical nails or pins to hold bone fragments together for fractures of tubercles. Usually only minimal external immobilization is necessary after surgery.
  Hanging cast for fractures of the neck of the humerus. A hanging cast is one placed on the lower arm to provide weight to overcome muscle spasms so the fractured bones will realign themselves.
  Shoulder-to wrist rigid cast for uncomplicated shaft fractures.
• If a cast is not necessary, continue R.I.C.E. instructions for 96 hours.

• After 96 hours, apply heat. Localized heat promotes healing by increasing blood circulation in the injured area. If no cast is necessary, use hot baths, showers, compresses, heating ointments and liniments or whirlpools. If a cast is necessary, use a heat lamp or heating pad so heat can penetrate the cast.
• After the cast is removed, use frequent ice massage. Fill a large styrofoam cup with water and freeze. Tear a small amount of foam from the top so ice protrudes. Massage firmly over the injured area in a circle about the size of a baseball. Do this for 15 minutes at a time 3 or 4 times a day.

MEDICATION—Your doctor may prescribe:
• General anesthesia, local anesthesia or muscle relaxants to make bone manipulation and fixation of bone fragments possible.
• Pain relievers for severe pain.
• Acetaminophen for mild pain.
• Stool softeners to prevent constipation due to inactivity.

ACTIVITY
• Actively exercise all muscle groups not immobilized. Muscle contractions promote fracture alignment and hasten healing.
• Begin reconditioning the arm after clearance from your doctor.
• Resume you normal activities gradually after treatment.

DIET
• Do not eat or drink before manipulation or surgery to treat the fracture. Fluid or solid food in your stomach makes vomiting while under anesthesia more hazardous.
• During recovery, balance the amount of food you eat with any change in your level of physical activity.

REHABILITATION—Begin daily rehabilitation exercises when movement is comfortable. Use ice massage for 10 minutes prior to exercise. See Rehabilitation section for elbow exercises and for wrist and hand exercises.

 ## CALL YOUR DOCTOR IF

• You have symptoms of a fractured arm.
• Any of the following occurs after surgery or other treatment:
  Blue or gray skin color beyond the cast, particularly under the fingernails.
  Loss of feeling below the fracture site.
  Increased pain, swelling or drainage in the surgical area.
  Signs of infection (headache, muscle aches, dizziness or a general ill feeling and fever).
  Swelling above or below the cast.
  Nausea or vomiting; constipation.

ARM STRAIN, BICEPS
(Biceps Tendon Rupture, Partial or Complete)

GENERAL INFORMATION

DEFINITION—Injury to the biceps muscle or tendon. The biceps muscle is a large muscle in the front of the upper arm. The muscle, tendons and bones comprise a contractile unit. The unit stabilizes the elbow and shoulder joints and allows their motion. A strain occurs at the weakest part of a unit. Strains are of 3 types:
- Mild (Grade I)—Slightly pulled muscle without tearing of muscle or tendon fibers. There is no loss of strength.
- Moderate (Grade II)—Tearing of fibers in a muscle or tendon or at the attachment to bone. Strength is diminished.
- Severe (Grade III)—Rupture of the muscle-tendon-bone attachment, with separation of fibers. Severe strains may require surgical repair. Chronic strains are caused by overuse. Acute strains are caused by direct injury or overstress.

BODY PARTS INVOLVED
- Biceps muscle.
- Biceps tendon.
- Humerus and bones of the shoulder.
- Soft tissues surrounding the strain, including nerves, periosteum (covering of bone), blood vessels and lymph vessels.

SIGNS & SYMPTOMS
- Pain when moving or stretching the biceps muscle.
- Muscle spasm.
- Swelling over the injury.
- Loss of strength (moderate or severe strain).
- Crepitation ("crackling" feeling and sound when pressed with fingers).
- Popeye sign (bulging deformity of biceps muscle) in severe strains.
- Calcification of the muscle or tendon (visible with x-rays).
- Inflammation of the sheath covering the tendon.

CAUSES
- Prolonged overuse of muscle-tendon units in the biceps of the upper arm.
- Spur formation near the shoulder.
- Single violent injury or force applied to the biceps.

RISK INCREASES WITH
- Contact sports such as boxing, football or wrestling.
- Throwing sports; weightlifting.
- Any cardiovascular medical problem that results in decreased circulation.
- Medical history of any bleeding disorder.
- Obesity.
- Poor nutrition.
- Previous upper arm injury.
- Poor muscle conditioning.

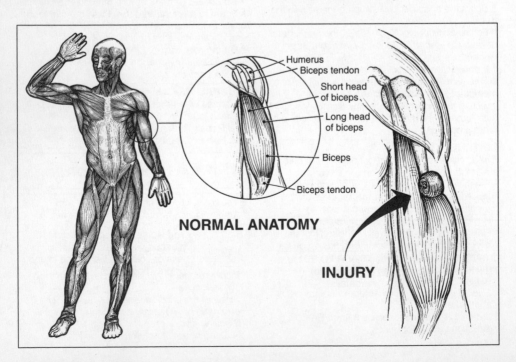

Humerus
Biceps tendon
Short head of biceps
Long head of biceps
Biceps
Biceps tendon

NORMAL ANATOMY

INJURY

HOW TO PREVENT
• Participate in a strengthening, flexibility and conditioning program appropriate for your sport.
• Warm up before practice or competition.
• Wear proper protective equipment.

 WHAT TO EXPECT

APPROPRIATE HEALTH CARE
• Doctor's diagnosis.
• Application of tape, plaster splints or casts (sometimes).
• Self-care during rehabilitation.
• Physical therapy (moderate or severe strain).
• Surgery (severe strain) to repair rupture.

DIAGNOSTIC MEASURES
• Your own observation of symptoms.
• Medical history and exam by a doctor.
• X-rays of the shoulder, arm and elbow to rule out fractures.
• Diagnostic ultrasound or MRI (see Glossary for both) to confirm diagnosis and to rule out rotator cuff tear.

POSSIBLE COMPLICATIONS
• Prolonged healing time if activity is resumed too soon.
• Proneness to repeated injury.
• Unstable or arthritic shoulder or elbow following repeated injury.
• Inflammation at the attachment to bone (periostitis).
• Prolonged disability (sometimes).
• This injury frequently occurs with a rotator cuff tear, which may be missed.

PROBABLE OUTCOME—If this is a first-time injury, proper care and sufficient healing time before resuming activity should prevent permanent disability. Torn ligaments and tendons require as long to heal as fractured bones. Average healing times are:
• Mild strain—2 to 10 days.
• Moderate strain—10 days to 6 weeks.
• Severe strain—6 to 10 weeks.
If this is a repeat injury, complications listed above are more likely to occur.

 HOW TO TREAT

NOTE—Follow your doctor's instructions. These instructions are supplemental.

FIRST AID—Use instructions for R.I.C.E., the first letters of *rest, ice, compression* and *elevation*. See Appendix 1 for details.

CONTINUING CARE
• Use ice massage 3 or 4 times a day for 15 minutes at a time. Fill a large styrofoam cup with water and freeze. Tear a small amount of foam from the top so ice protrudes. Massage firmly over the injured area in a circle about the size of a softball.
• After the first 96 hours, apply heat instead of ice if it feels better. Use heat lamps, hot soaks, hot showers, heating pads or heat liniments and ointments.
• Take whirlpool treatments, if available.
• Wrap the injured arm with an elasticized bandage between treatments.
• Massage gently and often to provide comfort and decrease swelling.

MEDICATION
• For minor discomfort, you may use:
  Aspirin, acetaminophen or ibuprofen.
  Topical liniments and ointments.
• Your doctor may prescribe:
  Stronger pain relievers.
  Injection of a long-acting local anesthetic to reduce pain.
  Injections of a corticosteroid, such as triamcinolone, to reduce inflammation.

ACTIVITY
• For a moderate or severe strain, use a sling for at least 72 hours—longer with a cast or splints.
• Resume your normal activities gradually.

DIET—During recovery, balance the amount of food you eat with any change in your level of physical activity. Eat a variety of foods to get the energy, protein, vitamins, minerals and fiber you need for good health and healing.

REHABILITATION
• Begin daily rehabilitation exercises when supportive wrapping is no longer needed. Use ice massage for 10 minutes prior to exercise.
• See Rehabilitation section for elbow exercises and shoulder exercises.
• Begin a supervised weightlifting program.

 CALL YOUR DOCTOR IF

• You have symptoms of a moderate or severe biceps strain, or a mild strain persists longer than 10 days.
• Pain or swelling worsens despite treatment.
• The following occur with a cast or splints:
  Pain, numbness or coldness below the injury.
  Dusky, blue or gray fingernails.

ARM STRAIN, FOREARM

GENERAL INFORMATION

DEFINITION—Injury to the muscles or tendons connected to the bones in the lower arm. Forearm strain is common because of the many tendons that glide together in the same or separate sheaths. Muscles, tendons and their attached bones comprise contractile units. These units stabilize the elbow and wrist joints and allows their motion. A strain occurs at the weakest part of a unit. Strains are of 3 types:
* Mild (Grade I)—Slightly pulled muscle without tearing of muscle or tendon fibers. There is no loss of strength.
* Moderate (Grade II)—Tearing of fibers in a muscle or tendon or at the attachment to bone. Strength is diminished.
* Severe (Grade III)—Rupture of the muscle-tendon-bone attachment, with separation of fibers. Severe strains may require surgical repair. Chronic strains are caused by overuse. Acute strains are caused by direct injury or overstress.

BODY PARTS INVOLVED
* Muscles and tendons of the forearm.
* Ulna and radius, the bones attached to the lower arm muscles and tendons.
* Soft tissues surrounding the strain, including nerves, periosteum (covering of bone), blood vessels and lymph vessels.

SIGNS & SYMPTOMS
* Pain when moving or stretching the forearm.
* Muscle spasm.
* Swelling over the injury.
* Loss of strength (moderate or severe strain).
* Crepitation ("crackling" feeling and sound when pressed with fingers).
* Calcification of the muscle or tendon (visible with x-rays).
* Inflammation of the sheath covering the tendon.

CAUSES
* Prolonged overuse of muscle-tendon units in the forearm and wrist.
* Single violent injury or force applied to the forearm.

RISK INCREASES WITH
* Contact sports such as football, wrestling or hockey.
* Any cardiovascular medical problem that results in decreased circulation.
* Medical history of any bleeding disorder.
* Obesity.
* Poor nutrition.
* Previous injury to the forearm, wrist or elbow.
* Poor muscle conditioning.

HOW TO PREVENT
* Participate in a strengthening, flexibility and conditioning program appropriate for your sport.
* Warm up before practice or competition.
* Decrease repetitive forearm and hand movements when pain or soreness begins.
* Use proper protective equipment.

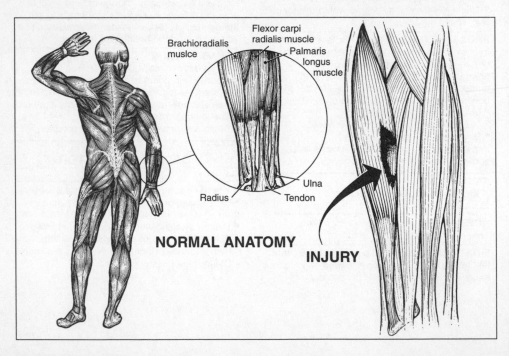

Brachioradialis muslce
Flexor carpi radialis muscle
Palmaris longus muscle
Radius
Ulna
Tendon

NORMAL ANATOMY

INJURY

? WHAT TO EXPECT

APPROPRIATE HEALTH CARE
- Doctor's diagnosis.
- Application of tape, plaster splints or casts (sometimes).
- Self-care during rehabilitation.
- Physical therapy (moderate or severe strain).
- Surgery (severe strain).

DIAGNOSTIC MEASURES
- Your own observation of symptoms.
- Medical history and exam by a doctor.
- X-rays of the forearm, wrist and elbow to rule out fractures.

POSSIBLE COMPLICATIONS
- Prolonged healing time if activity is resumed too soon.
- Proneness to repeated injury.
- Unstable or arthritic elbow or wrist following repeated injury.
- Inflammation at the attachment to bone (periostitis).
- Prolonged disability (sometimes), especially weakness.

PROBABLE OUTCOME—If this is a first-time injury, proper care and sufficient healing time before resuming activity should prevent permanent disability. Torn ligaments and tendons require as long to heal as fractured bones do. Average healing times are:
- Mild strain—2 to 10 days.
- Moderate strain—10 days to 6 weeks.
- Severe strain—6 to 10 weeks.

If this is a repeat injury, complications listed above are more likely to occur.

HOW TO TREAT

NOTE—Follow your doctor's instructions. These instructions are supplemental.

FIRST AID—Follow instructions for R.I.C.E., the first letters of *rest, ice, compression* and *elevation*. See Appendix 1 for details.

CONTINUING CARE
If casts or splints are necessary:
- Keep fingers free, and exercise them frequently.
- Begin daily rehabilitation exercises when casts or splints are no longer needed. Use ice massage for 10 minutes prior to exercise.
- See Appendix 2 (Care of Casts).

If cast or splints are not necessary:
- Use ice massage 3 or 4 times a day for 15 minutes at a time. Fill a large styrofoam cup with water and freeze. Tear a small amount of foam from the top so ice protrudes. Massage firmly over the injured area in a circle about the size of a softball.
- After the first 96 hours, apply heat instead of ice if it feels better. Use heat lamps, hot soaks, hot showers, heating pads or heat liniments and ointments.
- Take whirlpool treatments, if available.
- Wrap the injured forearm with an elasticized bandage between treatments.
- Begin daily rehabilitation exercises when supportive wrapping is no longer needed. Use ice massage for 10 minutes prior to exercise.
- Massage gently and often to provide comfort and decrease swelling.

MEDICATION
- For minor discomfort, you may use:
  Aspirin, acetaminophen or ibuprofen.
  Topical liniments and ointments.
- Your doctor may prescribe:
  Stronger pain relievers.
  Injection of a long-acting local anesthetic to reduce pain (rare).
  Injections of a corticosteroid, such as triamcinolone, to reduce inflammation (rare).

ACTIVITY
- For a moderate or severe strain, use a sling for at least 72 hours—longer with a cast or splints.
- Resume your normal activities gradually.

DIET—During recovery, balance the amount of food you eat with any change in your level of physical activity. Eat a variety of foods to get the energy, protein, vitamins, minerals and fiber you need for good health and healing.

REHABILITATION—See Rehabilitation section for elbow exercises and wrist and hand exercises.

CALL YOUR DOCTOR IF

- You have symptoms of a moderate or severe forearm strain or a mild strain persists longer than 10 days.
- Pain or swelling worsens despite treatment.
- The following occur with a cast or splints:
  Pain, numbness or coldness below the injury.
  Dusky, blue or gray fingernails.

ARM STRAIN, TRICEPS

GENERAL INFORMATION

DEFINITION—Injury to the triceps muscle or tendon. The triceps muscle is the large muscle at the back of the upper arm. The muscle, tendon and attached bones comprise a contractile unit. The unit stabilizes the elbow and shoulder joints and allows their motion. A strain occurs at the weakest part of a unit. Strains are of 3 types:
- Mild (Grade I)—Slightly pulled muscle without tearing of muscle or tendon fibers. There is no loss of strength.
- Moderate (Grade II)—Tearing of fibers in a muscle or tendon or at the attachment to bone. Strength is diminished.
- Severe (Grade III)—Rupture of the muscle-tendon-bone attachment, with separation of fibers. A severe strain may require surgical repair. Chronic strains are caused by overuse. Acute strains are caused by direct injury or overstress.

BODY PARTS INVOLVED
- Triceps muscle.
- Tendon of the triceps.
- Bones in the shoulder and arm.
- Soft tissues surrounding the strain, including nerves, periosteum (covering of bone), blood vessels and lymph vessels.

SIGNS & SYMPTOMS
- Pain with motion or stretching, especially forceful extension of the forearm at the elbow joint.
- Muscle spasm.
- Swelling around the injury.
- Loss of strength (moderate or severe strain).
- Crepitation ("crackling" feeling and sound when the injured area is pressed with fingers).
- Calcification of the muscle or tendon (visible with x-rays).
- inflammation of the sheath covering the tendon.

CAUSES
- Prolonged overuse of muscle-tendon units in the arm and elbow.
- Single violent injury or force applied to the upper arm and elbow.

RISK INCREASES WITH
- Contact sports such as football, baseball or boxing.
- Throwing sports.
- Weightlifting.
- Any cardiovascular medical problem that results in decreased circulation.
- Medical history of any bleeding disorder.
- Obesity.
- Poor nutrition.
- Previous upper arm injury.
- Poor muscle conditioning.

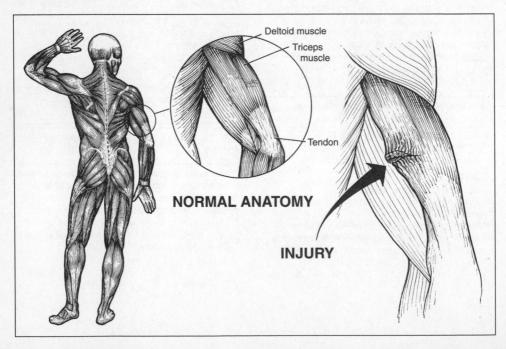

Deltoid muscle
Triceps muscle
Tendon

NORMAL ANATOMY

INJURY

HOW TO PREVENT
• Participate in a strengthening, flexibility and conditioning program appropriate for your sport.
• Warm up before practice or competition.
• Use proper protective equipment, such as shoulder pads.

 ## WHAT TO EXPECT

APPROPRIATE HEALTH CARE
• Doctor's diagnosis.
• Application of tape, plaster splints or casts (sometimes).
• Self-care during rehabilitation.
• Physical therapy (moderate or severe strain).
• Surgery (severe strain).

DIAGNOSTIC MEASURES
• Your own observation of symptoms.
• Medical history and exam by a doctor.
• X-rays of the shoulder, arm and elbow to rule out fractures.

POSSIBLE COMPLICATIONS
• Prolonged healing time if activity is resumed too soon.
• Proneness to repeated injury.
• Unstable or arthritic shoulder or elbow following repeated injury.
• Inflammation at the attachment to bone (periostitis).
• Prolonged disability (sometimes), especially weakness.

PROBABLE OUTCOME—If this is a first-time injury, proper care and sufficient healing time before resuming activity should prevent permanent disability. Torn ligaments and tendons require as long to heal as fractured bones do. Average healing times are:
• Mild strain—2 to 10 days.
• Moderate strain—10 days to 6 weeks.
• Severe strain—6 to 10 weeks.
If this is a repeat injury, complications listed above are more likely to occur.

 ## HOW TO TREAT

NOTE—Follow your doctor's instructions. These instructions are supplemental

FIRST AID—Use instructions for R.I.C.E., the first letters of *rest, ice, compression* and *elevation*. See Appendix 1 for details.

CONTINUING CARE.
• Use ice massage 3 or 4 times a day for 15 minutes at a time. Fill a large styrofoam cup with water and freeze. Tear a small amount of foam from the top so ice protrudes. Massage firmly over the injured area in a circle about the size of a softball.
• After the first 96 hours, apply heat instead of ice if it feels better. Use heat lamps, hot soaks, hot showers, heating pads or heat liniments and ointments.
• Take whirlpool treatments, if available.
• Wrap the injured arm with an elasticized bandage between treatments.
• Massage gently and often to provide comfort and decrease swelling.

MEDICATION
• For minor discomfort, you may use: Aspirin, acetaminophen or ibuprofen. Topical liniments and ointments.
• Your doctor may prescribe: Stronger pain relievers. Injection of a long-acting local anesthetic to reduce pain (rare).

ACTIVITY
• For a moderate or severe strain, use a sling for at least 72 hours—longer with a cast or splints.
• Resume your normal activities.

DIET—During recovery, balance the amount of food you eat with any change in your level of physical activity. Eat a variety of foods to get the energy, protein, vitamins, minerals and fiber you need for good health and healing.

REHABILITATION—Begin daily rehabilitation exercises when supportive wrapping is no longer needed. Use ice massage for 10 minutes prior to exercise. See Rehabilitation section for elbow exercises and shoulder exercises.

 ## CALL YOUR DOCTOR IF

• You have symptoms of a moderate or severe triceps strain or a mild strain persists longer than 10 days.
• Pain or swelling worsens despite treatment.
• The following occur with a cast or splints: Pain, numbness or coldness below the injury. Dusky, blue or gray fingernails.

ARM STRAIN, UPPER ARM

GENERAL INFORMATION

DEFINITION—Injury to the muscles or tendons connected to the humerus, the bone in the upper arm. Muscles, tendons and their attached bones comprise contractile units. These units stabilize the elbow and shoulder joints and allow their motion. A strain occurs at the weakest part of a unit. Strains are of 3 types:
- Mild (Grade I)—Slightly pulled muscle without tearing of muscle or tendon fibers. There is no loss of strength.
- Moderate (Grade II)—Tearing of fibers in a muscle or tendon or at the attachment to bone. Strength is diminished.
- Severe (Grade III)—Rupture of the muscle-tendon-bone attachment, with separation of fibers. A severe strain may require surgical repair. Chronic strains are caused by overuse. Acute strains are caused by direct injury or overstress.

BODY PARTS INVOLVED
- Muscles of the upper arm.
- Tendons of the upper arm muscles.
- Humerus, the bone of the upper arm.
- Soft tissues surrounding the strain, including nerves, periosteum (covering of bone), blood vessels and lymph vessels.

SIGNS & SYMPTOMS
- Pain when moving or stretching upper arm.
- Muscle spasm of the injured muscles.
- Swelling in the upper arm.
- Loss of strength in the upper arm (moderate or severe strain).
- Crepitation ("crackling" feeling and sound when the injured area is pressed with fingers).
- Calcification of the muscle or its tendon (visible with x-rays).
- Inflammation of the tendon sheath.

CAUSES
- Prolonged overuse of muscle-tendon units in the upper arm.
- Single violent injury or force applied to the upper arm.

RISK INCREASES WITH
- Contact sports.
- Throwing sports.
- Any cardiovascular medical problem that results in decreased circulation.
- Medical history of any bleeding disorder.
- Obesity.
- Poor nutrition.
- Previous elbow, upper arm or shoulder injury.
- Poor muscle conditioning or muscle overuse.

HOW TO PREVENT
- Participate in a strengthening, flexibility and conditioning program appropriate for your sport.
- Warm up before practice or competition.
- Use proper protective equipment, such as shoulder pads.

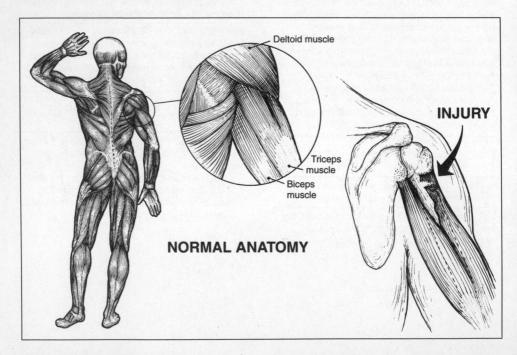

Deltoid muscle

Triceps muscle

Biceps muscle

NORMAL ANATOMY

INJURY

WHAT TO EXPECT

APPROPRIATE HEALTH CARE
- Doctor's diagnosis.
- Application of tape, plaster splints or casts (sometimes).
- Self-care during rehabilitation.
- Physical therapy (moderate or severe strain).
- Surgery (severe strain).

DIAGNOSTIC MEASURES
- Your own observation of symptoms.
- Medical history and exam by a doctor.
- X-rays of the elbow, arm and shoulder to rule out fractures.

POSSIBLE COMPLICATIONS
- Prolonged healing time if activity is resumed too soon.
- Proneness to repeated injury.
- Unstable or arthritic shoulder or elbow following repeated injury.
- Inflammation at the attachment to bone (periostitis).
- Prolonged disability (sometimes), especially weakness.

PROBABLE OUTCOME
- If this is a first-time injury, proper care and sufficient healing time before resuming activity should prevent permanent disability. Torn ligaments and tendons require as long to heal as fractured bones do. Average healing times are:
- Mild strain—2 to 10 days.
- Moderate strain—10 days to 6 weeks.
- Severe strain—6 to 10 weeks.
If this is a repeat injury, complications listed above are more likely to occur.

HOW TO TREAT

NOTE—Follow your doctor's instructions. These instructions are supplemental.

FIRST AID—Use instructions for R.I.C.E., the first letters of *rest, ice, compression* and *elevation*. See Appendix 1 for details.

CONTINUING CARE
- Use ice massage 3 or 4 times a day for 15 minutes at a time. Fill a large styrofoam cup with water and freeze. Tear a small amount of foam from the top so ice protrudes. Massage firmly over the injured area in a circle about the size of a softball.

- After the first 96 hours, apply heat instead of ice if it feels better. Use heat lamps, hot soaks, hot showers, heating pads or heat liniments and ointments.
- Take whirlpool treatments, if available.
- Wrap the injured arm with an elasticized bandage between treatments.
- Massage gently and often to provide comfort and decrease swelling.

MEDICATION
- For minor discomfort, you may use:
  Aspirin, acetaminophen or ibuprofen.
  Topical liniments and ointments.
- Your doctor may prescribe:
  Stronger pain relievers.
  Injection of a long-acting local anesthetic to reduce pain.
  Injection of a corticosteroid, such as triamcinolone, to reduce inflammation.

ACTIVITY
- For a moderate or severe strain, use a sling for at least 72 hours—longer with a cast or splints.
- Resume your normal activities gradually.

DIET—During recovery, balance the amount of food you eat with any change in your level of physical activity. Eat a variety of foods to get the energy, protein, vitamins, minerals and fiber you need for good health and healing.

REHABILITATION—Begin daily rehabilitation exercises when supportive wrapping is no longer needed. Use ice massage for 10 minutes prior to exercise. See Rehabilitation section for elbow exercises and shoulder exercises.

CALL YOUR DOCTOR IF

- You have symptoms of a moderate or severe upper arm strain or a mild strain persists longer than 10 days.
- Pain or swelling worsens despite treatment.
- The following occur with a cast or splints:
  Dusky, blue or gray fingernails.
  Pain, numbness or coldness below the injury.

BACK, RUPTURED DISK
(Herniated Disk; Slipped Disk;
Herniated Nucleus Pulposus)

 ## GENERAL INFORMATION

DEFINITION—Sudden or gradual break in the supportive ligaments surrounding a spinal disk (a cushion separating bony spinal vertebrae), with extrusion of the disk contents, usually backward toward the spinal nerves.

BODY PARTS INVOLVED—Disks of the neck or lower spine are the most common sites, especially between the 4th and 5th lumbar vertebrae (L4 and L5).

SIGNS & SYMPTOMS
In the lower back:
● Severe pain in the low back or in the back of one leg, buttock or foot (sciatica). Pain usually affects one side and worsens with movement, coughing, sneezing, lifting or straining.
● Weakness, numbness or muscular wasting of the affected leg.
In the neck:
● Pain in the neck or shoulder or down one arm. Pain worsens with movement.
● Weakness, numbness or muscular wasting of the affected arm.

CAUSES—Weakening and rupture of the disk material, creating pressure on nearby spinal nerves. Rupture of the disk is caused by sudden injury or chronic stress, such as from constant lifting or obesity.

RISK INCREASES WITH
● Any sport in which movement causes downward or twisting pressure on the neck or spine. The most common include bowling, tennis, jogging, track, football, racquetball, weightlifting or gymnastics.
● Poor muscle conditioning and inadequate warmup.
● Family history of low back pain or disk disorders. Genetic factors apparently play a poorly understood role in increasing risk.
● Preexisting spondylolisthesis (see Glossary).

HOW TO PREVENT
● Practice proper posture when lifting.
● Exercise regularly to maintain good muscle tone, especially in abdominal and back muscles.
● If previously injured, avoid any vigorous physical activity that requires twisting of the body under uncontrollable conditions.

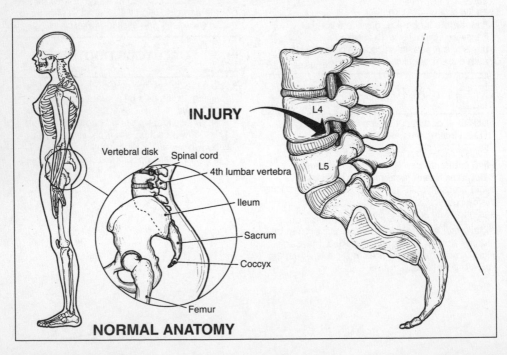

INJURY

L4

L5

Vertebral disk

Spinal cord

4th lumbar vertebra

Ileum

Sacrum

Coccyx

Femur

NORMAL ANATOMY

WHAT TO EXPECT

APPROPRIATE HEALTH CARE
- Self-care after diagnosis.
- Doctor's treatment.
- Traction at home or in the hospital (sometimes) for neck disk ruptures.
- Surgery to relieve nerve pressure if conservative methods do not relieve symptoms and special studies confirm the diagnosis and location of a protruding ruptured disk.
- Injection of epidural steroids to decrease swelling.
- Rehabilitation to strengthen muscles.
- Psychotherapy, counseling or biofeedback training to learn coping methods for enduring pain when pain persists despite treatment.

DIAGNOSTIC MEASURES
- Your own observation of symptoms.
- Medical history and physical exam by a doctor.
- X-rays of the neck or lower spine, including myelogram (see Glossary).
- CT scan or MRI (see Glossary for both).

POSSIBLE COMPLICATIONS
- Loss of bladder and bowel function.
- Paralysis of the arm (neck disk rupture) or leg (lower back disk rupture).
- Muscle wasting and weakness.
- Decreased sexual function.
- Surgical wound infection if surgery is required.

PROBABLE OUTCOME—Spontaneous recovery in many cases. Bed rest for as much as 2 weeks should be tried before considering other therapy (unless complications occur). When necessary, surgery with or without spinal fusion may cure the problem.

HOW TO TREAT

NOTE—Follow your doctor's instructions. These instructions are supplemental

FIRST AID
- Don't move any person with a neck or back injury unless his or her life is at risk. Don't twist the back, neck or head. Support the whole back and neck with splints of some sort, or await a litter or spine board.

- Keep the person warm with blankets to decrease the possibility of shock.
- Seek emergency medical help immediately.

CONTINUING CARE—Apply ice packs to the painful area during the first 72 hours and occasionally thereafter if they provide relief. Alternately, try to relieve pain with a heat lamp, hot showers, hot baths, warm compresses or a heating pad.

MEDICATION
- For minor discomfort, you may use non-prescription drugs such as aspirin or ibuprofen.
- Your doctor may prescribe:
  Prescription pain relievers for severe pain.
  Muscle relaxants.
  Nonsteroidal anti-inflammatory drugs to reduce inflammation around the rupture.
  Laxatives or stool softeners to prevent constipation.

ACTIVITY—Rest in bed for as much as 2 weeks during the acute phase. Resume your normal activities when symptoms improve or after recovery from surgery. Resume athletic activities after clearance from your doctor.

REHABILITATION—See Rehabilitation section for exercises, depending on the area of injury. Begin rehabilitation after clearance from your doctor.

DIET—During recovery, balance the amount of food you eat with any change in your level of physical activity. Eat a variety of foods to get the energy, protein, vitamins, minerals and fiber you need for good health and healing.

CALL YOUR DOCTOR IF

- You have symptoms of a ruptured disk.
- The following occur during treatment:
  Increased pain or weakness in the extremities.
  Loss of bladder or bowel control.
  New, unexplained symptoms. Drugs used in treatment may produce side effects.
- After treatment, weakness, numbness or pain in the back, buttocks, legs or arms returns.

BACK SPRAIN, LUMBODORSAL REGION
(Mechanical Low Back Pain)

 GENERAL INFORMATION

DEFINITION—Violent overstretching of one or more ligaments in the lumbodorsal vertebrae of the spine. This is the most stable section of the vertebral column. Sprains involving two or more ligaments cause considerably more disability than single-ligament sprains. When the ligament is overstretched, it becomes tense and gives way at its weakest point, either where it attaches to bone or within the ligament itself. If the ligament pulls loose a fragment of bone, it is called an avulsion fracture. There are 3 types of sprains:
- Mild (Grade I)—Tearing of some ligament fibers, with associated muscle spasm. There is no loss of function.
- Moderate (Grade II)—Rupture of a portion of the ligament, resulting in some loss of function.
- Severe (Grade III)—Complete rupture of the ligament or complete separation of ligament from bone. There is total loss of function. Severe sprains may require surgical repair.

BODY PARTS INVOLVED
- Any of the many ligaments connecting the vertebrae in the lumbodorsal spine.
- Tissues surrounding the sprain, including blood vessels, tendons, bone, periosteum (covering of bone) and muscles.

SIGNS & SYMPTOMS
- Severe pain at the time of injury.
- Popping or feeling of tearing in the back.
- Tenderness at the injury site.
- Swelling in the back.
- Bruising that appears soon after injury.

CAUSES—Stress on a ligament that then forces the lumbodorsal vertebrae out of their normal location. A sprain of the lumbodorsal vertebrae will frequently occur when a stressful act is performed, while an athlete is off balance or malpositioned or during repeated stressful activity involving muscles in the lumbodorsal area.

RISK INCREASES WITH
- Contact, throwing and lifting sports.
- Gymnastics or diving.
- Previous spine injury.
- Obesity.
- Poor muscle conditioning.

HOW TO PREVENT
- Participate in a strengthening, flexibility and conditioning program appropriate for your sport.
- Warm up before practice or competition.
- Tape vulnerable joints before practice or competition to prevent reinjury.
- Employ the proper technique for the physical activity, especially for lifting sports.

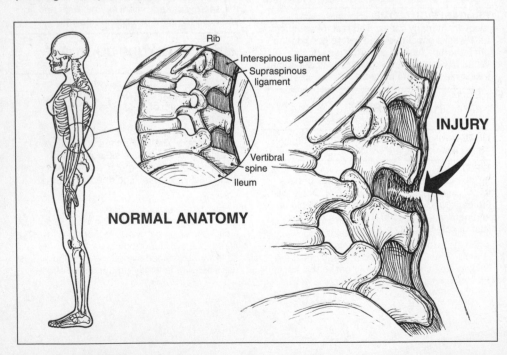

NORMAL ANATOMY

INJURY

WHAT TO EXPECT

APPROPRIATE HEALTH CARE
- Doctor's diagnosis.
- Application of tape, cast (rare) or elastic corset or brace.
- Self-care during rehabilitation.
- Physical therapy (moderate or severe sprain).
- Bed rest for severe sprain.

DIAGNOSTIC MEASURES
- Your own observation of symptoms.
- Medical history and exam by a doctor.
- X-rays of the spine to rule out fractures.

POSSIBLE COMPLICATIONS
- Prolonged healing time if usual activities are resumed too soon.
- Proneness to repeated back injury.
- Inflammation at the ligament attachment to bone (periostitis).
- Prolonged disability (sometimes).
- Unstable or arthritic spine following repeated injury.

PROBABLE OUTCOME—If this is a first-time injury, proper care and sufficient healing time before resuming activity should prevent permanent disability. Ligaments have a poor blood supply, and torn ligaments require as much healing time as fractures. Average healing times are :
- Mild sprains—2 to 4 weeks.
- Moderate sprains—4 to 6 weeks.
- Severe sprains—6 to 10 weeks.

HOW TO TREAT

NOTE—Follow your doctor's instructions. These instructions are supplemental.

FIRST AID—Use instructions for R.I.C.E., the first letters of *rest, ice, compression* and *elevation*. See Appendix 1 for details.

CONTINUING CARE—If your doctor does not apply a cast, tape or elastic bandage:
- Continue using an ice pack 3 or 4 times a day. Place ice chips or cubes in a plastic bag. Wrap the bag in a moist towel, and place it over the injured area. Use for 20 minutes at a time.
- Wrap the injured area from the top of the hip to the lower rib cage with an elasticized bandage between ice treatments.
- After 72 hours, apply heat instead of ice if it feels better. Use heat lamps, hot soaks, hot showers, heating pads or heat liniments and ointments.

- Take whirlpool treatments, if available.
- Massage gently and often to provide comfort and decrease swelling.
- Ask your doctor about the advisability of using a special corset.

MEDICATION
- For minor discomfort, you may use:
  Aspirin, acetaminophen or ibuprofen.
  Topical liniments and ointments.
- Your doctor may prescribe:
  Muscle relaxants.
  Stronger pain relievers.
  Injection of a long-acting local anesthetic to reduce pain.
  Injection of a corticosteroid, such as triamcinolone, to reduce inflammation.

ACTIVITY—Resume your normal activities gradually after clearance from your doctor.

DIET—During recovery, balance the amount of food you eat with any change in your level of physical activity. Eat a variety of foods to get the energy, protein, vitamins, minerals and fiber you need for good health and healing.

REHABILITATION
- Begin daily rehabilitation exercises when the cast or supportive wrapping is no longer necessary.
- Use ice massage for 10 minutes before and after exercise. Fill a large styrofoam cup with water and freeze. Tear a small amount of foam from the top so ice protrudes. Massage firmly over the injured area in a circle about the size of a softball.
- See Rehabilitation section for low back exercises and upper back exercises.

CALL YOUR DOCTOR IF

- You have symptoms of a moderate or severe lumbodorsal back sprain or a mild sprain persists longer than 2 weeks.
- Pain, swelling or bruising worsens despite treatment.
- Pain develops in the leg or radiates to the leg, with coughing or sneezing.
- Any of the following occurs after surgery:
  Increased pain, swelling, redness, drainage or bleeding in the surgical area.
  Signs of infection (headache, muscle aches, dizziness or a general ill feeling with fever).
- You lose bladder or bowel control.
- New, unexplained symptoms develop. Drugs used in treatment may produce side effects.

BACK SPRAIN, SACROILIAC REGION

GENERAL INFORMATION

DEFINITION—Violent overstretching of one or more ligaments in the sacroiliac region of the spine. When the ligament is overstretched, it becomes tense and gives way at its weakest point, either where it attaches to bone or within the ligament itself. There are 3 types of sprains:
• Mild (Grade I)—Tearing of some ligament fibers, with associated muscle spasm. There is no loss of function.
• Moderate (Grade II)—Rupture of a portion of the ligament, resulting in some loss of function.
• Severe (Grade III)—Complete rupture of the ligament or complete separation of ligament from bone. There is total loss of function. A severe sprain may require surgical repair.

BODY PARTS INVOLVED
• Ligaments of the sacroiliac region.
• Sacrum (spinal region) and ilium (bones of the pelvis).
• Tissues surrounding the sprain, including blood vessels, tendons, bone, periosteum (covering of bone) and muscles.

SIGNS & SYMPTOMS
• Severe back pain at the time of injury, with radiation of pain into the buttocks or hip, but no lower.
• A feeling of popping or tearing in the sacroiliac area.
• Tenderness and swelling at the injury site.
• Bruising (sometimes) that appears soon after injury.

CAUSES—Direct blow or stress on a ligament that temporarily forces or pries the sacroiliac joint out of its normal configuration.

RISK INCREASES WITH
• Contact sports such as football or wrestling.
• Weightlifting.
• Sudden movement while one leg is in front and the other is behind.
• Previous back injury.
• Obesity.
• Poor muscle conditioning, especially in the low back, abdomen, buttock and hip.
• Inadequate protection from equipment.

HOW TO PREVENT
• Participate in a strengthening, flexibility and conditioning program appropriate for your sport.
• Warm up before practice or competition.
• Tape vulnerable joints before practice or competition if you have been injured previously.

WHAT TO EXPECT

APPROPRIATE HEALTH CARE
• Doctor's care.
• Physical therapy (moderate or severe sprain).

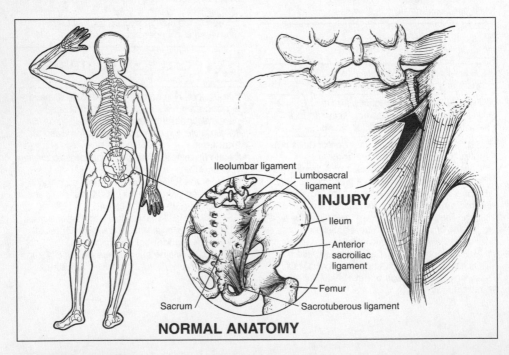

Ileolumbar ligament
Lumbosacral ligament
INJURY
Ileum
Anterior sacroiliac ligament
Femur
Sacrum
Sacrotuberous ligament

NORMAL ANATOMY

DIAGNOSTIC MEASURES
• Your own observation of symptoms.
• Medical history and exam by a doctor.
• X-rays of the lower spine, hip and pelvis to rule out fractures.

POSSIBLE COMPLICATIONS
• Prolonged healing time if usual activities are resumed too soon.
• Proneness to repeated sacroiliac injury.
• Inflammation at the ligament attachment to bone (periostitis).
• Prolonged disability (sometimes).
• Unstable or arthritic sacroiliac joint following repeated injury.

PROBABLE OUTCOME—If this is a first-time injury, proper care and sufficient healing time before resuming activity should prevent permanent disability. Ligaments have a poor blood supply, and torn ligaments require as much healing time as fractures. Average healing times are:
• Mild sprains—2 to 4 weeks.
• Moderate strains—4 to 6 weeks.
• Severe sprains—6 to 10 weeks.

 HOW TO TREAT

NOTE—Follow your doctor's instructions. These instructions are supplemental.

FIRST AID
• Use instructions for R.I.C.E., the first letters of *rest, ice, compression* and *elevation* (if possible). See Appendix 1 for detail.
• Don't move the person until a litter or spine board can be obtained for safe transport.
• Don't allow the person to walk until the diagnosis is confirmed. The spinal cord may be injured with movement.

CONTINUING CARE—If the doctor does not apply tape or an elastic bandage:
• Use an ice pack 3 or 4 times a day. Place ice chips or cubes in a plastic bag. Wrap the bag in a moist towel, and place it over the injured area. Use for 20 minutes at a time.
• Wrap the lower abdomen and hips with an elastic bandage between ice treatments.

• After 72 hours, apply heat instead of ice if it feels better. Use heat lamps, hot soaks, hot showers or heating pads.
• Take whirlpool treatments, if available.

MEDICATION
• For minor discomfort, you may use:
Aspirin, acetaminophen or ibuprofen.
Topical liniments and ointments.
• Your doctor may prescribe:
Muscle relaxants.
Stronger pain relievers.
Injection of a long-acting local anesthetic to reduce pain.
Injection of a corticosteroid, such as triamcinolone, to reduce inflammation.

ACTIVITY—Resume your normal activities gradually after clearance from your doctor.

DIET—During recovery, balance the amount of food you eat with any change in your level of physical activity. Eat a variety of foods to get the energy, protein, vitamins, minerals and fiber you need for good health and healing.

REHABILITATION
• Begin daily rehabilitation exercises when pain subsides and supportive wrapping is no longer needed. Use ice massage for 10 minutes before and after workouts. Fill a large styrofoam cup with water and freeze. Tear a small amount of foam from the top so ice protrudes. Massage firmly in a circle over the injured area.
• See Rehabilitation section for low back exercises.

 CALL YOUR DOCTOR IF

• You have symptoms of a moderate or severe sacroiliac sprain or mild sprain persists longer than 2 weeks.
• Pain, swelling or bruising worsen despite treatment.
• You experience pain, numbness or coldness in the legs.
• New, unexplained symptoms develop. Drugs used in treatment may produce side effects.

BACK STRAIN, DORSAL OR THORACIC SPINE REGION

GENERAL INFORMATION

DEFINITION—Injury to muscles or tendons that attach to the vertebral column at the dorsal or thoracic region of the back. The dorsal or thoracic spine is that part where ribs attach to surround the lungs. Muscles, tendons and their attached vertebrae comprise contractile units. The units stabilize the spine and allow its motion. A strain occurs at the weakest part of a unit. Strains are of 3 types:
- Mild (Grade I)—Slightly pulled muscle without tearing of muscle or tendon fibers. There is no loss of strength
- Moderate (Grade II)—Tearing of fibers in a muscle tendon or at the attachment to bone. Strength is diminished.
- Severe (grade III)—Rupture of the muscle-tendon-bone attachment, with separation of fibers.

Chronic strains are caused by overuse. Acute strains are caused by direct injury or overstress.

BODY PARTS INVOLVED
- Tendons and muscles of the dorsal or thoracic spine.
- One or more vertebral bones.
- Soft tissues surrounding the strain, including nerves, periosteum (covering of bone), blood vessels and lymph vessels.

SIGNS & SYMPTOMS
- Pain with motion or stretching of the back or generalized pain in the back.
- Muscle spasm when moving the back.
- Swelling along a muscle of the back.
- Loss of strength (moderate or severe strain).
- Calcification of the muscle or its tendon (visible with x-rays).
- Inflammation of the tendon sheath.

CAUSES
- Prolonged overuse or stretching of muscle-tendon units in the back.
- Single violent injury or force applied to the dorsal region of the back.

RISK INCREASES WITH
- Major exertion in an off-balance position, such as a shotputter's throwing from an imperfect stance.
- Sports such as gymnastics, golf, weightlifting or diving.
- Medical history of any bleeding disorder.
- Obesity.
- Poor nutrition.
- Previous back injury.
- Poor muscle conditioning.

HOW TO PREVENT
- Participate in a strengthening, flexibility and conditioning program appropriate for your sport.
- Warm up before practice or competition

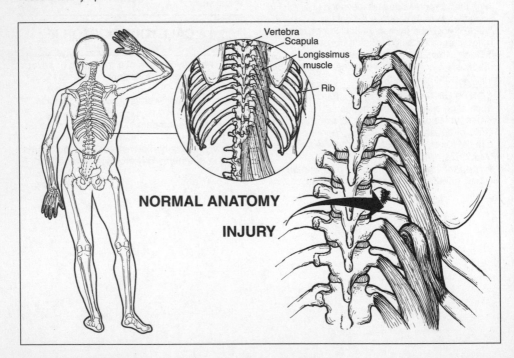

Vertebra
Scapula
Longissimus muscle
Rib

NORMAL ANATOMY

INJURY

WHAT TO EXPECT

APPROPRIATE HEALTH CARE
- Doctor's diagnosis.
- Application of tape (sometimes).
- Self-care during rehabilitation.
- Physical therapy (moderate or severe strain).

DIAGNOSTIC MEASURES
- Your own observation of symptoms.
- Medical history and exam by a doctor.
- X-rays of the back to rule out fractures.

POSSIBLE COMPLICATIONS
- Prolonged healing time if activity is resumed too soon.
- Proneness to repeated injury.
- Chronically painful or arthritic back following repeated injury.
- Inflammation at the attachment to bone (periostitis).
- Prolonged disability (sometimes).

PROBABLE OUTCOME—If this is a first-time injury, proper care and sufficient healing time before resuming activity should prevent permanent disability. Torn ligaments and tendons require as long to heal as fractured bones. Average healing times are:
- Mild strain—2 to 10 days.
- Moderate strain—10 days to 6 weeks.
- Severe strain—6 to 10 weeks.

If this is a repeat injury, complications listed above are more likely to occur.

 # HOW TO TREAT

NOTE—Follow your doctor's instructions. These instruction are supplemental.

FIRST AID—Use instructions for R.I.C.E., the first letters of *rest, ice, compression* and *elevation*. See Appendix 1 for details.

CONTINUING CARE
- Use ice massage 3 or 4 times a day for 15 minutes at a time. Fill a large styrofoam cup with water and freeze. Tear a small amount of foam from the top so ice protrudes. Massage firmly over the injured area in a circle about the size of a softball.
- After the first 72 hours, apply heat instead of ice if it feels better. Use heat lamps, hot soaks, hot showers, heating pads or heat liniments and ointments.
- Take whirlpool treatments, if available.
- Wrap the injured back with an elasticized bandage between treatments.
- Massage gently and often to provide comfort and decrease swelling.

MEDICATION
- For minor discomfort, you may use:
  Aspirin, acetaminophen or ibuprofen.
  Topical liniments and ointments.
- Your doctor may prescribe:
  Stronger pain relievers.
  Muscle relaxants.
  Injection of a long-acting local anesthetic to reduce pain.
  Injection of a corticosteroid, such as triamcinolone, to reduce inflammation.

ACTIVITY—Rest in bed until pain improves. Resume your normal activities gradually after treatment.

DIET—During recovery, balance the amount of food you eat with any change in your level of physical activity. Eat a variety of foods to get the energy, protein, vitamins, minerals and fiber you need for good health and healing.

REHABILITATION—Begin daily rehabilitation exercises when supportive wrapping is no longer needed. See Rehabilitation section for low back exercises and upper back exercises.

 # CALL YOUR DOCTOR IF

- You have symptoms of a moderate or severe back strain or a mild strain persists longer than 10 days.
- Pain or swelling worsens despite treatment.

BACK STRAIN, LUMBAR SPINE REGION

GENERAL INFORMATION

DEFINITION—Injury to muscles or tendons that attach to the vertebral column at the lumbar (lower midpoint) spine. Muscles, tendons and their attached vertebrae comprise contractile units. The units stabilize the spine and allow its motion. A strain occurs at the weakest point of a unit. Strains are of 3 types:
- Mild (Grade I)—Slightly pulled muscle without tearing of muscle or tendon fibers. There is no loss of strength.
- Moderate (Grade II)—Tearing of fibers in a muscle or tendon or at the attachment to bone. Strength is diminished.
- Severe (Grade III)—Rupture of the muscle-tendon-bone attachment, with separation of fibers. A severe strain may require surgical repair. Chronic strains are caused by overuse. Acute strains are caused by direct injury or overstress.

BODY PARTS INVOLVED
- Tendons and muscles of the lower midspine.
- One or more vertebral bones or bones of the pelvis.
- Soft tissues surrounding the strain, including nerves, periosteum (covering of bone), blood vessels and lymph vessels.

SIGNS AND SYMPTOMS
- Pain with motion or stretching of the lower back.
- Muscle spasm in the lower back.
- Swelling along muscles of the back.
- Calcification of the muscle or tendon (visible with x-rays).

CAUSES
- Prolonged overuse of muscle-tendon units in the lower back.
- Single violent injury or force applied to the lower back.

RISK INCREASES WITH
- Contact sports, especially football or hockey.
- Gymnastics, golf or diving.
- Improper lifting of heavy objects.
- Medical history of any bleeding disorder.
- Obesity.
- Poor nutrition.
- Previous back injury, especially if it resulted in loss of back mobility.
- Poor muscle conditioning.

HOW TO PREVENT
- Participate in a strengthening, flexibility and conditioning program appropriate for your sport. Include exercises to promote back flexibility.
- Warm up before practice or competition.
- Use proper lifting techniques. Don't bend over to lift. Squat to lift, and rise using leg muscles.
- Wear proper protective devices, such as a back brace or taping, to prevent a recurrence after you recover.

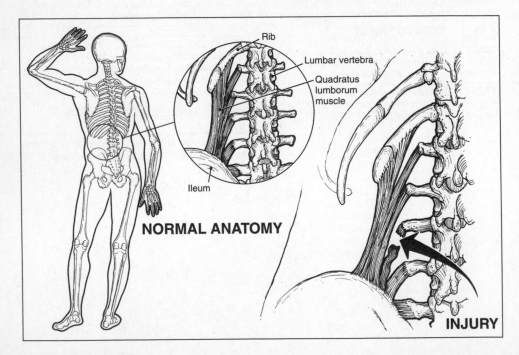

Rib

Lumbar vertebra

Quadratus lumborum muscle

Ileum

NORMAL ANATOMY

INJURY

WHAT TO EXPECT

APPROPRIATE HEALTH CARE
- Doctor's diagnosis
- Application of a cast (rare), brace or corset (sometimes).
- Self-care during rehabilitation.
- Physical therapy (moderate or severe strain).
- Surgery (severe strain).

DIAGNOSTIC MEASURES
- Your own observation of symptoms.
- Medical history and exam by a doctor.
- X-rays of the lumbar spine to rule out fractures or dislocations.

POSSIBLE COMPLICATIONS
- Prolonged healing time if activity is resumed too soon.
- Proneness to repeated lumbar spine injury.
- Unstable or arthritic vertebrae following repeated injury.
- Inflammation at the attachment to bone (periostitis).
- Prolonged disability (sometimes).

PROBABLE OUTCOME—If this is a first-time injury, proper care and sufficient healing time before resuming activity should prevent permanent disability. Recurrence is likely without adequate healing time. Torn ligaments and tendons require as long to heal as fractured bones. Average healing times are:
- Mild strain—2 to 10 days.
- Moderate strain—10 days to 6 weeks.
- Severe strain—6 to 10 weeks.

If this is a repeated injury, complications listed above are more likely to occur.

 # HOW TO TREAT

NOTE—Follow your doctor's instructions. These instructions are supplemental.

FIRST AID
- Rest the injured area at the first sign of severe symptoms. Rest in bed until pain decreases. Use a firm mattress.
- Use ice to help stop internal muscular bleeding. Prepare an ice pack of ice cubes or chips wrapped in plastic or in a container. Place towel over the injured area to prevent damage. Apply ice for 20 minutes, then rest 10 minutes. Repeat application for 24 to 48 hours after injury.

CONTINUING CARE
- When bed rest is discontinued, you may need cast or brace to allow the strain to heal completely. Later a special corset may be used.
- Use ice massage 3 or 4 times a day for 15 minutes at a time. Fill a large styrofoam cup with water and freeze. Tear a small amount of foam from the top so ice protrudes. Massage firmly over the injured area in a circle about the size of a softball.
- After 72 hours, apply heat instead of ice if it feels better. Use heat lamps, hot soaks, heating pads or heat liniments and ointments.
- Take whirlpool treatments, if available.
- Massage gently and often to provide comfort and decrease swelling.

MEDICATION
- For minor discomfort, you may use:
  Aspirin, acetaminophen or ibuprofen.
  Topical liniments and ointments.
- Your doctor may prescribe:
  Stronger pain relievers.
  Injection of a long-acting local anesthetic to reduce pain.
  Injection of a corticosteroid, such as triamcinolone, to reduce inflammation.

ACTIVITY—Rest in bed until pain subsides. If activities are resumed too early, recurrence is likely.

DIET—During recovery, balance the amount of food you eat with any change in your level of physical activity. Eat a variety of foods to get the energy, protein, vitamins, minerals and fiber you need for good health and healing.

REHABILITATION—Begin daily rehabilitation exercises when supportive devices are no longer needed. Use ice massage for 10 minutes prior to exercises. See Rehabilitation section for low back exercises and upper back exercises.

 # CALL YOUR DOCTOR IF

- You have persistent back pain.
- Pain or swelling worsens despite treatment.

BICYCLE SEAT NEUROPATHY

GENERAL INFORMATION

DEFINITION—A term used to describe certain problems experienced by bicycle riders (both male and female) who regularly ride a bicycle. Neuropathy refers to decreased nerve functioning. Numbness and other symptoms occur in the perineum area (the general region between the anus and the genital organs). The symptoms may last a few seconds to a few minutes or take days or weeks to resolve.

BODY PARTS INVOLVED
• Perineum; an area of skin that is located below the anus (the opening for bowel movements). For women, the perineum extends to the vaginal opening; for men it extends to the base of the testicles. The perineum includes the nerves and arteries to the genitals.
• Genital area and the rectum area.

SIGNS & SYMPTOMS
• Numbness, tingling or pain in the perineum area.
• Penile numbness.
• Male impotence (erectile dysfunction). There is some controversy over whether bicycle riding is linked to impotence.
• In females, the numbness may extend to the clitoris possibly causing sexual dysfunction.
• Pain when sitting.

CAUSES—A typical bicycle seat (unlike a chair) directs all the pressure to the perineum (crotch) area. There is chronic compression between the bicycle seat and the perineum. The compression can become acute when you hit a bump. Through the perineum runs an artery that supplies blood, and nerves (including the pudendal nerve and genital-femoral nerve) that provide sensation to the genitals. Sitting on the perineum puts pressure on the nerves and artery, which can lead to the symptoms.

RISK INCREASES WITH
• A cyclist supporting his or her body weight on a narrow seat.
• Long-distance cycling races and tours.
• Multiday bicycle rides.
• Frequent use of a stationary bicycle for exercising.

HOW TO PREVENT
• Ride a bike that is a proper fit for the individual rider (including frame size and handlebar height).
• Appropriate adjustment of the bicycle seat. Using a seat specifically designed to prevent excessive perineal pressure may help (such as seats with a center cutout or split nose).
• Wear padded bicycle shorts.
• Rider changing his or her riding position frequently. Stand up and pedal every 10 minutes to encourage blood flow in the perineum.
• Avoid lengthy rides and limit the amount of time spent biking each week.

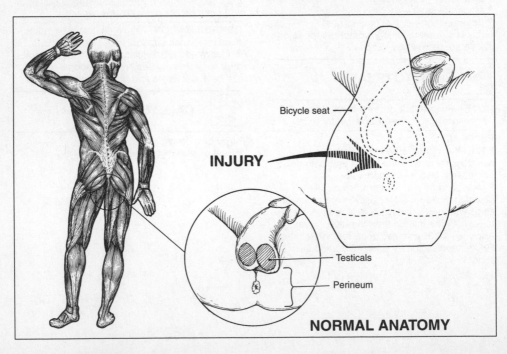

Bicycle seat

INJURY

Testicals

Perineum

NORMAL ANATOMY

- Use proper riding techniques for rides over rough and varied terrain, e.g. using the legs as shock absorbers.
- Cyclists may try a recumbent model, which puts less pressure on the perineum area because the rider sits on his or her buttocks and not with the seat between the legs.

 WHAT TO EXPECT

APPROPRIATE HEALTH CARE
- An affected rider should stop cycling until symptoms resolve.
- Doctor's treatment for recurring symptoms or ongoing problems with impotence.

DIAGNOSTIC MEASURES
- Your own observation of symptoms.
- Medical history and exam by a doctor.
- Rarely, an ultrasound, CT scan or x-rays may be recommended to rule out other medical problems such as a pelvic fracture.

POSSIBLE COMPLICATIONS—Complications are unlikely if recommended preventive measures are utilized.

PROBABLE OUTCOME
- The prognosis and recovery is very good. Cases of bicycle seat neuropathy and its resulting symptoms, such as impotence, usually resolve over time once the pressure is relieved from the perineal region.
- Rate of recovery is different for individuals and may be dependent on the amount of time previously spent cycling.

 HOW TO TREAT

NOTE—Follow your doctor's instructions. These instructions are supplemental.

FIRST AID—None. This condition will resolve itself.

CONTINUING CARE
- Main aspect of treatment is the adjustment of the bike seat and bike position, such as tilting the nose of the seat down or to lower the seat height to relieve pressure off of the perineum. Make sure that the bicycle seat, handlebars and pedals are correctly adjusted and that the bicycle is the appropriate size.
- Change position on the bike (e.g., ride with hands on the top of the handlebars instead of having hands down in the drops or riding with aerobars).
- Stand up intermittently to relieve pressure or stop cycling temporarily until the symptoms resolve.
- Review the section on How to Prevent for additional suggestions.

MEDICATION—For minor discomfort, you may use aspirin, acetaminophen or ibuprofen.

ACTIVITY—Usually there are no limits to normal activities or continued bicycle riding if preventive techniques are used.

DIET—Balance the amount of food you eat with any change in your level of physical activity. Eat a variety of foods to get the energy, protein, vitamins, minerals and fiber you need for good health and healing.

REHABILITATION—If you are unsure about proper riding techniques, consult an expert at a sports-medicine facility or a bike shop to learn how to safely enjoy the benefits of a cycling workout.

 CALL YOUR DOCTOR IF

- You have symptoms of bicycle seat neuropathy that last longer than a few days.
- Continued symptoms occur despite changes in the biking equipment you use and amount of time spent in riding. This may indicate a different source of the symptoms.

BLADDER OR URETHRA INJURY

GENERAL INFORMATION

DEFINITION—Damage to the urinary bladder (the organ that stores urine manufactured by the kidneys) or the urethra (the tube through which urine travels from the bladder to the outside).

BODY PARTS INVOLVED
* Bladder.
* Urethra.
* Muscles, tendons, blood vessels, nerves and connective tissues of the pelvic floor.

SIGNS & SYMPTOMS
* Severe abdominal pain and tenderness over the bladder.
* Shock (sweating; faintness; nausea; panting; rapid pulse; pale, cold, moist skin).
* Bloody discharge from the urethra or blood in the urine.

CAUSES—Fracture of a pelvic bone that punctures or bruises the bladder or urethra (usually).

RISK INCREASES WITH
* Contact sports such as football, rugby, soccer or hockey.
* Cycling, motor sports.
* Falls from heights.
* Full bladder during sports activities.
* Repeated injury to the lower pelvis.

HOW TO PREVENT
* Wear adequate protective equipment.
* Keep bladder empty during exercise or competitive sports.

WHAT TO EXPECT

APPROPRIATE HEALTH CARE
* Doctor's treatment.
* Hospitalization or emergency room care.
* Surgery (usually) to repair a punctured bladder. A damaged urethra may heal without surgery. However, usually urine must be diverted from the injury by passage of a tube through the urethra into the bladder.

DIAGNOSTIC MEASURES
* Your own observation of symptoms.
* Medical history and physical exam by a doctor.
* Laboratory urine studies.
* X-rays of the urinary tract.

POSSIBLE COMPLICATIONS
* Internal bleeding.
* Rupture of the bladder (rare).
* Urine leakage into the abdomen, causing abdominal inflammation or infection.
* Recurrent infections from scars in the urethra that narrow the urinary passage.

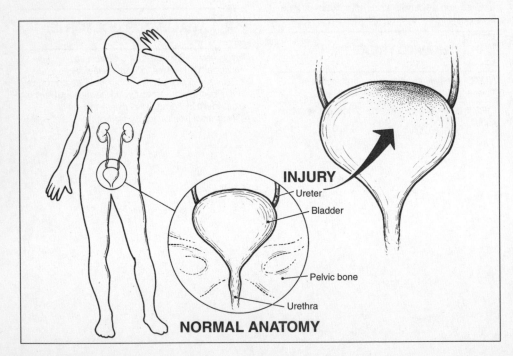

INJURY
- Ureter
- Bladder
- Pelvic bone
- Urethra

NORMAL ANATOMY

PROBABLE OUTCOME—A punctured bladder or urethra requires emergency treatment. Most bladder and urethra injuries heal completely with bed rest, time, supportive treatment or surgery.

HOW TO TREAT

NOTE—Follow your doctor's instructions. These instructions are supplemental.

FIRST AID
• Keep the person warm with blankets to decrease the possibility of shock.
• Immobilize the person on a stretcher or spine board.
• Elevate the lower extremities with pillows or blocks.
• Take the patient to the nearest emergency facility.

CONTINUING CARE—No specific instructions except those under other headings. If surgery is required, your doctor will supply postoperative instructions.

MEDICATION—Your doctor may prescribe antibiotics to prevent infection.

ACTIVITY—Stay as active as your strength allows. Allow 1 month for recovery. Don't return to work, exercise or competitive sports or resume sexual relations until healing is complete.

DIET
• No food or water before surgery.
• Drink 6 to 8 glasses of fluid daily.
• Don't drink alcohol.
• During recovery, balance the amount of food you eat with any change in your level of physical activity. Eat a variety of foods to get the energy, protein, vitamins, minerals and fiber you need for good health and healing.

REHABILITATION—Rehabilitation exercises must be individualized. Follow your doctor's or surgeon's directions.

CALL YOUR DOCTOR IF

• You have any symptoms of bladder or urethra injury.
• During or after treatment, you develop chills and fever of 101°F (38.3°C) or higher.
• New, unexplained symptoms develop. Drugs used in treatment may produce side effects.

BREAST CONTUSION

GENERAL INFORMATION

DEFINITION—Bruising of skin and underlying tissues of the breast or nipple. Contusions cause bleeding from ruptured small capillaries that allow blood to infiltrate fatty tissues, muscles, tendons, nerves or other soft tissues.

BODY PARTS INVOLVED
• Male or female breast.
• Skin, nipple, subcutaneous fatty tissues, blood vessels (both large vessels and capillaries), muscles and connective tissues.

SIGNS & SYMPTOMS
• Local swelling of the breast—either superficial or deep.
• Pain in the breast or nipple.
• Feeling of firmness when pressure is exerted on the injury area.
• Tenderness.
• Discoloration under the skin, beginning with redness and progressing to the characteristic "black-and-blue" bruise.
• Hard, tender ring surrounding the nipple.

CAUSES—Direct blow to the breast, usually by a blunt object.

RISK INCREASES WITH
• Contact sports such as wrestling, baseball, softball or boxing, especially if the breast area has inadequate protection.
• Medical history of any bleeding disorder.
• Poor nutrition.
• Obesity.

HOW TO PREVENT
• Wear appropriate protective gear for the chest during competition or other athletic activity if there is a risk of contusion.
• Women should wear breast support—a sport bra, elasticized binder or both—for participation in contact sports.

WHAT TO EXPECT

APPROPRIATE HEALTH CARE
• Doctor's care unless the contusion is quite small.
• Self-care during recovery.

DIAGNOSTIC MEASURES
• Your own observation of symptoms.
• Physical exam and medical history by a doctor for all except minor injuries. Total extent of the injury may not be apparent for 48 to 72 hours following injury.

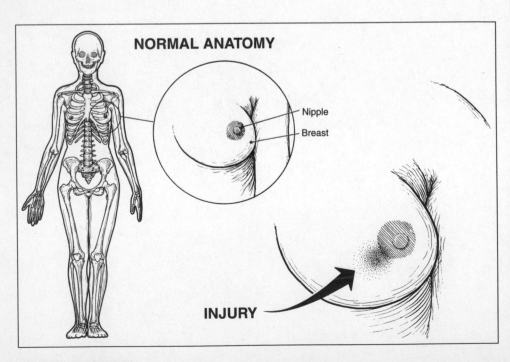

NORMAL ANATOMY

Nipple

Breast

INJURY

- X-rays of injured area to assess total injury to soft tissues and to rule out the possibility of underlying fracture.
- Follow-up exam to make sure that any lumps remaining 3 months after injury do not represent possible malignancy.

POSSIBLE COMPLICATIONS
- Excessive bleeding, leading to disability. Infiltrative-type bleeding can (rarely) lead to calcification.
- Prolonged healing time if usual activities are resumed too soon.
- Infection if skin over the injury is broken.

PROBABLE OUTCOME—Healing time varies from 2 to 6 weeks, depending on the extent of injury.

 # HOW TO TREAT

NOTE—Follow your doctor's instructions. These instructions are supplemental.

FIRST AID—Use instructions for R.I.C.E., the first letters of *rest, ice, compression* and *elevation*. See Appendix 1 for details.

CONTINUING CARE
- Continue to use ice massage. Fill a large styrofoam cup with water and freeze. Tear a small amount of foam from the top so ice protrudes. Massage firmly over the injured area in a circle about the size of a softball. Do this for 15 minutes at a time 3 or 4 times a day, and also before workouts or competition.

- After 72 hours, apply heat instead of ice if it feels better. Use heat lamps, hot soaks, hot showers, heating pads, or heat liniments and ointments.
- Take whirlpool treatments, if available.
- Protect the injured area with pads, or wrap with an elasticized bandage between treatments.

MEDICATIONS
- For minor discomfort, you may use non-prescription medicines such as acetaminophen or ibuprofen. Do not use aspirin for injuries involving bleeding.
- Your doctor may prescribe stronger medicine for pain, if needed.

ACTIVITY—Begin activities slowly, and stop exercise as soon as pain begins. Increase activity as healing progresses.

DIET—During recovery, balance the amount of food you eat with any change in your level of physical activity. Eat a variety of foods to get the energy, protein, vitamins, minerals and fiber you need for good health and healing.

REHABILITATION—None.

 # CALL YOUR DOCTOR IF

- A breast contusion doesn't improve within a day or two.
- Signs of infection (drainage from skin, headache, muscle aches, dizziness, fever or a general ill feeling) occur if skin was broken.
- Firm nodules that appear following injury do not disappear in 3 months.

BREASTBONE (STERNUM) SPRAIN AT THE COLLARBONE (CLAVICLE) (Sternoclavicular Sprain)

GENERAL INFORMATION

DEFINITION—Violent overstretching of one or more ligaments in the sternoclavicular joint where the collarbone meets the breastbone. Sprains involving two or more ligaments cause considerably more disability than single-ligament sprains. When the ligament is overstretched, it becomes tense and gives way at its weakest point, either where it attaches to bone or within the ligament itself. If the ligament pulls loose a fragment of bone, it is called an avulsion fracture. There are 3 types of sprains:
- Mild (Grade I)—Tearing of some ligament fibers. There is no loss of function.
- Moderate (Grade II)—Rupture of a portion of the ligament, resulting in some loss of function.
- Severe (Grade III)—Complete rupture of the ligament or complete separation of ligament from bone. There is total loss of function. A severe sprain may require surgical repair.

BODY PARTS INVOLVED
- Ligaments of the sternoclavicular joint.
- Tissues surrounding the sprain, including blood vessels, tendons, bone, periosteum (covering of bone) and muscles.

SIGNS & SYMPTOMS
- Severe pain at the time of injury.
- A feeling of popping or tearing in the collarbone area.
- Tenderness at the injury site.
- Swelling in the collarbone area.
- Bruising that appears soon after injury.

CAUSES
- Stress on a ligament by a force that thrusts the shoulder sharply forward, temporarily forcing the sternoclavicular joint out of its normal location.
- Falling on an outstretched hand.
- Falling directly onto the top of the shoulder or onto the collarbone.

RISK INCREASES WITH
- Contact sports such as boxing or football.
- Cycling.
- Weightlifting.
- Previous breastbone or collarbone injury.
- Obesity.
- Poor muscle conditioning.
- Inadequate protection from equipment.

HOW TO PREVENT
- Warm up before practice or competition.
- Wear proper protective equipment, such as shoulder and chest pads.

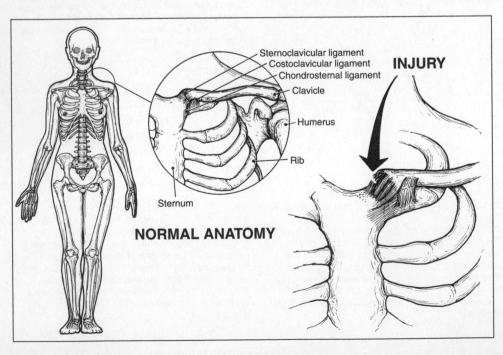

Sternoclavicular ligament
Costoclavicular ligament
Chondrosternal ligament
Clavicle
Humerus
Rib
Sternum

NORMAL ANATOMY

INJURY

WHAT TO EXPECT

APPROPRIATE HEALTH CARE
- Doctor's diagnosis.
- Application of a cast, tape, elastic bandage or special brace.
- Self-care during rehabilitation.
- Physical therapy (moderate or severe sprain).
- Surgery (severe sprain).

DIAGNOSTIC MEASURES
- Your own observation of symptoms.
- Medical history and exam by a doctor.
- X-rays of the shoulder, chest and clavicle to rule out fractures or dislocation of the sterno-clavicular joint.

POSSIBLE COMPLICATIONS
- Prolonged healing time if usual activities are resumed too soon.
- Proneness to repeated injury.
- Inflammation of the ligament attachment to bone (periostitis).
- Prolonged disability (sometimes).
- Unstable or arthritic joint following repeated injury.
- Dislocation of the sternoclavicular joint.

PROBABLE OUTCOME—If this is a first-time injury, proper care and sufficient healing time before resuming activity should prevent permanent disability. Ligaments have a poor blood supply, and torn ligaments require as much healing time as fractures. Average healing times are:
- Mild sprains—2 to 6 weeks.
- Moderate sprains—6 to 8 weeks.
- Severe sprains—8 to 10 weeks.

HOW TO TREAT

NOTE—Follow your doctor's instructions. These instructions are supplemental.

FIRST AID—Use instructions for R.I.C.E., the first letters of *rest, ice, compression* and *elevation*. See Appendix 1 for details

CONTINUING CARE—If the doctor does not apply a cast, tape or elastic bandage:
- Use of a sling to support and rest the injured limb.
- Continue using an ice pack 3 or 4 times a day. Place ice chips or cubes in a plastic bag. Wrap the bag in a moist towel, and place it over the injured area. Use for 20 minutes at a time.
- After 72 hours, apply heat instead of ice if it feels better. Use heat lamps, hot soaks, hot showers, heating pads or heat liniments and ointments.

- Take whirlpool treatments, if available.
- Massage gently and often to provide comfort and decrease swelling.

MEDICATION
- For minor discomfort, you may use:
  Aspirin, acetaminophen or ibuprofen.
  Topical liniments and ointments.
- Your doctor may prescribe:
  Stronger pain relievers.
  Injection of a long-acting local anesthetic to reduce pain.
  Injections of a corticosteroid, such as triamcinolone, to reduce inflammation.

ACTIVITY—Resume your normal activities gradually after clearance from your doctor.

DIET—During recovery, balance the amount of food you eat with any change in your level of physical activity. Eat a variety of foods to get the energy, protein, vitamins, minerals and fiber you need for good health and healing.

REHABILITATION
- Begin daily rehabilitation exercises when pain subsides.
- Use ice massage for 10 minutes before and 10 minutes after exercise. Fill a large styrofoam cup with water and freeze. Tear a small amount of foam from the top so ice protrudes. Massage firmly over the injured area in a circle about the size of a softball.
- See Rehabilitation section for upper back exercises and shoulder exercises.

CALL YOUR DOCTOR IF

- You have symptoms of a moderate or severe sternoclavicular sprain or a mild sprain persists longer than 2 weeks.
- Pain, swelling or bruising worsens despite treatment.
- You experience pain, numbness or coldness in the shoulder or the arm or below the injury site.
- Skin turns blue, gray or a dusky color beyond the cast or sling.
- The collarbone moves backward out of normal position (dislocation of the sterno-clavicular joint).
- Any of the following occurs after surgery:
  Increased pain, swelling, redness, drainage or bleeding in the surgical area.
  Signs of infection (headache, muscle aches, dizziness or a general ill feeling with fever).
- New, unexplained symptoms develop. Drugs used in treatment may produce side effects.
- You develop shortness of breath and difficulty swallowing associated with a sternoclavicular dislocation.

BURNER (STINGER)

GENERAL INFORMATION

DEFINITION—A burner is an injury to one or more nerves between the neck and shoulder. The names (burner or stinger) come from the typical symptoms an athlete experiences. Other terms used to describe the injury are pinched nerve or "hot shot." Burners are common injuries (especially with tackling in football). Symptoms often last less than 5 minutes.

BODY PARTS INVOLVED—Nerves that provide feeling to the arms and hands. The nerves originate from the cervical (neck) spinal cord. As these nerves leave the neck, they form the brachial plexus. They weave together then branch as they pass under the clavicle (collarbone) on the way to the shoulder.

SIGNS & SYMPTOMS
- Burning or stinging feeling between your neck and shoulder.
- Arm may feel painful, numb, tingly, weak or have a brief paralysis. The weakness often involves the muscles that allow you to lift the arm away from the body, to bend the elbow, and to grip. Affected athlete often tries to "shake off" the injury to restore feeling to the arm.
- Burners happen in only one arm at a time. If both of your arms or one arm and a leg are hurt, it may mean a serious neck injury.
- Burner symptoms usually resolve within a few minutes of the injury, they can also develop hours or days later, and may persist.

CAUSES
- The injury often results from a direct blow to the top of the shoulder which drives it down and causes the neck to bend toward the opposite side. This stretches nerves between your neck and shoulder.
- Nerves are bruised when the area above your collarbone is hit directly.

RISK INCREASES WITH
- Contact sports, such as football, wrestling and hockey.
- Athletic activities including cycling, snow skiing, gymnastics, and martial arts.

HOW TO PREVENT
- Use proper techniques in football tackling and blocking.
- Wear proper protective gear for the sport or activity. Be sure it fits properly and is in good condition. If you have had a burner previously, consider using special protective equipment.
- Before the season begins, participate in an exercise program to develop full range of motion and protective strength of the neck and shoulder muscles.

WHAT TO EXPECT

APPROPRIATE HEALTH CARE
- Self-care for some. Report the injury to the coach or trainer even if the symptoms disappear quickly.

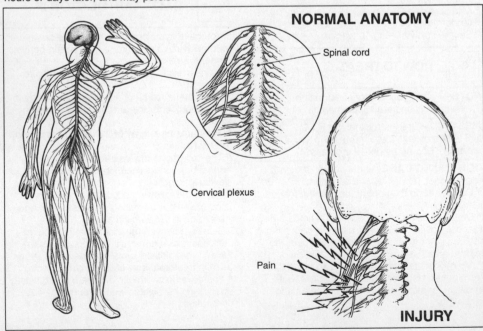

NORMAL ANATOMY

Spinal cord

Cervical plexus

Pain

INJURY

- In some cases, the injury could lead to more severe nerve damage if left undiagnosed and untreated.
- Doctor's care if symptoms persist or if burners recur during the same season.

DIAGNOSTIC MEASURES
- Your own observation of symptoms.
- Medical history and physical exam by a doctor.
- X-rays (or an MRI) of the spine may be performed in patients with severe neck pain, limited range of motion, weakness or recurrent injury.
- Electromyographic (EMG) may be recommended for patients with symptoms that last at least three weeks. The test can show that you have a burner and provide information about how long it will last.

POSSIBLE COMPLICATIONS
- Chronic symptoms may remain.
- You may need physical therapy to help stretch and strengthen your muscles.
- Burners recur frequently.

PROBABLE OUTCOME
- Burners are usually a brief injury with rapid recovery being the rule. The majority will get better on their own.
- Medical studies have found that most of the time, burner injuries go unreported and the injured player returns to the game without any further complication.

 ## HOW TO TREAT

NOTE—Follow your doctor's instructions. These instructions are supplemental.

FIRST AID
- If appropriate, the athletic trainer, physical therapist, or team doctor examines the cervical spine and will evaluates nerve function. Serious spine injuries need to be ruled out.
- Use instructions for R.I.C.E., the first letters of *rest, ice, compression* and *elevation*. See Appendix 1 for details.

CONTINUING CARE
- Rest your head and neck until the symptoms are gone.

- Continue using an ice pack 3 or 4 times a day. Place ice chips or cubes in a plastic bag. Wrap the bag in a moist towel, and place it over the injured area. Use for 20 minutes at a time.
- If the stiffness in the neck muscles continues, it may be treated with heat, massage or muscle stimulation.

MEDICATION—Generally, no medication is required for this injury. Nonsteroidal anti-inflammatory medications such as aspirin or ibuprofen may be used for pain and for reduction of swelling and inflammation.

ACTIVITY
- To return to your sport, you must have no pain, numbness or tingling. You must be able to move your neck in all directions. Your strength must be back to normal. You must be able to play your sport without problems from the injury.
- In the majority of cases, the athlete is able to return to the game or activity after the symptoms are resolved.An athlete may be examined frequently during the game for further problems including recurrence of symptoms.

DIET—During recovery, balance the amount of food you eat with any change in your level of physical activity. Eat a variety of foods to get the energy, protein, vitamins, minerals and fiber you need for good health and healing.

REHABILITATION
- For most athletes, there is no need for rehabilitation.
- If your symptoms persist, physical therapy and rehabilitation may be recommended to improve muscle function and soft tissue tightness in the neck and shoulder area. Return to play will be determined by the trainer or team doctor.

 ## CALL YOUR DOCTOR IF

- You have symptoms of a burner during a game, advise the trainer, doctor on the sidelines or the coach, before you go back in the game.
- You have symptoms of a burner that continue for an hour or more after the injury occurred.
- You experience repeated episodes of a burner injury.

BUTTOCK CONTUSION

GENERAL INFORMATION

DEFINITION—Bruising of skin and underlying tissues of the buttock caused by a direct blow. Contusions cause bleeding from ruptured small capillaries that allow blood to infiltrate muscles, tendons, nerves or other soft tissues.

BODY PARTS INVOLVED
• Buttock.
• Skin, subcutaneous tissues, tendons, ligaments, blood vessels (both large vessels and capillaries), periosteum (the outside lining of bone), muscles and connective tissues.

SIGNS & SYMPTOMS
• Swelling and a hard lump in the injured buttock—either superficial or deep.
• Pain and tenderness in the buttock.
• Feeling of firmness when pressure is exerted on the buttock.
• Discoloration under the skin, beginning with redness and progressing to the characteristic "black-and-blue" bruise.

CAUSES—Direct blow to the buttock, usually by a blunt object.

RISK INCREASES WITH
• Contact sports, especially football, ice hockey, basketball and baseball (sliding).
• Sports that make falling from a height likely, such as high jumping, pole vaulting, skating or gymnastics.
• Medical history of any bleeding disorder.
• Poor nutrition.
• Inadequate protection of exposed areas during contact sports.
• Obesity.

HOW TO PREVENT
• Wear protective equipment such as hip pads when appropriate.
• Build coordination prior to exercise, athletic practice or competition.

WHAT TO EXPECT

APPROPRIATE HEALTH CARE
• Doctor's care for precise diagnosis unless the injury is quite small.
• Self-care for minor contusions and during rehabilitation for serious contusions.
• Physical therapy for serious contusions.

DIAGNOSTIC MEASURES
• Your own observation of symptoms.
• Physical exam and medical history by a doctor for all except minor injuries.
• X-rays of the buttock to assess total injury to soft tissues and to rule out the possibility of underlying fracture. The total extent of injury may not be apparent for 48 to 72 hours following injury.

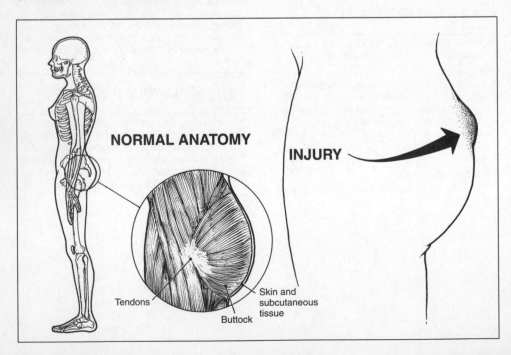

NORMAL ANATOMY

Tendons

Buttock

Skin and subcutaneous tissue

INJURY

POSSIBLE COMPLICATIONS
- Excessive bleeding into the buttock, leading to disability. Infiltrative-type bleeding can (rarely) lead to calcification and impaired function of injured muscle.
- Prolonged healing time if usual activities are resumed too soon.
- Infection if skin over the injury site is broken.
- Fracture of the underlying pelvic bone (frequent complication of buttock contusion).
- Injury to the sciatic nerve.

PROBABLE OUTCOME—Healing time varies from 1 to 4 weeks, depending on the extent of injury.

 ## HOW TO TREAT

NOTE—Follow your doctor's instructions. These instructions are supplemental.

FIRST AID—Use instructions for R.I.C.E., the first letters of *rest, ice, compression* and *elevation* (if possible). See Appendix 1 for details.

CONTINUING CARE
- Continue ice massage. Fill a large styrofoam cup with water and freeze. Tear a small amount of foam from the top so ice protrudes. Massage firmly over the injured area in a circle about the size of a softball. Do this for 15 minutes at a time 3 to 4 times a day, and also before workouts or competition.
- After 72 hours, apply heat instead of ice if it feels better. Use heat lamps, hot soaks, hot showers, heating pads or heat liniments and ointments.
- Take whirlpool treatments, if available.
- Protect the injured area with pads or an elasticized bandage wrap between treatments.
- Massage gently and often to provide comfort and decrease swelling.

MEDICATIONS
- For minor discomfort, you may use non-prescription medicines such as acetaminophen or ibuprofen. Do not use aspirin for injuries involving bleeding.
- Your doctor may prescribe stronger medicine for pain if needed.

ACTIVITY—Begin activities slowly, and stop exercise as soon as pain begins. Increase activity as healing progresses

DIET—During recovery, balance the amount of food you eat with any change in your level of physical activity. Eat a variety of foods to get the energy, protein, vitamins, minerals and fiber you need for good health and healing.

REHABILITATION—Rehabilitation exercises must be individualized. Follow your doctor's or surgeon's directions.

 ## CALL YOUR DOCTOR IF

- A buttock contusion doesn't improve within a day or two.
- Signs of infection (drainage from skin, headache, muscle aches, dizziness, fever or a general ill feeling) occur if skin was broken.

CHEST MUSCLE STRAIN

GENERAL INFORMATION

DEFINITION—Injury to the muscles and tendons that attach to the sternum (breastbone). Muscles, tendons and their attached bones comprise contractile units. The units stabilize the breastbone and ribs and also their motion. A strain occurs at the weakest part of a unit. Strains are of 3 types:
- Mild (grade I)—slightly pulled muscle without tearing of muscle or tendon fibers. There is no loss of strength.
- Moderate (grade II)—Tearing of fibers in a muscle tendon or at the attachment to a rib. Strength is diminished.
- Severe (Grade III)—Rupture of this muscle-tendon-rib attachment with separation of fibers. A severe strain may require surgical repair. Chronic strains are caused by overuse. Acute strains are caused by direct injury or overstress.

BODY PARTS INVOLVED.
- Muscles (pectoralis and intercostal muscles) and tendons that attach the ribs to the sternum.
- Sternum.
- Soft tissues surrounding the strain, including nerves, periosteum (covering of bone), blood vessels and lymph vessels.

SIGNS & SYMPTOMS
- Pain when moving or stretching, especially when making "pushing" movements of the arm.
- Muscle spasm.
- Swelling around the injury.
- Loss of strength (moderate or severe strain).
- Calcification of muscles or tendons (visible with x-rays).

CAUSES
- Prolonged overuse of muscle-tendon units attached to the sternum and ribs.
- Single violent injury or force applied to the muscle-tendon units around the sternum and ribs.

RISK INCREASES WITH
- Contact sports.
- Weightlifting.
- Medical history of any bleeding disorder.
- Obesity.
- Poor nutrition.
- Previous sternum or rib injury.
- Poor muscle conditioning.

HOW TO PREVENT
- Participate in a strengthening, flexibility and conditioning program appropriate for your sport.
- Warm up before practice or competition.
- Wear proper protective chest padding.

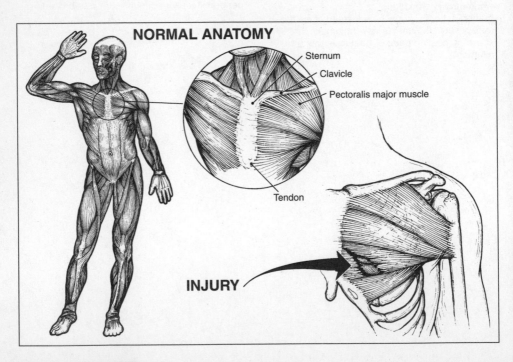

NORMAL ANATOMY

Sternum

Clavicle

Pectoralis major muscle

Tendon

INJURY

WHAT TO EXPECT

APPROPRIATE HEALTH CARE
- Doctor's diagnosis.
- Application of tape (sometimes).
- Self-care during rehabilitation.
- Physical therapy (moderate or severe strain).
- Surgery (severe strain).

DIAGNOSTIC MEASURES
- Your own observation of symptoms.
- Medical history and exam by a doctor.
- X-rays of the chest to rule out fractures.

POSSIBLE COMPLICATIONS
- Prolonged healing time if activity is resumed too soon.
- Proneness to repeated injury.
- Inflammation at the attachment to bone (periostitis).
- Prolonged disability (sometimes).

PROBABLE OUTCOME—If this is a first-time injury, proper care and sufficient healing time before resuming activity should prevent permanent disability. Torn ligaments and tendons require as long to heal as fractured bones do. Average healing times are:
- Mild strain—2 to 10 days.
- Moderate strain—10 days to 6 weeks.
- Severe strain—6 to 10 weeks.

 ## HOW TO TREAT

NOTE—Follow your doctor's instructions. These instructions are supplemental.

FIRST AID—Use instructions for R.I.C.E., the first letters of *rest, ice, compression* and *elevation*. See Appendix 1 for details.

CONTINUING CARE
- Use ice massage 3 or 4 times a day for 15 minutes at a time. Fill a large styrofoam cup with water and freeze. Tear a small amount of foam from the top so ice protrudes. Massage firmly over the injured area in a circle about the size of a softball.

- After the first 72 hours, apply heat instead of ice if it feels better. Use heat lamps, hot soaks, hot showers, heating pads or heat liniments and ointments.
- Take whirlpool treatments, if available.
- Wrap the chest with an elasticized bandage between treatments.
- Massage gently and often to provide comfort and decrease swelling.

MEDICATION
- For minor discomfort, you may use:
  Aspirin, acetaminophen or ibuprofen.
  Topical liniments and ointments.
- Your doctor may prescribe:
  Stronger pain relievers.
  Injection of a long-acting local anesthetic to reduce pain.
  Injections of corticosteroids, such as triamcinolone, to reduce inflammation.

ACTIVITY—Resume your normal activities gradually.

DIET—During recovery, balance the amount of food you eat with any change in your level of physical activity. Eat a variety of foods to get the energy, protein, vitamins, minerals and fiber you need for good health and healing.

REHABILITATION—Begin a supervised weightlifting program after clearance from your doctor.

 ## CALL YOUR DOCTOR IF

- Your have symptoms of a moderate or severe chest muscle strain or a mild strain persists longer than 10 days.
- Pain or swelling worsens despite treatment.

COLLARBONE (CLAVICLE) CONTUSION

GENERAL INFORMATION

DEFINITION—Bruising of skin and underlying tissues at the clavicle (collarbone) caused by a direct blow. Contusions cause bleeding from ruptured small capillaries that allow blood to infiltrate muscles, tendons or other soft tissues. A collarbone contusion is usually accompanied by injury to the sternum (breastbone) or shoulder bone.

BODY PARTS INVOLVED—Tissues over the clavicle, shoulder and breastbone, including blood vessels, muscles, tendons, nerves, covering of bone (periosteum) and connective tissues.

SIGNS AND SYMPTOMS
- Local swelling—either superficial or deep.
- Tenderness over the injury, but no additional pain when moving.
- Feeling of firmness when pressure is exerted at the injury site.
- Discoloration under the skin, beginning with redness and progressing to the characteristic "black-and-blue" bruises.
- Restricted shoulder and chest activity proportional to the extent of injury.

CAUSES—Direct blow to the clavicle, usually from a blunt object.

RISK INCREASES WITH
- Contact sports such as football, wrestling, ice hockey and basketball, especially if the shoulder and chest are not adequately protected.
- Medical history of any bleeding disorder.
- Poor nutrition, including vitamin deficiency.
- Use of anticoagulants or aspirin.

HOW TO PREVENT—Wear appropriate protective shoulder and chest pads during competition or other athletic activity if there is risk of a clavicle contusion.

WHAT TO EXPECT

APPROPRIATE HEALTH CARE
- Doctor's care unless the contusion is quite small.
- Self-care for minor contusions or for serious contusions during rehabilitation.
- Physical therapy for serious contusions.

DIAGNOSTIC MEASURES
- Your own observation of symptoms.
- Medical history and physical exam by a doctor for all except minor injuries.
- X-rays of the clavicle, shoulder and sternum to assess total injury to soft tissues and to rule out the possibility of an underlying fracture or shoulder separation. The total extent of injury may not be apparent for 45 to 72 hours.

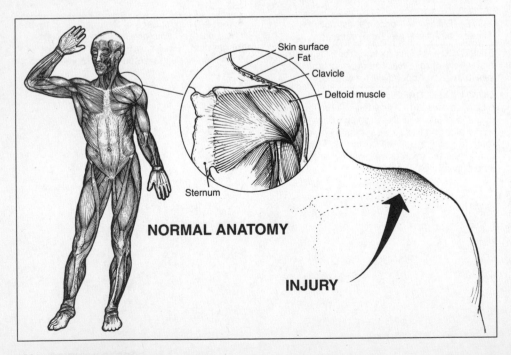

Skin surface
Fat
Clavicle
Deltoid muscle
Sternum

NORMAL ANATOMY

INJURY

POSSIBLE COMPLICATIONS
• Excessive bleeding, leading to disability. Infiltrative-type bleeding can (rarely) lead to calcification and impaired function of injured muscle.
• Prolonged healing time if usual activities are resumed too soon.
• Infection if skin over the contusion is broken.

PROBABLE OUTCOME—Healing time varies with the extent of injury, but all but the most serious contusions should heal in 6 to 10 days.

 ## HOW TO TREAT

NOTE—Follow your doctor's instructions. These instructions are supplemental.

FIRST AID—Use instructions for R.I.C.E., the first letters of *rest, ice, compression* and *elevation.* See Appendix 1 for details.

CONTINUING CARE
• Use a sling if it makes you more comfortable.
• Continue ice massage. Fill a large styrofoam cup with water and freeze. Tear a small amount of foam from the top so ice protrudes. Massage gently over the injured area in a circle about the size of a softball. Do this for 15 minutes at a time 3 or 4 times a day, and also before workouts or competition.
• After 72 hours, apply heat instead of ice if it feels better. Use heat lamps, hot soaks, hot showers, heating pads, heat liniments and ointments or whirlpool treatments.
• Massage gently and often to provide comfort and decrease swelling.

MEDICATION
• For minor discomfort, you may use:
Acetaminophen or ibuprofen.
Topical liniments and ointments.
• Your doctor may prescribe stronger medicine for pain.

ACTIVITY—Begin activities slowly, and stop exercise as soon as pain begins. Increase activity as healing progresses. Wear protective padding over contusion when you return to activity.

DIET—During recovery, balance the amount of food you eat with any change in your level of physical activity. Eat a variety of foods to get the energy, protein, vitamins, minerals and fiber you need for good health and healing.

REHABILITATION
• Begin daily rehabilitation exercises when movement is comfortable and a sling is no longer necessary.
• See Rehabilitation section for upper back exercises and shoulder exercises.

 ## CALL YOUR DOCTOR IF

• You have a clavicle contusion that doesn't improve in 1 or 2 days.
• Skin is broken and signs of infection (drainage, increasing pain, fever, headache, muscle aches, dizziness or a general ill feeling) occur.

COLLARBONE (CLAVICLE) DISLOCATION AT SHOULDER JOINT (Shoulder Separation; Acromioclavicular Separation)

GENERAL INFORMATION

DEFINITION—An injury in which adjoining bones of the clavicle (collarbone) are displaced from their normal positions and the joint is disrupted. A minor dislocation is called a subluxation. (A less severe injury to these same ligaments comprises a sprain of the acromio-clavicular joint).

BODY PARTS INVOLVED
● Clavicle, sternum (breastbone) and scapula (shoulder blade).
● Ligaments that hold the clavicle to the scapula.
● Soft tissues in the injury area, including nerves, periosteum (covering of bone), blood vessels and muscles.

SIGNS & SYMPTOMS
● Excruciating pain in the collarbone-shoulder area at the time of injury.
● Loss of shoulder function.
● Severe pain when attempting to move the tip of the shoulder.
● Visible deformity if the dislocated bones have locked in the dislocated position. Bones may spontaneously reposition themselves and leave no deformity, but damage is the same.
● Tenderness over the dislocation.
● Swelling and bruising over the injury.
● Numbness or paralysis in the arm below the dislocation caused by pressure on or bruising of the nearby nerve.

CAUSES
● Direct fall onto the tip of the shoulder.
● Pulling or jerking on the arm.
● Falling on an outstretched hand or flexed elbow (common in football and polo).
● End result of a severe shoulder sprain at the acromioclavicular joint.

RISK INCREASES WITH
● Contact sports.
● Previous shoulder-clavicle dislocation or sprain.
● Repeated shoulder injury of any type.
● Poor muscle conditioning.

HOW TO PREVENT
● Participate in a strengthening, flexibility and conditioning program appropriate for your sport.
● Warm up adequately before physical activity.
● Wear shoulder pads during contact sports to protect the shoulder-clavicle area from injury.
● Avoid contact sports if treatment does not restore a strong, stable shoulder.

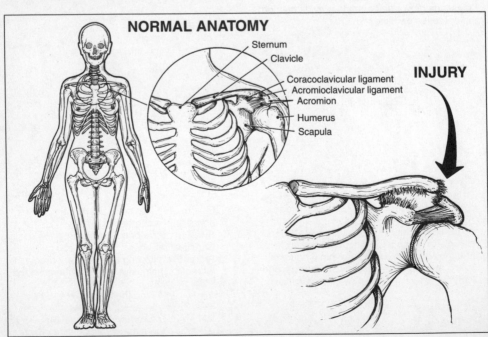

NORMAL ANATOMY

Sternum
Clavicle
Coracoclavicular ligament
Acromioclavicular ligament
Acromion
Humerus
Scapula

INJURY

WHAT TO EXPECT

APPROPRIATE HEALTH CARE
• Doctor's treatment, which includes manipulating the joint to reposition the bones or fitting a sling for support during healing.
• Surgery (sometimes) to restore the joint to its normal position and repair torn ligaments and tendons. Acute or recurring separations may require surgical reconstruction or resection of the joint.

DIAGNOSTIC MEASURES
• Your own observation of symptoms.
• Medical history and exam by a doctor.
• X-rays of the shoulder.

POSSIBLE COMPLICATIONS
At the time of injury:
• Shock.
• Pressure on or injury to nearby nerves, ligaments, tendons, muscles, blood vessels or connective tissues.
After treatment or surgery:
• Excessive internal bleeding.
• Impaired blood supply to the dislocated area.
• Death of bone cells due to interruption of the blood supply.
• Infection introduced during surgical treatment.
• Recurrent dislocations.
• Prolonged healing if activity is resumed too soon.
• Unstable or arthritic acromioclavicular joint following repeated injury.

PROBABLE OUTCOME—After the dislocation has been corrected, the shoulder may require immobilization with a semirigid dressing and sling for 2 to 4 weeks. Injured ligaments require a minimum of 6 weeks to heal, but range-of-motion exercises and general body conditioning can begin earlier.

 HOW TO TREAT

NOTE—Follow your doctor's instructions. These instructions are supplemental.

FIRST AID
• Use instructions for R.I.C.E., the first letters of *rest, ice, compression* and *elevation.* See Appendix 1 for details.
• The doctor may manipulate the separated clavicle to return it to its normal position. Manipulation should occur within 6 hours of injury, or shock may result. Also, many tissues lose their elasticity and may become difficult to return to their normal positions.

CONTINUING CARE
• At home, continue ice massage 3 or 4 times a day for 15 minutes at a time. Fill a large styrofoam cup with water and freeze. Tear a small amount of foam from the top so ice protrudes. Massage firmly over the injured area in a circle about the size of a softball.
• After 72 hours, apply heat instead of ice if it feels better. Use heat lamps, hot soaks, hot showers or heating pads.
• Massage gently and often to provide comfort and decrease swelling.
• Wrap the injured shoulder with an elasticized bandage between treatments.

MEDICATION—Your doctor may prescribe:
• General anesthesia or muscle relaxants to make joint manipulation possible or for fixation of the joint.
• Acetaminophen to relieve moderate pain.
• Prescription pain relievers for severe pain.
• Stool softeners to prevent constipation due to decreased activity.
• Antibiotics to fight infection if surgery is necessary.

ACTIVITY
• If surgery is not necessary, resume your normal conditioning program after clearance from your doctor.
• If surgery is necessary, resume activity gradually under your doctor's supervision.

DIET
• Do not eat or drink before surgery or manipulation to correct the dislocation. Fluid or solid food in your stomach makes vomiting while under general anesthesia more hazardous.
• During recovery, eat a well-balanced diet.

REHABILITATION—Begin daily rehabilitation exercises when pain subsides. Use ice massage for 10 minutes prior to exercise. See Rehabilitation section for upper back exercises and shoulder exercises.

 CALL YOUR DOCTOR IF

• You have symptoms of a dislocated clavicle.
• Any of the following occurs after injury or treatment:
  Numbness, loss of feeling, paleness or coldness in the arm. This is an emergency!
  Nausea or vomiting.
  Blue or gray skin color below the shoulder, especially under the fingernails.
  Swelling above or below the dressing or sling.
  Constipation.
• Any of the following occurs after surgery:
  Increasing pain, swelling or drainage in the surgical area.
  Signs of infection (headache, muscle aches, dizziness or a general ill feeling and fever).
• New, unexplained symptoms develop. Drugs used in treatment may produce side effects.

COLLARBONE (CLAVICLE) FRACTURE, OUTER END

GENERAL INFORMATION

DEFINITION—A complete or incomplete break in the outer third of the clavicle (collarbone). Frequently this fracture extends into the shoulder joint and is associated with rupture of the acromioclavicular ligaments.

BODY PARTS INVOLVED
- Clavicle (collarbone).
- Shoulder joint.
- Acromioclavicular joint (between the scapula and the collarbone).
- Soft tissues surrounding the site, including nerves, tendons, ligaments, blood vessels and bone attached to ligaments.

SIGNS & SYMPTOMS
- Severe pain at the fracture site.
- Swelling around the fracture.
- Visible deformity if the fracture is complete and bone fragments separate enough to distort normal contours.
- Tenderness to the touch.
- Numbness or coldness in the shoulder and arm on the affected side if the blood supply is impaired.

CAUSES—Direct blow or indirect stress to the bone. Indirect stress may be caused by twisting or a violent muscle contraction.

RISK INCREASES WITH
- Contact sports such as football or soccer.
- History of bone or joint disease, especially osteoporosis.
- Obesity.
- Poor nutrition, especially calcium deficiency.
- If surgery and/or anesthesia is needed, risk increases with smoking and use of drugs, including mind-altering drugs, muscle relaxants, antihypertensives, tranquilizers, sleep inducers, insulin. sedatives, beta-adrenergic blockers or corticosteroids.

HOW TO PREVENT
- Build adequate muscle strength and achieve good conditioning prior to exercise, athletic practice or competition. Increased muscle mass helps protect bones and underlying tissues.
- Use protective equipment such as shoulder pads when appropriate.

WHAT TO EXPECT

APPROPRIATE HEALTH CARE
- Doctor's treatment.
- Hospitalization (sometimes) for anesthesia and surgery to set the fracture.
- Special shoulder harness to promote healing (sometimes).

DIAGNOSTIC MEASURES
- Your own observation of symptoms.

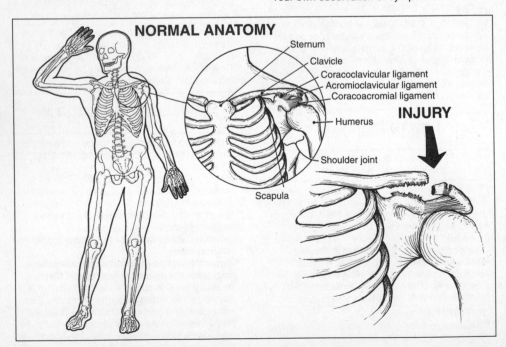

NORMAL ANATOMY

Sternum
Clavicle
Coracoclavicular ligament
Acromioclavicular ligament
Coracoacromial ligament
Humerus
Shoulder joint
Scapula

INJURY

- Medical history and exam by a doctor.
- X-rays of injured areas, including the shoulder joint and the joint between the shoulder and the clavicle.

POSSIBLE COMPLICATIONS
At the time of injury:
- Shock.
- Pressure on or injury to nearby nerves, ligaments, tendons, muscles, blood vessels or connective tissues.

After treatment or surgery:
- Delayed union or nonunion of the fracture (more common in open clavicle fractures).
- Avascular necrosis (death of bone cells due to interruption of the blood supply).
- Excessive scar tissues at the fracture site, causing compression of nerves and blood vessels in the neck. This may lead to pain, numbness and tingling in the neck, shoulder, arms and hands.
- Arrest of normal bone growth in children.
- Infection in open fractures (skin broken over fracture site) or at the incision if surgical setting was necessary.
- Shortening of the injured bones.
- Proneness to repeated collarbone injury.
- Unstable or arthritic acromioclavicular joint following repeated injury.
- Prolonged healing time if activity is resumed too soon.

PROBABLE OUTCOME—Plates and screws implanted in surgery may be in place permanently (can be removed if they cause symptoms). However, try to resume full function and normal range of motion within 3 or 4 weeks. Healing is complete when there is no motion at the fracture site and when x-rays show complete bone union.

 HOW TO TREAT

NOTE—Follow your doctor's instructions. These instructions are supplemental.

FIRST AID
- Keep the person warm with blankets to decrease the possibility of shock.
- Cut away clothing, if possible. Don't move the injured area to remove clothing.
- Follow instructions for R.I.C.E., the first letters of *rest, ice, compression* and *elevation*. See Appendix 1 for details.
- The doctor will realign and set the broken bones with surgery or, if possible, without. Manipulation should be done as soon as possible after injury. Also, many tissues lose their elasticity and become difficult to return to their normal positions.

CONTINUING CARE
- Immobilization will be necessary. For this fracture, a sling usually works quite well.
- Use frequent ice massage. Fill a large styrofoam cup with water and freeze. Tear a small amount of foam from the top so ice protrudes. Massage firmly over the injured area in a circle about the size of a baseball. Do this for 15 minutes at a time 3 or 4 times a day, and also before workouts or competition.
- After 72 hours, localized application of heat promotes healing by increasing blood circulation in the injured area. Use a heating pad, hot soaks, hot showers, heating pads or heat liniments and ointments.

MEDICATION—Your doctor may prescribe:
- General anesthesia, local anesthesia or muscle relaxants to make bone manipulation and fixation of bone fragments possible.
- Prescription pain relievers for severe pain.
- Stool softeners to prevent constipation due to inactivity.
- Acetaminophen or aspirin for mild pain.

ACTIVITY
- Actively exercise all muscle groups not immobilized. Muscle contractions promote fracture alignment and hasten healing.
- Resume normal activities gradually after treatment.

DIET
- Do not eat or drink before manipulation or surgery to treat the fracture. Fluid or solid food in your stomach makes vomiting while under anesthesia more hazardous.
- During recovery, balance the amount of food you eat with any change in your level of physical activity. Eat a variety of foods to get the energy, protein, vitamins, minerals and fiber you need for good health and healing.

REHABILITATION
- Circumduction exercises (see Glossary) should begin the first day after surgery.
- Begin reconditioning the injured area after clearance from your doctor.

 CALL YOUR DOCTOR IF

- You have symptoms of a collarbone fracture.
- Any of the following occurs after surgery or other treatment:
  Increased pain, swelling or drainage in the surgical area.
  Signs of infection (headache, muscle aches, dizziness or a general ill feeling and fever).
  Blue or gray skin color beyond the sling, especially under the fingernails.
  Loss of feeling below the fracture site.
  Nausea or vomiting; constipation.

COLLARBONE (CLAVICLE) FRACTURE, SHAFT MIDPORTION

GENERAL INFORMATION

DEFINITION—A complete or incomplete break in the middle third of the clavicle (collarbone). This is the most common collarbone fracture.

BODY PARTS INVOLVED
- Clavicle (collarbone).
- Shoulder joint.
- Soft tissues surrounding the fracture site, including nerves, tendons, ligaments, blood vessels and bone attached to ligaments.

SIGNS & SYMPTOMS
- Severe pain at the fracture site.
- Swelling around the fracture.
- Visible deformity if the fracture is complete and bone fragments separate enough to distort normal body contours.
- Tenderness to the touch.
- Numbness or coldness in the shoulder and arm on the affected side if the blood supply is impaired.

CAUSES—Direct blow or indirect stress to the clavicle, either at the shoulder or at the collarbone midpoint.

RISK INCREASES WITH
- Contact sports such as football or hockey.
- History of bone or joint disease, especially osteoporosis.
- Poor nutrition, especially calcium deficiency.
- Age under 12.
- Obesity.
- If surgery is needed, surgical risk increases with smoking and use of drugs, including mind-altering drugs, muscle relaxants, antihypertensives, tranquilizers, sleep inducers, insulin. sedatives, beta-adrenergic blockers or corticosteroids.

HOW TO PREVENT
- Build adequate muscle strength and achieve good conditioning prior to exercise, athletic practice or competition. Increased muscle mass helps protect bones and underlying tissues.
- Use appropriate protective equipment when participating in contact sports.

WHAT TO EXPECT

APPROPRIATE HEALTH CARE
- Doctor's treatment.
- Hospitalization (sometimes) for anesthesia and surgery to set the fracture.

DIAGNOSTIC MEASURES
- Your own observation of symptoms.
- Medical history and exam by a doctor.
- X-rays of injured areas, including the shoulder joint and the joint between the shoulder blade (scapula) and the clavicle.

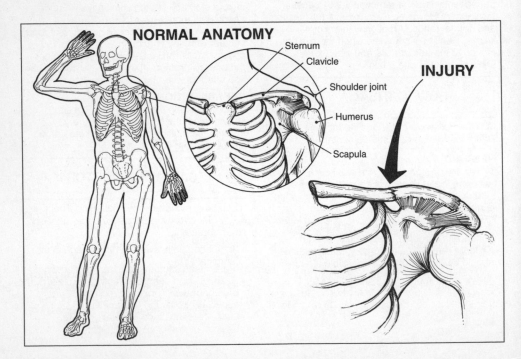

NORMAL ANATOMY

Sternum
Clavicle
Shoulder joint
Humerus
Scapula

INJURY

POSSIBLE COMPLICATIONS
At the time of injury:
- Shock.
- Pressure on or injury to nearby nerves, ligaments, tendons, muscles, blood vessels or connective tissues.

After treatment or surgery:
- Delayed union or nonunion of the fracture (more common in open fractures).
- Avascular necrosis (death of bone cells due to interruption of the blood supply).
- Excessive scar tissues at the fracture site, causing compression of nerves and blood vessels in the neck. This may lead to pain, numbness and tingling in the neck, shoulder, arms and hands.
- Arrest of normal bone growth in children.
- Infection in open fractures (skin broken over fracture site) or at the incision if surgical setting was necessary.
- Shortening of the injured bones.
- Proneness to repeated collarbone injury if healing is incomplete.
- Prolonged healing time if activity is resumed too soon.

PROBABLE OUTCOME—Plates and screws implanted in surgery may be in place permanently. However, try to resume full function and normal range of motion by 3 or 4 weeks. Healing is complete when there is no motion at the fracture site and when x-rays show complete bone union.

 ## HOW TO TREAT

NOTE—Follow your doctor's instructions. These instructions are supplemental.

FIRST AID
- Keep the person warm with blankets to decrease the possibility of shock.
- Cut away clothing, if possible. Don't move the injured area to remove clothing.
- Use instructions for R.I.C.E., the first letters of *rest, ice, compression* and *elevation*. See Appendix 1 for details.
- Use a sling to immobilize the injured area and surrounding joints before taking the injured person to a medical facility.

CONTINUING CARE
- The doctor will realign and set the broken bones with surgery or, if possible, without. Children rarely require surgery. Manipulation should be done as soon as possible after injury. Also, many tissues lose their elasticity and become difficult to return to their normal positions.
- Immobilization will be necessary. For this fracture, a sling usually works quite well. However, a "figure of eight" dressing may be used.

- After 72 hours, localized application of heat promotes healing by increasing blood circulation in the injured area. Use heat lamps, hot soaks, hot showers or heating pads.
- Use frequent ice massage. Fill a large styrofoam cup with water and freeze. Tear a small amount of foam from the top so ice protrudes. Massage firmly over the injured area in a circle about the size of a baseball. Do this for 15 minutes at a time 3 or 4 times a day.
- Take whirlpool treatments, if available.

MEDICATION—Your doctor may prescribe:
- General anesthesia, local anesthesia or muscle relaxants to make bone manipulation and fixation of bone fragments possible.
- Prescription pain relievers for severe pain.
- Stool softeners to prevent constipation due to inactivity.
- Acetaminophen for moderate pain.

ACTIVITY
- Actively exercise all muscle groups not immobilized. Muscle contractions promote fracture alignment and hasten healing.
- Resume normal activities gradually after treatment.
- Begin reconditioning the injured area after clearance from your doctor.

DIET
- Do not eat or drink before manipulation or surgery to treat the fracture. Fluid or solid food in your stomach makes vomiting while under anesthesia more hazardous.
- During recovery, balance the amount of food you eat with any change in your level of physical activity. Eat a variety of foods to get the energy, protein, vitamins, minerals and fiber you need for good health and healing.

REHABILITATION
- Circumduction exercises (see Glossary) should begin the first day after surgery.
- Begin daily rehabilitation exercises when movement is comfortable. Use ice massage for 10 minutes following exercise.

 ## CALL YOUR DOCTOR IF

- You have signs or symptoms of a collarbone fracture.
- Any of the following occurs after surgery or other treatment:
  Increased pain, swelling or drainage in the surgical area.
  Signs of infection (headache, muscle aches, dizziness or a general ill feeling and fever).
  Change in skin color beyond the sling to blue or gray, particularly under the fingernails.
  Loss of feeling below the fracture site.
  Nausea or vomiting; constipation.

COLLARBONE-AREA STRAIN, DELTOID MUSCLE

GENERAL INFORMATION

DEFINITION—Injury to the deltoid muscle or tendon that attaches to the collarbone (clavicle). Muscles, tendons and their attached bones comprise a contractile unit. The unit stabilizes the shoulder and allows its motion. A strain occurs at the unit's weakest part. Strains are of 3 types:
- Mild (Grade I)—Slightly pulled muscle without tearing of muscle or tendon fibers. There is no loss of strength.
- Moderate (Grade II)—Tearing of fibers in the muscle or tendon or at the attachment, to bone. Strength is diminished.
- Severe (Grade III)—Rupture of the muscle-tendon-bone attachment, with separation of fibers. A severe strain may require surgical repair.

BODY PARTS INVOLVED
- Deltoid muscle and deltoid tendon in the collarbone area.
- Collarbone area (clavicle).
- Soft tissues surrounding the strain, including nerves, periosteum (covering of bone), blood vessels and lymph vessels.

SIGNS & SYMPTOMS
- Pain with motion or stretching, particularly throwing.
- Muscle spasm.
- Swelling in the collarbone area.
- Loss of strength (moderate or severe strain).
- Calcification of the muscle or tendon (visible with x-rays).

CAUSES
- Prolonged overuse of the deltoid muscle-tendon unit.
- Single violent injury or force applied to the collarbone area.

RISK INCREASES WITH
- Contact sports.
- Weightlifting.
- Throwing sports.
- Medical history of any bleeding disorder.
- Obesity.
- Poor nutrition.
- Previous shoulder or collarbone injury.
- Poor muscle conditioning.

HOW TO PREVENT
- Participate in a strengthening, flexibility and conditioning program appropriate for your sport.
- Warm up before practice or competition.
- Use proper protective equipment, such as shoulder pads, when appropriate.

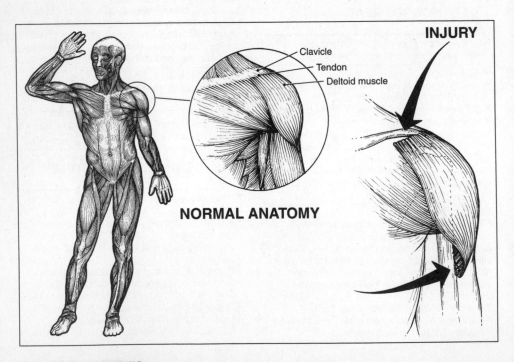

Clavicle
Tendon
Deltoid muscle

NORMAL ANATOMY

INJURY

WHAT TO EXPECT

APPROPRIATE HEALTH CARE
- Doctor's diagnosis.
- Self-care during rehabilitation.
- Physical therapy (moderate or severe strain).
- Surgery (severe strain).

DIAGNOSTIC MEASURES
- Your own observation of symptoms.
- Medical history and exam by a doctor.
- X-rays of the collarbone area to rule out fractures.

POSSIBLE COMPLICATIONS
- Prolonged healing time if activity is resumed too soon.
- Proneness to repeated injury.
- Inflammation at the attachment to bone (periostitis).
- Prolonged disability (sometimes), especially weakness.

PROBABLE OUTCOME—If this is a first-time injury, proper care and sufficient healing time before resuming activity should prevent permanent disability. Torn ligaments and tendons require as long to heal as fractured bones. Average healing times are:
- Mild strain—2 to 10 days.
- Moderate strain—10 days to 6 weeks.
- Severe strain—6 to 10 weeks.

If this is a repeat injury, complications listed above are more likely to occur.

HOW TO TREAT

NOTE—Follow your doctor's instructions. These instructions are supplemental.

FIRST AID—Use instructions for R.I.C.E., the first letters of *rest, ice, compression* and *elevation*. See Appendix 1 for details.

CONTINUING CARE
- Use ice massage 3 or 4 times a day for 15 minutes at a time. Fill a large styrofoam cup with water and freeze. Tear a small amount of foam from the top so ice protrudes. Massage firmly over the injured area in a circle about the size of a baseball.
- After the first 72 hours, apply heat instead of ice if it feels better. Use heat lamps, hot soaks, hot showers, heating pads or heat liniments and ointments.
- Massage gently and often to provide comfort and decrease swelling.

MEDICATION
- For minor discomfort, you may use:
  Aspirin, acetaminophen or ibuprofen.
  Topical liniments and ointments.
- Your doctor may prescribe:
  Stronger pain relievers.
  Injection of a long-acting local anesthetic to reduce pain.
  Injections of corticosteroids, such as triamcinolone, to reduce inflammation.

ACTIVITY
- For a moderate or severe strain, use a sling for at least 72 hours.
- Resume your normal activities gradually.

DIET—During recovery, balance the amount of food you eat with any change in your level of physical activity. Eat a variety of foods to get the energy, protein, vitamins, minerals and fiber you need for good health and healing.

REHABILITATION—Begin daily rehabilitation exercises when pain subsides. Use ice massage for 10 minutes prior to exercise. See Rehabilitation section for upper back exercises and shoulder exercises.

CALL YOUR DOCTOR IF

- You have symptoms of a moderate or severe deltoid strain or a mild strain persists longer than 10 days.
- Pain or swelling worsens despite treatment.

DELAYED ONSET MUSCLE SORENESS (DOMS)

GENERAL INFORMATION

DEFINITION—Delayed onset muscle soreness (DOMS) occurs hours after an exercise is over. DOMS is not an injury as such, but can be painful and sometimes incapacitating. Nearly every healthy adult has experienced DOMS no matter what the person's general fitness level is. The symptoms of DOMS are a normal response to unusual exertion and are part of an adaptation process that leads to greater strength once the muscles recover. A certain amount of DOMS is a reasonable and expected consequence of getting in shape.

BODY PARTS INVOLVED—DOMS affects only the muscles that are attached to the skeleton (e.g., biceps muscle). It does not affect cardiac (heart muscle) or smooth muscle (which lines the blood vessels).

SIGNS & SYMPTOMS
- Symptoms appear approximately 8-24 hours after a workout, usually peak between 24-48 hours, and normally disappear within 3-7 days.
- Muscle pain, soreness, swelling, and loss of muscle function.
- Muscles are sensitive upon touching or with movement.
- Decreased range of motion and flexibility in the muscles.

CAUSES—Different theories exist to explain the cause of DOMS—microscopic tears in the muscles themselves; damage to the connective tissue attached to muscle; and the inflammation theory states that the pain felt during DOMS is simply a by-product of our bodies attempt to fix the damage that has been caused by a workout. The accumulation of lactic acid in the muscles is not a cause of DOMS.
- DOMS results from overuse of the muscle. With DOMS, the intensity of an exercise seems to be more important than the duration.
- Activities that require muscles to forcefully contract while they are lengthening—eccentric contractions (rather than concentric muscle contractions in which muscle works while it shortens) seem to cause the most soreness. Eccentric contractions occur when lowering weights, in the downward movements of squats and push-ups, when descending stairs, and running downhill.

RISK INCREASES WITH
- Strenuous exercise.
- Too much activity, too soon, or a change in activity (from non-impact, such as cycling) to high impact (such as running).
- Heavy unaccustomed exercises. Even if you're exercising regularly, any unaccustomed activity may cause delayed soreness.

HOW TO PREVENT
- There are no proven effective preventive measures. There are some ways that may help minimize the amount of discomfort.

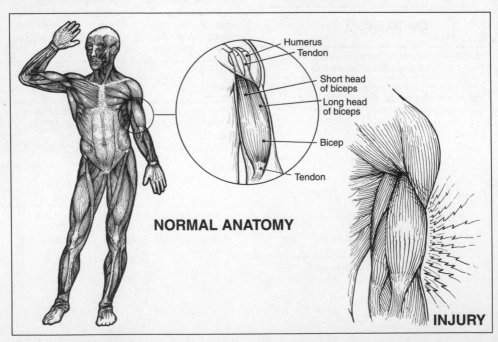

Humerus
Tendon
Short head of biceps
Long head of biceps
Bicep
Tendon

NORMAL ANATOMY

INJURY

- Studies linking DOMS to stretching have been conducted and have mixed results—some report that stretching causes DOMS and others say it doesn't. If you do stretch before or after exercising, do so slowly, and only to the point at which you feel slight discomfort and hold the stretch for anywhere between 10-30 seconds.
- Warm-up properly before you start an activity. Do a few minutes of light, low-impact aerobic activity, such as walking or biking.
- Give your muscles time to adapt to an activity. Make changes gradually (over several weeks if needed) to a new exercise program or new or different sports activity.
- Cool down after a workout.
- If starting a new weightlifting program, begin with weights you can lift fairly easily and increase the weight slowly in subsequent workouts.
- Avoid making sudden major changes in the type of exercise you do and sudden major increases in the time you spend in exercising.
- Research to date does not support the use of anti-inflammatory drugs, antioxidant supplements, ointments or creams in the prevention of DOMS.

 WHAT TO EXPECT

APPROPRIATE HEALTH CARE
- Self-care for most cases of DOMS.
- Doctor's treatment if you experience severe or continuing pain.

DIAGNOSTIC MEASURES
- Your own observation of symptoms.
- Medical history and exam by a doctor.

POSSIBLE COMPLICATIONS—There is no associated long-term damage or reduced function in the muscles involved.

PROBABLE OUTCOME
- Mild to moderate DOMS usually resolves itself within 3–7 days.
- The exercise that initially caused DOMS appears to trigger a protective effect and subsequent regular and frequent exercise (at least twice weekly) will no longer result in this condition. The protection is lost if there is too great a time lapse (10–14 days) between vigorous exercise sessions.

 HOW TO TREAT

NOTE—If you received medical care, follow your doctor's instructions. These instructions are supplemental.

FIRST AID—None.

CONTINUING CARE
- Avoid any vigorous activity that increases pain.
- Use ice massage. Fill a large styrofoam cup with water and freeze. Tear a small amount of foam from the top so ice protrudes. Massage gently over the painful area in a circle about the size of a softball. Do this for 15 minutes at a time 3 or 4 times a day, and also before workouts or competition.
- After 72 hours if discomfort persists, apply heat instead of ice if it feels better. Use heat lamps, hot soaks, hot showers, heating pads, heat liniments and ointments or whirlpool treatments.
- Massage gently and often to provide comfort and decrease any swelling. Massage may reduce DOMS, but doesn't seem to speed the recovery.

MEDICATION
- For minor pain and inflammation, you may try aspirin or ibuprofen, but they are not always effective for DOMS.
- Some reports show that vitamin C supplements help DOMS, but the evidence is unclear.
- Over-the-counter topical products are often used to soothe aching muscles.

ACTIVITY
- Perform low-impact aerobic exercise to increase blood flow to the affected muscles, which may help diminish soreness.
- Although the relief is temporary, exercise of the sore muscle probably is the best way to reduce DOMS.
- If muscle soreness or pain increases after you begin exercising, stop and use ice on the muscles.

DIET—Balance the amount of food you eat with any change in your level of physical activity. Eat a variety of foods to get the energy, protein, vitamins, minerals and fiber you need for good health and healing.

REHABILITATION—None required.

 CALL YOUR DOCTOR IF

- You have severe or continued pain due to delayed onset muscle soreness.
- Symptoms don't improve after treatment.

EAR INJURY

GENERAL INFORMATION

DEFINITION—Ear injuries may include:
- Contusion (bruising).
- Laceration from a sharp instrument.
- Injury to the eardrum or internal ear.

BODY PARTS INVOLVED
- Skin of the ear.
- Cartilage of the ear.
- Perichondrium (thin membrane layer between the cartilage and the skin).
- Nerves, blood vessels and connective tissues.
- Parts of the internal ear—eardrum, middle ear and inner ear.

SIGNS & SYMPTOMS
- Contusion or laceration—Pain, swelling, bleeding and bruising of skin around the ear.
- Internal injury—Loss of hearing, ringing in the ear, loss of equilibrium or bleeding from a ruptured eardrum.

CAUSES
- Direct blow to the ear.
- Accidental insertion of a sharp object into the ear.
- Sudden excessive changes in pressure.

RISK INCREASES WITH
- Contact sports, especially wrestling or boxing.
- Diving.

HOW TO PREVENT—Wear protective headgear for contact sports. Some ear injuries cannot be prevented.

WHAT TO EXPECT

APPROPRIATE HEALTH CARE
- Doctor's examination and treatment.
- Emergency room care for laceration or internal ear injury.
- Self-care during healing.

DIAGNOSTIC MEASURES
- Your own observation of symptoms.
- Medical history and physical exam by a doctor, including consultation with an ear specialist or plastic surgeon if necessary.
- X-rays of the skull to detect an accompanying skull fracture.

POSSIBLE COMPLICATIONS
- Chronic infection of the injured ear cartilage if the skin is broken from laceration or abrasion.
- "Cauliflower ear" resulting from repeated contusions with bleeding through soft tissues. The tissues under the skin and the lining of the ear cartilage thicken permanently. (There is no treatment for this condition—only prevention.)
- Infection from abrasion, laceration or other injury to the eardrum or other internal ear structures.
- Temporary or permanent hearing loss.

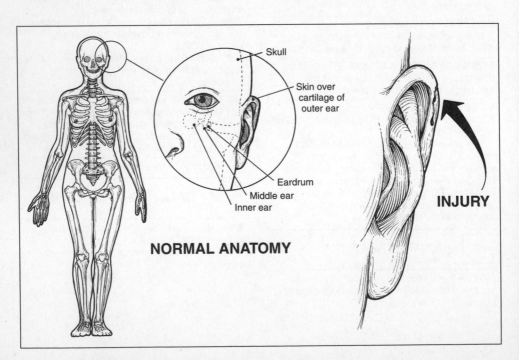

Skull

Skin over cartilage of outer ear

Eardrum

Middle ear

Inner ear

NORMAL ANATOMY

INJURY

PROBABLE OUTCOME—Contusions and lacerations may require 10 to 14 days to heal. Sutures from lacerations are usually removed in about 10 days. Other types of ear injuries usually heal without complications if they are diagnosed and treated quickly. In some cases, hearing loss after injury is permanent.

 ## HOW TO TREAT

NOTE—Follow your doctor's instructions. These instructions are supplemental.

FIRST AID
- Don't try to stop bleeding from inside the ear.
- Don't allow the injured person to hit or thump the head to try to restore hearing.
- Cover the external ear with a clean cloth or sterile bandage.
- Apply an ice pack of ice cubes or chips in a plastic bag or moist towel.
- Compress the area loosely with an elastic wrap. Don't wrap too tightly.
- Keep the injured person in a partial reclining position while transporting him or her to an emergency facility.

CONTINUING CARE
For contusions:
- The doctor will aspirate blood from between the skin and ear cartilage if needed. If swelling persists, multiple small incisions may prevent a cauliflower ear from developing.
- Use ice packs or warm compresses to relieve discomfort.
- Sleep with your head elevated using 2 pillows until symptoms subside.
- Change bulky bandages often to keep them soft and protective.

For lacerations:
- Your doctor must carefully repair the cut to prevent deformity.
- Keep the wound dry and covered for 48 hours.
- After 48 hours, replace the bandage when it gets wet.
- When you change the bandage, apply a small amount of petroleum jelly or nonprescription antibiotic ointment to the bandage.
- Ignore small amounts of bleeding. Control heavier bleeding by firmly pressing a facial tissues or clean cloth to the bleeding spot for 10 minutes.

MEDICATION—Your doctor may prescribe:
- Antibiotics to treat infection.
- Pain relievers.

ACTIVITY—Resume your normal activities as soon as you are able.

DIET—During recovery, balance the amount of food you eat with any change in your level of physical activity. Eat a variety of foods to get the energy, protein, vitamins, minerals and fiber you need for good health and healing.

REHABILITATION—None.

 ## CALL YOUR DOCTOR IF

- You have any ear injury.
- Any of the following occurs after treatment:
  Increased pain or pain that persists longer than 2 days.
  Hearing loss.
  Increased bleeding or swelling.
  Signs of infection (headache, muscle aches, dizziness, fever or general ill feeling).
- New, unexplained symptoms. Drugs used in treatment may produce side effects.

ELBOW BURSITIS

GENERAL INFORMATION

DEFINITION—Inflammation of the radio-humeral bursa in the elbow. Bursitis may vary in degree from mild irritation to an abscess formation that causes excruciating pain. In acute bursitis at the elbow, blood from an injury usually causes the inflammation. Bursitis will continue until the blood is removed or reabsorbed. Chronic bursitis results from undertreated acute bursitis and usually requires surgery to repair.

BODY PARTS INVOLVED
- Bursa between the radius and humerus (arm bones) where they meet in the elbow. This bursa is a soft sac filled with lubricating fluid that facilitates motion between the radius and humerus.
- Soft tissue surrounding the elbow, including nerves, tendons, ligaments, blood vessels (both large vessels and capillaries), periosteum (the outside lining of bone) and muscles.

SIGNS & SYMPTOMS
- Pain at the elbow.
- Tenderness.
- Swelling.
- Redness (sometimes) over the affected bursa.
- Fever, if infection is present.
- Limited elbow movement.

CAUSES
- Direct blow to the elbow or forearm.
- Acute or chronic infection.
- Arthritis.
- Gout.
- Unknown (frequently).

RISK INCREASES WITH
- Participating in competitive athletics, particularly contact sports.
- Previous history of bursitis in any joint.
- Exposure to cold weather.
- Poor conditioning and inadequate warmup before exercise.
- Inadequate protective equipment in contact sports.

HOW TO PREVENT
- Use protective elbow pads for contact sports.
- Wear warm clothing in cold weather.
- To prevent recurrence, continue to wear extra protection over the elbow until healing is complete.

WHAT TO EXPECT

APPROPRIATE HEALTH CARE
- Doctor's treatment.
- Surgery (sometimes), particularly for a frozen elbow or for a severely infected joint that drains to the outside.

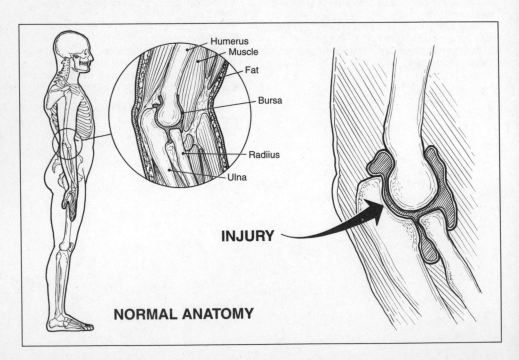

Humerus
Muscle
Fat
Bursa
Radiius
Ulna

INJURY

NORMAL ANATOMY

DIAGNOSTIC MEASURES
• Your own observation of symptoms.
• Medical history and physical exam by a doctor.
• X-rays of the elbow and wrist.

POSSIBLE COMPLICATIONS
• Temporary or permanent limitation of elbow's normal mobility.
• Prolonged healing time if activity is resumed too soon.
• Proneness to repeated flare-ups.
• Unstable or arthritic elbow following repeated episodes of bursitis.
• Spontaneous rupture of bursa if severe infection is present.

PROBABLE OUTCOME—Radio-humeral bursitis is a common problem. Symptoms usually subside in 3 to 4 weeks with treatment. If serious infection occurs and surgery is needed, allow 6 to 8 weeks for healing.

 HOW TO TREAT

NOTE—Follow your doctor's instructions. These instructions are supplemental.

FIRST AID—None. This problem develops slowly.

CONTINUING CARE
• Use frequent ice massage. Fill a large styrofoam cup with water and freeze. Tear a small amount of foam from the top so ice protrudes. Massage firmly over the injured area in a circle about the size of a softball. Do this for 15 minutes at a time, 3 or 4 times a day, and before workouts or competition.
• After 72 hours, apply heat instead of ice, if it feels better. Use heat lamps, hot soaks, hot showers, heating pads, or heat liniments and ointments.
• Take whirlpool treatments, if available.
• Use a sling to support the elbow joint, if needed. Don't exercise the elbow with the palm turned up or down.
• Elevate the elbow above the level of the heart to reduce swelling and prevent accumulation of fluid. Use pillows for propping.
• Massage gently and often to provide comfort and decrease swelling.

MEDICATION—Your doctor may prescribe:
• Non-steroidal anti-inflammatory drugs.
• Corticosteroid injections into the bursa to reduce inflammation.
• Prescription pain relievers for severe pain. Use non-prescription acetaminophen or ibuprofen (available under many trade names) for mild pain.
• Injection into the inflamed bursa of a long-lasting local anesthetic mixed with a corticosteroid drug, such as triamcinolone.
• Antibiotics if the bursa is infected.

ACTIVITY—Rest the inflamed area as much as possible. If you must resume normal activity immediately, wear a sling until the pain becomes more bearable. To prevent a frozen elbow, begin normal, slow joint movement as soon as possible.

DIET—Eat a well-balanced diet that includes extra protein, such as meat, fish, poultry, cheese, milk and eggs. Increase fiber and fluid intake to prevent constipation that may result from decreased activity. Your doctor may suggest vitamin and mineral supplements to promote healing.

REHABILITATION—See section on rehabilitation exercises.

 CALL YOUR DOCTOR IF

• You have symptoms of elbow bursitis.
• Pain increases despite treatment.
• Any of the following occur after surgery: Pain, swelling, tenderness, drainage or bleeding increases in the surgical area. You develop signs of infection (headache, muscle aches, dizziness or a general ill feeling and fever). New, unexplained symptoms develop. Drugs used in treatment may produce side effects.

ELBOW CONTUSION

GENERAL INFORMATION

DEFINITION—Bruising of the skin and underlying tissues of the elbow due to a direct blow. Contusions cause bleeding from ruptured small capillaries that allow blood to infiltrate muscles, tendons or other soft tissues. Because skin is so close to bone in this area, contusion of the elbow is a common injury to athletes.

BODY PARTS INVOLVED—Elbow tissues, including blood vessels, muscles, tendons, nerves, connective tissues and covering of bone (periosteum). Periosteum injury is particularly common in elbow contusions.

SIGNS & SYMPTOMS
* Swelling in the elbow—either superficial or deep.
* Pain and tenderness over the elbow.
* Feeling of firmness when pressure is exerted at the injury site.
* Discoloration under the skin, beginning with redness and progressing to the characteristic "black-and-blue" bruise.
* Restricted elbow activity proportional to the extent of injury.

CAUSES
* Direct blow to the elbow, usually from a blunt object.
* Falling on the elbow.

RISK INCREASES WITH
* Contact supports such as football, hockey basketball or soccer, especially if the elbows are not adequately protected.
* Medical history of any bleeding disorder.
* Poor nutrition, including vitamin deficiency.
* Use of anticoagulants or aspirin.

HOW TO PREVENT—Wear appropriate protective gear and equipment, such as elbow pads, during competition or other athletic activity if there is risk of an elbow contusion.

WHAT TO EXPECT

APPROPRIATE HEALTH CARE
* Doctor's care unless the contusion is quite small.
* Self-care for minor contusions or for serious contusions during rehabilitation.
* Physical therapy for serious elbow contusions.

DIAGNOSTIC MEASURES
* Your own observation of symptoms.
* Medical history and physical exam by a doctor for all except minor injuries.
* X-rays of the elbow, wrist and shoulder to assess total injury to soft tissues and to rule out the possibility of underlying fractures. The total extent of injury may not be apparent for 48 to 72 hours

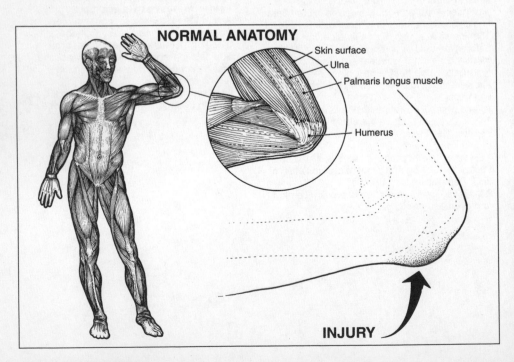

NORMAL ANATOMY

Skin surface
Ulna
Palmaris longus muscle
Humerus

INJURY

POSSIBLE COMPLICATIONS
- Excessive bleeding, leading to disability. Infiltrative-type bleeding can (rarely) lead to calcification and impaired function of injured muscle.
- Prolonged healing time if usual activities are resumed too soon.
- Infection if skin over the contusion is broken.

PROBABLE OUTCOME—Complete healing without complications. Most elbow contusions will heal in 6 to 10 days.

 ## HOW TO TREAT

NOTE—Follow your doctor's instructions. These instructions are supplemental.

FIRST AID—Use instructions for R.I.C.E., the first letters of *rest, ice, compression* and *elevation*. See Appendix 1 for details.

CONTINUING CARE
- Wrap an elasticized bandage over a felt pad on the injured area. Keep the area compressed for about 72 hours.
- Immobilize the arm in a sling.
- Use ice soaks 3 or 4 times a day. Fill a bucket with ice water, and soak the injured area for 20 minutes at a time.
- After 72 hours, apply heat instead of ice if it feels better. Use heat lamps, hot soaks, hot showers, heating pads, heat liniments and ointments or whirlpool treatments.
- Massage gently and often from wrist toward shoulder to provide comfort and decrease swelling.

MEDICATION
- For minor discomfort, you may use:
  Acetaminophen or ibuprofen.
  Topical liniments and ointments.
- Your doctor may prescribe stronger medicine for severe pain.

ACTIVITY—Begin activities slowly, and stop exercise as soon as pain begins. Increase activity as healing progresses.

DIET—During recovery, balance the amount of food you eat with any change in your level of physical activity. Eat a variety of foods to get the energy, protein, vitamins, minerals and fiber you need for good health and healing.

REHABILITATION
- Begin daily rehabilitation exercises when supportive wrapping is no longer needed.
- Use ice massage for 10 minutes before and after workouts. Fill a large styrofoam cup with water and freeze. Tear a small amount of foam from the top so ice protrudes. Massage firmly over the injured area in a circle about the size of a softball.
- See Rehabilitation section for elbow exercises.

 ## CALL YOUR DOCTOR IF

- You have an elbow contusion that doesn't improve in 1 or 2 days.
- Skin is broken and signs of infection (drainage, increasing pain, fever, headache muscle aches, dizziness or a general ill feeling) occur.

ELBOW CONTUSION, ULNAR NERVE
("Crazy Bone" or "Crazy Nerve" Contusion)

GENERAL INFORMATION

DEFINITION—Bruising injury from a direct blow to the ulnar nerve where it lies close to the surface at the elbow. Contusions cause bleeding from ruptured small capillaries that allow blood to infiltrate the nerve. Direct injury to the nerve causes damage even if bleeding of capillaries is not a factor.

BODY PARTS INVOLVED
- Ulnar nerve.
- Ulnar groove in the elbow portion of the humerus (bone of the upper arm).

SIGNS & SYMPTOMS
- Swelling in the elbow—either superficial or deep.
- Immediate pain in the elbow.
- Shocking, electric sensations extending down to the ring finger and little finger.
- Gradually increasing numbness and pain along the route of the ulnar nerve in the forearm and hand.
- Atrophy of muscles in the hand.

CAUSES
- Direct blow to the elbow area from a blunt object.
- Falling on the elbow.

RISK INCREASES WITH
- Contact sports such as football, soccer or hockey, especially when elbows are not adequately protected.
- Medical history of any bleeding disorder.
- Poor nutrition, including vitamin deficiency.

HOW TO PREVENT—Wear appropriate protective gear, such as elbow pads, during competition or other athletic activity if there is risk of an elbow injury.

WHAT TO EXPECT

APPROPRIATE HEALTH CARE
- Doctor's care unless the contusion is quite small.
- Surgery to treat the contused nerve in chronic cases. This may involve transferring and transplanting the nerve into muscle where it is sutured in place.
- Self-care for minor contusion or during rehabilitation following surgery for serious ulnar nerve contusions.
- Physical therapy following surgery.

DIAGNOSTIC MEASURES
- Your own observation of symptoms.
- Medical history and physical exam by a doctor for all except minor injuries.

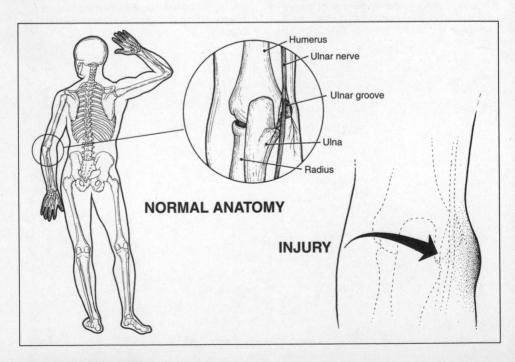

NORMAL ANATOMY

- Humerus
- Ulnar nerve
- Ulnar groove
- Ulna
- Radius

INJURY

- X-rays of the elbow to assess total injury to soft tissues and to rule out the possibility of underlying fractures. The total extent of injury may not be apparent for 48 to 72 hours.

POSSIBLE COMPLICATIONS
- Permanent damage to the ulnar nerve, leading to disability in the forearm and hand.
- Prolonged healing time if usual activities are resumed too soon.
- Infection if skin over the contusion is broken.

PROBABLE OUTCOME—Healing time varies from 2 to 6 weeks, depending on the extent of injury and whether surgery is required. In a few cases, some symptoms may be permanent.

HOW TO TREAT

NOTE—Follow your doctor's instructions. These instructions are supplemental.

FIRST AID—Use instructions for R.I.C.E., the first letters of *rest, ice, compression* and *elevation*. See Appendix 1 for details.

CONTINUING CARE
- Wrap an elasticized bandage over a felt pad on the injured area. Keep the area compressed for about 72 hours.
- Immobilize the arm in a sling.
- Use ice soaks 3 or 4 times a day. Fill a bucket with ice water, and soak the injured area for 20 minutes at a time.
- After 72 hours, apply heat instead of ice if it feels better. Use heat lamps, hot soaks, hot showers, heating pads, heat liniments and ointments or whirlpool treatments.

MEDICATION
- For minor discomfort, you may use: Acetaminophen or ibuprofen. Topical liniments and ointments.
- Your doctor may prescribe stronger medicine for pain.

ACTIVITY—Begin activities slowly, and stop exercise as soon as pain begins. Increase activity as healing progresses.

DIET—During recovery, balance the amount of food you eat with any change in your level of physical activity. Eat a variety of foods to get the energy, protein, vitamins, minerals and fiber you need for good health and healing.

REHABILITATION
- Begin daily rehabilitation exercises when movement is comfortable and sling is no longer needed.
- Use ice massage for 10 minutes before and after workouts. Fill a large styrofoam cup with water and freeze. Tear a small amount of foam from the top so ice protrudes. Massage firmly over the injured area in a circle about the size of a softball.
- See Rehabilitation section for elbow exercises.

CALL YOUR DOCTOR IF

- You have symptoms of an elbow or ulnar nerve contusion.
- Any of the following occurs after surgery: Increasing pain, swelling, redness, drainage or bleeding in the surgical area. Signs of infection, headache, muscle aches, dizziness, fever or a general ill feeling. Nausea or vomiting Constipation.
- New, unexplained symptoms develop. Drugs used in treatment may produce side effects.

ELBOW DISLOCATION

GENERAL INFORMATION

DEFINITION—An injury to the elbow joint so that adjoining bones are displaced from their normal positions and no longer touch each other. An elbow dislocation requires urgent medical attention, because damage to nerves and blood vessels can occur and must be relieved.

BODY PARTS INVOLVED
- Elbow joint.
- Adjoining arm bones (ulna, radius and humerus).
- Collateral ligaments of the elbow.
- Soft tissues surrounding the dislocation, including nerves, tendons. muscles and blood vessels.

SIGNS & SYMPTOMS
- Excruciating pain at the time of injury.
- Loss of elbow function.
- Severe pain when trying to move the elbow.
- Visible deformity if the dislocated bones have locked in the dislocated position. Bones may spontaneously reposition themselves and leave no deformity, but damage is the same.
- Tenderness over the dislocation.
- Swelling and bruising around the elbow.
- Numbness or paralysis in the arm below the dislocation caused by pressure on nerves.
- Decreased or absent pulse at the wrist, coolness and dusky bluish color of the hand (due to blood vessel damage).

CAUSES
- Direct blow to the elbow.
- Falling onto an outstretched hand.
- End result of a severe elbow sprain.
- Congenital elbow abnormality, such as shallow or malformed joint surfaces.
- Powerful muscle contractions.

RISK INCREASES WITH
- Contact sports such as football, soccer or basketball.
- Field or track events that involve jumping, such as the high jump or pole vault.
- Previous elbow dislocations or sprains.
- Repeated elbow injury of any kind.
- Poor muscle conditioning.

HOW TO PREVENT
- Build your overall strength and muscle tone with a long-term conditioning program appropriate for your sport.
- Wear elbow pads for contact sports.

WHAT TO EXPECT

APPROPRIATE HEALTH CARE
- Doctor's treatment to reposition the bones with manipulation and examination to ensure that no fracture has occurred.
- Surgery (sometimes) to restore the elbow to its normal position and repair tendons and collateral ligaments. Acute or recurring dislocations may require surgical reconstruction or replacement of the elbow.

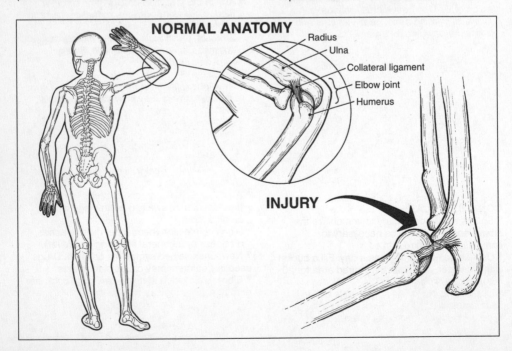

NORMAL ANATOMY

Radius
Ulna
Collateral ligament
Elbow joint
Humerus

INJURY

• Application of splints or a cast and sling.

DIAGNOSTIC MEASURES
• Your own observation of symptoms.
• Medical history and exam by a doctor.
• X-rays of the elbow and adjacent bones.

POSSIBLE COMPLICATIONS
• Damage to nearby nerves or major blood vessels.
• Elbow fracture.
• Excessive internal bleeding.
• Shock or loss of consciousness.
• Recurrent dislocations (rarely), if a previous dislocation has not healed completely.
• Proneness to repeated injury.
• Unstable or arthritic elbow following repeated injury.

PROBABLE OUTCOME—After the dislocation has been corrected, the elbow will require immobilization with anterior and posterior splints and a sling for 5 to 10 days. There will be marked stiffness after all elbow dislocations, but with competent medical care, motion should be unrestricted after 2 to 6 months. Injured ligaments require a minimum of 6 weeks to heal.

 ## HOW TO TREAT

NOTE—Follow your doctor's instructions. These instructions are supplemental.

FIRST AID
• Keep the person warm with blankets to decrease the possibility of shock.
• Cut away clothing if possible, but don't move the injured area to do so.
• Immobilize the elbow, shoulder and wrist with padded splints in the position they are in. Don't try to manipulate the elbow.
• Follow instructions for R.I.C.E., the first letters of *rest, ice, compression* and *elevation*. See Appendix 1 for details.
• The doctor will manipulate and realign the dislocated bones. Surgery may be required to do this. Manipulation should be done within 6 hours of injury or shock may occur. Also, many tissues lose their elasticity and may become difficult to return to their normal functional positions.

CONTINUING CARE
• Splints will be necessary to immobilize the elbow, and a sling will be necessary to immobilize the entire arm.
• Use ice soaks 3 or 4 times a day. Fill a bucket with ice water, and soak the injured area for 20 minutes at a time.
• Use heat applications if heat feels better. Use heat lamps, hot showers or heating pads.
• Take whirlpool treatments if available.

MEDICATION—Your doctor may prescribe:
• General anesthesia or muscle relaxants to make joint manipulation possible.
• Acetaminophen to relieve moderate pain.
• Prescription pain relievers for severe pain.
• Antibiotics to fight infection if surgery is necessary.

ACTIVITY
• Actively exercise all muscle groups not immobilized. Muscle contractions promote proper bone alignment and hasten healing.
• Resume your normal activities gradually.

DIET
• Do not eat or drink before manipulation or surgery to correct the dislocation. Fluid or solid food in your stomach makes vomiting under general anesthesia more hazardous.
• During recovery, balance the amount of food you eat with any change in your level of physical activity. Eat a variety of foods to get the energy, protein, vitamins, minerals and fiber you need for good health and healing.

REHABILITATION
• Begin daily rehabilitation exercises when supportive wrapping is no longer needed.
• Use ice massage for 10 minutes before and after workouts. Fill a large styrofoam cup with water and freeze. Tear a small amount of foam from the top so ice protrudes. Massage firmly in a circle over the injured area.
• See Rehabilitation section for elbow exercises.

 ## CALL YOUR DOCTOR IF

• Any of the following occurs after injury:
  Numbness, paleness or coldness in the elbow. This is an emergency!
  Elbow deformity.
  Difficulty moving the elbow joint.
  Nausea or vomiting.
  Numbness or complete loss of feeling below the elbow.
• Any of the following occurs after treatment:
  Swelling above or below the splints.
  Blue or gray skin color under the fingernails.
  Constipation.
• Any of the following occurs after surgery:
  Increased pain, swelling or drainage in the surgical area.
  Signs of infection (headache, muscle aches, dizziness or a general ill feeling and fever).
• New, unexplained symptoms develop. Drugs used in treatment may cause side effects.
• Elbow dislocation that you can "pop" back into normal position occurs repeatedly.

ELBOW FRACTURE, CORONOID PROCESS

GENERAL INFORMATION

DEFINITION—A complete or incomplete break in the coronoid process of the ulna (a part of a bone in the forearm). It usually accompanies an elbow dislocation.

BODY PARTS INVOLVED
- Elbow joint.
- Coronoid process of the ulna, a curved portion of the bone that forms part of the joint.
- Soft tissues surrounding the fracture site, including nerves, tendons, ligaments, blood vessels, cartilage and muscle.

SIGNS & SYMPTOMS
- Severe pain at the fracture site.
- Swelling around the fracture.
- Visible deformity if the fracture is complete and bone fragments separate enough to distort normal body contours.
- Tenderness to the touch.
- Numbness or coldness in the lower arm and hand if the blood supply is impaired.

CAUSES
- Direct blow to the elbow.
- Indirect injury due to falling on an outstretched hand with the elbow stiff.
- Any injury that causes dislocation of the elbow.

RISK INCREASES WITH
- Activities such as gymnastics or cheerleading.
- History of bone or joint disease, especially osteoporosis.
- Age under 12 and over 60.
- Obesity.
- If surgery is necessary, surgical risk increases with smoking and use of certain drugs.

HOW TO PREVENT
- Build adequate muscle strength and achieve good conditioning prior to exercise, athletic practice or competition. Increased muscle mass helps protect bones and underlying tissues.
- Use appropriate protective equipment, such as padded elbow pads, when participating in contact sports.

WHAT TO EXPECT

APPROPRIATE HEALTH CARE
- Doctor's treatment to reposition the dislocated elbow and to remove the coronoid process surgically or reattach it in its normal position.
- Surgery to set the fracture and repair soft tissues of the elbow and fix or remove any bone fragments.
- Whirlpool, ultrasound or massage (to displace excess fluid from the injured joint space).

DIAGNOSTIC MEASURES
- Your own observation of symptoms.
- Medical history and exam by a doctor.

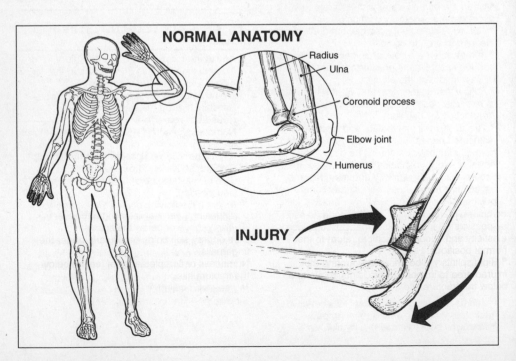

NORMAL ANATOMY

Radius
Ulna
Coronoid process
Elbow joint
Humerus

INJURY

- X-rays of injured areas, including joints above and below the primary injury site.
- Repeat x-rays after approximately 1 week if first x-rays were negative and pain continues.

POSSIBLE COMPLICATIONS
At the time of injury:
- Shock.
- Pressure on or injury to nearby nerves, ligaments, tendons, muscles, blood vessels or connective tissues.

After treatment or surgery:
- Delayed union or nonunion of the fracture.
- Impaired blood supply to the fracture site.
- Arrest of normal bone growth in children.
- Infection in open fractures (skin broken over fracture site) or at the incision if surgical setting was necessary.
- Shortening of the injured bones.
- Unstable or arthritic joint following repeated injury.
- Proneness to repeated injury.
- Prolonged healing time if activity is resumed too soon.

PROBABLE OUTCOME—The average time for healing of this fracture is 6 to 8 weeks in adults and 4 to 6 weeks in children. Healing is considered complete when there is no motion at the fracture site and when x-rays show complete bone union.

 ## HOW TO TREAT

NOTE—Follow your doctor's instructions. These instructions are supplemental.

FIRST AID
- Keep the person warm with blankets to decrease the possibility of shock.
- Cut away clothing, if possible. don't move the injured elbow to remove clothing.
- Use instructions for R.I.C.E., the first letters of *rest, ice, compression* and *elevation*. See Appendix 1 for details.

CONTINUING CARE
- The doctor will set the broken bones and repair soft tissues and bone with surgery. Surgery is necessary to ensure normal motion and stability of the forearm after healing is complete. Manipulation should be done as soon as possible after injury. Also, many tissues lose elasticity and become difficult to return to their normal positions.
- Rigid splints will be necessary around the injured area to immobilize the joints above and below the fracture site.
- After 96 hours, application of localized heat promotes healing by increasing blood circulation in the injured area. Use heat lamps or heating pads so heat can penetrate splints.
- After splints are removed, use frequent ice massage. Fill a large styrofoam cup with water and freeze. Tear a small amount of foam from the top so ice protrudes. Massage firmly over the injured area in a circle about the size of a baseball. Do this for 15 minutes at a time 3 or 4 times a day.
- Apply heat instead of ice if it feels better. Use heat lamps, hot soaks, hot showers, heating pads or heat liniments and ointments.
- Take whirlpool treatments, if available.

MEDICATION—Your doctor may prescribe:
- General anesthesia for surgery.
- Prescription pain relievers for severe pain.
- Stool softeners to prevent constipation due to inactivity.
- Acetaminophen (available without prescription) for mild pain after initial treatment.

ACTIVITY
- Resume normal activities gradually after treatment.
- Begin reconditioning the injured area after clearance from your doctor.

DIET
- Do not drink or eat before manipulation or surgery to treat the fracture. Fluid or solid food in your stomach makes vomiting while under anesthesia more hazardous.
- During recovery, balance the amount of food you eat with any change in your level of physical activity. Eat a variety of foods to get the energy, protein, vitamins, minerals and fiber you need for good health and healing.

REHABILITATION—Begin daily rehabilitation exercises when movement is comfortable. Use ice massage for 10 minutes prior to exercise. See Rehabilitation section for elbow exercises.

 ## CALL YOUR DOCTOR IF

- You have signs or symptoms of an elbow fracture.
- Any of the following occurs after surgery or other treatment:
  Increased pain, swelling or drainage in the surgical area.
  Signs of infection (headache, muscle aches, dizziness or a general ill feeling and fever).
  Swelling above or below the splints.
  Blue or gray skin color, particularly under the fingernails.
  Numbness or complete loss of feeling below the fracture site.
  Nausea or vomiting.
  Constipation.

ELBOW FRACTURE, EPICONDYLE

GENERAL INFORMATION

DEFINITION—A complete or incomplete break in the epicondyle of the humerus (the large bone in the arm between the elbow and shoulder). The epicondyle is located on the outside of the humerus at its lower end and forms a part of the elbow joint. This fracture often accompanies an elbow dislocation.

BODY PARTS INVOLVED
- Epicondyle of the humerus.
- Elbow joint.
- Soft tissues around the fracture site, including nerves, tendons, ligaments, joint membranes and blood vessels.

SIGNS & SYMPTOMS
- Severe elbow pain at the time of injury.
- Swelling of soft tissues around the fracture.
- Visible deformity if the fracture is complete and the bone fragments separate enough to distort normal arm contours.
- Tenderness to the touch.
- Numbness and coldness in the hand and lower arm if the blood supply is impaired.

CAUSES—Direct blow or indirect stress to the elbow. Indirect stress may be caused by twisting or violent muscle contraction.

RISK INCREASES WITH
- Contact sports such as football or hockey.
- History of bone or joint disease, especially osteoporosis.
- Age under 12 or over 60.
- Obesity.
- If surgery or anesthesia is needed, risk increases with smoking and use of drugs, including mind-altering drugs, muscle relaxants, antihypertensives, tranquilizers, sleep inducers, insulin, sedatives, beta-adrenergic blockers or corticosteroids.

HOW TO PREVENT
- Participate in a strengthening, flexibility and conditioning program appropriate for your sport. Increased muscle mass helps protect bones and underlying tissues.
- Use appropriate protective equipment, such as foam rubber elbow pads, during participation in contact sports.

WHAT TO EXPECT

APPROPRIATE HEALTH CARE
- Doctor's treatment to reposition the dislocated elbow and manipulate the fractured elbow.
- Hospitalization (sometimes) for surgical setting of the fracture.
- Whirlpool, ultrasound or massage (to displace excess fluid from the injured joint space).

DIAGNOSTIC MEASURES
- Your own observation of symptoms.
- Medical history and exam by a doctor.
- X-rays of the arm from shoulder to wrist.

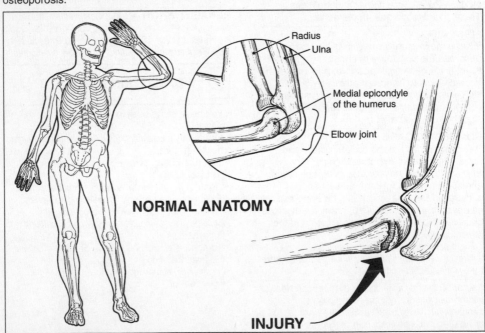

Radius
Ulna
Medial epicondyle of the humerus
Elbow joint

NORMAL ANATOMY

INJURY

POSSIBLE COMPLICATIONS

At the time of injury:
- Shock.
- Pressure on or injury to nearby nerves, ligaments, tendons, muscles, blood vessels or connective tissues.

After treatment or surgery:
- Delayed union or nonunion of the fracture.
- Impaired blood supply to the fracture site.
- Avascular necrosis (death of bone cells due to interruption of the blood supply).
- Arrest of normal bone growth in children.
- Infection in open fractures (skin broken over fracture site) or at the incision if surgical setting was necessary.
- Shortening of the injured bones.
- Prolonged healing time if activity is resumed too soon.
- Proneness to repeated elbow injury.
- Unstable or arthritic elbow following repeated injury.

PROBABLE OUTCOME—The average healing time for this fracture is 6 to 8 weeks in adults and 4 to 6 weeks in children. Healing is complete when there is no motion at the fracture site and when x-rays show complete bone union.

 HOW TO TREAT

NOTE—Follow your doctor's instructions. These instructions are supplemental.

FIRST AID
- Keep the person warm with blankets to decrease the possibility of shock.
- Cut away clothing, if possible, but don't move the injured elbow to do so.
- Follow instructions for R.I.C.E., the first letters of *rest, ice, compression and elevation*. See Appendix 1 for details.
- The doctor will set the broken bones with surgery or, if possible, without. The setting lines up the broken bones as close to their normal positions as possible. Manipulation should be done as soon as possible after injury. Also, many tissues lose their elasticity and become difficult to return to their normal positions.

CONTINUING CARE
- Immobilization will be necessary, usually with plaster splints around the injured area to immobilize the elbow and wrist.
- After 96 hours, application of localized heat promotes healing by increasing blood circulation in the injured area. Use a heat lamp or a heating pad for 30 minutes at a time so heat can penetrate the cast or splints.
- After the cast or splints are removed, use frequent ice massage. Fill a large styrofoam cup with water and freeze. Tear a small amount of foam from the top so ice protrudes. Massage firmly over the injured area in a circle about the size of a baseball. Do this for 15 minutes at a time 3 or 4 times a day.
- Apply heat instead of ice if it feels better. Use heat lamps, hot soaks, hot showers, heating pads or heat liniments and ointments.
- Take whirlpool treatments, if available.

MEDICATION—Your doctor may prescribe:
- General anesthesia, local anesthesia or muscle relaxants to make bone manipulation and fixation of bone fragments possible.
- Prescription pain relievers for severe pain.
- Stool softeners to prevent constipation due to inactivity.
- Acetaminophen for mild pain.

ACTIVITY
- Actively exercise all muscle groups not immobilized. Muscle contractions promote fracture alignment and hasten healing.
- Begin reconditioning the elbow area after clearance from your doctor.
- Resume normal activities gradually after treatment.

DIET
- Do not drink or eat before manipulation or surgery to treat the fracture. Fluid or solid food in your stomach makes vomiting while under anesthesia more hazardous.
- During recovery, balance the amount of food you eat with any change in your level of physical activity. Eat a variety of foods to get the energy, protein, vitamins, minerals and fiber you need for good health and healing.

REHABILITATION—Begin daily rehabilitation exercises when movement is comfortable. Use ice massage for 10 minutes prior to exercise. See Rehabilitation section for elbow exercises.

 CALL YOUR DOCTOR IF

- You have signs or symptoms of an elbow fracture.
- Any of the following occurs after surgery or other treatment:
    Increased pain, swelling or drainage in the surgical area.
    Signs of infection (headache, muscle aches, dizziness or a general ill feeling and fever).
    Swelling above or below the splints.
    Blue or gray skin color beyond the cast or splints, particularly under the fingernails.
    Numbness or complete loss of feeling below the fracture site.
    Nausea or vomiting.
    Constipation.

ELBOW FRACTURE, LOWER HUMERUS
(Supracondylar Humerus Fracture)

GENERAL INFORMATION

DEFINITION—A complete or incomplete break in the lower end of the humerus just above the elbow joint.

BODY PARTS INVOLVED
- Lower end of the humerus (upper arm bone).
- Elbow joint.
- Soft tissues surrounding the fracture site, including nerves, tendons, ligaments, blood vessels, cartilage and muscles.

SIGNS & SYMPTOMS
- Severe elbow and arm pain at the time of injury.
- Swelling around the fracture.
- Visible deformity if the fracture is complete and bone fragments separate enough to distort normal body contours.
- Tenderness to the touch.
- Numbness or coldness in the elbow, lower arm and hand if the blood supply is impaired.

CAUSES
- Direct blow to the elbow.
- Indirect stress due to falling on an outstretched hand with the elbow locked.

RISK INCREASES WITH
- Contact sports such as football.
- Monkey bars, roller skates and skateboards.
- Age under 10 years.
- History of bone or joint disease, especially osteoporosis.
- Obesity.
- Surgical risk increases with smoking and use of drugs, including mind-altering drugs, muscle relaxants, antihypertensives, tranquilizers, sleep inducers, insulin, sedatives, beta-adrenergic blockers or corticosteroids.

HOW TO PREVENT
- Participate in a strengthening, flexibility and conditioning program appropriate for your sport.
- Use appropriate protective equipment, such as padded elbow pads, for contact sports.

WHAT TO EXPECT

APPROPRIATE HEALTH CARE
- Doctor's treatment to manipulate the broken bones and repair soft tissues of the elbow.
- Anesthesia and surgery to set the fracture and repair soft tissues (usually requires placement of pins). Also, application of a cast or splints after bone healing is complete.
- Whirlpool, ultrasound or massage (to displace excess fluid from the injured joint space).

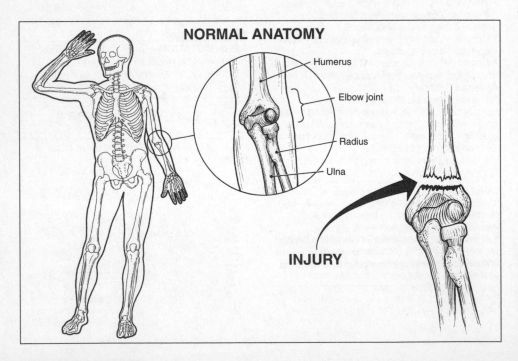

NORMAL ANATOMY

- Humerus
- Elbow joint
- Radius
- Ulna

INJURY

DIAGNOSTIC MEASURES
- Your own observation of symptoms.
- Medical history and exam by a doctor.
- X-rays of injured areas, including joints above and below the primary injury site.

POSSIBLE COMPLICATIONS
At the time of injury:
- Shock.
- Pressure on or injury to nearby nerves, ligaments, tendons, muscles, blood vessels or connective tissues.

After treatment or surgery:
- Delayed union or nonunion of the fracture.
- Angulated healing with abnormal rotation or alignment of the elbow and arm.
- Impaired blood supply to the fracture site.
- Avascular necrosis (death of bone cells due to interruption of the blood supply).
- Arrest of normal bone growth in children.
- Infection in open fractures (skin broken over fracture site) or at the incision if surgical setting was necessary.
- Shortening of the injured bones.
- Prolonged healing time if activity is resumed too soon; proneness to repeated injury.
- Atrophy of forearm muscles and poor hand control due to damage to blood vessels or nerves. (This may result from abnormally tense swelling of the forearm or injury to the artery.)

PROBABLE OUTCOME—The average healing time for this fracture is 6 to 8 weeks in adults and 4 to 6 weeks in children. Healing is considered complete when there is no motion at the fracture site and when x-rays show complete bone union.

 HOW TO TREAT

NOTE—Follow your doctor's instructions. These instructions are supplemental.

FIRST AID
- Keep the person warm with blankets to decrease the possibility of shock.
- Cut away clothing, if possible. Don't move the injured area to remove clothing.
- Follow instructions for R.I.C.E., the first letters of *rest, ice, compression* and *elevation*. See Appendix 1 for details.
- The doctor will realign and set the broken bones either with surgery or, if possible, without. Manipulation should be done as soon as possible after injury. Also, many tissues lose their elasticity and become difficult to return to their normal positions.

CONTINUING CARE
- Immobilization will be necessary, usually with rigid splints around the elbow and wrist.

- After 96 hours, localized heat promotes healing by increasing blood circulation in the injured area. Use a heating pad or heat lamp for 30 minutes at a time so heat can penetrate the splints.
- After the splints are removed, use frequent ice massage. Fill a large styrofoam cup with water and freeze. Tear a small amount of foam from the top so ice protrudes. Massage firmly over injured area in a circle about the size of a baseball for 15 minutes at a time 3 or 4 times a day.
- Apply heat instead of ice if it feels better. Use heat lamps, hot soaks, hot showers or heating pads. Take whirlpool treatments, if available.

MEDICATION—Your doctor may prescribe:
- General anesthesia for surgery.
- Prescription pain relievers for severe pain.
- Stool softeners to prevent constipation.
- Acetaminophen for mild pain.

ACTIVITY
- Actively exercise all muscle groups not immobilized. Muscle contractions promote fracture alignment and hasten healing.
- Resume normal activities gradually after treatment.
- Begin reconditioning the injured area after clearance from your doctor.

DIET
- Do not eat or drink before manipulation or surgery to treat the fracture. Fluid or solid food in your stomach makes vomiting while under anesthesia more hazardous.
- Balance the amount of food you eat with any change in your level of physical activity.

REHABILITATION—Begin daily rehabilitation exercises when movement is comfortable. Use ice massage for 10 minutes prior to exercise. See Rehabilitation section for elbow exercises.

 CALL YOUR DOCTOR IF

- You have signs or symptoms of an elbow fracture.
- Any of the following occurs after surgery or other treatment:
  Increased pain, swelling or drainage in the surgical area.
  Signs of infection (headache, muscle aches, dizziness or a general ill feeling and fever).
  Swelling above or below the cast.
  Blue or gray skin color beyond the cast, particularly under the fingernails.
  Numbness or complete loss of feeling below the fracture site.
  Nausea or vomiting; constipation.
- Inability to actively move fingers and wrist or excessive pain when they are moved passively.

ELBOW FRACTURE, RADIUS
(Radial Head Fracture)

 GENERAL INFORMATION

DEFINITION—A complete or incomplete break in the head of the radius, one of the bones of the forearm.

BODY PARTS INVOLVED
- Head of the radius.
- Elbow joint; soft tissues surrounding the fracture site, including nerves, tendons, ligaments, blood vessels, cartilage and muscles.

SIGNS & SYMPTOMS
- Severe pain at the fracture site.
- Swelling around the elbow joint.
- Visible deformity if the fracture is complete and bone fragments separate enough to distort normal arm contours.
- Tenderness to the touch.
- Numbness and coldness in the lower arm and hand if the blood supply is impaired.

CAUSES
- Direct blow to the elbow.
- Indirect injury due to falling on an outstretched hand with the elbow stiff, or any injury that causes dislocation of the elbow.

RISK INCREASES WITH
- Contact sports such as football.
- History of bone or joint disease, especially osteoporosis.
- Poor nutrition, especially calcium deficiency.
- Age under 12 or over 60.
- Obesity.
- If surgery is necessary, surgical risk increases with smoking and use of drugs, including mind-altering drugs, muscle relaxants, antihypertensives, tranquilizers, sleep inducers, insulin, sedatives, beta-adrenergic blockers or corticosteroids

HOW TO PREVENT
- Build adequate muscle strength and achieve good conditioning prior to exercise, athletic practice or competition. Increased muscle mass helps protect bones and underlying tissues.
- Use appropriate protective equipment, such as padded elbow pads, when participating in contact sports.

 WHAT TO EXPECT

APPROPRIATE HEALTH CARE
- Doctor's treatment to aspirate blood from the elbow joint and to remove the radial head surgically if it is shattered beyond repair or to return the fractured pieces to their normal positions.
- Surgery to set the fracture and repair the soft tissues and bones of the elbow.
- Whirlpool, ultrasound or massage (to displace excess fluid from the injured joint space).

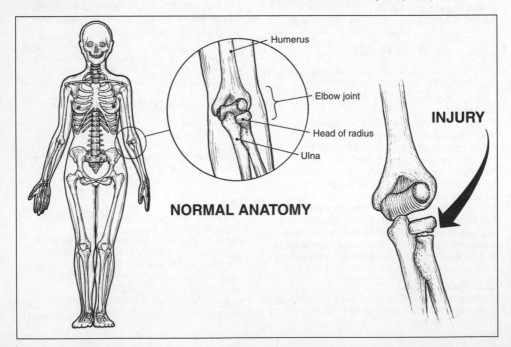

Humerus

Elbow joint

Head of radius

Ulna

NORMAL ANATOMY

INJURY

DIAGNOSTIC MEASURES
- Your own observation of symptoms.
- Medical history and exam by a doctor.
- X-rays of injured areas, including joints above and below the primary injury site.
- Additional x-rays a week later if pain persists despite a normal x-ray just after injury.

POSSIBLE COMPLICATIONS
At the time of injury:
- Shock.
- Pressure on or injury to nearby nerves, ligaments, tendons, muscles, blood vessels, cartilage or connective tissues.

After treatment or surgery:
- Delayed union or nonunion of the fracture.
- Impaired blood supply to the fracture site.
- Avascular necrosis (death of bone cells due to interruption of the blood supply).
- Arrest of normal bone growth in children.
- Infection in open fractures (skin broken over fracture site) or at the incision if surgical setting was necessary.
- Shortening of the injured bones.
- Proneness to repeated elbow injury.
- Unstable or arthritic elbow following repeated injury.
- Prolonged healing time if activity is resumed too soon.

PROBABLE OUTCOME—The average healing time for this fracture is 6 to 8 weeks in adults and 4 to 6 weeks in children. Healing is considered complete when there is no motion at the fracture site and when x-rays show complete bone union.

HOW TO TREAT

NOTE—Follow your doctor's instructions. These instructions are supplemental.

FIRST AID
- Keep the person warm with blankets to decrease the possibility of shock.
- Cut away clothing, if possible. Don't move the injured area to remove clothing.
- Use instructions for R.I.C.E., the first letters of *rest, ice, compression* and *elevation*. See Appendix 1 for details.
- The doctor will realign and set the broken bones and repair damaged soft tissues with surgery. Surgery to fix or remove bone fragments may be necessary for this injury to ensure normal rotation of the forearm after healing is complete. Manipulation should be done as soon as possible after injury. Also, many tissues lose their elasticity and become difficult to return to their normal positions.

CONTINUING CARE
- Immobilization of the elbow with rigid splints will be necessary.

- After 96 hours, application of localized heat promotes healing by increasing blood circulation in the injured area. Use a heating pad or heat lamp so heat can penetrate the splints.
- After splints are removed, use an ice pack 3 or 4 times a day. Place ice chips or cubes in a plastic bag, and wrap the bag in a moist towel. Place it over the injured area for 20 minutes at a time.
- Apply heat instead of ice if it feels better. Use heat lamps, hot soaks, hot showers, heating pads or heat liniments and ointments.
- Take whirlpool treatments, if available.

MEDICATION—Your doctor may prescribe:
- General anesthesia for surgery.
- Prescription pain relievers for severe pain.
- Stool softeners to prevent constipation due to inactivity.
- Acetaminophen for mild pain.

ACTIVITY
- Actively exercise all muscle groups not immobilized. Muscle contractions promote fracture alignment and hasten healing.
- Resume normal activities gradually after treatment.

DIET
- Do not drink or eat before manipulation or surgery to treat the fracture. Fluid or solid food in your stomach makes vomiting while under anesthesia more hazardous.
- Balance the amount of food you eat with any change in your level of physical activity.

REHABILITATION
- Begin reconditioning the injured area after clearance from your doctor.
- Use ice massage for 10 minutes before and after workouts. Fill a large styrofoam cup with water and freeze. Tear a small amount of foam from the top so ice protrudes. Massage firmly in a circle over the injured area. See Rehabilitation section for elbow exercises.

CALL YOUR DOCTOR IF

- You have signs or symptoms of an elbow fracture.
- Any of the following occurs after surgery or other treatment:
  Increased pain, swelling or drainage in the surgical area.
  Signs of infection (headache, muscle aches, dizziness or a general ill feeling and fever).
  Swelling above or below the splints.
  Blue or gray skin color beyond the splints, particularly under the fingernails.
  Loss of feeling below the fracture site.
  Nausea or vomiting; constipation.

ELBOW FRACTURE, ULNA
(Olecranon Fracture)

GENERAL INFORMATION

DEFINITION—A complete or incomplete break in the olecranon process, the head of the ulna (one of the bones of the forearm). This fracture is often associated with an elbow dislocation.

BODY PARTS INVOLVED
● Head of the ulna, which forms part of the elbow.
● Elbow joint.
● Soft tissues surrounding the fracture site, including nerves, tendons, ligaments, blood vessels, cartilage and muscles.

SIGNS & SYMPTOMS
● Severe pain at the fracture site.
● Swelling around the fracture.
● Visible deformity if the fracture is complete and bone fragments separate enough to distort normal arm contours.
● Tenderness to the touch.
● Numbness or coldness in the lower arm and hand if the blood supply is impaired.

CAUSES
● Direct blow to the elbow.
● Indirect stress due to falling on an outstretched hand with the elbow stiff, or any injury that causes dislocation of the elbow.

RISK INCREASES WITH
● Contact sports such as football.
● Anterior (backward) dislocation of the elbow joint.
● History of bone or joint disease, especially osteoporosis.
● Poor nutrition, especially calcium deficiency.
● Age under 12 or over 60.
● Obesity.
● If surgery is necessary, surgical risk increases with smoking and use of drugs, including mind-altering drugs, muscle relaxants, antihypertensives, tranquilizers, sleep inducers, insulin, sedatives, beta-adrenergic blockers or corticosteroids.

HOW TO PREVENT
● Build adequate muscle strength and achieve good conditioning prior to exercise, athletic practice or competition. Increased muscle mass helps protect bones and underlying tissues.
● Use appropriate protective equipment, such as padded elbow pads, for contact sports.

WHAT TO EXPECT

APPROPRIATE HEALTH CARE
● Doctor's treatment to remove the olecranon process surgically (if it is shattered) or to reattach it to its normal position and fix the bone with pins and screws.

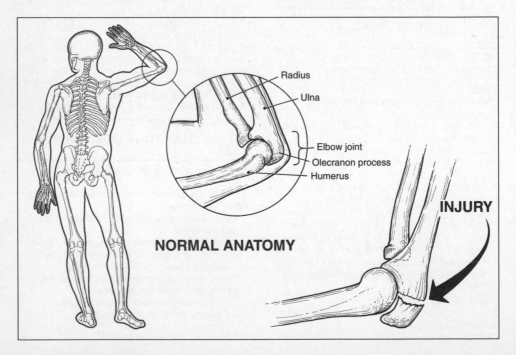

Radius
Ulna
Elbow joint
Olecranon process
Humerus

NORMAL ANATOMY

INJURY

- Surgery to set the fracture and repair the soft tissues and bones of the elbow.
- Whirlpool, ultrasound or massage (to displace excess fluid from the injured joint space).

DIAGNOSTIC MEASURES
- Your own observation of symptoms.
- Medical history and exam by a doctor.
- X-rays of injured areas, including joints above and below the primary injury site.
- Repeat x-rays after approximately 1 week if first x-rays were normal but pain continues.

POSSIBLE COMPLICATIONS
At the time of injury:
- Shock.
- Pressure on or injury to nearby nerves, ligaments, tendons, muscles, blood vessels or connective tissues.
After treatment or surgery:
- Delayed union or nonunion of the fracture.
- Avascular necrosis (death of bone cells due to interruption of the blood supply).
- Arrest of normal bone growth in children.
- Infection in open fractures (skin broken over fracture site) or at the incision if surgical setting was necessary.
- Shortening of the injured bones.
- Proneness to repeated elbow injury.
- Unstable or arthritic joint following repeated injury.
- Prolonged healing time if activity is resumed too soon.

PROBABLE OUTCOME—The average healing time for this fracture is 6 to 8 weeks in adults and 4 to 6 weeks in children. Healing is considered complete when there is no motion at the fracture site and when x-rays show complete bone union.

 HOW TO TREAT

NOTE—Follow your doctor's instructions. These instructions are supplemental.
- Keep the person warm with blankets to decrease the possibility of shock.
- Cut away clothing, if possible. Don't move the injured area to remove clothing.
- Use instructions for R.I.C.E., the first letters of *rest, ice, compression,* and *elevation*. See Appendix 1 for details.
- The doctor will realign and set the broken bones and repair damaged soft tissues and bone with surgery. Manipulation should be done as soon as possible after injury. Also, many tissues lose their elasticity and become difficult to return to their normal positions.

CONTINUING CARE
- Immobilization will be necessary. Rigid splints are used to immobilize the elbow and wrist.
- After 96 hours, application of localized heat promotes healing by increasing blood circulation in the injured area. Use a heating pad or heat lamp so heat can penetrate the splints.
- After the splints are removed, use frequent ice massage. Fill a large styrofoam cup with water and freeze. Tear a small amount of foam from the top so ice protrudes. Massage firmly over the injured area in a circle about the size of a baseball. Do this for 15 minutes at a time 3 or 4 times a day, and also before workouts or competition.
- Apply heat instead of ice if it feels better. Use heat lamps, hot soaks, hot showers, heating pads or heat liniments and ointments.
- Take whirlpool treatments, if available.

MEDICATION—Your doctor may prescribe:
- General anesthesia for surgery.
- Narcotic pain relievers for severe pain.
- Stool softeners to prevent constipation due to inactivity.
- Acetaminophen for mild pain.

ACTIVITY—Actively exercise all muscle groups not immobilized. Muscle contractions promote fracture alignment and hasten healing. Resume normal activities gradually after treatment.

DIET
- Do not eat or drink before manipulation or surgery to treat the fracture. Fluid or solid food in your stomach makes vomiting while under anesthesia more hazardous.
- During recovery, balance the amount of food you eat with any change in your level of physical activity. Eat a variety of foods to get the energy, protein, vitamins, minerals and fiber you need for good health and healing.

REHABILITATION—Begin reconditioning the injured area after clearance from your doctor. See Rehabilitation section for elbow exercises.

 CALL YOUR DOCTOR IF

- You have signs or symptoms of an elbow fracture.
- Any of the following occurs after surgery or other treatment:
  Increased pain, swelling or drainage in the surgical area.
  Signs of infection (headache, muscle aches, dizziness or a general ill feeling and fever).
  Swelling above or below the splints.
  Blue or gray skin color beyond the splints, particularly under the fingernails.
  Loss of feeling below the fracture site.
  Nausea or vomiting; constipation.

ELBOW SPRAIN

GENERAL INFORMATION

DEFINITION—Violent overstretching of one or more ligaments in the elbow joint. Elbow sprains are relatively uncommon. Sprains involving two or more ligaments cause considerably more disability than single-ligament sprains. When the ligament is overstretched, it becomes tense and gives way and its weakest point, either where it attaches to bone or within the ligament itself. If the ligament pulls loose a fragment of bone, it is called an avulsion fracture. There are three types of sprains:
- Mild (Grade I)—Tearing of some ligament fibers. There is no loss of function.
- Moderate (Grade II)—Rupture of a portion of the ligament, resulting in some loss of function.
- Severe (Grade III)—Complete rupture of the ligament or complete separation of ligament from bone. There is total loss of function. A severe sprain may require surgical repair, especially in a throwing athlete.

BODY PARTS INVOLVED
- Ligaments of the elbow joint.
- Tissues surrounding the sprain, including blood vessels, tendon, bone, periosteum (covering of bone) and muscle.

SIGNS AND SYMPTOMS
- Severe pain at the time of injury.
- A feeling of popping or tearing inside the elbow.
- Tenderness at the injury site.
- Swelling around the elbow.
- Bruising that appears soon after injury.

CAUSES—Sharp force that bends the elbow sideways or backwards, causing stress on a ligament and temporarily forcing or prying the elbow joint out of its normal location.

RISK INCREASES WITH
- Contact sports as football, basketball, hockey and soccer.
- Throwing sports such as baseball or javelin throwing.
- Previous elbow injury.
- Obesity.
- Poor muscle conditioning.

HOW TO PREVENT
- Long-term strengthening and conditioning appropriate for sport.
- Warm up before practice or competition.
- Tape vulnerable joints before practice or competition.

WHAT TO EXPECT

APPROPRIATE HEALTH CARE
- Doctor's diagnosis.
- Application of a cast, tape, elastic bandage or sling.
- Self-care during rehabilitation.
- Physical therapy (moderate or severe sprain).
- Surgery (severe sprain).

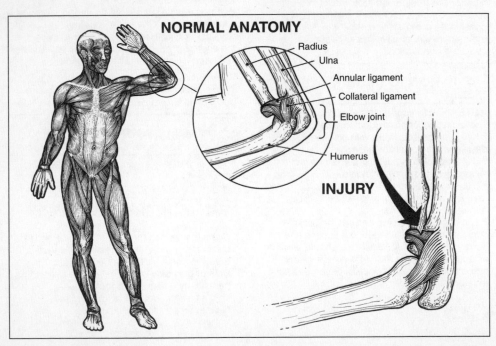

NORMAL ANATOMY

Radius
Ulna
Annular ligament
Collateral ligament
Elbow joint
Humerus

INJURY

DIAGNOSTIC MEASURES
- Your own observation of symptoms.
- Medical history and exam by a doctor.
- X-rays of the elbow, wrist and shoulder to rule out fractures.
- MRI to define severe sprain (especially in throwing athletes).

POSSIBLE COMPLICATIONS
- Prolonged healing time if usual activities are resumed too soon.
- Proneness to repeated injury.
- Inflammation at the ligament attachment to bone (periostitis).
- Prolonged disability (sometimes).
- Unstable or arthritic elbow following repeated injury.

PROBABLE OUTCOME—If this is a first-time injury, proper care and sufficient healing time before resuming activity should prevent permanent disability. Ligaments have a poor blood supply, and torn ligaments require as much healing time as fractures. Average healing times are:
- Mild sprains—2 to 6 weeks.
- Moderate sprains—6 to 8 weeks.
- Severe sprains—8 to 10 weeks.

 HOW TO TREAT

NOTE—Follow your doctor's instructions. These instructions are supplemental.

FIRST AID—Use instructions for R.I.C.E, the first letters of *rest, ice, compression* and *elevation*. See Appendix 1 for details.

CONTINUING CARE—If the doctor does not apply a cast, tape or elastic bandage:
- Continue using an ice pack 3 or 4 times a day. Place ice chips or cubes in a plastic bag. Wrap the bag in a moist towel, and place it over the injured area. Use for 20 minutes at a time.
- After 72 hours, apply heat instead of ice if it feels better. Use heat lamps, hot soaks, hot showers, heating pads or heat liniments and ointments.
- Take whirlpool treatments, if available.
- Massage gently and often to provide comfort and decrease swelling.

MEDICATION
- For minor discomfort, you may use:
Aspirin, acetaminophen or ibuprofen.
Topical liniments and ointments.
- Your doctor may prescribe:
Stronger pain relievers.
Injection of a long-acting local anesthetic to reduce pain.
Injections of a corticosteroid, such as triamcinolone, to reduce inflammation (rarely).
Nonsteroidal anti-inflammatory medications.

ACTIVITY—Resume your normal activities gradually after clearance from your doctor.

DIET—During recovery, balance the amount of food you eat with any change in your level of physical activity. Eat a variety of foods to get the energy, protein, vitamins, minerals and fiber you need for good health and healing.

REHABILITATION
- Begin daily rehabilitation exercises when the cast or supportive wrapping is no longer necessary.
- Use ice massage for 10 minutes before and after exercise. Fill a large styrofoam cup with water and freeze. Tear a small amount of foam from the top so ice protrudes. Massage firmly over the injured area in a circle about the size of a softball.
- See Rehabilitation section for elbow exercises.

 CALL YOUR DOCTOR IF

- You have symptoms of a moderate or severe elbow sprain or a mild sprain persists longer than 2 weeks.
- Pain, swelling or bruising worsens despite treatment.
- Any of the following occurs after casting or splinting:
Pain, numbness or coldness below the elbow.
Blue, gray or dusky fingernails.
- Any of the following occurs after surgery:
Increased pain, swelling, redness, drainage or bleeding in the surgical area.
Signs of infection (headache, muscle aches, dizziness or a general ill feeling with fever).
- New, unexplained symptoms develop. Drugs used in treatment may produce side effects.

ELBOW STRAIN

GENERAL INFORMATION

DEFINITION—Injury to the muscles or tendons that attach to bones in the elbow. Muscles, tendons and their attached bones comprise contractile units. These units stabilize the elbow joint and allow its motion. A strain occurs at a unit's weakest part. Strains are of 3 types:
- Mild (Grade I)—Slightly pulled muscle without tearing of muscle or tendon fibers. There is no loss of strength.
- Moderate (Grade II)—Tearing of fibers in a muscle or tendon or at the attachment to bone. Strength is diminished.
- Severe (Grade III)—Rupture of the muscle-tendon-bone attachment, with separation of fibers. Severe strains may require surgical repair. Chronic strains are caused by overuse. Acute strains are caused by direct injury or overstress.

SIGNS & SYMPTOMS
- Pain when moving or stretching the elbow.
- Muscle spasm in the elbow area.
- Swelling over the injury.
- Loss of strength (moderate or severe strain).
- Crepitation ("crackling" feeling and sound when the injured area is pressed with fingers).
- Calcification of muscles or tendons (visible with x-rays).
- Inflammation of a tendon sheath.

CAUSES
- Prolonged overuse of muscle-tendon units in the elbow.
- Sudden, forceful hyperextension of the elbow.
- Single violent injury or force applied to the elbow.

RISK INCREASES WITH
- Contact sports.
- Racquet sports.
- Throwing sports.
- Weightlifting.
- Medical history of any bleeding disorder.
- Obesity.
- Poor nutrition.
- Previous elbow injury.
- Poor muscle conditioning.

HOW TO PREVENT
- Participate in a strengthening, flexibility and conditioning program appropriate for your sport.
- Warm up before practice or competition. Include adequate stretching.
- Tape the elbow area before practice or competition to prevent recurrence of injury.
- Wear proper protective equipment, such as elbow pads, for participation in contact sports.

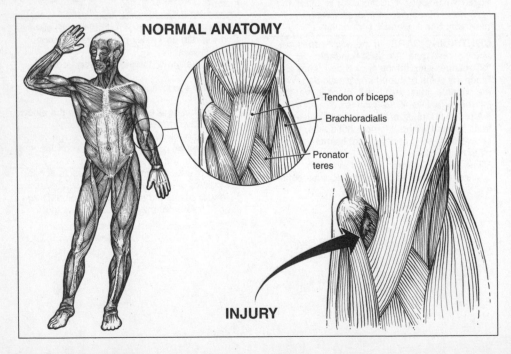

NORMAL ANATOMY

Tendon of biceps

Brachioradialis

Pronator teres

INJURY

WHAT TO EXPECT

APPROPRIATE HEALTH CARE
- Doctor's diagnosis.
- Application of tape, plaster splints or cast (sometimes).
- Self-care during rehabilitation.
- Physical therapy (moderate or severe strain).
- Surgery (severe strain).

DIAGNOSTIC MEASURES
- Your own observation of symptoms.
- Medical history and exam by a doctor.
- X-rays of the elbow and wrist to rule out fractures.

POSSIBLE COMPLICATIONS
- Prolonged healing time if activity is resumed too soon.
- Proneness to repeated elbow injury.
- Inflammation at the attachment to bone (periostitis).
- Prolonged disability (sometimes), especially weakness.

PROBABLE OUTCOME—If this is a first-time injury, proper care and sufficient healing time before resuming activity should prevent permanent disability. Torn ligaments and tendons require as long to heal as fractured bones. Average healing times are:
- Mild strain—2 to 10 days.
- Moderate strain—10 days to 6 weeks.
- Severe strain—6 to 10 weeks.
If this is a repeat injury, complications listed above are more likely to occur.

 # HOW TO TREAT

NOTE—Follow your doctor's instructions. These instructions are supplemental.

FIRST AID—Use instructions for R.I.C.E., the first letters of *rest, ice, compression* and *elevation*. See Appendix 1 for details.

CONTINUING CARE
If splints are used:
- Be sure to keep fingers free, and exercise them frequently.
- See Appendix 2 (Care of Casts).

If casts or splints are not used:
- Use ice massage 3 or 4 times a day for 15 minutes at a time. Fill a large styrofoam cup with water and freeze. Tear a small amount of foam from the top so ice protrudes. Massage firmly over the injured area in a circle about the size of a softball.
- After the first 24 hours, apply heat instead of ice if it feels better. Use heat lamps, hot soaks, hot showers, heating pads or heat liniments and ointments.
- Take whirlpool treatments, if available.
- Wrap the injured elbow with an elasticized bandage between treatments.
- Massage gently and often to provide comfort and decrease swelling.

MEDICATION
- For minor discomfort, you may use:
  Aspirin, acetaminophen or ibuprofen.
  Topical liniments and ointments.
- Your doctor may prescribe:
  Stronger pain relievers.
  Injection of a long-acting local anesthetic to reduce pain.
  Injections of corticosteroids, such as triamcinolone, to reduce inflammation.

ACTIVITY
- For a moderate or severe strain, use a sling for at least 72 hours—longer with a cast or splints.
- Resume your normal activities gradually.

DIET—During recovery, balance the amount of food you eat with any change in your level of physical activity. Eat a variety of foods to get the energy, protein, vitamins, minerals and fiber you need for good health and healing.

REHABILITATION
- Begin daily rehabilitation exercises when supportive wrapping is no longer needed. Use ice massage for 10 minutes prior to exercise.
- See Rehabilitation section for elbow exercises.

 # CALL YOUR DOCTOR IF

- You have symptoms of a moderate or severe elbow strain or a mild strain persists longer than 10 days.
- Pain or swelling worsens despite treatment.
- The following occur with a cast or splints:
  Pain, numbness or coldness below the injury.
  Dusky, blue or gray fingernails.

ELBOW SYNOVITIS, RADIOHUMERAL

 GENERAL INFORMATION

DEFINITION—Inflammation of the synovial lining of the elbow joint. Synovitis may vary in degree from mild irritation to an abscess that causes excruciating pain. In acute synovitis at the elbow, blood from an injury usually causes the inflammation. Irritation will continue until the blood is removed or reabsorbed. Chronic synovitis results from undertreated acute synovitis and may require surgery to repair.

BODY PARTS INVOLVED
- Joint between the radius, ulna and humerus (arm bones) where they meet in the elbow. The synovial lining of the joint is a soft sac filed with lubricating fluid that facilitates motion between the radius and the humerus.
- Soft tissues surrounding the elbow, including nerves, tendons, ligaments, blood vessels (both large vessels and capillaries), periosteum (the outside lining of bone) and muscles.

SIGNS & SYMPTOMS
- Pain at the elbow.
- Tenderness.
- Swelling.
- Redness (sometimes) over the affected joint.
- Fever if infection is present.
- Limited elbow movement.

CAUSES
- Direct blow to the elbow or forearm.
- Acute or chronic infection.
- Arthritis.
- Gout.
- Unknown (frequently).

RISK INCREASES WITH
- Participating in competitive athletics, particularly contact sports.
- Previous history of synovitis in any joint.
- Exposure to cold weather.
- Poor conditioning and inadequate warmup before exercise.
- Inadequate protective equipment in contact sports.

HOW TO PREVENT
- Use protective elbow pads for contact sports.
- Wear warm clothing in cold weather.
- To prevent recurrence, continue to wear extra protection over the elbow until healing is complete.

 WHAT TO EXPECT

APPROPRIATE HEALTH CARE
- Doctor's treatment.
- Surgery (sometimes), particularly for a frozen elbow or for a severely infected joint that drains to the outside.

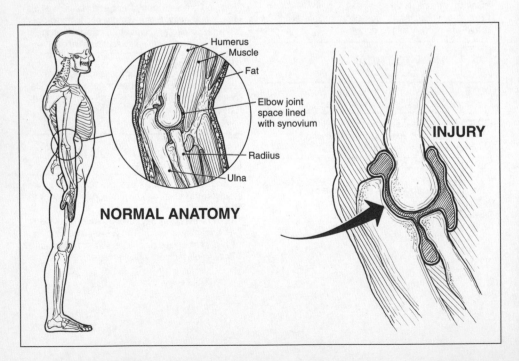

Humerus
Muscle
Fat
Elbow joint space lined with synovium
Radiius
Ulna

NORMAL ANATOMY

INJURY

DIAGNOSTIC MEASURES
- Your own observation of symptoms.
- Medical history and physical exam by a doctor.
- X-rays of the elbow and wrist.

POSSIBLE COMPLICATIONS
- Temporary or permanent limitation of elbow's normal mobility.
- Prolonged healing time if activity is resumed too soon.
- Proneness to repeated flare-ups.
- Unstable or arthritic elbow following repeated episodes of synovitis.
- Spontaneous rupture of the joint if severe infection is present.

PROBABLE OUTCOME—Radiohumeral synovitis is a common problem. Symptoms usually subside in 3 to 4 weeks with treatment. If serious infection occurs and surgery is needed, allow 6 to 8 weeks for healing.

 HOW TO TREAT

NOTE—Follow your doctor's instructions. These instructions are supplemental.

FIRST AID—None. This problem develops slowly.

CONTINUING CARE
- Use frequent ice massage. Fill a large styrofoam cup with water and freeze. Tear a small amount of foam from the top so ice protrudes. Massage firmly over the injured area in a circle about the size of a softball. Do this for 15 minutes at a time 3 or 4 times a day, and also before workouts or competition.
- After 72 hours, apply heat instead of ice if it feels better. Use heat lamps, hot soaks, hot showers, heating pads or heat liniments and ointments.
- Take whirlpool treatments, if available.
- Use a sling to support the elbow joint, if needed.
- Elevate the elbow above the level of the heart to reduce swelling and prevent accumulation of fluid. Use pillows for propping.
- Massage gently and often to provide comfort and decrease swelling.

MEDICATION—Your doctor may prescribe:
- Nonsteroidal anti-inflammatory drugs.
- Corticosteroid injections into the joint to reduce inflammation (if infection is not the cause of the synovitis).
- Prescription pain relievers for severe pain. Use nonprescription acetaminophen or ibuprofen for mild pain.
- Injection into the inflamed joint of a long-lasting local anesthetic mixed with a corticosteroid drug, such as triamcinolone.
- Antibiotics for infection.

ACTIVITY—Rest the inflamed area as much as possible. If you must resume normal activity immediately, wear a sling until the pain becomes more bearable. To prevent frozen elbow, begin normal, slow joint movement as soon as possible.

DIET—During recovery, balance the amount of food you eat with any change in your level of physical activity. Eat a variety of foods to get the energy, protein, vitamins, minerals and fiber you need for good health and healing. Your doctor may suggest vitamin and mineral supplements to promote healing.

REHABILITATION—See Rehabilitation section for elbow exercises.

 CALL YOUR DOCTOR IF

- You have symptoms of elbow synovitis.
- Pain increases despite treatment.
- Any of the following occurs after surgery: Pain, swelling, tenderness, drainage or bleeding increases in the surgical area. You develop signs of infection (headache, muscle aches, dizziness or a general ill feeling and fever).
- New, unexplained symptoms develop. Drugs used in treatment may produce side effects.

ELBOW TENDINITIS OR EPICONDYLITIS
(Tennis Elbow; Golfer's Elbow)

GENERAL INFORMATION

DEFINITION—Inflammation of muscles, tendons, bursa, or covering of bones (periosteum) at the elbow (tennis elbow when it is on the outside and golfer's elbow when it is on the inside).

BODY PARTS INVOLVED—Elbow muscles, tendons and one or both of the epicondyles (bony prominences on the sides of the elbow where muscles of the forearm attach to the bone of the upper arm).

SIGNS & SYMPTOMS
- Pain and tenderness over the epicondyle(s). Pain worsens with gripping or rotation of the forearm.
- Weak grip.
- Pain when twisting the hand and arm, as when playing tennis, throwing a ball with a twist, bowling, golfing, pushing off while skiing or using a screwdriver.

CAUSES—Partial tear of the tendon and attached covering of the bone caused by:
- Chronic stress on the tissues that attaches the forearm muscles to the elbow area.
- Sudden stress on the forearm.
- Wrist snap when serving balls in racquet sports.
- Wrist snap to make up for poor positioning and preparation in racquet sports.
- Incorrect grip.
- Incorrect hitting positions.
- Using a racquet or club that is too heavy.
- Using an oversized grip.

RISK INCREASES WITH
- Participation in sports that require strenuous forearm movement, such as tennis and racquetball.
- Poor conditioning of forearm muscles prior to vigorous exercise.
- Returning to activity before healing is complete.

HOW TO PREVENT
- Don't play sports such as tennis for long periods until your forearm muscles are strong and limber. Take frequent rest periods.
- Do forearm conditioning exercises to build your strength gradually prior to play.
- Warm up slowly and completely before participating in sports—especially before competition.
- Get lessons from a professional if you are a novice.
- Use a tennis elbow/golfer's elbow strap when you resume normal activity after treatment.

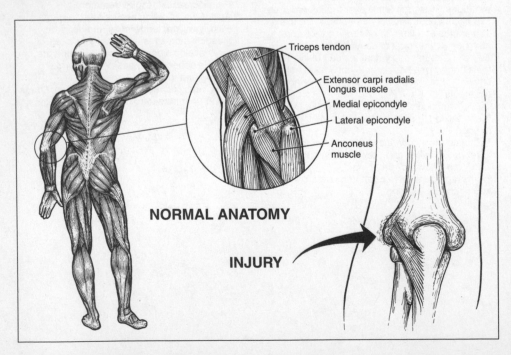

Triceps tendon
Extensor carpi radialis longus muscle
Medial epicondyle
Lateral epicondyle
Anconeus muscle

NORMAL ANATOMY

INJURY

WHAT TO EXPECT

APPROPRIATE HEALTH CARE
• Self-care after diagnosis.
• Doctor's treatment.
• Physical therapy.
• Surgery (rare).

DIAGNOSTIC MEASURES
• Your own observation of symptoms.
• Medical history and physical exam by a doctor.
• X-rays of the elbow.

POSSIBLE COMPLICATIONS
• Complete ligament tear, requiring surgery to repair.
• Slow healing.
• Frequent recurrence.

PROBABLE OUTCOME—Tennis elbow/golfer's elbow usually heals with heat treatments, corticosteroid injections and rest of the elbow. Surgery is occasionally necessary to partially release muscle, explore muscle origin (where it attaches to the bone) and relieve pain. Treatment may require 3 to 6 months.

 # HOW TO TREAT

NOTE—Follow your doctor's instructions. These instructions are supplemental.

FIRST AID—None. This problem develops slowly.

CONTINUING CARE
• Use heat to relieve pain. Use warm soaks, a heating pad or a heat lamp. You may receive diathermy or ultrasound (see Glossary) or whirlpool or massage treatments in your doctor's office or a physical therapy facility. These may bring quicker symptom relief and healing.

• You may need to wear a forearm splint to immobilize the elbow.

MEDICATION—Your doctor may prescribe:
• Nonsteroidal anti-inflammatory drugs to reduce inflammation.
• Injections of anesthetics to temporarily relieve pain.
• Injections of corticosteroids to reduce inflammation. *Caution:* Repeated injections may weaken the muscle tendon and increase the risk of tendon rupture.

ACTIVITY—Don't repeat the activity that caused tennis elbow/golfer's elbow until symptoms disappear. Then resume your normal activities gradually after proper conditioning.

DIET—During recovery, balance the amount of food you eat with any change in your level of physical activity. Eat a variety of foods to get the energy, protein, vitamins, minerals and fiber you need for good health and healing.

REHABILITATION
• Do the following exercise 3 or 4 times a day: Straighten the elbow fully; rotate arm inward at both the shoulder and forearm; fully flex the wrist. Press the back of the hand against a wall or table, and hold for 30 seconds. Repeat 4 to 5 times per session.
• See Rehabilitation section for additional elbow exercises.

 # CALL YOUR DOCTOR IF

• You have symptoms of tennis elbow or golfer's elbow.
• Symptoms don't improve in 2 weeks, despite treatment.

EXERTIONAL RHABDOMYOLYSIS

GENERAL INFORMATION

DEFINITION—Exertional rhabdomyolysis occurs when strenuous physical exercise results in damage to skeletal muscle causing cell breakdown and release of the contents of muscle cells into the bloodstream. The symptoms vary greatly from athlete to athlete and may be nonspecific. Males are more often affected than females. Rhabdomyolysis also occurs from crush injuries, alcohol abuse, use of certain medications or illicit drugs, infection, burns, hereditary disorders, seizures, trauma and other diseases and disorders.

BODY PARTS INVOLVED
• Specific groups of skeletal muscles or more generalized muscle groups. Most frequently, the affected muscle are the calves and lower back.
• If complications occur, the kidneys, heart and other body organ systems are involved.

SIGNS & SYMPTOMS
• Muscle pain (myalgias).
• Muscle weakness.
• Swelling or bruising.
• Fever; tiredness.
• Nausea or vomiting.
• Confusion, agitation, or delirium.
• Tea-colored or brown urine (called myoglobinuria).
• May be asymptomatic (no symptoms).

CAUSES—Rhabdomyolysis means striated muscle dissolution or disintegration. It is not clearly understood why this happens. The muscle injury causes a release of myoglobin, potassium, phosphate, creatine phosphokinase and uric acid inside the muscles to pour out into the blood and surrounding tissue spaces. Sodium and calcium tend to flow inward. The excess potassium affects the heart, the myoglobin causes kidney problems and calcium can destroys muscle fiber.

RISK INCREASES WITH
For exertional rhabdomyolysis:
• Unaccustomed, excessive, repetitive exercises such as push-ups, squat-jumps and leapfrogs, pull-ups; weightlifting; other strenuous exercise during the first days of a new training program.
• Marathon running and hiking.
• Genetic traits may predispose some athletes (with normal exercise, this condition would go unnoticed).
• Presence of cold or flu-like symptoms.
• Hot weather (causing profuse sweating or heat stroke).
• Dehydration.
• Heavy alcohol consumption.

HOW TO PREVENT
• Gradually increase exercise intensity.
• Because dehydration is implicated in rhabdomyolysis, adequate fluid should be available and ingested before and during exercise.

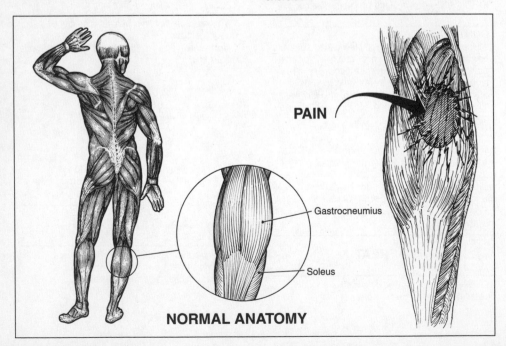

PAIN

Gastrocneumius

Soleus

NORMAL ANATOMY

- Avoiding exercise in extremely hot or humid environments.
- Don't try any new diet changes for the first time prior to a strenuous competitive event or practice.
- Don't use drugs which can exacerbate muscle damage.
- Exercise carefully and cautiously if you have an infection or a viral illness.

 ## WHAT TO EXPECT

APPROPRIATE HEALTH CARE
- Doctor's care.
- Hospitalization for intravenous (IV) fluids. Early and aggressive hydration flushes out the myoglobin from the kidneys and will help prevent complications.
- Kidney dialysis if severe renal failure occurs.

DIAGNOSTIC MEASURES
- Your own observation of symptoms.
- Medical history and physical exam by a doctor.
- Laboratory blood and urine studies.

POSSIBLE COMPLICATIONS
- Electrolyte imbalances such as hyperkalemia (excessive potassium).
- Acute renal failure (ARF) that may require dialysis.
- Compartment syndrome—muscle swelling that causes obstructed blood flow (may require surgery to resolve).
- Other complications that could be life-threatening include liver problems, metabolic acidosis, respiratory failure, heart rhythm problems and disseminated intravascular coagulation (DIC).

PROBABLE OUTCOME
- Patients can expect to recover completely from rhabdomyolysis if the syndrome is recognized and treated promptly so that complications are prevented. Mild cases may resolve in a few days.
- Recovery time and return to normal activities and exercising or athletic endeavors will depend on the individual. Two to three weeks will probably be necessary for recovery of muscle function for most individuals.
- For others, it may require six weeks to several months.

 ## HOW TO TREAT

NOTE—Follow your doctor's instructions. These instructions are supplemental.

FIRST AID—If symptoms develop, seek medical help right away. Call the doctor or take affected person to a doctor, urgent care facility or emergency room.

CONTINUING CARE
- The initial care in the hospital involves high volumes of IV fluids to flush out the kidneys and keep urine flow at certain levels.
- If fluid overload occurs or the kidneys have already started to fail, dialysis (kidney machine) may be used to remove the wastes and give the kidneys a rest until they recover. Recovery may take weeks to months.
- Treatment will be provided for any underlying condition that is diagnosed.
- Laboratory studies will be repeated until blood electrolytes are within the normal range.
- Close monitoring of all body systems (lungs, heart, nervous, gastrointestinal, urinary) will continue until recovery is complete.

MEDICATION
- Intravenous medications will be utilized to bring electrolytes to acceptable levels.
- Once recovery is complete, further medications are normally not required.

ACTIVITY
- After you return home, begin activities slowly. Increase activity as healing progresses.
- If surgery is required for compartment syndrome, your doctor will advise you of any activity restrictions and physical therapy that will be needed.

DIET
- Your doctor may restrict your diet during hospitalization.
- During recovery, balance the amount of food you eat with any change in your level of physical activity. Eat a variety of foods to get the energy, protein, vitamins, minerals and fiber you need for good health and healing.

REHABILITATION
- Rehabilitation exercises will need to be individualized. Follow your doctor's or surgeon's instructions.
- Rehabilitation exercises usually progress from active and gentle range of motion, to low intensity exercising (such as a stationary bike riding), to modified workouts and weightlifting.

 ## CALL YOUR DOCTOR IF

- You have symptoms of rhabdomyolysis.
- Following treatment, symptoms recur. Rhabdomyolysis may occur again.

EYE INJURY

GENERAL INFORMATION

DEFINITION—Injuries to the eye include:
* Contusions and fractures of bones that form the eye socket or orbit.
* Contusions and lacerations of the eyelids.
* Abrasions of the cornea (the transparent covering of the pupil of the eye) or other injuries to the eyeball.

BODY PARTS INVOLVED
* Bones that form the orbit.
* Eyelids.
* Eyeball—cornea, conjunctiva (white of the eye), iris (colored part of the eye) and aqueous humor (fluid in the eyeball).
* Muscles, tendons, periosteum (covering of bone), nerves, blood vessels, skin and connective tissues in the vicinity of the eye.

SIGNS & SYMPTOMS
Injury to the orbit:
* Pain.
* Swollen lid.
* Protruding eyeball if bleeding occurs in back of the eye.
* Numbness around the eye.
* Inability to move the eye normally.
* Decreased vision or double vision.

Injury to the lid:
* Pain.
* A cut, laceration or contusion with swelling, redness, tenderness, pain, bleeding or bruising ("black eye") in or around the eye.
* Change in ability to see clearly.

Injury to the eyeball:
* Eye pain.
* Sensitively to bright light.
* Eyelid spasm.
* Tearing.
* Blurred vision.
* Redness in the white of the eye.
* Irregular size of pupil.

CAUSES
* Direct blow in the vicinity of the eye.
* Irritation from many different materials, such as pesticides on grass, lime used for lines, gravel or dust.
* Foreign body imbedded in the eye, such as a small piece of gravel, sand or glass.
* Scratching of the cornea, either by a fingernail or by a rough foreign body.

RISK INCREASES WITH
* Contact sports such as football or soccer.
* Racquet sports.
* Windy weather.
* Rough terrains for workouts or competition.

HOW TO PREVENT
* Wear a face mask for contact sports where appropriate.
* Wear protective glasses for racquet sports.

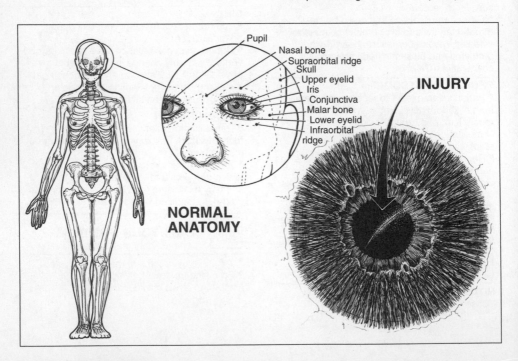

Pupil
Nasal bone
Supraorbital ridge
Skull
Upper eyelid
Iris
Conjunctiva
Malar bone
Lower eyelid
Infraorbital ridge

INJURY

NORMAL ANATOMY

WHAT TO EXPECT

APPROPRIATE HEALTH CARE
• Doctor's examination and treatment.
• Emergency room care.
• Repair of facial bones that affect the orbit.

DIAGNOSTIC MEASURES
• Your own observation of symptoms.
• Medical history and physical exam by a doctor, usually an ophthalmologist (eye specialist) or a surgeon specializing in facial injury.
• Vision examination.
• X-rays of the skull to detect possible fractures.

POSSIBLE COMPLICATIONS
• Infection, especially when an imbedded foreign body is not completely removed from the cornea.
• Permanent (sometimes total) loss of vision if infection penetrates the eyeball from the cornea.
• Bleeding into the eye as a result of a blunt injury.
• Scarring if eyelid lacerations are unattended.

PROBABLE OUTCOME
• Cornea injury with infection—This serious eye problem is usually curable in 2 to 3 weeks with special care from an ophthalmologist.
• Eyelid injury—Eyelid lacerations usually heal in 1 to 2 weeks if they are carefully closed surgically. Sutures are usually removed in 7 to 10 days.
• Orbit (bone) injury—Facial surgery by a cosmetic surgeon usually improves appearance. Bones require 6 to 8 weeks to heal.
• Injury due to foreign body—This type of injury heals easily if the foreign body is removed and antibiotic medication is used to fight infection.

 HOW TO TREAT

NOTE—Follow your doctor's instructions. These instructions are supplemental.

FIRST AID
• Don't try to remove contact lens.
• Don't rub or wash the eye.
• Cover both eyes with loose cloth pads. The eyes move together, so both eyes must be covered to prevent movement of the injured eye.
• Apply crushed ice in a soft cloth bag or a towel—not a heavy ice bag.
• Avoid any pressure on the eye. Bleeding from an eyelid is usually inconsequential, but pressure can cause further damage.
• Keep the injured person in a partial reclining position while en route to an emergency facility.

CONTINUING CARE
After emergency treatment:
• Protect eyes from bright light or sunlight by wearing dark glasses.
• Use ice packs or warm moist compresses to relieve discomfort. Prepare a compress by folding a clean cloth in several layers. Dip in warm water, wring out slightly and apply to the eye. Dip the compress often to keep it moist. Apply the compress for an hour, rest an hour and repeat.
• Sleep with the head elevated with 2 pillows until symptoms subside.
• Don't rub the eye.
For a laceration after suturing:
• Keep the wound dry and covered for 48 hours.
• If you change the bandage, apply a small amount of petroleum jelly or nonprescription antibiotic ointment to the bandage.
• After 48 hours, replace the bandage if it gets wet.
• Ignore small amounts of bleeding. Control heavier bleeding by firmly pressing a facial tissues or clean cloth to the bleeding spot, avoiding pressure on the eyeball itself.

MEDICATION—Your doctor may prescribe:
• Antibiotic eye drops or ointment to prevent infection.
• Pain relievers.
• Local anesthetic eye drops or drops to dilate the pupil and rest the eye muscle.

ACTIVITY—Resume your normal activities gradually after treatment.

DIET—Eat a well-balanced diet.

REHABILITATION—Rehabilitation exercises must be individualized. Follow your doctor's or surgeon's directions.

 CALL YOUR DOCTOR IF

• You have a foreign body in your eye.
• You have a cut or other eye injury.
• The following occur during or after treatment:
Pain increases or does not disappear in 2 days.
Your vision changes.
You cannot move the eye up and down normally.
You have a fever of 101°F (38.3°C).
You experience pain that is not relieved by acetaminophen.
New, unexplained symptoms develop. Drugs used in treatment may produce side effects.

FACE CONTUSION

GENERAL INFORMATION

DEFINITION—Bruising of skin and underlying tissues of the face caused by a direct blow. Contusions cause bleeding from ruptured small capillaries that allow blood to infiltrate muscles, tendons or other soft tissues. The face is particularly vulnerable to contusions because the skin is so close to hard underlying bone. (Note: Contusions and other injuries of the eyes, nose and ears require special consideration and care. They are addressed separately in this book.)

BODY PARTS INVOLVED—Face tissues, including blood vessels, muscles, tendons, nerves, covering of bone (periosteum) and connective tissues.

SIGNS & SYMPTOMS
* Local swelling at the contusion site. The swelling may be round or egg-shaped, superficial or deep.
* Pain and tenderness over the injury.
* Feeling of firmness when pressure is exerted on the injured area.
* Discoloration under the skin, beginning with redness and progressing to the characteristic "black-and-blue" bruise.

CAUSES—Direct blow to the skin, usually from a blunt object.

RISK INCREASES WITH
* Violent contact sports such as boxing or hockey, especially if the face is not adequately protected. Also common in baseball and fencing.
* Racquet sports.
* Medical history of any bleeding disorder.
* Poor nutrition, including vitamin deficiency.
* Use of anticoagulants or aspirin.

HOW TO PREVENT—Wear an appropriate face mask during competition or other athletic activity if a face contusion is likely.

WHAT TO EXPECT

APPROPRIATE HEALTH CARE
* Doctor's care unless the contusion is quite small.
* Self-care for minor contusions.

DIAGNOSTIC MEASURES
* Your own observation of symptoms.
* Medical history and physical exam by a doctor for all except minor injuries.
* X-ray of the facial area to rule out the possibility of underlying fracture. The total extent of injury may not be apparent for 48 to 72 hours.

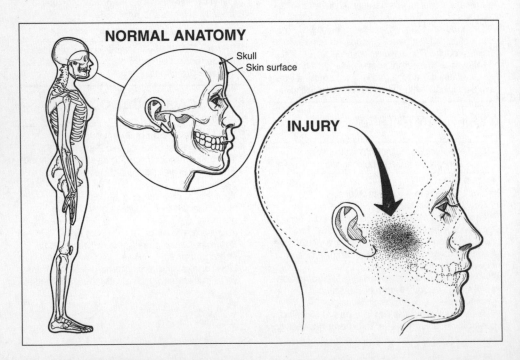

NORMAL ANATOMY

Skull
Skin surface

INJURY

POSSIBLE COMPLICATIONS
• Excessive bleeding. Infiltrative-type bleeding can (rarely) lead to calcification, impaired function and facial disfiguration.
• Prolonged healing time if usual activities are resumed too soon.
• Infection if skin over the contusion is broken.

PROBABLE OUTCOME—Healing time varies with the extent of injury, but all but the most serious face contusions should heal in 6 to 10 days.

 HOW TO TREAT

NOTE—Follow your doctor's instructions. These instructions are supplemental.

FIRST AID—Use instructions for R.I.C.E., the first letters of *rest, ice, compression* and *elevation*. See Appendix 1 for details.

CONTINUING CARE
• Use an ice pack 3 or 4 times a day. Wrap ice chips or cubes in a plastic bag, and wrap the bag in a moist towel. Place it over the injured area for 20 minutes at time.
• After 72 hours, apply heat instead of ice if it feels better. Use heat lamps, hot soaks, hot showers, heating pads or heat liniments and ointments.
• Massage gently and often to provide comfort and decrease swelling.

MEDICATION
• For minor discomfort, you may use: Acetaminophen or ibuprofen.
Topical liniments and ointments.
• Your doctor may prescribe stronger medicine for pain.

ACTIVITY—Begin activities slowly, and stop exercise as soon as pain begins. Increase activity as healing progresses.

DIET—During recovery, balance the amount of food you eat with any change in your level of physical activity. Eat a variety of foods to get the energy, protein, vitamins, minerals and fiber you need for good health and healing.

REHABILITATION—Rehabilitation exercises must be individualized. Follow your doctor's or surgeon's directions.

 CALL YOUR DOCTOR IF

• You have a face contusion that doesn't improve in 1 or 2 days.
• Skin is broken and signs of infection (drainage, increasing pain, fever, headache, muscle aches, dizziness or a general ill feeling) occur.

FACIAL BONE FRACTURE

GENERAL INFORMATION

DEFINITION—A complete or incomplete break in one or several bones in the face.

BODY PARTS INVOLVED
• Facial bones—upper jaw (maxilla), cheek bones (malar bones) and other bones that form the eye sockets (orbits) and nose. See also Jaw Fracture.
• Teeth.
• Joints between bones listed above.
• Eyes and nose.
• Soft tissues around the fracture site, including nerves, tendons, ligaments, periosteum (covering of bone), blood vessels and connective tissues.

SIGNS & SYMPTOMS
• Severe pain at the injury site.
• Swelling and bruising of soft tissues around the fracture, including black eye(s).
• Visible deformity if the fracture is complete and bone fragments separate enough to distort normal facial contours.
• Tenderness to the touch.
• Numbness around the fracture site.
• Bleeding from the nose or eye(s).

CAUSES—Direct blow to the face.

RISK INCREASES WITH
• Contact sports, especially boxing, wrestling and baseball.

• Cycling.
• Poor nutrition, especially calcium deficiency.
• If surgery or anesthesia is needed, risk increases with smoking and use of drugs, including mind-altering drugs, muscle relaxants, antihypertensives, tranquilizers, sleep inducers, insulin, sedatives, beta-adrenergic blockers or corticosteroids.

HOW TO PREVENT—Wear protective face masks and headgear when cycling or competing in contact sports. The use of protective equipment has significantly decreased the incidence of facial fractures.

WHAT TO EXPECT

APPROPRIATE HEALTH CARE
• Doctor's treatment. A plastic surgeon, oral surgeon, ophthalmologist or ear, nose and throat specialist may be consulted.
• Surgery (sometimes) to realign fractured bones and reconstruct normal facial contours.
• Self-care during rehabilitation.

DIAGNOSTIC MEASURES
• Your own observation of symptoms.
• Medical history and physical exam by a doctor.
• X-rays of the skull and facial bones.
• Laboratory studies to measure blood loss.
• CT scan (see Glossary) to rule out brain injury.
• Vision examination.

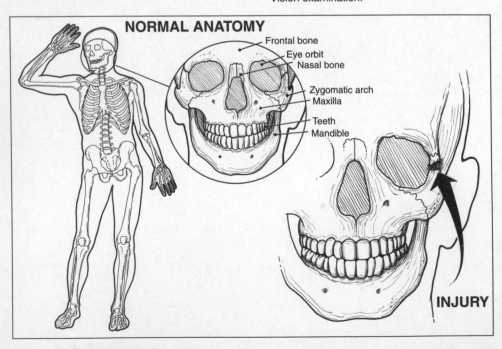

NORMAL ANATOMY

Frontal bone
Eye orbit
Nasal bone
Zygomatic arch
Maxilla
Teeth
Mandible

INJURY

POSSIBLE COMPLICATIONS
At the time of fracture:
- Shock.
- Pressure on or injury to eyes, nose, nearby nerves, ligaments, tendons, blood vessels or connective tissues.
- Breathing obstruction.

After treatment or surgery:
- Excessive bleeding.
- Impaired blood supply to the healing bone.
- Avascular necrosis (death of bone cells due to interruption of the blood supply).
- Infection introduced during surgical treatment.
- Unstable or arthritic jaw or neck joints following repeated injury.
- Malocclusion—improper bite due to displacement of teeth or jaws.

PROBABLE OUTCOME
- Surgery usually restores normal features and facial function.
- Teeth that have been knocked out can sometimes be replanted (see Tooth Injury & Loss, page 356). Speech will be changed while the wires are in place, but it should return to normal when they are removed.
- Normal vision should return if the eye is not injured.
- Recovery usually takes about 6 weeks. Healing is considered complete when there is no pain at the fractured site and when x-rays show complete bone union.

 HOW TO TREAT

NOTE—Follow your doctor's instructions. These instructions are supplemental.

FIRST AID
- If the victim is wearing a face mask, cut it away.
- Check for excessive bleeding and swelling that may cause breathing obstruction. If the victim is not breathing, administer cardiopulmonary resuscitation (CPR).
- Apply ice packs to the face to decrease swelling and pain.
- Elevate the upper body so the face is above the level of the heart. This reduces swelling and prevents accumulation of excess fluid. Use pillows to prop the head if you are sure there is no neck injury.
- Keep the person warm with blankets to decrease the possibility of shock.

CONTINUING CARE
Soon after injury:
- A broken jaw is frequently corrected by securing the teeth with wire or plastic splints so the jaw will heal in its proper position.
- Surgery is frequently necessary to realign facial bones and restore a normal appearance. Plates and screws are sometimes used. For best results, it should be done as soon as possible after injury.

During convalescence:
- Don't exercise to the point that you must pant for breath, because breathing may be difficult for a while.
- Protect the face from pressure. Sleep on your back.
- Don't blow your nose hard or use makeup until healing is complete.
- If your jaws are wired, learn how to release them quickly in case of emergency, such as severe coughing or vomiting.

MEDICATION—Your doctor may prescribe:
- Pain relievers.
- Antibiotics to fight infection if necessary.

ACTIVITY—Rest quietly for about 2 days, then resume your normal activities as strength returns.

DIET
- Do not eat or drink before manipulation or surgery to treat the fracture. Fluid or solid food in your stomach makes vomiting while under anesthesia more hazardous.
- You may need a liquid diet for several days. If your jaw is wired, an ongoing liquid diet will be necessary for up to 8 weeks. Add soft solid foods as you are able.

REHABILITATION—None.

 CALL YOUR DOCTOR IF

- You or someone else has signs or symptoms of a facial bone fracture.
- The following occur after treatment:
  Fever.
  Impaired or double vision.
  Severe headache.
  Loss of sensation in the face.
  Intolerable pain.
  Upper respiratory illness of any kind during healing. This increases the danger of infection.
  Loosening of wires or splints.
  New, unexplained symptoms. Drugs used in treatment may produce side effects.

FINGER DISLOCATION

GENERAL INFORMATION

DEFINITION—Injury to any finger joint so that adjoining bones are displaced from their normal positions and no longer touch each other. Fractures and ligament sprains frequently accompany this dislocation. Finger dislocations are a common problem for athletes.

BODY PARTS INVOLVED
- Any of the many finger bones.
- Ligaments that hold finger bones in place.
- Soft tissues surrounding the dislocation site, including periosteum (covering of bone), nerves, tendons, blood vessels and connective tissues.

SIGNS & SYMPTOMS
- Excruciating pain in the finger at the time of injury.
- Loss of function in the dislocated joint.
- Severe pain when attempting to move the injured finger.
- Visible deformity if the dislocated finger has locked in the dislocated position. Bones may spontaneously reposition themselves and leave no deformity, but damage is the same.
- Tenderness over the dislocation.
- Swelling and bruising at the injury site.
- Numbness or paralysis beyond the dislocation from pinching, cutting or pressure on blood vessels or nerves.

CAUSES
- Direct or indirect blow to the hand, finger or thumb.
- End result of a severe finger sprain.
- Congenital abnormality, such as a shallow or malformed joint surface.

RISK INCREASES WITH
- Contact sports, especially basketball, baseball and soccer.
- Previous finger or hand dislocation or sprain.
- Repeated injury to any part of the hand.
- Poor muscle conditioning in the hand.

HOW TO PREVENT
- To prevent a recurrence, protect vulnerable joints after healing with protective devices or tape.
- Develop a high level of muscle strength and conditioning, including the hand area.

WHAT TO EXPECT

APPROPRIATE HEALTH CARE
- Doctor's treatment. This will include manipulating the joint to reposition the bones.
- Surgery (sometimes) to restore the joint to its normal position and repair torn ligaments and tendons. Acute or recurring dislocations may require surgical reconstruction.
- Self-care during rehabilitation.

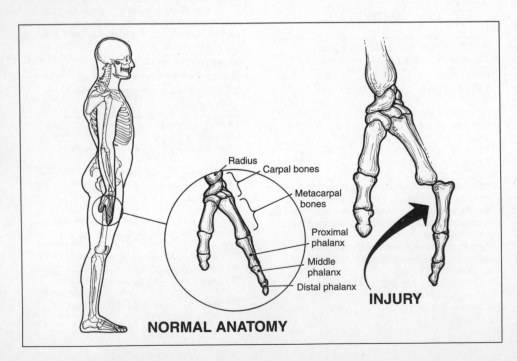

Radius
Carpal bones
Metacarpal bones
Proximal phalanx
Middle phalanx
Distal phalanx

INJURY

NORMAL ANATOMY

DIAGNOSTIC MEASURES
- Your own observation of symptoms.
- Medical history and exam by a doctor.
- X-rays of the hand and wrist.

POSSIBLE COMPLICATIONS
At the time of injury:
- Shock.
- Pressure on or injury to nearby nerves, ligaments, tendons, muscles, blood vessels and connective tissues.

After treatment or surgery:
- Impaired blood supply to the dislocated area.
- Death of bone cells due to interruption of the blood supply (avascular necrosis).
- Infection introduced during surgical treatment.
- Excessive bleeding around the dislocation site.
- Continuing recurrent dislocations with progressively less severe injuries (rare).
- Prolonged healing if activity is resumed too soon.
- Permanent limitation of range of motion.
- Unstable or arthritic joint following repeated injury or surgery.

PROBABLE OUTCOME—After the dislocation has been corrected, the hand may require immobilization with a cast or splint for 2 to 3 weeks. Complete healing of injured ligaments requires a minimum of 6 weeks. However, swelling may require 3 to 6 months to resolve.

 HOW TO TREAT

NOTE—Follow your doctor's instructions. These instructions are supplemental.

FIRST AID
- Use instructions for R.I.C.E., the first letters of *rest, ice, compression* and *elevation*. See Appendix 1 for details.
- The doctor will manipulate the dislocated finger to return bones to their normal positions. Manipulation should be done within 6 hours of injury. If not, many tissues lose their elasticity and become difficult to return to their normal positions.

CONTINUING CARE—After removal of the splint or cast:
- Use ice soaks 3 or 4 times a day. Fill a bucket with ice water, and soak the injured area for 20 minutes at a time.
- Apply heat if it feels better. Use heat lamps, hot soaks, hot showers, heating pads or heat liniments and ointments.
- Tape the injured finger to adjacent fingers.
- Massage gently and often to provide comfort and decrease swelling.

MEDICATION—Your doctor may prescribe:
- General anesthesia or local anesthesia to make joint manipulation possible.
- Acetaminophen or aspirin to relieve moderate pain.
- Pain relievers for severe pain.
- Antibiotics to fight infection if surgery is necessary.

ACTIVITY
- If surgery is not necessary, activity is not restricted except for limitations imposed by immobilization of the hand.
- If surgery is necessary, resume normal activities and reconditioning.

DIET
- Do not eat or drink before manipulation or surgery to correct the dislocation. Fluid or solid food in your stomach makes vomiting while under general anesthesia more hazardous.
- During recovery, balance the amount of food you eat with any change in your level of physical activity. Eat a variety of foods to get the energy, protein, vitamins, minerals and fiber you need for good health and healing.

REHABILITATION
- Begin daily rehabilitation exercises when supportive wrapping is no longer needed.
- Use ice massage for 10 minutes before and after workouts. Fill a large styrofoam cup with water and freeze. Tear a small amount of foam from the top so ice protrudes. Massage firmly over the injured area in a circle about the size of a softball.
- Rehabilitation exercises must be individualized. Follow your doctor's or surgeon's directions.

 CALL YOUR DOCTOR IF

- You have signs or symptoms of a dislocated finger.
- Any of the following occurs after treatment: Numbness, paleness or coldness in the finger. This is an emergency!
  Swelling above or below the splint or cast. Blue or gray skin color, particularly under the fingernails.
- Any of the following occurs after surgery: Increased pain, swelling or drainage in the surgical area.
  Signs of infection (headache, muscle aches, dizziness or a general ill feeling and fever).
- New, unexplained symptoms develop. Drugs used in treatment may produce side effects.
- Finger dislocations that you can "pop" back into normal position occur repeatedly.

FINGER FRACTURE

GENERAL INFORMATION

DEFINITION—A complete or incomplete break in a finger bone.

BODY PARTS INVOLVED
- Any of the bones of a finger, but usually the bone closest to the hand.
- Any of the joints of the fingers or the joints between the fingers and the hand.
- Soft tissues surrounding the fracture site, including nerves, tendons, ligaments and blood vessels.

SIGNS & SYMPTOMS
- Severe pain at the fracture site.
- Swelling of soft tissues surrounding the fracture.
- Visible deformity if the fracture is complete and bone fragments separate enough to distort normal finger contours.
- Tenderness to the touch.
- Numb or cold finger or fingertip if the blood supply is impaired.

CAUSES—Direct blow to or indirect stress on the finger bones.

RISK INCREASES WITH
- Dislocation of a finger joint or of a joint between the finger and hand.
- Contact sports such as boxing or baseball.
- History of bone or joint disease, especially osteoporosis.
- Poor nutrition, especially calcium deficiency.

- If surgery or anesthesia is needed, risk increases with smoking and use of drugs, including mind-altering drugs, muscle relaxants, antihypertensives, tranquilizers, sleep inducers, insulin, sedatives, beta-adrenergic blockers or corticosteroids.

HOW TO PREVENT—It you have had a previous finger injury, use tape or padding to protect the finger when participating in contact sports.

WHAT TO EXPECT

APPROPRIATE HEALTH CARE
- Doctor's treatment to manipulate the broken bones.
- Anesthesia and surgery to set the fracture.
- Self-care during rehabilitation.
- Whirlpool, ultrasound or massage (to displace excess fluid from the injured joint space).

DIAGNOSTIC MEASURES
- Your own observation of symptoms.
- Medical history and physical exam by a doctor.
- X-rays of injured areas, including joints above and below the primary injury site.

POSSIBLE COMPLICATIONS
- Pressure on or injury to nearby nerves, ligaments, tendons, muscles, blood vessels or connective tissues.
- Delayed union or nonunion of the fracture.

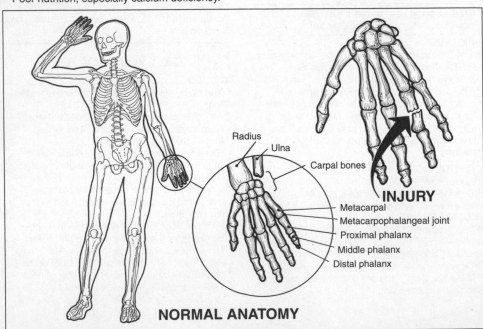

Radius
Ulna
Carpal bones
INJURY
Metacarpal
Metacarpophalangeal joint
Proximal phalanx
Middle phalanx
Distal phalanx

NORMAL ANATOMY

- Impaired blood supply to the fracture site.
- Avascular necrosis (death of bone cells due to interruption of the blood supply).
- Arrest of normal bone growth in children.
- Infection in open fractures (skin broken over fracture site) or at the incision if surgical setting was necessary.
- Shortening of the injured bones.
- Unstable or arthritic joint following repeated injury.
- Prolonged healing time if activity is resumed too soon.
- Weakness or stiffness of finger joints, which results in weakened grip strength.

PROBABLE OUTCOME—It is impossible to predict exactly how long it will take for any fracture to heal. Variable factors include age, sex and previous state of health and conditioning. The average healing time for this fracture is 4 to 6 weeks. Healing is considered complete when there is no motion at the fracture site and when x-rays show complete bone union.

 ## HOW TO TREAT

NOTE—Follow your doctor's instructions. These instructions are supplemental.

FIRST AID
- Use a padded splint or sling to immobilize the hand and wrist before transporting the injured person to the doctor's office or emergency facility.
- Use instructions for R.I.C.E., the first letters of *rest, ice, compression* and *elevation*. See Appendix 1 for details.
- The doctor will realign and set the broken bones either with surgery or, if possible, without. Manipulation should be done as soon as possible after injury. Also, many tissues lose their elasticity and become difficult to return to their normal positions.

CONTINUING CARE
- Immobilization will be necessary. A splint is placed on the injured finger, extending beyond the finger-hand joint.
- After 96 hours, application of localized heat promotes healing by increasing blood circulation in the injured area. Use a heating pad or heat lamp.
- After the splint is removed, use ice soaks 3 or 4 times a day. Fill a bucket with ice water, and soak the injured area for 20 minutes at a time.

- Apply heat instead of ice if it feels better. Use heat lamps, hot soaks, hot showers, heating pads or heat liniments and ointments.
- Take whirlpool treatments, if available.

MEDICATION—Your doctor may prescribe:
- General anesthesia, local anesthesia or muscle relaxants to make bone manipulation possible.
- Prescription pain relievers for severe pain.
- Acetaminophen (available without prescription) for mild pain after initial treatment.

ACTIVITY
- Actively exercise all muscle groups not immobilized. Muscle contractions in the hand and arm promote fracture alignment and hasten healing.
- Resume normal activities gradually after treatment.
- Begin reconditioning the injured area after clearance from your doctor.

DIET
- Do not eat or drink before manipulation or surgery to treat the fracture. Fluid or solid food in your stomach makes vomiting while under anesthesia more hazardous.
- During recovery, balance the amount of food you eat with any change in your level of physical activity. Eat a variety of foods to get the energy, protein, vitamins, minerals and fiber you need for good health and healing.

REHABILITATION
- Begin daily rehabilitation exercises when movement is comfortable. Use ice soaks for 10 minutes prior to exercise.
- See Rehabilitation section for wrist and hand exercises.

 ## CALL YOUR DOCTOR IF

- You have signs or symptoms of a finger fracture.
- Any of the following occurs after surgery or other treatment:
    Increased pain, swelling or drainage in the surgical area.
    Signs of infection (headache, muscle aches, dizziness or a general ill feeling and fever).
    Nausea or vomiting.
    Swelling or irritation above or below the splint.
    Blue or gray skin color beyond the splint, particularly in the fingertip or under the fingernail.
    Numbness or complete loss of feeling in the injured finger.

FINGER SPRAIN

GENERAL INFORMATION

DEFINITION—Violent overstretching of one or more ligaments that hold the finger joints together. Sprains involving two or more ligaments cause considerably more disability than single-ligament sprains. When the ligament is overstretched, it becomes tense and gives way at its weakest point, either where it attaches to bone or within the ligament itself. There are 3 types of sprains:
- Mild (Grade I)—Tearing of some ligament fibers. There is no loss of function.
- Moderate (Grade II)—Rupture of a portion of the ligament, resulting in some loss of function.
- Severe (Grade III)—Complete rupture of the ligament or complete separation of ligament from bone. There is total loss of function. A severe sprain may require surgical repair.

BODY PARTS INVOLVED
- Ligaments holding the joints of the fingers together.
- Tissues surrounding the sprain, including blood vessels, tendons, bone, periosteum (covering of bone) and muscles.

SIGNS & SYMPTOMS
- Severe pain at the time of injury.
- A feeling of popping or tearing inside a finger or fingers.
- Tenderness at the injury site.
- Swelling in the finger.
- Bruising that appears soon after injury.

CAUSES—Stress on a ligament that temporarily forces or pries finger joints out of their normal location. Finger sprains occur frequently in football, baseball, basketball and other exercises or sports activities.

RISK INCREASES WITH
- Contact sports, especially "catching" and "throwing" sports.
- Previous hand injury.
- Poor muscle conditioning.
- Inadequate protection from equipment.

HOW TO PREVENT—Tape vulnerable joints before athletic practice or competition.

WHAT TO EXPECT

APPROPRIATE HEALTH CARE
- Doctor's diagnosis.
- Application of a splint, tape or elastic bandage.
- Self-care during rehabilitation.
- Physical therapy (moderate or severe sprain).
- Surgery (severe sprain).

DIAGNOSTIC MEASURES
- Your own observations of symptoms.
- Medical history and exam by a doctor.
- X-rays of the hand and wrist to rule out fractures. Also, stress x-rays to demonstrate ligament looseness.

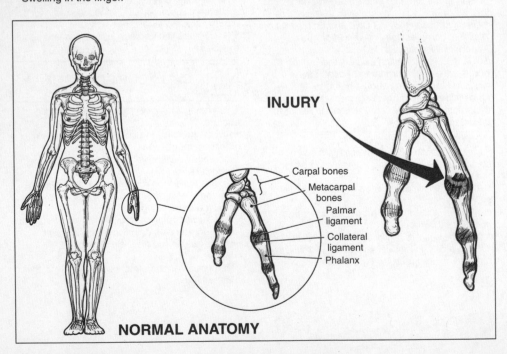

INJURY

Carpal bones
Metacarpal bones
Palmar ligament
Collateral ligament
Phalanx

NORMAL ANATOMY

POSSIBLE COMPLICATIONS
- Prolonged healing time if usual activities are resumed too soon.
- Proneness to repeated finger injury.
- Inflammation at the ligament attachment to bone (periostitis).
- Prolonged disability (sometimes).
- Unstable or arthritic finger following repeated injury.

PROBABLE OUTCOME—If this is a first-time injury, proper care and sufficient healing time before resuming activity should prevent permanent disability. Ligaments have a poor blood supply, and torn ligaments require as much healing time as fractures. Average healing times are:
- Mild sprains—2 to 6 weeks.
- Moderate sprains—6 to 8 weeks.
- Severe sprains—8 to 10 weeks.

Swelling around finger sprains may require 3 to 6 months to resolve.

 HOW TO TREAT

NOTE—Follow your doctor's instructions. These instructions are supplemental.

FIRST AID—Use instructions for R.I.C.E., the first letters of *rest, ice, compression* and *elevation*. See Appendix 1 for details.

CONTINUING CARE—If the doctor does not apply a splint, tape or elastic bandage:
- Continue using an ice pack 3 or 4 times a day. Put ice chips or cubes in a plastic bag. Wrap the bag in a moist towel, and place it over the injured area. Use for 20 minutes at a time.
- After 72 hours, apply heat instead of ice if it feels better. Use heat lamps, hot soaks, hot showers, heating pads or heat liniments and ointments.
- Take whirlpool treatments, if available.
- Massage gently and often to provide comfort and decrease swelling.

MEDICATION
- For minor discomfort, you may use:
Aspirin, acetaminophen or ibuprofen.
Topical liniments and ointments.
- Your doctor may prescribe:
Stronger pain relievers.
Injection of a long-acting local anesthetic to reduce pain.
Injections of a corticosteroid, such as triamcinolone, to reduce inflammation.

ACTIVITY—Resume your normal activities gradually after clearance from your doctor.

DIET—During recovery, balance the amount of food you eat with any change in your level of physical activity. Eat a variety of foods to get the energy, protein, vitamins, minerals and fiber you need for good health and healing.

REHABILITATION
- Begin daily rehabilitation exercises when the splint or supportive wrapping is no longer necessary.
- Use ice soaks 3 or 4 times a day. Fill a bucket with ice water, and soak the injured area for 20 minutes at a time.
- See Rehabilitation section for wrist and hand exercises.

 CALL YOUR DOCTOR IF

- You have symptoms of a moderate or severe finger sprain or a mild sprain persists longer than 2 weeks.
- Pain, swelling or bruising worsens despite treatment.
- Any of the following occurs after splinting:
Pain, numbness or coldness in the finger.
Blue, gray or dusky fingernail.
- Any of the following occurs after surgery:
Increased pain, swelling, redness, drainage or bleeding in the surgical area.
Signs of infection (headache, muscle aches, dizziness or a general ill feeling with fever).
- New, unexplained symptoms develop. Drugs used in treatment may produce side effects.

FINGERTIP INJURY

GENERAL INFORMATION

DEFINITION—Fingertip injuries include:
* Contusion or bruise with hemorrhage under the fingernail or in the tip of the finger.
* Lacerated fingernail.
* Avulsion injury (tearing away of part of the fingertip).

BODY PARTS INVOLVED
* Last phalanx (section of bone) of any finger or thumb.
* Skin on finger.
* Fingernail.
* Blood vessels, nerves, tendons, ligaments, subcutaneous tissues and connective tissues.

SIGNS & SYMPTOMS—Fingertip injuries may include any of these signs:
* Pain in the fingertip.
* Torn fingernail.
* Jagged cut in the tip of the finger.
* Tearing away (avulsion) of a part of the fingertip.
* Crushed or broken bone in the fingertip.
* Numbness if the nerve is damaged.
* Bleeding under the fingernail or external bleeding.
* Swelling of the fingertip.
* Bruising of the injured finger.

CAUSES
* Direct violence to the fingertip.
* Crushing blow to the fingertip.
* Jamming of the fingertip, as happens when catching balls.

RISK INCREASES WITH
* Contact sports such as football or baseball.
* Sports involving bats or balls moving at high speed.

HOW TO PREVENT—No preventive measures.

WHAT TO EXPECT

APPROPRIATE HEALTH CARE
* Self-care for mild injury.
* Doctor's treatment for serious injury.

DIAGNOSTIC MEASURES
* Your own observation of symptoms.
* Description of circumstances of injury to a doctor for serious injuries.
* Physical exam by doctor to establish a diagnosis. Your doctor will need a description of the circumstances of injury.
* X-rays of the hand to disclose the extent of injury and to rule out fractures.

POSSIBLE COMPLICATIONS
* Excessive bleeding.
* Loss of function in the fingertip from damage to tissues, the fingernail, nerve endings or bone.

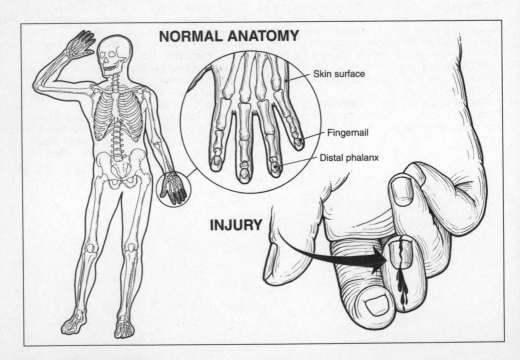

NORMAL ANATOMY

Skin surface

Fingernail

Distal phalanx

INJURY

- Arthritic changes in any finger joint injured simultaneously.
- Prolonged disability if the injured finger is used before healing is complete.
- Inflammation at the tendon's attachment to bone (periostitis).

PROBABLE OUTCOME
- Contusions—Complete healing in 2 to 3 weeks.
- Lacerated fingernail—Injured nail usually requires surgical removal in a hospital or hospital outpatient facility. Expect complete healing in about 3 weeks if no complications occur. The nail will regrow in a period of months if the nail bed is not damaged.
- Avulsion injury—Sometimes requires surgical repair or skin grafting. Frequently will heal by secondary intention (wound may close on its own) with dressing changes. Allow 6 weeks for healing.

 ## HOW TO TREAT

NOTE—Follow your doctor's instructions. These instructions are supplemental.

FIRST AID—Use instructions for R.I.C.E., the first letters of *rest, ice, compression* and *elevation.* See Appendix 1 for details.

CONTINUING CARE:
Care after surgery to repair a damaged fingertip:
- Keep the hand elevated to relieve pain and throbbing.
- Change bandages frequently. Keep bandages dry between baths. If the bandage gets wet, change it promptly.
If a cast is required:
- Do not allow pressure on any part of the cast until it is completely dry. Drying times vary depending on the thickness of the cast, temperature and humidity.

- If the cast gets wet and a soft area appears, return to your doctor's office to have it repaired.
- Whenever possible, raise the hand. Propping on pillows will keep swelling and discomfort at a minimum.

MEDICATION—Your doctor may prescribe:
- Prescription pain relievers for severe pain.
- Antibiotics to fight infection.
- You may use nonprescription drugs such as acetaminophen for minor pain.

ACTIVITY
- Resume work and normal activity as soon as possible.
- Avoid vigorous exercise for 6 weeks following surgery.

DIET—During recovery, balance the amount of food you eat with any change in your level of physical activity. Eat a variety of foods to get the energy, protein, vitamins, minerals and fiber you need for good health and healing.

REHABILITATION—See Rehabilitation section for wrist and hand exercises.

 ## CALL YOUR DOCTOR IF

Any of the following occurs:
- Severe, persistent pain under the cast.
- Color change, coldness or numbness in tissues beyond the cast.
- Tissues swelling greater than before the cast was applied.
- Signs of infection (headache, muscle aches, dizziness or a general ill feeling and fever).
- Pain, swelling, redness, drainage or bleeding in the surgical area.
- New, unexplained symptoms develop. Drugs used in treatment may produce side effects.

FOOT BURSITIS

GENERAL INFORMATION

DEFINITION—Inflammation of one of the bursas in the foot. Bursitis may vary in degree, from mild irritation to an abscess formation that causes excruciating pain. The most significant bursas are about the Achilles tendon and the heel bone. Another common site is next to the base of the big toe.

BODY PARTS INVOLVED
- Foot bursas (soft sacs filled with lubricating fluid that facilitate motion in the foot).
- Soft tissues surrounding the joints in the foot, including nerves, tendons, ligaments, blood vessels (both large vessels and capillaries), periosteum (the outside lining of bone) and muscles.

SIGNS AND SYMPTOMS
- Pain.
- Tenderness.
- Swelling.
- Redness (sometimes) over the affected bursa.
- Fever if infection is present.
- Restriction of motion of the foot.

CAUSES
- Direct blow or other injury to a foot joint.
- Acute or chronic infection.
- Arthritis.
- Gout.
- Chronic pressure over bony prominences and bursas due to footwear.
- Unknown (frequently).

RISK INCREASES WITH
- Participating in competitive athletics, particularly contact sports such as football, soccer or hockey.
- Previous history of bursitis in any joint.
- Exposure to cold weather.
- Poor conditioning and inadequate warmup.
- Inadequate protective equipment in contact sports.
- Ill-fitting footwear.

HOW TO PREVENT
- Wear well-fitting athletic shoes for contact sports.
- Warm up adequately before athletic practice or competition.
- Wear warm socks in cold weather.
- To prevent recurrence, continue to wear extra protection over the involved bursa in the foot.

WHAT TO EXPECT

APPROPRIATE HEALTH CARE
- Doctor's diagnosis and treatment.
- Surgery (sometimes), particularly for a frozen foot joint or chronic pain.

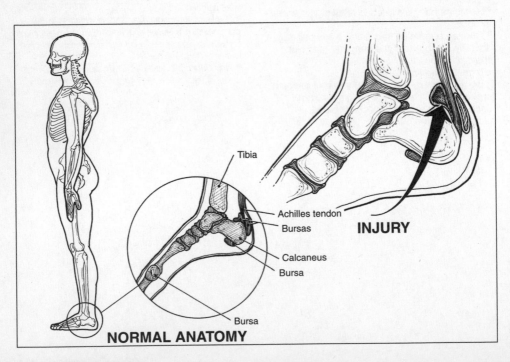

Tibia

Achilles tendon

Bursas

Calcaneus

Bursa

INJURY

Bursa

NORMAL ANATOMY

DIAGNOSTIC MEASURES
- Your own observation of symptoms.
- Medical history and physical exam by a doctor.
- X-rays of the foot and ankle.

POSSIBLE COMPLICATIONS
- Permanent limitation of the joint's normal mobility.
- Prolonged healing time if activity is resumed too soon.
- Proneness to repeated flare-ups.
- Potential Achilles tendon rupture.
- Spontaneous rupture of the bursa if severe infection is present.

PROBABLE OUTCOME—Foot bursitis is a common—but usually not serious—problem. Symptoms usually subside in 7 to 14 days with treatment if there is no infection present. Infection or the need for surgery may dictate 6 to 8 weeks to heal.

 HOW TO TREAT

NOTE—Follow your doctor's instructions. These instructions are supplemental.

FIRST AID—None. This problem develops slowly.

CONTINUING CARE
- Use frequent ice massage. Fill a large styrofoam cup with water and freeze. Tear a small amount of foam from the top so ice protrudes. Massage firmly over the injured area in a circle about the size of a softball. Do this for 15 minutes at a time 3 or 4 times a day, and also before workouts or competition.
- After 72 hours, apply heat instead of ice if it feels better. Use heat lamps, hot soaks, hot showers, heating pads or heat liniments and ointments.
- Take whirlpool treatments, if available.
- Use crutches to prevent weight-bearing, if needed.

- Elevate the foot above the level of the heart to reduce swelling and prevent accumulation of fluid. Use pillows for propping, or elevate the foot of the bed.
- Gentle massage will frequently provide comfort and decrease swelling.

MEDICATION—Your doctor may prescribe:
- Nonsteroidal anti-inflammatory drugs or creams.
- Antibiotics if the bursa is infected.
- Prescription pain relievers for severe pain. Use nonprescription acetaminophen or ibuprofen for mild pain.
- Injection with a long-lasting local anesthetic mixed with a corticosteroid drug, such as triamcinolone.

ACTIVITY—Rest the inflamed area as much as possible. If you must resume normal activity immediately, use crutches until the pain becomes more bearable. To prevent a frozen joint, begin normal, slow joint movement as soon as possible.

DIET—During recovery, balance the amount of food you eat with any change in your level of physical activity. Eat a variety of foods to get the energy, protein, vitamins, minerals and fiber you need for good health and healing. Your doctor may suggest vitamin and mineral supplements to promote healing.

REHABILITATION—See Rehabilitation section for ankle and foot exercises.

 CALL YOUR DOCTOR IF

- You have symptoms of foot bursitis.
- Pain increases, despite treatment.
- Pain, swelling, tenderness, drainage or bleeding increases in the surgical area.
- You develop signs of infection (headache, muscle aches, dizziness or a general ill feeling and fever).
- New, unexplained symptoms develop. Drugs used in treatment may produce side effects.

FOOT CONTUSION

GENERAL INFORMATION

DEFINITION—Bruising of the skin and underlying tissues of the foot caused by a direct blow. Contusions cause bleeding from ruptured small capillaries that allow blood to infiltrate muscles, tendons or other soft tissues.

BODY PARTS INVOLVED—Foot tissues including blood vessels, muscles, tendons, nerves, covering of bone (periosteum) and connective tissues.

SIGNS AND SYMPTOMS
- Local swelling—either superficial or deep.
- Pain and tenderness over the injury.
- Feeling of firmness when pressure is exerted at the injury site.
- Discoloration under the skin, beginning with redness and progressing to the characteristic "black-and-blue" bruise.
- Restricted foot activity proportional to the extent of injury.

CAUSES
- Direct blow to the foot, usually from a blunt object.
- Wearing a shoe that has faulty cleats or spikes or wearing a wrinkled sock. This will cause a "stone bruise."

RISK INCREASES WITH
- Contact sports such as football, basketball or baseball, especially if the foot is not adequately protected.
- Medical history of any bleeding disorder.
- Poor nutrition, including vitamin deficiency.
- Use of anticoagulants or aspirin.

HOW TO PREVENT—Wear appropriate protective footgear during competition or other athletic activity.

WHAT TO EXPECT

APPROPRIATE HEALTH CARE
- Doctor's care for serious or extensive contusions.
- Self-care for minor contusions or for serious contusions during rehabilitation.
- Physical therapy for serious contusions.

DIAGNOSTIC MEASURES
- Your own observation of symptoms.
- Medical history and physical exam by a doctor for all except minor injuries.
- X-rays of the foot and ankle to assess total injury to soft tissues and to rule out the possibility of underlying fractures. The total extent of injury may mot be apparent for 48 to 72 hours.

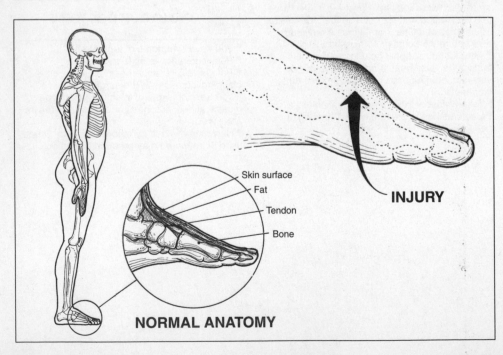

Skin surface
Fat
Tendon
Bone

INJURY

NORMAL ANATOMY

POSSIBLE COMPLICATIONS
• Excessive bleeding leading to disability. Infiltrate-type bleeding can (rarely) lead to calcification and impaired function of injured muscle.
• Prolonged healing time if usual activities are resumed too soon.
• Infection if skin over the contusion is broken.

PROBABLE OUTCOME—Healing time varies with the extent of injury, but average healing time for foot contusions is 1 to 2 weeks.

 ## HOW TO TREAT

NOTE—Follow your doctor's instructions. These instructions are supplemental.

FIRST AID—Use instructions for R.I.C.E., the first letters of *rest, ice, compression* and *elevation*. See Appendix 1 for details.

CONTINUING CARE
• Wrap an elasticized bandage over a sponge rubber pad placed on the injured area. Keep the area compressed for about 72 hours.
• Continue ice massage. Fill a large styrofoam cup with water and freeze. Tear a small amount of foam from the top so ice protrudes. Massage gently over the injured area in a circle about the size of a softball. Do this for 15 minutes at a time 3 or 4 times a day, and also before workouts or competition.
• After 72 hours, apply heat instead of ice if it feels better. Use heat lamps, hot soaks, hot showers, heating pads, heat liniments and ointments or whirlpool treatments.
• Massage gently and often to provide comfort and decrease swelling.

MEDICATION
• For minor discomfort, you may use: Acetaminophen or ibuprofen. Topical liniments and ointments.
• Your doctor may prescribe stronger medicine for pain.

ACTIVITY—Begin activity slowly, and stop exercise as soon as pain begins. Increase activity as healing progresses.

DIET—During recovery, balance the amount of food you eat with any change in your level of physical activity. Eat a variety of foods to get the energy, protein, vitamins, minerals and fiber you need for good health and healing.

REHABILITATION
• Begin daily rehabilitation exercises when supportive wrapping is no longer needed.
• See Rehabilitation section for ankle and foot exercises.

 ## CALL YOUR DOCTOR IF

• You have a foot contusion that doesn't improve in 1 or 2 days.
• Skin is broken and signs of infection (drainage, increasing pain, fever, headache, muscle aches, dizziness or a general ill feeling) occur.

FOOT DISLOCATION, SUBTALAR

 GENERAL INFORMATION

DEFINITION—Injury to a joint in the foot below the talus so that the calcaneus is displaced from its normal position and no longer touches the talus. A minor dislocation is called a subluxation. Joint surfaces still touch, but not in normal relation to each other.

BODY PARTS INVOLVED
- Any of the foot bones below the talus.
- Ligaments that hold foot bones in place.
- Soft tissues surrounding the dislocated bones, including nerves, tendons, muscles and blood vessels.

SIGNS & SYMPTOMS
- Excruciating pain at the time of injury.
- Inability to bear weight and walk.
- Severe pain when attempting to move the foot.
- Visible deformity if the dislocation remains locked in position.
- Tenderness over the dislocation.
- Swelling and bruising at the injury site.
- Numbness or paralysis below the dislocation from pinching, cutting or pressure on blood vessels or nerves.

CAUSES
- Direct blow to the foot.
- End result of a severe foot sprain.
- Congenital abnormality, such as a shallow or malformed joint surface.

RISK INCREASES WITH
- Participation in contact sports and jumping sports such as basketball and volleyball.
- Running or fast walking on uneven terrain or surfaces.
- Previous foot sprains or dislocations.
- Repeated injury to any joint in the foot.
- Poor muscle condition.

HOW TO PREVENT
- For participation in contact sports, protect vulnerable joints with supportive devices such as wrapped elastic bandages, tape or high-top athletic shoes.
- Warm up adequately before physical activity.
- Build your overall strength and muscle tone with a long-term conditioning program appropriate for your sport.
- Avoid irregular surfaces for running, fast walking or track and field events.

 WHAT TO EXPECT

APPROPRIATE HEALTH CARE
- Doctor's treatment, which includes manipulation of the joint to reposition the bones.
- Surgery (sometimes) to restore the joint to its normal position and repair torn ligaments and tendons or to repair or remove fracture fragments.
- Self-care during rehabilitation.

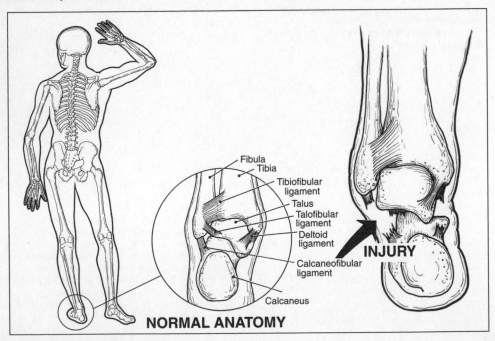

Fibula
Tibia
Tibiofibular ligament
Talus
Talofibular ligament
Deltoid ligament
Calcaneofibular ligament
Calcaneus

NORMAL ANATOMY

INJURY

DIAGNOSTIC MEASURES
- Your own observation of symptoms.
- Medical history and exam by a doctor.
- X-rays of the foot, ankle and adjacent bones.

POSSIBLE COMPLICATIONS
- Damage to nearby nerves or major blood vessels.
- Death of bone cells caused by interruption of the blood supply.
- Excessive internal bleeding at the dislocation site.
- Shock or loss of consciousness.
- Prolonged healing if activity is resumed too soon.
- Recurrent dislocations, particularly if a previous dislocation has not healed completely.
- Unstable or arthritic joint following repeated injury.

PROBABLE OUTCOME—After the dislocation has been corrected, the joint may require immobilization for 4 to 6 weeks with a cast from knee to toes. Complete healing of injured ligaments requires a minimum of 6 weeks, and swelling may continue for 3 to 6 months.

HOW TO TREAT

NOTE—Follow your doctor's instructions. These instructions are supplemental.

FIRST AID
- Keep the person warm with blankets to decrease the possibility of shock.
- Cut away clothing and shoe, if possible, but don't move the injured area to do so.
- Immobilize the foot and ankle with padded splints.
- Follow instructions for R.I.C.E., the first letters of *rest, ice, compression* and *elevation.* See Appendix 1 for details.

CONTINUING CARE
If a cast is not necessary:
- Use ice soaks 3 or 4 times a day. Fill a bucket with ice water, and soak the injured area for 20 minutes at a time.
- After 96 hours, application of localized heat promotes healing by increasing blood circulation in the injured area. Use hot baths, showers, compresses, heat lamps, heating pads, heat ointments and liniments or whirlpools.
- Wrap the foot with an elasticized bandage between treatments.
- Massage gently and often to provide comfort and decrease swelling.
If a cast is necessary:
- See Appendix 2 (Care of Casts).
- See Appendix 3 (Safe Use of Crutches).

MEDICATION—You doctor may prescribe:
- General anesthesia or muscle relaxants to make joint manipulation possible.

- Acetaminophen to relieve moderate pain.
- Narcotic pain relievers for severe pain.
- Stool softeners to prevent constipation due to decreased activity.
- Antibiotics to fight infection.

ACTIVITY
If surgery is not necessary:
- Resume sports participation after clearance from your doctor.
If surgery is necessary:
- Avoid vigorous exercise for 6 weeks after surgery. Then resume normal activities gradually after a mobility and strengthening program.
- Don't drive until healing is complete.

DIET
- Do not eat or drink before manipulation or surgery to correct the dislocation. Fluid or solid food in your stomach makes vomiting under general anesthesia more hazardous.
- During recovery, balance the amount of food you eat with any change in your level of physical activity. Eat a variety of foods to get the energy, protein, vitamins, minerals and fiber you need for good health and healing.

REHABILITATION
- Begin daily rehabilitation exercises when supportive wrapping is no longer needed.
- Use ice massage for 10 minutes before and after workouts. Fill a large styrofoam cup with water and freeze. Tear a small amount of foam from the top so ice protrudes. Massage firmly over the injured area in a circle about the size of a softball.
- See Rehabilitation section for ankle and foot exercises.

CALL YOUR DOCTOR IF

- Any of the following occurs after injury:
  Numbness, paleness or coldness in the foot. This is an emergency!
  Foot deformity.
  Difficulty moving the foot.
  Nausea or vomiting.
- Any of the following occurs after treatment:
  Swelling above or below the cast.
  Blue or gray skin color, particularly under the toenails.
  Constipation.
- Any of the following occurs after surgery:
  Increased pain, swelling or drainage in the surgical area.
  Signs of infection (headache, muscle aches, dizziness or a general ill feeling and fever).
- New, unexplained symptoms develop. Drugs used in treatment may cause side effects.
- Foot dislocations that you can "pop" back into normal position occur repeatedly.

FOOT DISLOCATION, TALUS

GENERAL INFORMATION

DEFINITION—Injury and displacement of the talus so it no longer touches adjoining bones. Fractures and ligament tears frequently accompany this dislocation.

BODY PARTS INVOLVED
- Talus and adjacent foot bones (tibia, fibula, navicular, calcaneus).
- Ligaments that hold foot bones together.
- Soft tissues surrounding the dislocation site, including periosteum (covering of bone), nerves, tendons, blood vessels and connective tissues.

SIGNS & SYMPTOMS
- Excruciating pain in the foot at time of injury.
- Loss of function in the foot and ankle and severe pain when attempting to move them.
- Visible deformity if the dislocated bones have locked in the dislocated positions. Bones may spontaneously reposition themselves and leave no deformity, but damage is the same.
- Tenderness over the dislocation.
- Swelling and bruising at the injury site.
- Numbness or paralysis below the dislocation from pressure on or pinching or cutting of blood vessels or nerves.

CAUSES
- Direct or indirect blow to the foot and ankle.
- End result of a severe foot sprain.

- Congenital abnormality, such as abnormal arches or shallow or malformed joint surfaces.

RISK INCREASES WITH
- Contact sports.
- Running and jumping events.
- Exercise on uneven surfaces.
- Previous foot dislocation or sprain.
- Repeated injury to any joint in the foot.
- Poor muscle conditioning.

HOW TO PREVENT
- For participation in contact sports or activities involving running and jumping, protect vulnerable joints. Wear protective devices, such as high-top athletic shoes, and use tape.
- Avoid irregular surfaces for running, fast walking and track and field events.
- Warm up adequately before physical activity.
- Build your overall strength, flexibility and muscle tone with a conditioning program.
- Avoid contact sports if treatment does not restore a strong, stable foot and ankle.

WHAT TO EXPECT

APPROPRIATE HEALTH CARE
- Doctor's treatment. This will include manipulating the joint to restore the bones.
- Surgery (sometimes) to restore the joint to its normal position and repair torn ligaments and tendons. Acute or recurring dislocations may require surgical reconstruction or replacement of the joint.

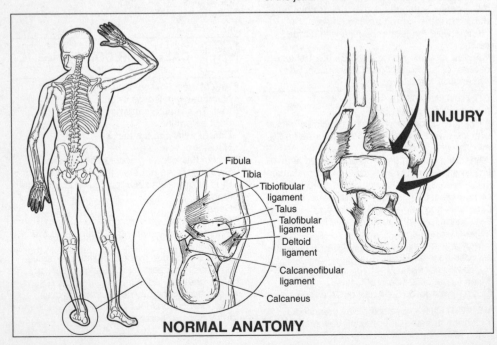

Fibula
Tibia
Tibiofibular ligament
Talus
Talofibular ligament
Deltoid ligament
Calcaneofibular ligament
Calcaneus

NORMAL ANATOMY

INJURY

DIAGNOSTIC MEASURES
- Your own observation of symptoms.
- Medical history and exam by a doctor.
- X-rays.

POSSIBLE COMPLICATIONS
At the time of injury:
- Shock.
- Pressure on or injury to nearby nerves, ligaments, tendons, muscles, blood vessels and connective tissues.

After treatment or surgery:
- Excessive internal bleeding.
- Impaired blood supply to the talus.
- Death of bone cells due to interruption of the blood supply (avascular necrosis of talus).
- Infection introduced during surgical treatment.
- Prolonged healing if activity is resumed too soon.
- Recurrent dislocations.
- Unstable or arthritic joint following repeated injury.

PROBABLE OUTCOME
- After the dislocation has been corrected, the joint may require immobilization with a cast or splint covering the foot and ankle for 4 to 6 weeks. Injured ligaments require a minimum of 6 weeks to heal.
- If avascular necrosis develops, it can require 6 months or more of non-weight-bearing with crutches.

 ## HOW TO TREAT

NOTE—Follow your doctor's instructions. These instructions are supplemental.

FIRST AID
- Keep the person warm with blankets to decrease the possibility of shock.
- Cut away clothing and shoe if possible, but don't move the injured area to do so.
- Immobilize the foot and ankle with padded splints.
- Follow instructions for R.I.C.E., the first letters of *rest, ice, compression* and *elevation*. See Appendix 1 for details.

CONTINUING CARE
If a cast is not necessary:
- Use ice soaks 3 or 4 times a day. Fill a bucket with ice water, and soak the injured area for 20 minutes at a time.
- After 96 hours, application of localized heat promotes healing by increasing blood circulation in the injured area. Use hot baths, showers, compresses, heat lamps, heating pads, heat ointments and liniments or whirlpools.
- Wrap the foot and ankle with an elasticized bandage between treatments.
- Massage gently and often to provide comfort and decrease swelling.

If a cast is necessary:
- See Appendix 2 (Care of Casts).
- See Appendix 3 (Safe Use of Crutches).

MEDICATION—Your doctor may prescribe:
- General anesthesia or muscle relaxants to make joint manipulation possible.
- Acetaminophen to relieve moderate pain.
- Prescription pain relievers for severe pain.
- Stool softeners to prevent constipation due to decreased activity.
- Antibiotics to fight infection.

ACTIVITY
If surgery is not necessary:
- Resume sports participation after clearance from your doctor.

If surgery is necessary:
- Avoid vigorous exercise for 6 weeks after surgery. Then resume normal activities gradually.
- Don't drive until healing is complete.

DIET
- Do not eat or drink before manipulation or surgery to correct the dislocation. Fluid or solid food in your stomach makes vomiting while under general anesthesia more hazardous.
- During recovery, balance the amount of food you eat with any change in your level of physical activity.

REHABILITATION
- Begin daily rehabilitation exercises when supportive wrapping is no longer needed.
- Use ice massage for 10 minutes before and after workouts. Fill a large styrofoam cup with water and freeze. Tear a small amount of foam from the top so ice protrudes. Massage firmly in a circle over the injured area.
- See Rehabilitation section for ankle and foot exercises.

 ## CALL YOUR DOCTOR IF

- Any of the following occurs after injury:
  Foot deformity.
  Difficulty moving the foot.
  Numbness, paleness or coldness in the foot. This is an emergency!
  Nausea or vomiting.
- Any of the following occurs after treatment:
  Swelling above or below the cast.
  Blue or gray skin color under the toenails.
  Constipation.
  Any of the following occurs after surgery:
  Increased pain, swelling or drainage in the surgical area.
  Signs of infection (headache, muscle aches, dizziness or a general ill feeling and fever).
- New, unexplained symptoms develop. Drugs used in treatment may cause side effects.
- Foot dislocations that you can "pop" back into normal position occur repeatedly.

FOOT FRACTURE

GENERAL INFORMATION

DEFINITION—A complete or incomplete break in bones of the foot. The many bones of the central and front portions of the foot are the most susceptible to fracture.

BODY PARTS INVOLVED
- Bones of the foot.
- Ankle joint and the many joints of the foot.
- Soft tissues surrounding the fracture site, including nerves, tendons, ligaments and blood vessels.

SIGNS & SYMPTOMS
- Severe foot pain at the time of injury.
- Swelling of soft tissues surrounding the fracture.
- Visible deformity if the fracture is complete and bone fragments separate enough to distort normal foot contours.
- Tenderness to the touch.
- Numbness and coldness in the foot and toes if the blood supply is impaired.

CAUSES—Direct blow or indirect stress to the bone. Indirect stress may be caused by twisting or violent muscle contractions, such as kicking.

RISK INCREASES WITH
- Contact sports, especially football and soccer.
- History of bone or joint disease, especially osteoporosis.
- Obesity.
- Poor nutrition, especially calcium deficiency.
- If surgery or anesthesia is needed, risk increases with smoking and use of drugs such as mind-altering drugs, muscle relaxants, tranquilizers, sleep induces, insulin, sedatives, beta-adrenergic blockers or corticosteroids.

HOW TO PREVENT—Use athletic shoes especially designed for the sport in which you are involved.

WHAT TO EXPECT

APPROPRIATE HEALTH CARE
- Doctor's treatment to manipulate and set the broken bones.
- Anesthesia and surgery to set the fracture.
- Self-care during rehabilitation.
- Whirlpool, ultrasound or massage (to displace fluid from the injured joint space).

DIAGNOSTIC MEASURES
- Your own observation of symptoms.
- Medical history and physical exam by a doctor.
- X-rays of injured areas, including joints above and below the primary injury site.

POSSIBLE COMPLICATIONS
At the time of injury:
- Shock.
- Pressure on or injury to nearby nerves, ligaments, tendons, muscles, blood vessels or connective tissues.

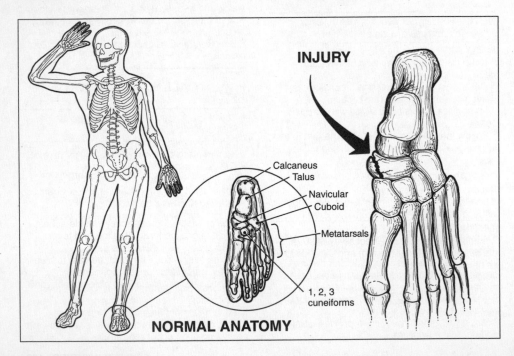

INJURY

Calcaneus
Talus
Navicular
Cuboid
Metatarsals
1, 2, 3 cuneiforms

NORMAL ANATOMY

After treatment or surgery:
- Delayed union or nonunion of the fracture.
- Impaired blood supply to the fracture site.
- Avascular necrosis (death of bone cells due to interruption of the blood supply).
- Arrest of normal bone growth in children.
- Infection in open fractures (skin broken over fracture site) or at the incision if surgical setting was necessary.
- Shortening of the injured bones.
- Proneness to repeated foot injury.
- Unstable or arthritic joint following repeated injury.
- Prolonged healing time if activity is resumed too soon.
- Problems caused by casts. See Appendix 2 (Care of Casts).

PROBABLE OUTCOME—It is impossible to predict exactly how long it will take for any fracture to heal. Variable factors include age, sex and previous state of health and conditioning. The average healing time for this fracture is 6 to 8 weeks. Healing is considered complete when there is no motion at the fracture site and when x-rays show complete bone union.

 HOW TO TREAT

NOTE—Follow your doctor's instructions. These instructions are supplemental.

FIRST AID
- Keep the person warm with blankets to decrease the possibility of shock.
- Use instructions for R.I.C.E., the first letters of *rest, ice, compression* and *elevation*. See Appendix 1 for details.
- The doctor will probably realign and set the broken bones in the following manner:
  Hind-portion fracture: Large fragments are repositioned surgically. Otherwise the fracture is treated as a moderate sprain.
  Central-portion fracture: These uncommon compression fractures require surgery.
  Front-portion fracture: These are treated like toe fractures (see Toe Fracture).
Manipulation should be done as soon as possible after injury. Also, many tissues lose their elasticity and become difficult to return to their normal positions.

CONTINUING CARE
- Immobilization is usually necessary. If so, a rigid cast covers the entire foot and extends to just below the knee.
- After cast removal, use frequent ice massage. Fill a large styrofoam cup with water and freeze. Tear a small amount of foam from the top so ice protrudes. Massage firmly over the injury area in a circle about the size of a softball. Do this for 15 minutes at a time 3 or 4 times a day, and also before workouts or competition.
- Apply heat instead of ice if it feels better. Use heat lamps, hot soaks, hot showers, heating pads or heat liniments and ointments.
- Take whirlpool treatments, if available.

MEDICATION—Your doctor may prescribe:
- General anesthesia, local anesthesia or muscle relaxants to make bone manipulation and fixation of bone fragments possible.
- Narcotic or synthetic narcotic pain relievers for severe pain.
- Stool softeners to prevent constipation due to inactivity.
- Acetaminophen (available without prescription) for mild pain after initial treatment.

ACTIVITY
- Actively exercise all muscle groups not immobilized. The resulting muscle contractions promote fracture alignment and hasten healing.
- Resume normal activities gradually after treatment.
- Begin reconditioning the injured area after clearance from your doctor.

DIET
- Do not drink or eat before manipulation or surgery to treat the fracture. Fluid or solid food in your stomach makes vomiting while under anesthesia more hazardous.
- During recovery, balance the amount of food you eat with any change in your level of physical activity. Eat a variety of foods to get the energy, protein, vitamins, minerals and fiber you need for good health and healing.

REHABILITATION—Begin daily rehabilitation exercises when supportive wrapping is no longer needed. Use ice massage for 10 minutes prior to exercise. See Rehabilitation section for ankle and foot exercises.

 CALL YOUR DOCTOR IF

- You have signs or symptoms of a foot fracture.
- Any of the following occurs after surgery or other treatment:
  Increased pain, swelling or drainage in the surgical area.
  Signs of infection (headache, muscle aches, dizziness or a general ill feeling and fever).
  Swelling above or below the cast.
  Change in skin color beyond the cast to blue or gray, particularly under the toenails.
  Numbness or complete loss of feeling beyond the fracture site.
  Nausea or vomiting; constipation.

FOOT GANGLION
(Synovial Hernia; Ganglion Cyst)

GENERAL INFORMATION

DEFINITION—A small, usually hard nodule lying directly over a tendon or a joint capsule on the top or bottom of the foot. Occasionally the nodule may become quite large. Sometimes a foot ganglion may regress and disappear altogether, only to reappear later.

BODY PARTS INVOLVED
- Top or sole of the foot.
- Tendon sheath (a thin membranous covering of any tendon).
- Any of many joint spaces in the foot.

SIGNS & SYMPTOMS
- Hard lump over a tendon or joint capsule in the foot. The nodule "yields" to heavy pressure because it is not solid.
- No pain usually, but overuse of the foot may cause mild pain and aching.
- Tenderness if the lump is pressed hard.
- Discomfort with extremes of motion (flexing or extending) and with repetition of the exercise that produced the ganglion.

CAUSES
- Mild or chronic sprains in a foot joint, causing weakness of the joint capsule.
- Defect in the fibrous sheath of the joint or tendon, permitting part of the underlying synovium (thin membrane that lines the tendon sheath) to protrude. Irritation of the protruding synovium causes it to produce thickened fluid. Continued irritation makes it enlarge and harden, forming the ganglion.

RISK INCREASES WITH
- Repeated injury, especially mild sprains. Foot ganglions frequently occur in runners, jumpers, skiers and participants in contact sports.
- Inadequate warmup prior to practice or competition.
- Poor muscle strength or conditioning.
- If surgery is necessary, surgical risk increases with smoking, poor nutrition, alcoholism and recent or chronic illness.

HOW TO PREVENT
- Build your strength in a long-term conditioning program appropriate for your sport.
- Warmup before practice or competition.

WHAT TO EXPECT

APPROPRIATE HEALTH CARE
- Doctor's care for diagnosis and possible injections of local anesthetics or corticosteroids.
- Surgery to remove cyst. Surgery will be conducted under general or local anesthesia in an outpatient surgical facility or hospital operating room.

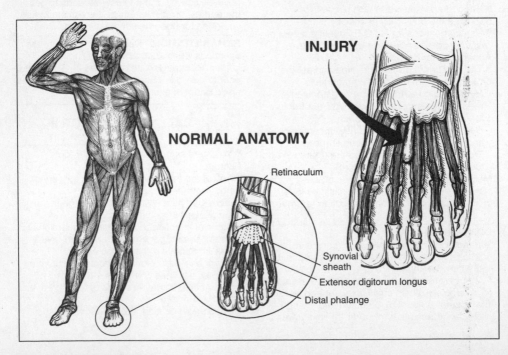

INJURY

NORMAL ANATOMY

Retinaculum

Synovial sheath

Extensor digitorum longus

Distal phalange

DIAGNOSTIC MEASURES
- Your own observation of signs and symptoms.
- Medical history and physical examination by a doctor.
- X-rays of the area.
- Needle aspiration of the cyst.

POSSIBLE COMPLICATIONS
- After surgery:
  Excessive bleeding.
  Surgical wound infection.
  Recurrence if surgical removal is incomplete.
- Calcification of ganglion (rare).

PROBABLE OUTCOME—Ganglions sometimes disappear spontaneously, only to recur later. Surgery is frequently necessary. After surgery, allow about 3 weeks for recovery if no complications occur.

 HOW TO TREAT

NOTE—Follow your doctor's instructions. These instructions are supplemental.

FIRST AID—None. This condition develops gradually.

CONTINUING CARE
Immediately after surgery:
- The affected area is usually immobilized in a splint or boot for 1 to 2 weeks following surgery.
After the bandage or splint is removed by the doctor:
- Bathe and shower as usual. You may wash the incision gently with mild unscented soap.
- Apply nonprescription antibiotic ointment to the wound before applying new bandages.
- Wrap the foot with an elasticized bandage until healing is complete.
- Use an ice pack 3 or 4 times a day. Wrap ice chips or cubes in a plastic bag, and wrap the bag in a moist towel. Place it over the injured area for 20 minutes at a time.
- You may apply heat instead of ice if it feels better. Use heat lamps, hot soaks, hot showers, heating pads or heat liniments and ointments.
- Take whirlpool treatments, if available.

MEDICATION
- Your doctor may prescribe pain relievers. Don't take prescription pain medication longer than 4 to 7 days. Use only as much as you need.
- You may use nonprescription drugs, such as acetaminophen, for minor pain.

ACTIVITY
- Return to work and normal activity as soon as possible.
- Avoid vigorous exercise for 3 weeks after surgery.

DIET—During recovery, balance the amount of food you eat with any change in your level of physical activity. Eat a variety of foods to get the energy, protein, vitamins, minerals and fiber you need for good health and healing.

REHABILITATION
- Begin daily rehabilitation exercises when supportive wrapping is no longer needed.
- Use ice massage for 10 minutes before and after workouts. Fill a large styrofoam cup with water and freeze. Tear a small amount of foam from the top so ice protrudes. Massage firmly over the injured area in a circle about the size of a softball.
- See Rehabilitation section for ankle and foot exercises.

 CALL YOUR DOCTOR IF

- You have signs or symptoms of a foot ganglion.
- Any of the following occurs after surgery:
  Increased pain, swelling, redness, drainage or bleeding in the surgical area.
  Signs of infection (headache, muscle aches, dizziness or a general ill feeling and fever).
  New, unexplained symptoms. Drugs used in treatment may produce side effects.

FOOT HEMATOMA

GENERAL INFORMATION

DEFINITION—A collection of pooled blood within constricted space on the top of the foot (dorsum) or bottom of the foot (plantar area).

BODY PARTS INVOLVED
- Dorsum or plantar area of the foot, especially alongside the heel pad.
- Soft tissues surrounding the hematoma, including nerves, tendons, ligaments, muscles and blood vessels.

SIGNS & SYMPTOMS
- Swelling over the injured area.
- Fluctuance (feeling of mobile fluid beneath the skin).
- Tenderness.
- Redness that progresses through several color changes—purple, green-yellow, yellow—before it completely heals.

CAUSES—Direct injury, usually from a blunt object or from landing on a hard surface. Bleeding into tissues then causes the surrounding tissues to be pushed away. An injury may occur above the foot or as high as the knee, but gravity will move the blood to the sides of the heel pad.

RISK INCREASES WITH
- Contact sports, especially if the foot is not adequately protected.
- Medical history of any bleeding disorder.
- Poor nutrition, including vitamin deficiency.
- Use of anticoagulants or aspirin.

HOW TO PREVENT—Wear appropriate, well-designed shoes during competition or other athletic activity to decrease the risk of foot injury.

WHAT TO EXPECT

APPROPRIATE HEALTH CARE
- Doctor's care unless the hematoma is very small.
- Needle aspiration of blood from the hematoma (sometimes) if the hematoma is accessible. At the same time, hyaluronidase (an enzyme) can be injected into the hematoma space. Hyaluronidase hastens absorption of the blood.
- Self-care for minor hematomas or following serious hematomas during the rehabilitation phase.
- Physical therapy following serious hematomas.

DIAGNOSTIC MEASURES
- Your own observation of symptoms.
- Physical exam and medical history by a doctor for all except minor injuries.

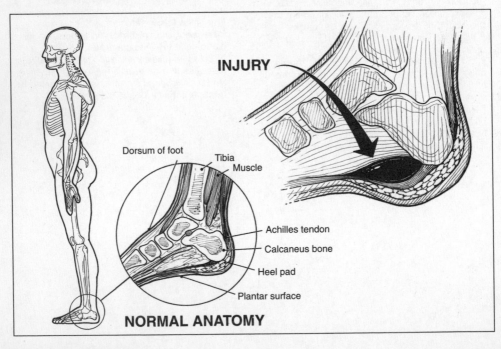

INJURY

Dorsum of foot

Tibia
Muscle

Achilles tendon

Calcaneus bone

Heel pad

Plantar surface

NORMAL ANATOMY

- X-rays of the injured area to assess total injury to the foot and to rule out the possibility of an underlying bone fracture. Total extent of the injury may not be apparent for 48 to 72 hours.

POSSIBLE COMPLICATIONS
- Infection introduced through a break in the skin at the time of injury or during aspiration of the hematoma.
- Prolonged healing time if activity is resumed too soon.
- Calcification of the blood remaining in the hematoma if the blood is not completely removed or absorbed.

PROBABLE OUTCOME—Average healing time is 2 weeks to 2 months unless the blood is removed with aspiration. Healing time may be lessened with this treatment.

 # HOW TO TREAT

NOTE—Follow your doctor's instructions. These instructions are supplemental.

FIRST AID—Use instructions for R.I.C.E., the first letters of *rest, ice, compression* and *elevation*. See Appendix 1 for details.

CONTINUING CARE
- Continue ice massage 3 or 4 times a day for 15 minutes at a time. Fill a large styrofoam cup with water and freeze. Tear a small amount of foam from the top so ice protrudes. Massage firmly over the injured area in a circle about the size of a softball.
- After 72 hours, application of localized heat promotes healing by increasing blood circulation in the injured area. Use hot baths, showers, ointments and liniments or whirlpools.
- Don't massage the foot. You may trigger bleeding again.
- Wrap an elastic bandage over a sponge rubber pad placed on the injured area. Keep compressed for 72 hours, especially after a needle aspiration of blood.

MEDICATION
- For minor discomfort, you may use: Nonprescription medicines such as acetaminophen or ibuprofen. Topical liniments and ointments.
- Your doctor may prescribe stronger medicine for pain if needed.

ACTIVITY—Begin activities slowly, and stop exercise as soon as pain begins. Increase activity as healing progresses. To prevent a delay in healing, protect the hematoma area against excessive motion soon after injury. Motion breaks down the clot and causes irritation throughout the foot, leading to possible scar formation, calcification and restricted movement after healing.

DIET—During recovery, balance the amount of food you eat with any change in your level of physical activity. Eat a variety of foods to get the energy, protein, vitamins, minerals and fiber you need for good health and healing.

REHABILITATION
- Begin daily rehabilitation exercises when supportive wrapping is no longer needed. Use gentle ice massage for 10 minutes prior to exercise.
- See Rehabilitation section for ankle and foot exercises.

 # CALL YOUR DOCTOR IF

- You have signs or symptoms of a foot hematoma that doesn't begin to improve in 1 to 2 days.
- Skin is broken and signs of infection (drainage, increasing pain, fever, headache, muscle aches, dizziness or a general ill feeling) occur.

FOOT SPRAIN

GENERAL INFORMATION

DEFINITION—Violent overstretching of one or more ligaments in the foot. Sprains involving two or more ligaments cause considerably more disability than single-ligament sprains. When the ligament is overstretched, it becomes tense and gives way at its weakest point, either where it attaches to bone or within the ligament itself. If the ligament pulls loose a fragment of bone, it is called an avulsion fracture. There are 3 types of sprains:
- Mild (Grade I)—Tearing of some ligament fibers. There is no loss of function.
- Moderate (Grade II)—Rupture of a portion of the ligament, resulting in some loss of function.
- Severe (Grade III)—Complete rupture of the ligament or complete separation of ligament from bone. There is total loss of function. A severe sprain requires surgical repair.

BODY PARTS INVOLVED
- Any ligament in the foot.
- Tissues surrounding the sprain, including blood vessels, tendons, bone, periosteum (covering of bone) and muscles.

SIGNS & SYMPTOMS
- Severe pain at the time of injury.
- A feeling of popping or tearing inside the foot.
- Tenderness at the injury site.
- Swelling in the foot.
- Bruising that appears soon after injury.

CAUSES—Stress on a ligament that temporarily forces or pries a joint in the foot out of its normal location.

RISK INCREASES WITH
- Running, walking and jumping in such sports as basketball, soccer, volleyball, skiing, distance jumping or high jumping. Athletes in these sports often accidentally land on the side of the foot.
- Previous foot injury.
- Poor muscle strength or conditioning.
- Inadequate protection from equipment.

HOW TO PREVENT
- Build your strength with a conditioning program appropriate for your sport.
- Warm up before practice or competition.
- Tape vulnerable joints before practice or competition.
- Use protective equipment, such as appropriate shoes with good support.

WHAT TO EXPECT

APPROPRIATE HEALTH CARE
- Doctor's care.
- Application of a cast, tape or elastic bandage.
- Surgery (sometimes) to repair severe sprains.
- Physical therapy for rehabilitation.
- Self-care during and after rehabilitation.

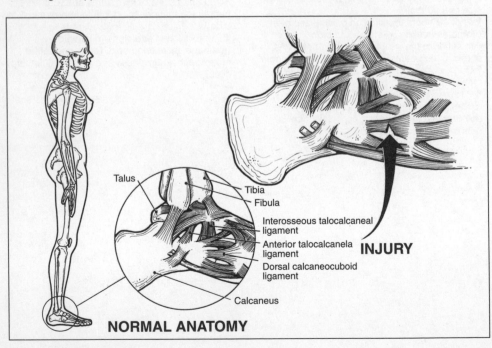

Talus
Tibia
Fibula
Interosseous talocalcaneal ligament
Anterior talocalcanela ligament
Dorsal calcaneocuboid ligament
Calcaneus

INJURY

NORMAL ANATOMY

DIAGNOSTIC MEASURES
- Your own observation of symptoms.
- Medical history and exam by a doctor.
- X-rays of the foot and ankle to rule out fractures.

POSSIBLE COMPLICATIONS
- Prolonged healing time if usual activities are resumed too soon.
- Proneness to repeated foot injury.
- Inflammation at the ligament's attachment to bone (periostitis).
- Prolonged disability (sometimes).
- Unstable or permanently arthritic foot joints following repeated injury.

PROBABLE OUTCOME—If this is a first-time injury, proper care and sufficient healing time before resuming activity should prevent permanent disability. Ligaments have a poor blood supply, and torn ligaments require as much healing time as fractures. Average healing times are:
- Mild sprains—2 to 6 weeks.
- Moderate sprains—6 to 8 weeks.
- Severe sprains—8 to 10 weeks.

 ## HOW TO TREAT

NOTE—Follow your doctor's instructions. These instructions are supplemental.

FIRST AID—Use instructions for R.I.C.E., the first letters of *rest, ice, compression* and *elevation*. See Appendix 1 for details.

CONTINUING CARE—If the doctor does not apply a cast, tape or elastic bandage:
- Continue using an ice pack 3 or 4 times a day. Place ice chips or cubes in a plastic bag. Wrap the bag in a moist towel, and place it over the injured area. Use for 20 minutes at a time.
- Wrap the injured foot with an elasticized bandage between ice treatments.
- After 72 hours, apply heat instead of ice if it feels better. Use heat lamps, hot soaks, hot showers, heating pads or heat liniments and ointments.
- Take whirlpool treatments, if available.
- Massage the foot gently and often to provide comfort and decrease swelling.

MEDICATION
- For minor discomfort, you may use:
  Aspirin, acetaminophen or ibuprofen.
  Topical liniments and ointments.
- Your doctor may prescribe:
  Stronger pain relievers.
  Injection of a long-acting local anesthetic to reduce pain.
  Injections of a corticosteroid, such as triamcinolone, to reduce inflammation (rarely).

ACTIVITY—Resume your normal activities gradually after clearance from your doctor.

DIET—During recovery, balance the amount of food you eat with any change in your level of physical activity. Eat a variety of foods to get the energy, protein, vitamins, minerals and fiber you need for good health and healing.

REHABILITATION
- Begin daily rehabilitation exercises when the cast or supportive wrapping is no longer necessary.
- Use ice massage for 10 minutes before and after exercise. Fill a large styrofoam cup with water and freeze. Tear a small amount of foam from the top so ice protrudes. Massage firmly over the injured area in a circle about the size of a softball.
- See Rehabilitation section for ankle and foot exercises.

 ## CALL YOUR DOCTOR IF

You have symptoms of a moderate or severe foot sprain or a mild sprain persists longer than 2 weeks.
- Pain, swelling or bruising worsens despite treatment.
- Any of the following occurs after casting or splinting:
  Pain, numbness or coldness below the cast or splint.
  Blue, gray or dusky toenails.
- Any of the following occurs after surgery:
  Increased pain, swelling, redness, drainage or bleeding in the surgical area.
  Signs of infection (headache, muscle aches, dizziness or a general ill feeling with fever).
- New, unexplained symptoms develop. Drugs used in treatment may produce side effects.

FOOT STRAIN

GENERAL INFORMATION

DEFINITION—Injury to the muscles or tendons that surround the foot. Muscles, tendons and their attached bones comprise contractile units. These units stabilize the foot and allow its motion. A strain occurs at the weakest part of a unit. Strains are of 3 types:
- Mild (Grade)—Slightly pulled muscle without tearing of muscle or tendon fibers. There is no loss of strength.
- Moderate (Grade II)—Tearing of fibers in a muscle or tendon or at the attachment to bone. Strength is diminished.
- Severe (Grade III)—Rupture of the muscle-tendon-bone attachment, with separation of fibers. A severe strain may require surgical repair. Chronic strains are caused by overuse. Acute strains are caused by direct injury or overstress.

BODY PARTS INVOLVED
- Tendon and muscles of the foot.
- Foot bones.
- Soft tissues surrounding the strain, including nerves, periosteum (covering of bone), blood vessels and lymph vessels.

SIGNS & SYMPTOMS
- Pain when moving or stretching the foot.
- Muscle spasm in the foot.
- Tenderness and swelling at the injury site.
- Loss of strength (moderate or severe strain).

- Calcification of the muscle or its tendon (visible with x-ray).
- Inflammation of the tendon sheath.

CAUSES
- Prolonged overuse of muscle-tendon units in the ankle or foot.
- Single violent injury or force applied to the foot or ankle.

RISK INCREASES WITH
- Contact sports such as football, soccer or hockey.
- Sports that require quick starts, such as starting a race.
- Medical history of any bleeding disorder.
- Obesity.
- Poor nutrition.
- Previous foot or ankle injury.
- Poor muscle conditioning.

HOW TO PREVENT
- Participation in a strengthening, flexibility and conditioning program appropriate for your sport.
- Warm up before practice or competition.
- Wear well-fitting athletic shoes appropriate for your sport.

WHAT TO EXPECT

APPROPRIATE HEALTH CARE
- Doctor's diagnosis.
- Application of tape, plaster splints or casts (sometimes).

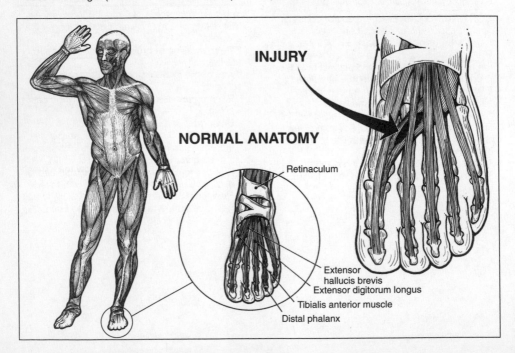

INJURY

NORMAL ANATOMY

Retinaculum

Extensor hallucis brevis
Extensor digitorum longus
Tibialis anterior muscle
Distal phalanx

- Self-care during rehabilitation.
- Physical therapy (moderate or severe strain).
- Surgery (severe strain).

DIAGNOSTIC MEASURES
- Your own observation of symptoms.
- Medical history and exam by a doctor.
- X-rays of the foot and ankle to rule out fractures.

POSSIBLE COMPLICATIONS
- Prolonged healing time if activity is resumed too soon.
- Proneness to repeated injury.
- Unstable or arthritic foot joints following repeated injury.
- Inflammation at the attachment to bone (periostitis).
- Prolonged disability (sometimes), especially weakness.

PROBABLE OUTCOME—If this is a first-time injury, proper care and sufficient healing time before resuming activity should prevent permanent disability. Torn ligaments and tendons require as long to heal as fractured bones. Average healing times are:
- Mild strain—2 to 10 days.
- Moderate strain—10 days to 6 weeks.
- Severe strain—6 to 10 weeks.

 HOW TO TREAT

NOTE—Follow your doctor's instructions. These instructions are supplemental.

FIRST AID—Use instructions for R.I.C.E., the first letters of *rest, ice, compression* and *elevation*. See Appendix 1 for details.

CONTINUING CARE—If a cast or splints are used, leave toes free and exercise them occasionally. If a cast or splints are not used:
- Use ice massage 3 or 4 times a day for 15 minutes at a time. Fill a large styrofoam cup with water and freeze. Tear a small amount of foam from the top so ice protrudes. Massage firmly over the injured area in a circle about the size of a softball.

- After the first 72 hours, apply heat instead of ice if it feels better. Use heat lamps, hot soaks, hot showers, heating pads or heat liniments and ointments.
- Take whirlpool treatments, if available.
- Wrap the injured ankle with an elasticized bandage between treatments.
- Massage gently and often to provide comfort and decrease swelling.

MEDICATION
- For minor discomfort, you may use:
  Aspirin, acetaminophen or nonsteroidal anti-inflammatories.
  Topical liniments and ointments.
- Your doctor may prescribe:
  Stronger pain relievers.
  Injection of a long-acting local anesthetic to reduce pain.
  Injections of a corticosteroid, such as triamcinolone, to reduce inflammation.

ACTIVITY
- For a moderate or severe strain, walk with crutches for at least 72 hours—longer with a cast or splints. See Appendix 3 (Safe Use of Crutches).
- Resume normal activities gradually after pain has subsided.

DIET—During recovery, balance the amount of food you eat with any change in your level of physical activity. Eat a variety of foods to get the energy, protein, vitamins, minerals and fiber you need for good health and healing.

REHABILITATION—Begin daily rehabilitation exercises when supportive wrapping is no longer needed. See Rehabilitation section for ankle and foot exercises.

 CALL YOUR DOCTOR IF

- You have symptoms of a moderate or severe foot strain or a mild strain persists longer than 10 days.
- Pain or swelling worsens despite treatment.
- The following occur with casts or splints:
  Pain, numbness or coldness below the injury site.
  Dusky, blue or gray toenails.

FOOT STRESS FRACTURE
(March Fracture; Fatigue Fracture)

GENERAL INFORMATION

DEFINITION—A complete or incomplete hairline break in a foot (metatarsal) bone. The term *march fracture* arose during World War I, when many young soldiers not conditioned for stress were put into ill-fitting shoes and required to take long hikes over rough terrain. The x-ray appearance may be similar to that of a bone tumor. Stress fractures may not appear clearly on x-rays for several weeks after pain begins in the foot.

BODY PARTS INVOLVED
- Metatarsal bones of the foot.
- Metatarsal joints.
- Soft tissues around the fracture site, including muscles, nerves, tendons, ligaments, periosteum (covering of bone), blood vessels and connective tissues.

SIGNS & SYMPTOMS
- Pain in the foot when walking or running. Pain diminishes or disappears when the load is taken off the feet.
- Tenderness to the touch in the fracture area.

CAUSES—Fatigue of the foot bone(s) caused by repeated overload, as with marching, walking, running or jogging.

RISK INCREASES WITH
- Age over 60.
- Walking, running, jogging or standing for prolonged periods.
- Hiking carrying a heavy pack.
- History of bone or joint disease, especially osteoporosis.
- Oligomenorrhea or amenorrhea (irregular or absent menstrual periods) in female athletes.
- Obesity.
- Poor nutrition, especially calcium deficiency.

HOW TO PREVENT
- Heed early warnings of an impending stress fracture, such as foot pain after extended standing or walking. Adjust activities before a fracture occurs.
- Ensure an adequate calcium intake (1000 mg to 1500 mg a day) with milk and milk products or calcium supplements.
- Avoid such strenuous exercise or so low-calorie a diet that oligomenorrhea or amenorrhea develops.
- Do not rapidly increase running distance, change to a harder running surface or begin carrying a heavier pack for long hikes. These changes require a planned training progression.

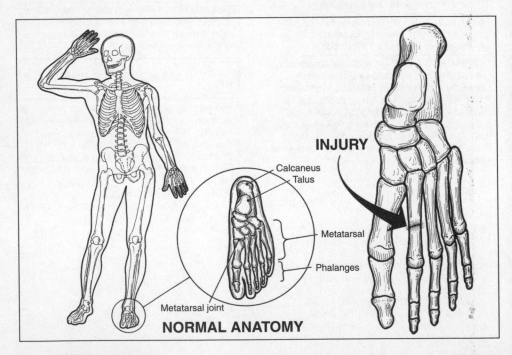

INJURY

Calcaneus
Talus

Metatarsal

Phalanges

Metatarsal joint

NORMAL ANATOMY

WHAT TO EXPECT

APPROPRIATE HEALTH CARE
- Doctor's diagnosis and care.
- Physical therapy and rehabilitation.
- Self-care during rehabilitation.

DIAGNOSTIC MEASURES
- Your own observation of symptoms.
- Medical history and physical exam by a doctor.
- X-rays of both feet and ankles. X-rays are often normal for the first 10 to 24 days after symptoms begin.
- Radioactive technetium 99 scan (see Glossary) or MRI if symptoms are typical, but x-rays are negative.

POSSIBLE COMPLICATIONS
- Complete fracture due to continued stress on the foot after symptoms begin.
- Pressure on or injury to nearby nerves, ligaments, tendons, blood vessels or connective tissues.
- Problems arising from plaster casts, splints or other immobilizing materials. See Appendix 2 (Care of Casts).
- Unstable or arthritic joint following repeated injury.
- Prolonged foot pain.

PROBABLE OUTCOME—It is impossible to predict exactly how long it will take for any fracture to heal. Variable factors include age, sex and previous state of health and conditioning. The average healing time for this fracture is 6 to 8 weeks with adequate treatment. Healing is considered complete when there is no pain at the fracture site and when x-rays show complete bone union. After healing is complete, slowly return to previous activity level.

 HOW TO TREAT

NOTE—Follow your doctor's instructions. These instructions are supplemental.

FIRST AID—None. This injury develops gradually.

CONTINUING CARE
- This fracture does not require setting (realignment), because the fractured bone is not displaced.
- Immobilization may be necessary. If so, a rigid walking cast will be placed around the foot, ankle and lower leg for 3 weeks, followed by a supportive shoe. Sometimes a removable cast boot or stiff-soled shoe provides enough support and immobilization to allow healing.

- Use frequent ice massage after the cast is removed. Fill a large styrofoam cup with water and freeze. Tear a small amount of foam from the top so ice protrudes. Massage firmly over the injured area in a circle about the size of a baseball. Do this for 15 minutes at a time 3 or 4 times a day, and also before workouts or competition.
- Apply heat instead of ice if it feels better. Use heat lamps, hot soaks, hot showers, heating pads or heat liniments and ointments.
- Take whirlpool treatments, if available.
- Massage gently and often to provide comfort and decrease swelling.

MEDICATION—Your doctor may prescribe:
- Prescription pain relievers for severe pain.
- Stool softeners to prevent constipation due to inactivity.
- Acetaminophen or ibuprofen (available without prescription) for mild pain after initial treatment.

ACTIVITY
- Don't bear weight on the injured foot. Learn to walk with crutches, and use them through the first week with your walking cast. See Appendix 3 (Safe Use of Crutches). Prop your foot up whenever possible.
- Begin reconditioning and rehabilitation after clearance from your doctor.
- Resume normal daily activities gradually after treatment.

DIET—During recovery, balance the amount of food you eat with any change in your level of physical activity. Eat a variety of foods to get the energy, protein, vitamins, minerals and fiber you need for good health and healing.

REHABILITATION—Begin daily rehabilitation exercises when movement is comfortable. Use ice massage for 10 minutes prior to exercise. See Rehabilitation section for ankle and foot exercises.

 CALL YOUR DOCTOR IF

- You have unexplained foot pain.
- Toes become dark, blue, cold or numb while the cast is on.
- Foot pain returns, despite treatment. This may indicate recurrence of stress fracture.

FOOT TENOSYNOVITIS

GENERAL INFORMATION

DEFINITION—Inflammation of the lining of a tendon sheath in the foot. This lining secretes a fluid that lubricates the tendon. When the lining becomes inflamed, the tendon cannot glide smoothly in its covering.

BODY PARTS INVOLVED
- Any foot tendon lining.
- Soft tissues in the surrounding area, including blood vessels, nerves, ligaments, periosteum (covering of bone) and connective tissues.

SIGNS & SYMPTOMS
- Constant pain or pain with motion.
- Limited motion of the foot and ankle.
- Crepitation (a "crackling" sound when the tendon moves or is touched).
- Redness and tenderness over the inflamed tendon.

CAUSES
- Strain from unusual use or overuse of muscles and tendons in the foot.
- Direct blow or injury to the foot. Tenosynovitis becomes more likely with repeated injury to the ankle or foot.
- Infection introduced through broken skin at the time of injury or through a surgical incision after injury.

- Constrictive footwear that causes pressure over the course of a tendon under repetitive use.

RISK INCREASES WITH
- Contact sports, especially kicking sports such as soccer or football.
- Skiing.
- If surgery is needed, surgical risk increases with smoking, poor nutrition, alcoholism or drug abuse and recent or chronic illness.

HOW TO PREVENT
- Engage in a program of physical conditioning before beginning regular sports participation.
- Warm up adequately before practice or competition.
- Wear protective gear appropriate for your sport.
- Learn proper moves and techniques for your sport.

WHAT TO EXPECT

APPROPRIATE HEALTH CARE
- Doctor's examination and diagnosis.
- Surgery (sometimes) to enlarge the tendon's covering and restore a smooth gliding motion. The surgical procedure is performed under general anesthesia in an outpatient surgical facility or hospital operating room.

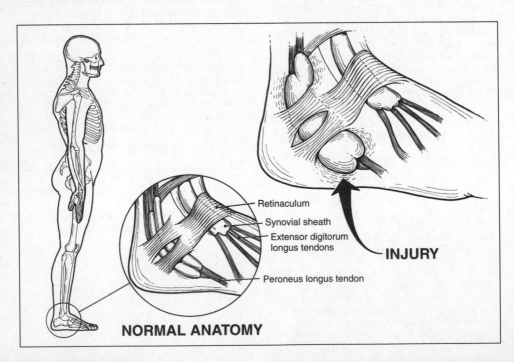

Retinaculum
Synovial sheath
Extensor digitorum longus tendons
Peroneus longus tendon

INJURY

NORMAL ANATOMY

DIAGNOSTIC MEASURES
• Your own observations of symptoms and signs.
• Medical history and physical examination by your doctor.
• X-rays of the area to rule out other abnormalities.
• Laboratory studies:
  Blood and urine studies before surgery.
  Tissues examination after surgery.

POSSIBLE COMPLICATIONS
• Prolonged healing time if activity is resumed too soon.
• Proneness to repeated injury of foot tendons.
• Adhesive tenosynovitis—The tendon and its covering become bound together. Restriction of motion may be complete or partial. Surgery is necessary to remove the covering or transfer the tendon to a less constrictive area.
• Constrictive tenosynovitis—The walls of the covering thicken and narrow its opening, preventing the tendon from sliding through. Surgery is necessary to cut away part of the covering.

PROBABLE OUTCOME—Tenosynovitis is usually curable in about 6 weeks with heat treatments, corticosteroid injections and rest of the inflamed area. Recovery is usually quicker if the inflammation is caused by a direct blow rather than by a strain or sprain.

 ## HOW TO TREAT

NOTE—Follow your doctor's instructions. These instructions are supplemental.

FIRST AID—None. This problem develops slowly.

CONTINUING CARE
• Wrap the foot and ankle with an elasticized bandage until healing is complete.
• Apply heat frequently. Use heat lamps, hot soaks, hot showers, heating pads or heat liniments and ointments.
• Take whirlpool treatments, if available.

MEDICATION—You may use nonprescription drugs such as acetaminophen or nonsteroidal anti-inflammatories for minor pain.
Your doctor may prescribe:
• Stronger pain relievers for severe pain.
• Injection of the tendon's covering with a combination of a long-acting local anesthetic and a nonabsorbable corticosteroid to relieve pain and inflammation.

ACTIVITY—Resume normal activity slowly.

DIET—During recovery, balance the amount of food you eat with any change in your level of physical activity. Eat a variety of foods to get the energy, protein, vitamins, minerals and fiber you need for good health and healing. Your doctor may suggest vitamin and mineral supplements to promote healing.

REHABILITATION
• Begin daily rehabilitation exercises when supportive wrapping is no longer needed.
• Use ice massage for 10 minutes before and after exercise. Fill a large styrofoam cup with water and freeze. Tear a small amount of foam from the top so ice protrudes. Massage firmly over the injured area in a circle about the size of a softball.
• See Rehabilitation section for ankle and foot exercises.

 ## CALL YOUR DOCTOR IF

• You have symptoms of foot tenosynovitis.
• Any of the following occurs after surgery:
  Increased pain, swelling, redness, drainage or bleeding in the surgical area.
  Signs of infection (headache, muscle aches, dizziness or a general ill feeling and fever).
  New, unexplained symptoms. Drugs used in treatment may produce side effects.

GENITAL CONTUSION

GENERAL INFORMATION

DEFINITION—Bruising of the skin and underlying tissues of the external genitals of the male or female due to a direct blow. Contusions cause bleeding from ruptured small capillaries that allow blood to infiltrate skin, scrotum, vaginal lips (labia) or other soft tissues. See also Perineum Contusion.

BODY PARTS INVOLVED—Genitals, including penis, scrotum, spermatic cord and testicles—or vaginal labia and clitoris—urethra, blood vessels and covering of bones (periosteum) in the pelvis.

SIGNS & SYMPTOMS
* Local swelling in the genital area—either superficial or deep.
* Pain and tenderness over the injury.
* Feeling of firmness when pressure is exerted at the injury site.
* Discoloration under the skin, beginning with redness and progressing to the characteristic "black-and-blue" bruise.
* Restricted activity in the genital area depending on the extent of injury.

CAUSES—Direct blow to the genitals, usually from a blunt object.

RISK INCREASES WITH
* Contact sports.
* Gymnastics.
* Bicycling.
* Horseback riding.
* Medical history of any bleeding disorder.
* Poor nutrition, including vitamin deficiency.

HOW TO PREVENT—Wear appropriate protective gear, such as a padded athletic supporter or cup, during competition or other athletic activity if there is risk of a genital contusion.

WHAT TO EXPECT

APPROPRIATE HEALTH CARE
* Doctor's care unless the contusion is quite small. A doctor should evaluate any testicle injury.
* Self-care for minor contusions.
* Ultrasound studies to evaluate testicle injuries.

DIAGNOSTIC MEASURES
* Your own observation of symptoms.
* Medical history and physical exam by a doctor for all except minor injuries.
* X-rays of injured area to assess total injury to soft tissues and to rule out the possibility of underlying fractures. The total extent of injury may not be apparent for 48 to 72 hours.

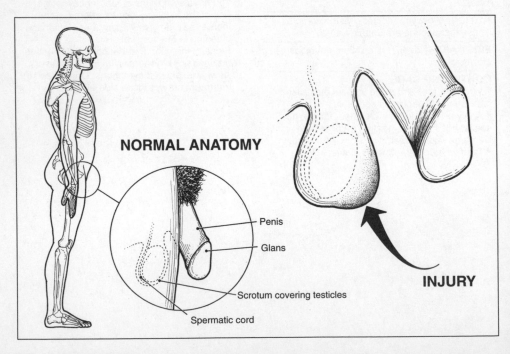

NORMAL ANATOMY

Penis

Glans

Scrotum covering testicles

Spermatic cord

INJURY

POSSIBLE COMPLICATIONS
- Excessive internal bleeding.
- Loss of testicle from injury.
- Prolonged healing time if usual activities are resumed too soon.
- Infection if skin over the contusion is broken.

PROBABLE OUTCOME—Despite severe pain at the time of injury, most genital contusions heal without complications. Reproductive capacity is rarely affected. Healing time varies with the extent of injury, from 3 to 14 days.

 ## HOW TO TREAT

NOTE—Follow your doctor's instructions. These instructions are supplemental.

FIRST AID—Use instructions for R.I.C.E., the first letters of *rest, ice, compression* and *elevation*. See Appendix 1 for details.

CONTINUING CARE
- Keep the area compressed and supported for 72 hours. Use an athletic supporter for compression for males and sanitary pads for females.
- Use an ice pack 3 or 4 times a day. Wrap ice chips or cubes in a plastic bag, and wrap the bag in a moist towel. Place it over the injured area for 20 minutes at a time.
- After 72 hours, apply heat instead of ice if it feels better. Use heat lamps, hot soaks, hot showers, heating pads, heat liniments and ointments or whirlpool treatments.
- Use crutches for a few days to avoid weight-bearing if the contusion is severe and hurts worse when walking.

MEDICATION
- For minor discomfort, you may use:
  Aspirin, acetaminophen or ibuprofen.
  Topical liniments and ointments.
- Your doctor may prescribe stronger medicine for pain.

ACTIVITY
- Avoid sexual intercourse and sexual excitement until healing is complete.
- Begin activities slowly, and stop exercise as soon as pain begins. Increase activity as healing progresses.
- Avoid contact sports if the function of one testicle is lost.

DIET—During recovery, balance the amount of food you eat with any change in your level of physical activity. Eat a variety of foods to get the energy, protein, vitamins, minerals and fiber you need for good health and healing.

REHABILITATION—None.

 ## CALL YOUR DOCTOR IF

- You have a genital contusion that does not improve in 1 or 2 days.
- Skin is broken and signs of infection (drainage, increasing pain, fever, headache, muscle aches, dizziness or a general ill feeling) occur.

GROIN STRAIN

GENERAL INFORMATION

DEFINITION—Injury to the muscles or tendons in the area of the groin where the abdomen meets the thigh. Muscles, tendons and their attached bones comprise contractile units. These units stabilize the pelvis and allow its motion. A strain occurs at a unit's weakest part. Strains are of 3 types:
- Mild (Grade I)—Slightly pulled muscle without tearing of muscle or tendon fibers. There is no loss of strength.
- Moderate (Grade II)—Tearing of fibers in a muscle or tendon or at the attachment to bone. Strength is diminished.
- Severe (Grade III)—Rupture of the muscle-tendon-bone attachment, with separation of fibers. A severe strain may require surgical repair. Chronic strains are caused by overuse. Acute strains are caused by direct injury or overstress.

BODY PARTS INVOLVED
- Tendons and muscles of the groin area, including abdominal, pelvic and thigh muscles.
- Bones of the groin area, including the pelvis, spine and upper leg bone (femur).
- Soft tissues surrounding the strain, including nerves, periosteum (covering of bone), blood vessels and lymph vessels.

SIGNS & SYMPTOMS
- Pain in the groin with motion or stretching of the leg at the hip joint.
- Muscle spasm in the abdomen or thigh.
- Swelling in the groin.
- Loss of strength (moderate or severe strain).
- Calcification of a muscle or its tendon (visible with x-ray).

CAUSES
- Prolonged overuse of muscle-tendon units in the groin.
- Single violent injury or force applied to the groin muscle-tendon unit.

RISK INCREASES WITH
- Contact sports.
- Sports that require quick starts, such as the start of a race.
- Medical history of any bleeding disorder.
- Obesity.
- Poor nutrition.
- Previous groin injury.
- Poor muscle conditioning.

HOW TO PREVENT
- Participate in a strengthening, flexibility and conditioning program appropriate for your sport.
- Warm up before practice or competition.

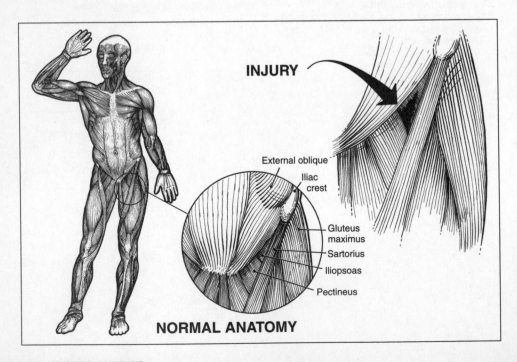

INJURY

External oblique
Iliac crest
Gluteus maximus
Sartorius
Iliopsoas
Pectineus

NORMAL ANATOMY

WHAT TO EXPECT

APPROPRIATE HEALTH CARE
- Doctor's diagnosis.
- Self-care during rehabilitation.
- Physical therapy (moderate or severe strain).
- Surgery (severe strain).

DIAGNOSTIC MEASURES
- Your own observation of symptoms.
- Medical history and exam by a doctor.
- X-rays of the injured hip, thigh and pelvis to rule out possible fractures.

POSSIBLE COMPLICATIONS
- Prolonged healing time if activity is resumed too soon.
- Proneness to repeated injury.
- Unstable or arthritic hip following repeated injury.
- Inflammation at the attachment to bone (periostitis).
- Prolonged disability (sometimes), especially weakness.

PROBABLE OUTCOME—If this is a first-time injury, proper care and sufficient healing time before resuming activity should prevent permanent disability. Average healing times are:
- Mild strain—2 to 10 days.
- Moderate strain—10 days to 6 weeks.
- Severe strain—6 to 10 weeks.

If this is a repeated injury, complications listed above are more likely to occur.

HOW TO TREAT

NOTE—Follow your doctor's instructions. These instructions are supplemental.

FIRST AID—Use instructions for R.I.C.E., the first letters of *rest, ice, compression* and *elevation* (if possible). See Appendix 1 for details.

CONTINUING CARE
- Use ice massage 3 or 4 times a day for 15 minutes at a time. Fill a large styrofoam cup with water and freeze. Tear a small amount of foam from the top so ice protrudes. Massage firmly over the injured area in a circle about the size of a softball.
- After the first 24 hours, apply heat instead of ice if it feels better. Use heat lamps, hot soaks, hot showers, heating pads or heat liniments and ointments.
- Support the injured groin area with an elasticized bandage between treatments.

MEDICATION
- For minor discomfort, you may use:
  Aspirin, acetaminophen or ibuprofen.
  Topical liniments and ointments.
- Your doctor may prescribe:
  Stronger pain relievers.
  Injection of a long-acting local anesthetic to reduce pain.
  Injections of a corticosteroid, such as triamcinolone, to reduce inflammation.

ACTIVITY
- For a moderate or severe strain, walk with crutches for at least 72 hours. See Appendix 3 (Safe Use of Crutches).
- Resume your normal activities gradually.

DIET—During recovery, balance the amount of food you eat with any change in your level of physical activity. Eat a variety of foods to get the energy, protein, vitamins, minerals and fiber you need for good health and healing.

REHABILITATION—Begin daily rehabilitation exercises when supportive wrapping is no longer needed. See Rehabilitation section for hip and pelvis exercises.

CALL YOUR DOCTOR IF

- You have symptoms of a groin strain.
- Pain or swelling worsens despite treatment.

GROWTH PLATE INJURIES

GENERAL INFORMATION

DEFINITION—An injury to the growth plate in a child or adolescent. A growth plate is soft tissue that grows on the end of long bones which is eventually replaced with solid bone. Long bones are those that contribute to height or length of an extremity (particularly the arms and legs). Adults don't have growth plates. An injury that would cause a sprain in an adult can be a potentially serious growth plate injury in a young child. The growth plate isn't as strong as bone, ligaments or tendons. Growth plates are the weakest areas in a child's skeleton and are the most susceptible to injury. Most growth plate injuries are fractures.

BODY PARTS INVOLVED
- Growth plate (known as the physis) is the area of developing tissue near the end of the long bones in children and adolescents. Each long bone has a growth plate at either end. The growth plate determines the future length and shape of the mature bone. Once growth is complete (in adolescence), growth plates are replaced by solid bone.
- Growth plate fractures occur most:
  In the long bones of the fingers (phalanges).
  Outer bone of the forearm (radius) at the wrist.
  Lower bones of the leg (the tibia and fibula).
  Upper leg bone (femur).
  Ankle, foot, or hip bone.

SIGNS & SYMPTOMS
- Pain, swelling, tenderness and limitation of motion.
- Unable to use an arm or leg, due to severe pain from an injury.
- Inability to continue to play after a sudden sports injury.
- Symptoms of a growth plate injury can mimic a sprain.

CAUSES
- A fall or blow to the body.
- Overuse injury.
- Twisting an ankle or knee.
- Accidents (motor vehicle, motorcycle, all terrain vehicle).
- Some growth plate injuries may be due to genetic disorders, existing medical problems or other miscellaneous causes.

RISK INCREASES WITH
- Participating in competitive sports (football, basketball, softball, track and field, gymnastics).
- Participating in recreational activities (biking, skiing, sledding, skateboarding).
- Lack of physical conditioning. It is a major contributor to overuse and acute injuries.
- Running or playing on furniture or playground equipment
- Girls' skeletons mature earlier than boys, so older boys are more likely to have a growth-plate injury than older girls.
- The highest rate of injury is among 14-year-old boys and girls ages 11 and 12.

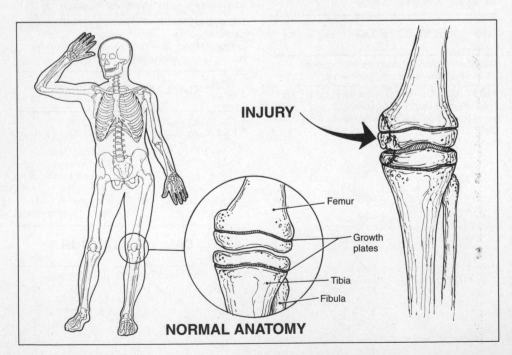

INJURY

Femur

Growth plates

Tibia

Fibula

NORMAL ANATOMY

HOW TO PREVENT
- Schedule a preseason medical exam to identify any problems or preexisting injuries.
- Be sure a child is in shape before participating in a sports activity.
- Be sure child knows and abides by the rules of the sport.
- Help child build overall strength, flexibility and muscle tone with a conditioning program.
- In contact sports or activities involving running and jumping, protect vulnerable joints. Wear proper protective gear and devices.
- Warm up adequately before physical activity.
- Parents or coaches should never require or allow a child to "play through" pain.

 WHAT TO EXPECT

APPROPRIATE HEALTH CARE
- Doctor's treatment.
- Surgery (sometimes).

DIAGNOSTIC MEASURES
- Your own observation of symptoms.
- Medical history and exam by a doctor.
- X-rays. Injuries to the growth plate may be hard to see on x-ray, so an x-ray of the noninjured side of the body may be taken so the two sides can be compared. In some cases, magnetic resonance imaging (MRI), computed tomography (CT), or ultrasound, will be used.

POSSIBLE COMPLICATIONS
- Complications can include recurring pain, arthritis, deformity and growth problems. The affected bone grows less than it would have without the injury. If only part of the growth plate is injured, growth may be lopsided and the limb may be crooked. Growth plate injuries at the knee are at greatest risk of complications.
- If these problems are detected and treated early, the possible long-term complications can be minimized or avoided.

PROBABLE OUTCOME
- Most growth plate fractures heal without any lasting harm.
- The majority of breaks heal in 1-2 months.

 HOW TO TREAT

NOTE—Follow your doctor's instructions. These instructions are supplemental.

FIRST AID
- Immobilize the injured area before transporting the child to the doctor's office or emergency facility.
- Use instructions for R.I.C.E., the first letters of *rest, ice, compression* and *elevation*. See Appendix 1 for details.

- The doctor will realign and set the broken bones (possibly with surgery). Manipulation should be done as soon as possible after injury.
- There are five basic types of growth plate injuries (Salter-Harris classification). A cast or splint is usually necessary for types 1, 2 and 3. Type 4 and 5 require surgery for proper alignment and healing.

CONTINUING CARE
- The doctor may suggest that ice be applied to the area.
- The growth of the bone must be watched closely for up to a year (or longer) with exams and x-rays to ensure the bone continues to grow and grow straight.

MEDICATION—Your doctor may prescribe:
- General anesthesia, local anesthesia or muscle relaxants to make bone manipulation possible.
- Prescription pain relievers for severe pain.
- Acetaminophen (available without prescription) for mild pain after initial treatment.

ACTIVITY
- Limit any activity that puts pressure on the injured area.
- Resume sports participation after clearance from the doctor (the muscles must have regained their original strength and the child can move the joint fully without pain). Resuming play too soon after a growth plate injury impedes healing, which can lead to long-term problems.
- Restrict vigorous activity for 6 weeks after surgery. Then resume normal activities gradually.

DIET
- Do not eat or drink before manipulation or surgery to treat the fracture. Fluid or solid food in the stomach makes vomiting while under anesthesia more hazardous.
- During recovery, eat a healthy diet.

REHABILITATION
- Your doctor will outline a program of rehabilitation for your child, either to be done at home or possibly a physical therapy facility.
- Rehabilitation begins as soon as the joint can be moved without pain. The goal is to restore normal range of motion and strength to the affected limb as quickly as possible, without aggravating the injury and slowing the healing.

 CALL YOUR DOCTOR IF

- Your child has symptoms of a growth plate injury.
- After treatment, your child has continued pain, swelling, bleeding or other problems.

HAND CONTUSION

GENERAL INFORMATION

DEFINITION—Bruising of the skin and underlying tissues of the hand due to a direct blow. Contusions cause bleeding from ruptured small capillaries that allow blood to infiltrate muscles, tendons or other soft tissues. The hand is especially vulnerable to contusions because of its exposure and use in almost all sports.

BODY PARTS INVOLVED—Hand tissues, including blood vessels, muscles, tendons, nerves, covering of bones (periosteum) and connective tissues.

SIGNS & SYMPTOMS
- Swelling on the back or in the palm of the hand. Swelling may be superficial or deep.
- Pain and tenderness over the injury.
- Feeling of numbness when pressure is exerted on the injured area.
- Discoloration under the skin, beginning with redness and progressing to the characteristic "black-and-blue" bruise.
- Restricted hand motion proportional to the extent of injury.

CAUSES—Direct blow to the hand, usually from a blunt object.

RISK INCREASES WITH
- Contact sports, especially when the hands are not adequately protected.
- Medical history of any bleeding disorder .
- Poor nutrition, including vitamin deficiency.
- Use of anticoagulants or aspirin.

HOW TO PREVENT—If possible, wear appropriate protective padding during competition or other athletic activity. If you must compete before a hand contusion heals, use padding, tape or a cast.

WHAT TO EXPECT

APPROPRIATE HEALTH CARE
- Doctor's care, unless the injury is quite small.
- Self-care for minor contusions and for serious contusions during the rehabilitation phase.
- Physical therapy for serious contusions.

DIAGNOSTIC MEASURES
- Your own observation of symptoms.
- Medical history and physical exam by a doctor for all except minor injuries.
- X-rays of the hand and wrist to assess total injury to soft tissues and to rule out the possibility of underlying fractures. The total extent of injury may not be apparent for 48 to 72 hours.

POSSIBLE COMPLICATIONS
- Excessive bleeding, leading to disability. Infiltrative-type bleeding can (rarely) lead to calcification and impaired function of injured muscles or tendons.

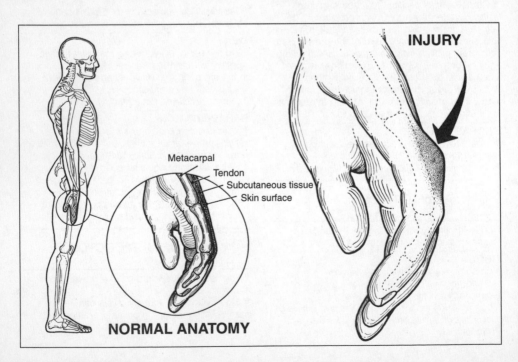

Metacarpal
Tendon
Subcutaneous tissue
Skin surface

NORMAL ANATOMY

INJURY

- Infection if skin over the contusion is broken.
- Infection of the tendon sheaths.
- Tendon rupture.

PROBABLE OUTCOME—Healing time varies with the extent of injury, but average healing time for hand contusions is 1 to 3 weeks.

 HOW TO TREAT

NOTE—Follow your doctor's instructions. These instructions are supplemental.

FIRST AID—Use instructions for R.I.C.E., the first letters of *rest, ice, compression* and *elevation*. See Appendix 1 for details.

CONTINUING CARE
- Wrap an elasticized bandage over a felt pad placed on the injured area. Keep the area compressed for about 72 hours.
- Continue ice massage. Fill a large styrofoam cup with water and freeze. Tear a small amount of foam from the top so ice protrudes. Massage firmly over the injured area in a circle about the size of a softball.
- After 72 hours, apply heat instead of ice if feels better. Use heat lamps, hot soaks, hot showers, heating pads, heat liniments and ointments or whirlpool treatments.
- Massage gently and often with light lubricating oil to provide comfort and decrease swelling. Stroke from the fingers toward the shoulder.

MEDICATION
- For minor discomfort, you may use:
  Aspirin, acetaminophen or ibuprofen.
  Topical liniments and ointments.
- Your doctor may prescribe stronger medicine for pain.

ACTIVITY—Begin activities slowly, and stop exercise as soon as pain begins. Increase activity as healing progresses.

DIET—During recovery, balance the amount of food you eat with any change in your level of physical activity. Eat a variety of foods to get the energy, protein, vitamins, minerals and fiber you need for good health and healing.

REHABILITATION
- Begin daily rehabilitation exercises when supportive wrapping is no longer needed.
- Use ice massage for 10 minutes before and after workouts.
- See Rehabilitation section for wrist and hand exercises.

 CALL YOUR DOCTOR IF

- You have a hand contusion that doesn't improve in 1 or 2 days.
- Skin is broken and signs of infection (drainage, increasing pain, fever, headache, muscle aches, dizziness or a general ill feeling) occur.

HAND DISLOCATION
(Carpometacarpal Dislocation)

 GENERAL INFORMATION

DEFINITION—Injury to the hand so that adjoining bones are displaced and no longer touch each other. The ulnar nerve is likely to be injured with this dislocation. If the ulnar nerve is involved, surgery is necessary to prevent permanent damage.

BODY PARTS INVOLVED
• Hand bones (carpal and metacarpal bones).
• Ligaments that hold the hand bones in the proper positions.
• Soft tissues surrounding the dislocation site, including periosteum (covering of bone), tendons, blood vessels and connective tissues.
• Ulnar nerve.

SIGNS & SYMPTOMS
• Excruciating pain at the time of injury.
• Loss of normal hand function.
• Severe pain when attempting to move hand.
• Visible deformity if the dislocated bones have locked in the dislocated positions. Bones may spontaneously reposition themselves and leave no deformity, but damage is the same.
• Tenderness over the dislocation.
• Much swelling and bruising at the injury site.
• Numbness or paralysis below the dislocation from pressure, pinching or cutting of blood vessels or nerves.

CAUSES
• Direct blow to the hand or falling on an outstretched hand (most common cause).
• End result of a severe hand sprain.

RISK INCREASES WITH
• Contact sports.
• Previous dislocation or sprain.
• Repeated injury to any hand joint.
• Poor muscle conditioning.
• Congenital abnormality.

HOW TO PREVENT—Initial injury usually cannot be prevented. After healing, protect vulnerable hand joints with wrapped elastic bandages, tape wraps, felt or foam rubber pads or plastic splints.

 WHAT TO EXPECT

APPROPRIATE HEALTH CARE
• Doctor's treatment. This will include manipulating the joint to reposition the bones.
• Surgery (sometimes) to restore the joint to its normal position and maintain the position with pins. Acute or recurring dislocations may require surgical reconstruction or fusion of the joint. Ulnar nerve involvement always requires surgery to salvage function in the muscles supplied by the ulnar nerve.
• Self-care during rehabilitation.

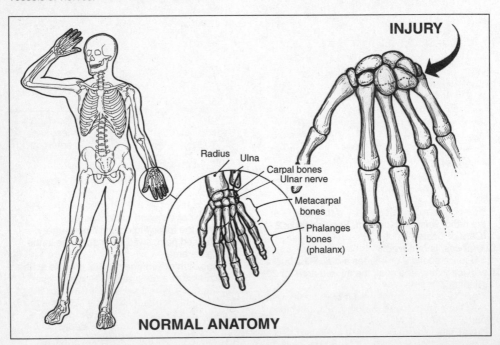

INJURY

Radius Ulna

Carpal bones
Ulnar nerve

Metacarpal bones

Phalanges bones (phalanx)

NORMAL ANATOMY

DIAGNOSTIC MEASURES
- Your own observation of symptoms.
- Medical history and exam by a doctor.
- X-rays of the wrist and hand.

POSSIBLE COMPLICATIONS
At the time of injury:
- Shock.
- Pressure on or injury to nearby nerves, ligaments, tendons, muscles, blood vessels or connective tissues.

After treatment or surgery:
- Excessive internal bleeding around the dislocation site.
- Impairment of blood supply to the dislocated area and muscles in the hand by excessive tense swelling (acute compartment syndrome).
- Death of bone cells due to interruption of the blood supply.
- Prolonged healing if activity is resumed too soon.
- Recurrent dislocations.
- Unstable or arthritic joint following repeated injury.

PROBABLE OUTCOME—After the dislocation has been corrected, the joint may require immobilization with a cast or splint for 2 to 8 weeks. Complete healing of injured ligaments requires a minimum of 6 weeks.

HOW TO TREAT

NOTE—Follow your doctor's instructions. These instructions are supplemental.

FIRST AID
- Use instructions for R.I.C.E., the first letters of *rest, ice, compression* and *elevation*. See Appendix 1 for details.
- The doctor will manipulate the dislocated bones in the hand to return them to their normal positions. Anesthesia and traction on fingers and countertraction on a flexed elbow are usually necessary to correct this dislocation. Manipulation should be done within 6 hours of injury or many tissues will lose elasticity and become difficult to return to their normal positions.

CONTINUING CARE
After injury:
- Immobilization is necessary with a cast over the hand, wrist and forearm. See Appendix 2 (Care of Casts).

After cast is removed:
- Use ice soaks 3 or 4 times a day. Fill a bucket with ice water, and soak the injured area for 20 minutes at a time.
- Apply heat instead of ice if it feels better. Use heat lamps, hot soaks, hot showers or heating pads.
- Take whirlpool treatments, if available.

- Wrap the hand with an elasticized bandage between treatments.
- Massage gently and often to provide comfort and decrease swelling.

MEDICATION—Your doctor may prescribe:
- General anesthesia or muscle relaxants to make joint manipulation possible.
- Acetaminophen to relieve moderate pain.
- Narcotic pain relievers for severe pain.
- Stool softeners to prevent constipation due to decreased activity.
- Antibiotics to fight infection if surgery is necessary.

ACTIVITY
If surgery is not necessary:
- Resume sports participation after clearance from your doctor.

If surgery is necessary:
- Resume normal activities gradually after surgery.
- Don't drive until healing is complete.

DIET
- Do not eat or drink before manipulation or surgery to correct the dislocation. Fluid or solid food in your stomach makes vomiting while under general anesthesia more hazardous.
- During recovery, eat a well-balanced diet.

REHABILITATION
- Begin daily rehabilitation exercises when supportive wrapping is no longer needed.
- Use ice message for 10 minutes before and after workouts. Fill a large styrofoam cup with water and freeze. Tear a small amount of foam from the top so ice protrudes. Massage firmly in a circle over the injured area.
- See Rehabilitation section for wrist and hand exercises.

CALL YOUR DOCTOR IF

- You have symptoms of a dislocated hand. Call immediately if the hand becomes numb, pale or cold after injury. This is an emergency!
- Any of the following occurs after treatment:
  Swelling above or below the cast.
  Blue or gray skin color beyond the cast, particularly under the fingernails.
  Loss of feeling in the hand.
  Nausea or vomiting; constipation.
- Any of the following occurs after surgery:
  Increased pain, swelling or drainage in the surgical area.
  Signs of infection (headache, muscle aches, dizziness or a general ill feeling and fever).
- New, unexplained symptoms develop. Drugs used in treatment may produce side effects.
- Hand dislocations that you can "pop" back into normal position occur repeatedly.

HAND FRACTURE, CARPAL

 GENERAL INFORMATION

DEFINITION—A complete or incomplete break in any one of several bones of the hand.

BODY PARTS INVOLVED
* Any carpal bone in the hand, but most frequently the carpal navicular bone.
* Wrist joint.
* Any of the joints between the hand and fingers.
* Soft tissues surrounding the fracture site, including nerves, tendons, ligaments and blood vessels.

SIGNS & SYMPTOMS
* Severe pain at the fracture site.
* Swelling of soft tissues surrounding the fracture.
* Tenderness to the touch.
* Numbness and coldness beyond the fracture site if the blood supply is impaired.

CAUSES—Direct blow or indirect stress to the bone. Indirect stress may be caused by twisting or violent muscle contraction.

RISK INCREASES WITH
* Contact sports, especially boxing.
* History of bone or joint disease, especially osteoporosis.
* Poor nutrition, especially calcium deficiency.

HOW TO PREVENT
* Use appropriate protective equipment, such as boxing gloves for boxing.
* If you have had a previous hand injury, protect the hand with taping and padding when participating in contact sports.

 WHAT TO EXPECT

APPROPRIATE HEALTH CARE
* Doctor's treatment to immobilize the broken bones.
* Surgery for most displaced fractures.
* Self-care during rehabilitation.

DIAGNOSTIC MEASURES
* Your own observation of symptoms.
* Medical history and physical exam by a doctor.
* X-rays of injured areas, including joints above and below the primary injury site.
* Repeat x-rays are frequently needed about 2 weeks after injury if the original x-rays were negative and pain continues.
* Technetium bone scan (see Glossary) to confirm presence of fracture when not visible on x-rays.

POSSIBLE COMPLICATIONS
At the time of injury:
* Misdiagnosis as a wrist sprain, delaying proper treatment.
* Shock.

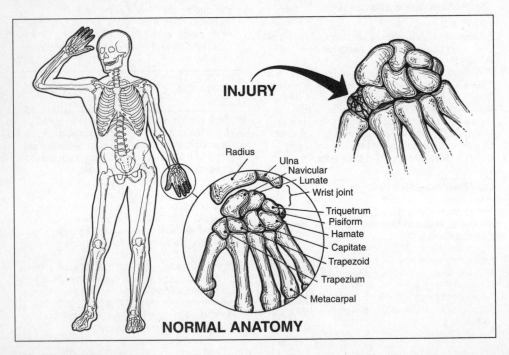

INJURY

Radius
Ulna
Navicular
Lunate
Wrist joint
Triquetrum
Pisiform
Hamate
Capitate
Trapezoid
Trapezium
Metacarpal

NORMAL ANATOMY

- Pressure on or injury to nearby nerves, ligaments, tendons, muscles, blood vessels or connective tissues.

After treatment or surgery:
- Delayed union or nonunion of the fracture.
- Impaired blood supply to the fracture site, with development of avascular necrosis (death of bone cells).
- Arrest of normal bone growth in children.
- Infection in open fractures (skin broken over fracture site).
- Shortening of the injured bones.
- Proneness to repeated hand injury.
- Unstable or arthritic joint following repeated injury.
- Prolonged healing time if activity is resumed too soon.
- Problems caused by casts. See Appendix 2 (Care of Casts).

PROBABLE OUTCOME—It is impossible to predict exactly how long it will take for any fracture to heal. Variable factors include age, sex and previous state of health and conditioning. The average healing time for this fracture is 2 to 4 months, depending on which bone is fractured (the navicular bone averages 4 months). Healing is considered complete when there is no motion at the fracture site and when x-rays show complete bone union.

 HOW TO TREAT

NOTE—Follow your doctor's instructions. These instructions are supplemental.

FIRST AID
- Use a padded splint or sling to immobilize the hand and wrist before transporting the injured person to the doctor's office or emergency facility.
- Keep the person warm with blankets to decrease the possibility of shock.
- Follow instructions for R.I.C.E., the first letters of *rest, ice, compression* and *elevation*. See Appendix 1 for details

CONTINUING CARE
- Immobilization will be necessary. Rigid casts or splints are placed around the hand to immobilize the joint above and the joint below the fracture site. After the cast has been removed, the hand needs protection with taping or with a leather gauntlet.

- After 96 hours, application of localized heat promotes healing by increasing blood circulation in the injured area. Use a heating pad or heat lamp so heat can penetrate the cast.
- After the cast is removed, use frequent ice massage. Fill a large styrofoam cup with water and freeze. Tear a small amount of foam from the top so ice protrudes. Massage firmly over the injured area in a circle about the size of a baseball. Do this for 15 minutes at a time 3 or 4 times a day, and also before workouts or competition.
- Apply heat instead of ice if it feels better. Use heat lamps, hot soaks, hot showers, heating pads or heat liniments and ointments.
- Take whirlpool treatments, if available.

MEDICATION—Your doctor may prescribe:
- Pain relievers for severe pain.
- Acetaminophen (available without prescription) for mild pain after initial treatment.

ACTIVITY
- Actively exercise all muscle groups not immobilized. Muscle contractions promote fracture alignment and hasten healing.
- Resume normal activities gradually after treatment.
- Begin reconditioning the injured area after clearance from your doctor.

DIET—During recovery, balance the amount of food you eat with any change in your level of physical activity. Eat a variety of foods to get the energy, protein, vitamins, minerals and fiber you need for good health and healing.

REHABILITATION—Begin daily rehabilitation exercises when movement is comfortable. Use ice message for 10 minutes prior to exercise. See Rehabilitation section for wrist and hand exercises.

 CALL YOUR DOCTOR IF

- You have signs or symptoms of a hand fracture.
- Any of the following occurs after treatment: Increased pain or swelling in the injured area. Swelling above or below the cast or splint. Change in skin color to blue or gray beyond the cast, particularly under the fingernails. Numbness or complete loss of feeling in the hand, fingers or thumb.

HAND FRACTURE, METACARPAL

GENERAL INFORMATION

DEFINITION—A complete or incomplete break in one of the metacarpal bones—the bones that connect the hand and wrist to the fingers.

BODY PARTS INVOLVED
- Metacarpal bones of the hand.
- Metacarpocarpal joints and metacarpophalangeal joints.
- Soft tissues around the fracture site, including nerves, tendons, ligaments and blood vessels.

SIGNS & SYMPTOMS
- Severe hand pain at the time of injury.
- Swelling of soft tissues around the fracture.
- Visible deformity if the fracture is complete.
- Tenderness to the touch.
- Numbness and coldness beyond the fracture site if the blood supply is impaired.

CAUSES
- Direct blow, such as a blow struck with the fist.
- Indirect stress to the bone. Indirect stress may be caused by twisting or violent muscle contraction.

RISK INCREASES WITH
- Contact sports, especially football and boxing.
- History of bone or joint disease, especially osteoporosis.
- Poor nutrition, especially calcium deficiency.

- If surgery or anesthesia is needed, surgical risk increases with smoking and use of drugs, including mind-altering drugs, muscle relaxants, antihypertensives, tranquilizers, sleep inducers, insulin, sedatives, beta-adrenergic blockers or corticosteroids.

HOW TO PREVENT
- Use appropriate protective equipment, such as padded gloves for boxing and hand pads for football.
- If you have had a previous hand fracture, use tape and padding to protect your hands before participating in contact sports.

WHAT TO EXPECT

APPROPRIATE HEALTH CARE
- Doctor's treatment to manipulate the broken bones.
- Anesthesia and surgery sometimes necessary to set the fracture and fix with pins or screws and plates.
- Self-care during rehabilitation.
- Whirlpool, ultrasound or massage (to displace excess fluid from the injured joint space).

DIAGNOSTIC MEASURES
- Your own observation of symptoms.
- Medical history and physical exam by a doctor.
- X-rays of injured areas, including joints above and below the primary injury site.

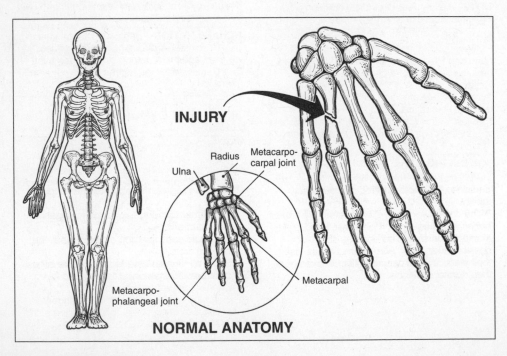

INJURY

Radius

Ulna

Metacarpo-carpal joint

Metacarpal

Metacarpo-phalangeal joint

NORMAL ANATOMY

POSSIBLE COMPLICATIONS

At the time of injury:
- Shock.
- Pressure on or injury to nearby nerves, ligaments, tendons, muscles, blood vessels or connective tissues.

After treatment or surgery:
- Delayed union or nonunion of the fracture.
- Impaired blood supply to the fracture site.
- Avascular necrosis (death of bone cells due to interruption of the blood supply).
- Arrest of normal bone growth in children.
- Infection in open fractures (skin broken over fracture site) or at the incision if surgical setting was necessary.
- Shortening or angulation of the injured bones.
- Rotational deformity can occur (fingers do not fold together when fist is clenched).
- Proneness to repeated hand injury.
- Unstable or arthritic joint following repeated injury.
- Prolonged healing time if activity is resumed too soon.
- Problems caused by casts. See Appendix 2 (Care of Casts).

PROBABLE OUTCOME—It is impossible to predict exactly how long it will take for any fracture to heal. Variable factors include age, sex and previous state of health and conditioning. The average healing time for this fracture is 4 to 6 weeks. Healing is considered complete when there is no motion at the fracture site and when x-rays show complete bone union.

 HOW TO TREAT

NOTE—Follow your doctor's instructions. These instructions are supplemental.

FIRST AID
- Keep the person warm with blankets to decrease the possibility of shock.
- Follow instructions for R.I.C.E., the first letters of *rest, ice, compression* and *elevation*. See Appendix 1 for details.
- Use a padded splint or sling to immobilize the hand and wrist before transporting the injured person to the doctor's office or emergency facility.
- The doctor will manipulate and set the broken bones with surgery or, if possible, without. Manipulation should be done as soon as possible after injury. Also, many tissues lose their elasticity and become difficult to return to their normal positions.

CONTINUING CARE
- Immobilization will be necessary. A rigid cast or splint will be placed around the injured area to immobilize the fingers and wrist.
- After 96 hours, application of localized heat promotes healing by increasing blood circulation in the injured area. Use a heat lamp or heating pad so heat can penetrate the cast.
- After the cast is removed, use frequent ice massage. Fill a large styrofoam cup with water and freeze. Tear a small amount of foam from the top so ice protrudes. Massage firmly over the injured area in a circle about the size of a baseball. Do this for 15 minutes at a time 3 or 4 times a day, and also before workouts or competition.

MEDICATION—Your doctor may prescribe:
- General anesthesia, local anesthesia or muscle relaxants to make bone manipulation possible.
- Pain relievers for severe pain.
- Acetaminophen (available without prescription) for mild pain after initial treatment.

ACTIVITY
- Actively exercise all muscle groups not immobilized. Muscle contractions promote fracture alignment and hasten healing.
- Begin reconditioning of the hand after clearance from your doctor.
- Resume normal activities gradually after treatment.

DIET
- Do not eat or drink before manipulation or surgery to treat the fracture. Fluid or solid food in your stomach makes vomiting while under anesthesia more hazardous.
- Balance the amount of food you eat with any change in your level of physical activity.

REHABILITATION—Begin daily rehabilitation exercises when movement is comfortable. Use ice massage for 10 minutes prior to exercise. See Rehabilitation section for wrist and hand exercises.

 CALL YOUR DOCTOR IF

- You have signs or symptoms of a hand fracture.
- Any of the following occurs after surgery or other treatment:
  Increased pain, swelling or drainage in the surgical area.
  Signs of infection (headache, muscle aches, dizziness or a general ill feeling and fever).
  Swelling above or below the cast.
  Blue or gray skin color under the fingernails.
  Numbness or complete loss of feeling in the fingers of the affected hand.
  Nausea or vomiting.

HAND FRACTURE, NAVICULAR
(Scaphoid Bone Fracture)

 GENERAL INFORMATION

DEFINITION—A complete or incomplete break in the navicular bone of the hand.

BODY PARTS INVOLVED
- Navicular (scaphoid) bone in the hand.
- Wrist joint.
- Soft tissues around the fracture site, including nerves, tendons, ligaments and blood vessels.

SIGNS & SYMPTOMS
- Severe pain at the fracture site.
- Swelling of soft tissues around the fracture.
- Tenderness to the touch over the navicular bone.
- Numbness and coldness in the hand and fingers if the blood supply is impaired.

CAUSES—Direct blow or indirect stress to the bone. The force is usually inflicted by a fall on an outstretched hand.

RISK INCREASES WITH
- Participation in contact sports, especially boxing, football and wrestling.
- History of bone or joint disease, especially osteoporosis; obesity.
- If surgery or anesthesia is needed, surgical risk increases with smoking and use of drugs, including mind-altering drugs, muscle relaxants, insulin, sedatives, beta-adrenergic blockers or corticosteroids.

HOW TO PREVENT
- Use appropriate protective equipment, such as wrist braces for inline skating or skateboarding.
- If you have had a previous injury, use tape and padding to protect you hand before participating in contact sports.

 WHAT TO EXPECT

APPROPRIATE HEALTH CARE
- Doctor's treatment to manipulate the broken bones and immobilize the injured area.
- Anesthesia and surgery with screw fixation when fracture is displaced.
- Self-care during rehabilitation.
- Whirlpool, ultrasound or massage (to displace excess fluid from the injured joint space).

DIAGNOSTIC MEASURES
- Your own observation of symptoms.
- Medical history and physical exam by a doctor.
- X-rays of injured areas, including the wrist joint above and the bones in the hand.
- Repeat x-rays may be needed after 2 to 8 weeks if the first set shows no injury but symptoms continue (this injury may not appear on x-rays for several weeks).
- Technetium bone scan (see Glossary) or MRI to confirm fracture prior to visibility on x-rays.

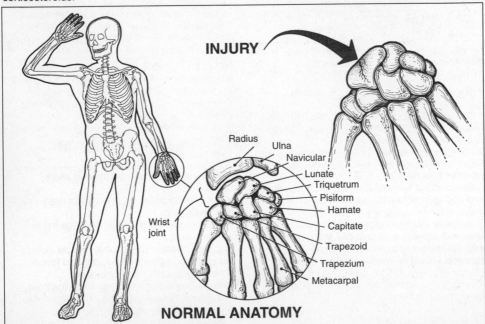

INJURY

Radius
Ulna
Navicular
Lunate
Triquetrum
Pisiform
Hamate
Capitate
Trapezoid
Trapezium
Metacarpal
Wrist joint

NORMAL ANATOMY

POSSIBLE COMPLICATIONS

At the time of injury:
- Shock.
- Pressure on or injury to nearby nerves, ligaments, tendons, muscles, blood vessels or connective tissues.

After treatment or surgery:
- Delayed union or nonunion of the fracture (frequently).
- Impaired blood supply to the fracture site, with development of avascular necrosis (death of bone) and even collapse of the bone, with subsequent arthritis.
- Arrest of normal bone growth in children.
- Infection in open fractures (skin broken over fracture site) or at the incision if surgical setting was necessary.
- Proneness to repeated hand injury.
- Unstable or arthritic joint following repeated injury
- Prolonged healing time if activity is resumed too soon.
- Problems caused by casts. See Appendix 2 (Care of Casts).

PROBABLE OUTCOME—It is impossible to predict exactly how long it will take for any fracture to heal. Variable factors include age, sex and previous state of health and conditioning. The average healing time for this fracture is 4 to 5 months (an unusually long time for a fracture to heal). Healing is considered complete when there is no motion at the fracture site and when x-rays show complete bone union. Sometimes this fracture never heals totally (this frequently leads to wrist arthritis).

 ## HOW TO TREAT

NOTE—Follow your doctor's instructions. These instructions are supplemental.

FIRST AID
- Keep the person warm with blankets to decrease the possibility of shock.
- Cut away clothing, if possible, but don't move the injured area to do so.
- Follow instructions for R.I.C.E., the first letters of *rest, ice, compression* and *elevation.* See Appendix 1 for details.
- Use a padded splint or sling to immobilize the hand and wrist before transporting the injured person to a medical facility.
- The doctor will manipulate and set the broken bones with surgery or, if possible, without. A navicular fracture with separated bone fragments should be manipulated as soon as possible after injury. Also, many tissues lose their elasticity and become difficult to return to their normal positions.

CONTINUING CARE
- Immobilization will be necessary. A rigid cast or plaster splints are placed around the injured area to immobilize the joint above and the joint below the fracture site.
- After 96 hours, application of localized heat promotes healing by increasing blood circulation in the injured area. Use a heat lamp or heating pad so heat can penetrate the cast.
- After the cast is removed, use frequent ice massage. Fill a large styrofoam cup with water and freeze. Tear a small amount of foam from the top so ice protrudes. Massage firmly over he injured area in a circle about the size of a baseball. Do this for 15 minutes at a time 3 or 4 times a day, and also before workouts or competition.

MEDICATION—Your doctor may prescribe:
- General anesthesia, local anesthesia or muscle relaxants to make bone manipulation possible.
- Pain relievers for severe pain.
- Acetaminophen (available without prescription) for mild pain after initial treatment.

ACTIVITY
- Actively exercise all muscle groups not immobilized. Muscle contractions of the arm and hand promote fracture alignment and hasten healing.
- Begin reconditioning the hand after clearance from your doctor.
- Resume normal activities gradually after treatment.

DIET
- Do not eat or drink before manipulation or surgery to treat the fracture. Fluid or solid food in your stomach makes vomiting while under anesthesia more hazardous.
- During recovery, eat a well-balanced diet.

REHABILITATION—Begin daily rehabilitation exercises when movement is comfortable. Use ice message for 10 minutes prior to exercise. See Rehabilitation section for wrist and hand exercises.

 ## CALL YOUR DOCTOR IF

- You have signs or symptoms of a hand fracture.
- Any of the following occurs after surgery or other treatment:
  Increased pain, swelling or drainage in the surgical area.
  Signs of infection (headache, muscle aches, dizziness or a general ill feeling and fever).
  Swelling above or below the cast.
  Blue or gray skin color under the fingernails.
  Numbness or complete loss of feeling in the fingers of the affected hand.
  Nausea or vomiting.

HAND GANGLION
(Synovial Hernia; Ganglion Cyst)

GENERAL INFORMATION

DEFINITION—A small, usually hard nodule lying directly over a tendon or a joint capsule on the back or palm of the hand. Occasionally the nodule may become quite large.

BODY PARTS INVOLVED
- Back or palm of the hand.
- Tendon sheath (a thin membranous covering of the tendon).
- Any of the joint spaces in the hand.

SIGNS & SYMPTOMS
- Hard lump over a tendon or joint capsule in the hand. The nodule "yields" to heavy pressure because it is not solid.
- No pain usually, but overuse of the hand may cause mild pain and aching.
- Tenderness if the lump is pressed hard.
- Discomfort with extremes of motion (flexing or extending) and with repetition of the exercise that produced the ganglion.

CAUSES
- Mild sprains and chronic sprains to a hand joint, causing weakness of the joint capsule.
- A defect in the fibrous sheath of the joint or tendon that permits a segment of the underlying synovium (the thin membrane that lines the tendon sheath) to herniate through it.

- Irritation accompanying the herniated synovium, causing continued production of thickened fluid. The sac gradually fills, enlarges, and becomes hard, forming the ganglion.

RISK INCREASES WITH
- Repeated injury, especially mild sprains. Hand ganglions frequently occur in bowlers, tennis players and handball, racquetball and squash players.
- Inadequate warmup prior to practice or competition.
- If surgery is necessary, surgical risk increases with smoking, poor nutrition, alcoholism and recent or chronic illness.

HOW TO PREVENT
- Build your strength with a long-term conditioning program appropriate for your sport.
- Warm up before practice or competition.

WHAT TO EXPECT

APPROPRIATE HEALTH CARE
- Doctor's care for diagnosis, possible aspiration of fluid and injections of local anesthetic or cortisone.
- Surgery (frequently). Surgery will be conducted under local or general anesthesia in an outpatient surgical facility or hospital operating room.

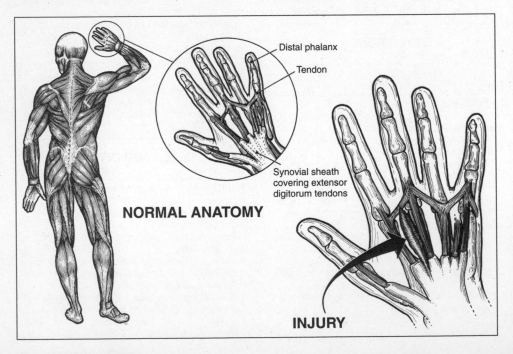

Distal phalanx

Tendon

NORMAL ANATOMY

Synovial sheath covering extensor digitorum tendons

INJURY

DIAGNOSTIC MEASURES
- Your own observation of signs and symptoms.
- Medical history and physical examination by a doctor.
- X-rays of the area.

POSSIBLE COMPLICATIONS
- After surgery:
  Excessive bleeding.
  Surgical wound infection.
  Recurrence if surgical removal is incomplete.
- Calcification of ganglion (rare).

PROBABLE OUTCOME—Ganglions
sometimes disappear spontaneously, only to recur later. Surgery is often the only treatment to offer a high likelihood of cure (although the recurrence rate is still 20%). After surgery, allow about 3 weeks for recovery if no complications occur.

 ## HOW TO TREAT

NOTE—Follow your doctor's instructions. These instructions are supplemental.

FIRST AID—None. This condition develops gradually.

CONTINUING CARE
Immediately after surgery:
- The affected area is usually immobilized in a splint for 1 to 2 weeks following surgery.
After bandage or splints removed by doctor:
- Bathe and shower as usual. You may wash the incision gently with mild unscented soap.
- Apply nonprescription antibiotic ointment to the wound before applying new bandages.
- Wrap the hand with an elasticized bandage until healing is complete.
- Use ice soaks 3 or 4 times a day. Fill a bucket with ice water, and soak the injured area for 20 minutes at a time.
- You may apply heat instead of ice if it feels better. Use heat lamps, hot soaks, hot showers, healing pads or heat liniments and ointments.
- Take whirlpool treatments, if available.

MEDICATION
- Your doctor may prescribe pain relievers.
- You may use nonprescription drugs, such as acetaminophen, for minor pain.

ACTIVITY
- Return to work and normal activity as soon as possible.
- Avoid vigorous exercise for 3 weeks after surgery.

DIET—During recovery, balance the amount of food you eat with any change in your level of physical activity. Eat a variety of foods to get the energy, protein, vitamins, minerals and fiber you need for good health and healing.

REHABILITATION
- Begin daily rehabilitation exercises when supportive wrapping is no longer needed.
- Use ice massage for 10 minutes before and after workouts. Fill a large styrofoam cup with water and freeze. Tear a small amount of foam from the top so ice protrudes. Massage firmly over the injured area in a circle about the size of a softball.
- See Rehabilitation section for wrist and hand exercises.

 ## CALL YOUR DOCTOR IF

- You have signs or symptoms of a hand ganglion.
- Any of the following occurs after surgery:
  Increased pain, swelling, redness, drainage or bleeding in the surgical area.
  Signs of infection (headache, muscle aches dizziness or a general ill feeling and fever).
  New, unexplained symptoms. Drugs used in treatment may produce side effects.

HAND HEMATOMA

GENERAL INFORMATION

DEFINITION—A collection of pooled blood in a small space on the back (or palm) of the hand.

BODY PARTS INVOLVED
- Back (or palm) of the hand.
- Soft tissues surrounding the hematoma, including nerves, tendons, ligaments, muscles and blood vessels.

SIGNS & SYMPTOMS
- Swelling over the injury site.
- Fluctuance (feeling of mobile fluid beneath the skin).
- Tenderness.
- Redness that progresses through several color changes—purple, green-yellow and yellow—before it completely heals.

CAUSES—Direct blow to the hand, usually with a blunt object. Bleeding into the tissues causes the surrounding tissues to be pushed away.

RISK INCREASES WITH
- Contact sports, especially if the hand is not adequately protected.
- Medical history of any bleeding disorder.
- Poor nutrition, including vitamin deficiency.
- Use of anticoagulants or aspirin.

HOW TO PREVENT
- Protect the hand with padding if there is a risk of hand injury during participation in athletic activity.
- If you must compete before healing, use tape, padding, splints or a cast to prevent injury.

WHAT TO EXPECT

APPROPRIATE HEALTH CARE
- Doctor's care unless the hematoma is very small.
- Needle aspiration of blood from the hematoma (sometimes) if the hematoma is accessible. At the same time, hyaluronidase (an enzyme) can be injected into the hematoma space. Hyaluronidase may hasten absorption of the blood.
- Self-care for minor hematomas or during the rehabilitation phase following serious hematomas.
- Physical therapy for serious hematomas.

DIAGNOSTIC MEASURES
- Your own observation of symptoms.
- Physical exam and medical history by a doctor for all except minor injuries.
- X-rays of the injured area to assess the total injury and to rule out underlying bone fractures. Total extent of the injury may not be apparent for 48 to 72 hours.

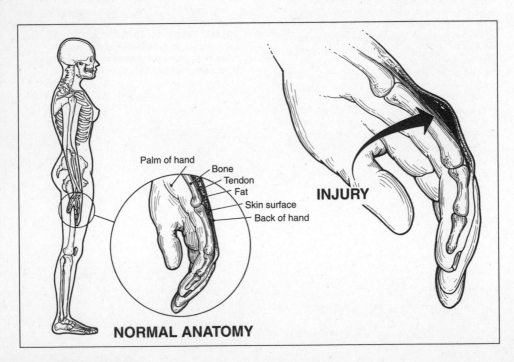

Palm of hand
Bone
Tendon
Fat
Skin surface
Back of hand

INJURY

NORMAL ANATOMY

POSSIBLE COMPLICATIONS
• Infection introduced through a break in the skin at the time of injury or during aspiration of the hematoma by a doctor.
• Prolonged healing time if activity is resumed too soon.
• Calcification of the blood remaining in the hematoma if blood has not been completely removed or absorbed.

PROBABLE OUTCOME—Average healing time is 2 to 6 weeks unless blood is removed with aspiration. Healing time may be lessened with this treatment.

 ## HOW TO TREAT

NOTE—Follow your doctor's instructions. These instructions are supplemental.

FIRST AID—Use instructions for R.I.C.E., the first letters of *rest, ice, compression* and *elevation*. See Appendix 1 for details.

CONTINUING CARE
• Use ice soaks 3 or 4 times a day. Fill a bucket with ice water, and soak the injured area for 20 minutes at a time.
• After 72 hours, application of localized heat promotes healing by increasing blood circulation in the injured area. Use hot baths, showers, compresses, heat lamps, heating pads, heat ointments and liniments, or whirlpools.
• Don't massage the hand, you may trigger bleeding again.
• Wrap an elastic bandage over a sponge rubber pad placed on the injured area. Keep area compressed for 72 hours, especially after aspiration of blood.

MEDICATION
• For minor discomfort, you may use:
Nonprescription medicines such as acetaminophen or ibuprofen.
Topical liniments and ointments.
• Your doctor may prescribe stronger medicine for pain if needed.

ACTIVITY—Begin activities slowly, and stop exercise as soon as pain begins. Increase activity as healing progresses. To prevent delayed healing, protect the hematoma area against excessive motion soon after injury. Motion breaks down the clot, leading to possible scar formation, calcification and limited movement after healing.

DIET—During recovery, balance the amount of food you eat with any change in your level of physical activity. Eat a variety of foods to get the energy, protein, vitamins, minerals and fiber you need for good health and healing.

REHABILITATION
• Begin daily rehabilitation exercise when supportive wrapping is no longer needed.
• Use a gentle ice massage for 10 minutes before and after workouts. Fill a large styrofoam cup with water and freeze. Tear a small amount of foam from the top so ice protrudes. Massage firmly over the injured area in a circle about the size of a softball.
• See Rehabilitation section for wrist and hand exercises.

 ## CALL YOUR DOCTOR IF

• You have signs or symptoms of a hand hematoma that doesn't improve in 1 or 2 days.
• Skin is broken and signs of infection (drainage, increasing pain, fever, headache, muscle aches, dizziness or a general ill feeling) occur.

HAND SPRAIN

GENERAL INFORMATION

DEFINITION—Violent overstretching of one or more ligaments in the hand. Sprains involving two or more ligaments cause considerably more disability than single-ligament sprains. When the ligament is overstretched, it becomes tense and gives way at its weakest point, either where it attaches to bone or within the ligament itself. If the ligament pulls loose a fragment of bone, it is called an avulsion fracture. There are 3 types of sprains:
- Mild (Grade I)—Tearing of some ligament fibers. There is no loss of function.
- Moderate (Grade II)—Rupture of a portion of the ligament, resulting in some loss of function.
- Severe (Grade III)—Complete rupture of the ligament or complete separation of ligament from bone. There is total loss of function. A severe sprain may require surgical repair.

BODY PARTS INVOLVED
- Ligaments connecting joints in the hand.
- Tissues surrounding the sprain, including blood vessels, tendons, bone, periosteum (covering of bone) and muscle.

SIGNS & SYMPTOMS
- Severe pain at the time of injury.
- A feeling of popping or tearing inside the hand.
- Tenderness at the injury site.
- Swelling in the hand.
- Bruising that appears soon after injury.

CAUSES—Stress on a ligament that temporarily forces or pries joints in the hand out of their normal locations. Hand sprains occur frequently in contact sports or sports in which falling on an overstretched hand is likely.

RISK INCREASES WITH
- Contact sports, especially boxing.
- Gymnastics.
- Previous hand injury.
- Obesity.
- Poor muscle conditioning.
- Inadequate protection from equipment.

HOW TO PREVENT
- Build your strength with a conditioning program appropriate for your sport.
- Warm up before practice or competition.
- Tape vulnerable joints before practice or competition.

WHAT TO EXPECT

APPROPRIATE HEALTH CARE
- Doctor's diagnosis.
- Application of a cast, tape or elastic bandage.
- Self-care during rehabilitation.
- Physical therapy (moderate or severe sprain).
- Surgery (severe sprain).

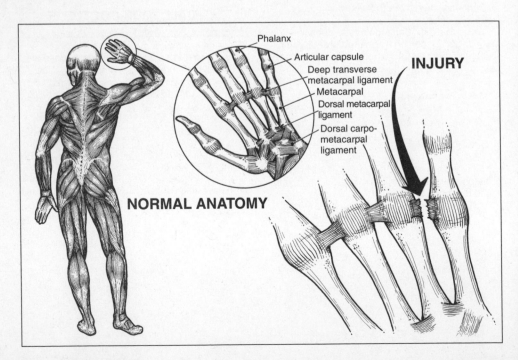

Phalanx
Articular capsule
Deep transverse metacarpal ligament
Metacarpal
Dorsal metacarpal ligament
Dorsal carpo-metacarpal ligament

INJURY

NORMAL ANATOMY

DIAGNOSTIC MEASURES
- Your own observation of symptoms.
- Medical history and exam by a doctor.
- X-rays of the hand and wrist to rule out fractures.

POSSIBLE COMPLICATIONS
- Prolonged healing time if usual activities are resumed too soon.
- Proneness to repeated injury.
- Inflammation at the ligament's attachment to bone (periostitis).
- Prolonged disability (sometimes).
- Unstable or arthritic hand joints following repeated injury (see Hand Dislocation).

PROBABLE OUTCOME—If this is a first-time injury, proper care and sufficient healing time before resuming activity should prevent permanent disability. Ligaments have a poor blood supply, and torn ligaments require as much healing time as fractures. Average healing times are:
- Mild sprains—2 to 6 weeks.
- Moderate sprains—6 to 8 weeks.
- Severe sprains—8 to 10 weeks.

 HOW TO TREAT

NOTE—Follow your doctor's instructions. These instructions are supplemental.

FIRST AID—Use instructions for R.I.C.E., the first letters of *rest, ice, compression* and *elevation.* See Appendix I for details.

CONTINUING CARE—If the doctor does not apply a cast, tape or elastic bandage:
- Continue using an ice pack 3 or 4 times a day. Place ice chips or cubes in a plastic bag. Wrap the bag in a moist towel, and place it over the injured area. Use for 20 minutes at a time.
- Wrap the hand with an elasticized bandage between ice treatments.
- After 72 hours, apply heat instead of ice if it feels better. Use heat lamps, hot soaks, hot showers, heating pads or heat liniments and ointments.
- Take whirlpool treatments, if available.
- Massage gently and often to provide comfort and decrease swelling.

MEDICATION
- For minor discomfort, you may use:
  Aspirin, acetaminophen, ibuprofen or other nonsteroidal anti-inflammatories.
  Topical liniments and ointments.
- Your doctor may prescribe:
  Stronger pain relievers.
  Injection of a long-acting local anesthetic to reduce pain.
  Injections of a corticosteroid, such as triamcinolone, to reduce inflammation.

ACTIVITY—Resume your normal activities gradually after clearance from your doctor.

DIET—During recovery, balance the amount of food you eat with any change in your level of physical activity. Eat a variety of foods to get the energy, protein, vitamins, minerals and fiber you need for good health and healing.

REHABILITATION
- Begin daily rehabilitation exercises when the cast or supportive wrapping is no longer necessary.
- Use ice massage for 10 minutes before and after exercise. Fill a large styrofoam cup with water and freeze. Tear a small amount of foam from the top so ice protrudes. Massage firmly over the injured area.
- See Rehabilitation section for wrist and hand exercises.

 CALL YOUR DOCTOR IF

- You have symptoms of a moderate or severe hand sprain or a mild sprain persists longer than 2 weeks.
- Pain, swelling or bruising worsens despite treatment.
- Any of the following occurs after casting or splinting:
  Pain, numbness or coldness in the hand.
  Blue, gray or dusky fingernails.
- Any of the following occurs after surgery:
  Increased pain, swelling, redness, drainage or bleeding in the surgical area.
  Signs of infection (headache, muscle aches, dizziness or a general ill feeling with fever).
- New, unexplained symptoms develop. Drugs used in treatment may produce side effects.

HAND STRAIN

GENERAL INFORMATION

DEFINITION—Injury to the muscles or tendons in the hand. Muscles, tendons and their attached bones comprise contractile units. The complex motions of the hand require many complex muscle-tendon units, so hand strains occur frequently. Strains are of 3 types:
- Mild (Grade I)—Slightly pulled muscle without tearing of muscle or tendon fibers. There is no loss of strength.
- Moderate (Grade II)—Tearing of fibers in a muscle or tendon or at the attachment to bone. Strength is diminished.
- Severe (Grade III)—Rupture of the muscle-tendon-bone attachment, with separation of fibers. A severe strain may require surgical repair. Chronic strains are caused by overuse. Acute strains are caused by direct injury or overstress.

BODY PARTS INVOLVED
- Tendons and muscles of the hand.
- Bones of the hand where they attach to muscles and tendons.
- Soft tissues surrounding the strain, including nerves, periosteum (covering of bone), blood vessels and lymph vessels.

SIGNS & SYMPTOMS
- Cramping and fatigue of hand muscles.
- Pain with motion or stretching.
- Crepitation ("crackling" feeling and sound when the injured area is pressed with fingers).
- Calcification of the muscle or tendon (visible with x-rays).
- Inflammation of the tendon sheath.

CAUSES
- Prolonged overuse of muscle-tendon units in the forearm, wrist or hand.
- Single violent injury or force applied to the forearm, wrist or hand.

RISK INCREASES WITH
- Contact sports such as wrestling.
- Sports that require constant gripping, such as rowing, tennis, golf or gymnastics.
- Medical history of any bleeding disorder.
- Poor nutrition.
- Previous hand injury.
- Poor muscle conditioning.

HOW TO PREVENT
- Participate in a strengthening, flexibility and conditioning program appropriate for your sport.
- Warm up before practice or competition.
- Protect the hands with taping and appropriate protective gear during participation in contact sports.

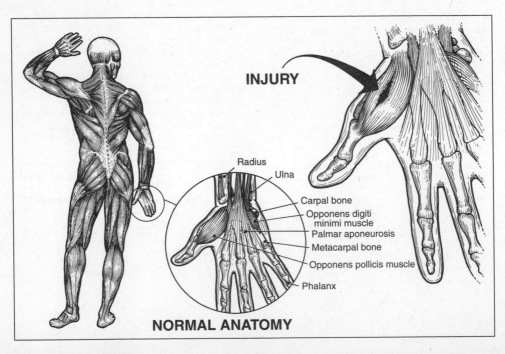

INJURY

Radius
Ulna
Carpal bone
Opponens digiti minimi muscle
Palmar aponeurosis
Metacarpal bone
Opponens pollicis muscle
Phalanx

NORMAL ANATOMY

WHAT TO EXPECT

APPROPRIATE HEALTH CARE
- Doctor's diagnosis.
- Self-care during rehabilitation.
- Physical therapy (moderate or severe strain).
- Surgery (severe strain).

DIAGNOSTIC MEASURES
- Your own observation of symptoms.
- Medical history and exam by a doctor.
- X-rays of the wrist, forearm and hand to rule out fractures.

POSSIBLE COMPLICATIONS
- Prolonged healing time if activity is resumed too soon.
- Proneness to repeated injury.
- Unstable or arthritic hand joints following repeated injury.
- Inflammation at the attachment to bone (periostitis).
- Prolonged disability (sometimes), especially weakness.

PROBABLE OUTCOME—If this is a first-time injury, proper care and sufficient healing time before resuming activity should prevent permanent disability. Torn ligaments and tendons require as long to heal as fractured bones. Average healing times are:
- Mild strain—2 to 10 days.
- Moderate strain—10 days to 6 weeks.
- Severe strain—6 to 10 weeks.

If this is a repeat injury, complications listed above are more likely to occur.

 # HOW TO TREAT

NOTE—Follow your doctor's instructions. These instructions are supplemental.

FIRST AID—Follow instructions for R.I.C.E., the first letters of *rest, ice, compression* and *elevation.* See Appendix 1 for details

CONTINUING CARE
- Use ice massage 3 or 4 times a day for 15 minutes at a time. Fill a large styrofoam cup with water and freeze. Tear a small amount of foam from the top so ice protrudes. Massage firmly over the injured area in a circle about the size of a softball.
- After the first 72 hours, apply heat instead of ice if it feels better. Use heat lamps, hot soaks, hot showers, heating pads or heat liniments and ointments.
- Take whirlpool treatments, if available.
- Wrap the injured wrist and hand with an elasticized bandage between treatments.
- Massage gently and often to provide comfort and decrease swelling.

MEDICATION
- For minor discomfort, you may use:
  Aspirin, acetaminophen or nonsteroidal anti-inflammatories.
  Topical liniments and ointments.
- Your doctor may prescribe:
  Stronger pain relievers.
  Injection of a long-acting local anesthetic to reduce pain (rare).
  Injections of corticosteroids, such as triamcinolone, to reduce inflammation (rare).

ACTIVITY
- For a moderate or severe strain, use a sling or splints for at least 72 hours.
- Resume your normal activities gradually.

DIET—During recovery, balance the amount of food you eat with any change in your level of physical activity. Eat a variety of foods to get the energy, protein, vitamins, minerals and fiber you need for good health and healing.

REHABILITATION—Begin daily rehabilitation exercises when supportive wrapping is no longer needed. Use ice massage for 10 minutes prior to exercise. See Rehabilitation section for wrist and hand exercises.

 # CALL YOUR DOCTOR IF

- You have symptoms of a moderate or severe hand strain or a mild strain persists longer than 10 days.
- Pain or swelling worsens despite treatment.

HAND TENDINITIS & TENOSYNOVITIS

GENERAL INFORMATION

DEFINITION—Inflammation of a tendon (tendinitis) or the lining of a tendon sheath (tenosynovitis) in the hand. This lining secretes a fluid that lubricates the tendon. When the lining becomes inflamed, the tendon cannot glide smoothly in its covering.

BODY PARTS INVOLVED
- Tendon in the hand.
- Lining and covering of the hand tendons.
- Soft tissues in the surrounding area, including blood vessels, nerves, ligaments, periosteum (covering of bone) and connective tissues.

SIGNS & SYMPTOMS
- Constant pain or pain with motion of the hand.
- Limited motion of the hand and wrist.
- Crepitation (a "crackling" sound when the tendon moves or is touched).
- Redness and tenderness over the injured tendon.

CAUSES
- Strain from unusual use or overuse of the wrist, hand or forearm.
- Direct blow or injury to the muscles and tendons of the wrist, hand and forearm. Tenosynovitis becomes more likely with repeated injury.

- Infection introduction through broken skin at the time of injury or through a surgical incision after surgery.

RISK INCREASES WITH
- Throwing sports and contact sports.
- Constrictive gloves or hand wraps that apply pressure over the course of a tendon in repetitive use.
- If surgery is needed, surgical risk increases with smoking, poor nutrition, alcoholism, drug abuse and recent or chronic illness.

HOW TO PREVENT
- Participate in a strengthening, flexibility and conditioning program appropriate for your sport.
- Warm up adequately before practice or competition.
- Wear protective gear appropriate for your sport.
- Learn proper moves and techniques for your sport.

WHAT TO EXPECT

APPROPRIATE HEALTH CARE
- Doctor's examination and diagnosis.
- Surgery (sometimes) to enlarge the tunnel of the tendon covering and restore a smooth gliding motion. The surgical procedure is performed under regional or general anesthesia in an outpatient surgical facility or hospital operating room.

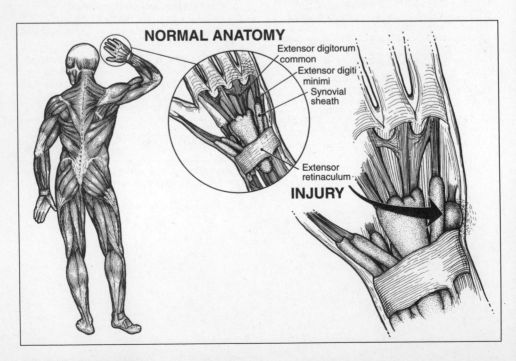

NORMAL ANATOMY

Extensor digitorum common
Extensor digiti minimi
Synovial sheath
Extensor retinaculum

INJURY

DIAGNOSTIC MEASURES
- Your own observation of symptoms and signs.
- Medical history and physical examination by your doctor.
- X-rays of the area to rule out other abnormalities.

POSSIBLE COMPLICATIONS
- Prolonged healing time if activity is resumed too soon.
- Adhesive tenosynovitis—The tendon and its covering become bound together. Loss of motion may be complete or partial. Surgery is necessary to remove the covering or transfer the tendon to a new area.
- Constrictive tenosynovitis—The walls of the covering thicken and narrow the opening, preventing the tendon from sliding through. Surgery is necessary to cut away part of the covering.

PROBABLE OUTCOME—Tenosynovitis is usually curable in about 6 weeks with heat treatments, corticosteroid injections and rest of the inflamed area. Recovery is usually quicker if the inflammation is caused by a direct blow rather than by a strain or sprain.

 HOW TO TREAT

NOTE—Follow your doctor's instructions. These instructions are supplemental.

FIRST AID—None. This problem develops slowly.

CONTINUING CARE
- Wrap the hand and wrist with an elasticized bandage until healing is complete.
- Apply heat frequently. Use heat lamps, hot soaks, hot showers, heating pads or heat liniments and ointments.
- Take whirlpool treatments if available.

MEDICATION—You may use nonprescription drugs, such as acetaminophen or nonsteroidal anti-inflammatories, for minor pain.
Your doctor may prescribe:
- Stronger pain relievers. Don't take prescription pain medication longer than 4 to 7 days. Use only as much as you need.
- Injection of the tendon covering with a combination of a long-acting local anesthetic and a nonabsorbable corticosteroid such as triamcinolone.

ACTIVITY—Resume normal activities gradually.

DIET—During recovery, balance the amount of food you eat with any change in your level of physical activity. Eat a variety of foods to get the energy, protein, vitamins, minerals and fiber you need for good health and healing.

REHABILITATION
- Begin daily rehabilitation exercises after pain disappears when supportive wrapping is no longer needed.
- Use ice massage for 10 minutes before and after exercise. Fill a large styrofoam cup with water and freeze. Tear a small amount of foam from the top so ice protrudes. Massage firmly over the injured area in a circle about the size of a baseball.
- See Rehabilitation section for wrist and hand exercises.

 CALL YOUR DOCTOR IF

- You have symptoms of hand tenosynovitis.
- Any of the following occurs after surgery:
Increased pain, swelling, redness, drainage or bleeding in the surgical area.
Signs of infection (headache, muscle aches, dizziness or a general ill feeling and fever).
New, unexplained symptoms. Drugs used in treatment may produce side effects.

HEAD INJURY, CEREBRAL CONCUSSION

GENERAL INFORMATION

DEFINITION—A violent jar or shock to the brain that causes an immediate change in brain function, including possible loss of consciousness.

BODY PARTS INVOLVED
- Head.
- Skull.
- Brain.

SIGNS & SYMPTOMS
Mild concussion:
- Temporary loss of consciousness.
- Memory loss (amnesia).
- Emotional instability.

Severe concussion:
- Prolonged unconsciousness.
- Dilated pupils.
- Change in breathing.
- Disturbed vision.
- Disturbed equilibrium.
- Memory loss.

CAUSES—Blow to the head.

RISK INCREASES WITH
- Contact sports.
- Activities with a risk of falling.
- Auto, motorcycle or bike racing.

HOW TO PREVENT—Wear a protective helmet for any activity with risk of head injury.

WHAT TO EXPECT

APPROPRIATE HEALTH CARE
- Doctor's diagnosis and care.
- Hospitalization for a serious brain concussion.
- Home care if the initial evaluation doesn't dictate hospitalization.

DIAGNOSTIC MEASURES
- Your own observation of symptoms.
- Physical exam and medical history by a doctor. The total extent of injury may not be apparent for 48 to 72 hours.
- X-rays of the head and neck to assess total injury to soft tissues and to rule out the possibility of a skull fracture.
- CT scan (see Glossary) of the head.
- Laboratory studies of blood and cerebrospinal fluid.

POSSIBLE COMPLICATIONS
- Permanent brain damage, depending on the extent of injury. Repeated concussions can cause slurred speech, slow movement, slow thought process and tremor.
- Excessive cerebral bleeding, causing a clot that puts pressure on the brain.

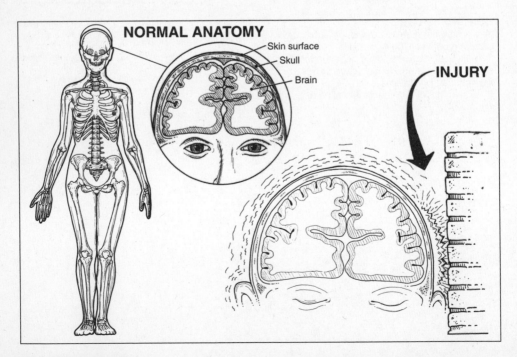

NORMAL ANATOMY

Skin surface
Skull
Brain

INJURY

• Infection if skin over the concussion site is broken.
• Postconcussion syndrome—recurring headache, memory loss, emotional changes, confusion and personality changes within first 6 months after concussion.
• Return to activity too soon carries the risk of repeat blows to the head, which may result in more extensive brain injury or even permanent loss of function.

PROBABLE OUTCOME—Complete recovery is likely with early diagnosis and treatment. Complications can be life-threatening or cause permanent brain damage.

 ## HOW TO TREAT

NOTE—Follow your doctor's instructions. These instructions are supplemental.

FIRST AID
• Ice helps stop bleeding from any scalp wound. Prepare an ice pack of ice cubes or chips wrapped in plastic or placed in a container. Place a towel over the injured area to prevent skin damage. Apply ice for 20 minutes, then rest 10 minutes. Repeat applications for 24 to 48 hours after injury.
• Elevate the head above the level of the heart to reduce swelling and prevent accumulation of fluid.

CONTINUING CARE—The extent of injury can be determined only with careful examination and observation. After a doctor's examination, the injured person may be sent home, but a responsible person must stay with the person and watch for serious symptoms. The first 24 hours after injury are critical, although serious aftereffects can appear later. If you are watching the patient, awaken him or her every hour for 24 hours. Report to the doctor immediately if you can't awake or arouse the person. Also report any of the following:
• Vomiting.
• Inability to move the arms and legs equally well on both sides.
• Temperature above 100°F (37.8°C).
• Stiff neck.
• Convulsions.
• Pupils of unequal sizes or shapes.
• Severe headache that persists longer than 4 hours after injury.
• Confusion.

MEDICATION—Don't use any medicine except nonprescription acetaminophen until the extent of injury is certain.

ACTIVITY—Rest in bed until the doctor determines the danger of brain injury is over. Normal activity may then be resumed as symptoms improve.

DIET—Follow a full liquid diet until the danger passes.

REHABILITATION—Depends on the possibility of brain damage. Consult your doctor.

 ## CALL YOUR DOCTOR IF

You have had a head injury and develop symptoms of a concussion or you observe the signs and symptoms in someone else.

HEAD INJURY, CEREBRAL CONTUSION

GENERAL INFORMATION

DEFINITION—Bruising of the brain following a blow. Contusions cause bleeding from ruptured small capillaries that allow blood to infiltrate brain tissues.

BODY PARTS INVOLVED
- Brain.
- Skin, subcutaneous tissues, blood vessels (both large vessels and capillaries), periosteum (the outside lining of the skull), muscles of the scalp and connective tissues.

SIGNS & SYMPTOMS—Depends on the extent of injury. The presence or absence of swelling at the injury site is not related to the seriousness of injury. Signs and symptoms include any or all of the following:
- Drowsiness or confusion.
- Vomiting and nausea.
- Blurred vision.
- Pupils of different sizes.
- Loss of consciousness—either temporarily or for long periods.
- Amnesia or memory lapses.
- Irritability.
- Headache.
- Bleeding of the scalp if the skin is broken.

CAUSES—Direct blow to the head, usually from a blunt object.

RISK INCREASES WITH
- Contact sports such as boxing, football or wrestling.
- Activities with a risk of falling.
- Auto, motorcycle or bike racing.

HOW TO PREVENT—Wear a protective helmet for any activity with risk of head injury.

WHAT TO EXPECT

APPROPRIATE HEALTH CARE
- Doctor's diagnosis and care
- Hospitalization for a serious brain contusion.
- Home care if the initial evaluation doesn't dictate hospitalization.

DIAGNOSTIC MEASURES
- Your own observation of symptoms.
- Physical exam and medical history by a doctor. The total extent of injury may not be apparent for 48 to 72 hours.
- X-rays of the head and neck to assess total injury to soft tissues and to rule out the possibility of a skull fracture.
- CT scan or MRI (see Glossary for both) of the head.
- Laboratory studies of blood and cerebrospinal fluid.

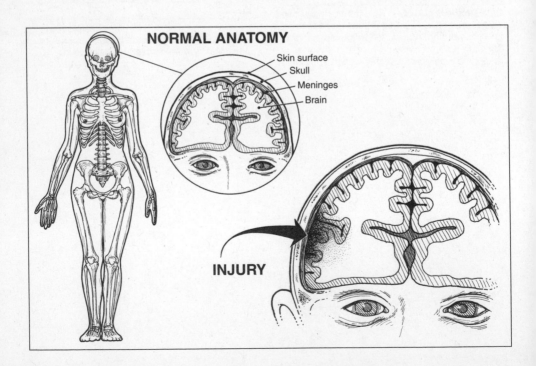

NORMAL ANATOMY

Skin surface
Skull
Meninges
Brain

INJURY

POSSIBLE COMPLICATIONS
- Permanent brain damage, depending on the extent of injury.
- Excessive cerebral bleeding, causing a clot that puts pressure on the brain.
- Return to activity too soon carries the risk of repeat blows to the head, which may result in more extensive brain injury or even permanent loss of function.
- Infection if skin over the contusion site is broken.

PROBABLE OUTCOME—Complete recovery is likely with early diagnosis and treatment. Complications can be life-threatening or cause permanent brain damage.

 HOW TO TREAT

NOTE—Follow your doctor's instructions. These instructions are supplemental.

FIRST AID
- Ice helps stop internal bleeding. Prepare an ice pack of ice cubes or chips wrapped in plastic or placed in a container. Place a towel over the injured area to prevent skin damage. Apply ice for 20 minutes, then rest 10 minutes. Repeat application for 24 or 48 hours after injury.
- Elevate the head above the level of the heart to reduce swelling and prevent accumulation of fluid.
- Avoid repeat blows.

CONTINUING CARE—The extent of injury can be determined only with careful examination and observation. After a doctor's examination, the injured person may be sent home, but a responsible person must stay with the person and watch for serious symptoms. The first 24 hours after injury are critical, although serious aftereffects can appear later. If you are watching the patient, awaken him or her every hour for 24 hours. Report to the doctor immediately if you can't awaken or arouse the person. Also report any of the following:
- Vomiting.
- Inability to move the arms and legs equally well on both sides.
- Temperature above 100°F (37.8°C).
- Stiff neck.
- Pupils of unequal sizes or shapes.
- Convulsions.
- Noticeable restlessness.
- Severe headache that persists longer than 4 hours after injury.
- Confusion.

MEDICATION—Don't use any medicine except nonprescription acetaminophen until the extent of injury is certain.

ACTIVITY—Bed rest is necessary until the doctor determines the danger of brain injury is over. Normal activity may then be resumed as symptoms improve.

DIET—A full liquid diet should be followed until the danger passes.

REHABILITATION—Rehabilitation exercises must be individualized. Follow your doctor's or surgeon's directions.

 CALL YOUR DOCTOR IF

You have had a head injury and develop symptoms of a contusion or you observe the signs and symptoms in someone else.

HEAD INJURY,
EXTRADURAL HEMORRHAGE & HEMATOMA
(Epidural Hemorrhage & Hematoma)

 GENERAL INFORMATION

DEFINITION—Bleeding (hemorrhage) between the skull and the outermost of 3 membranes (meninges) that cover the brain, resulting in a pooling of blood (hematoma) that causes pressure on the brain.

BODY PARTS INVOLVED
- Brain.
- Skull.
- Blood vessels to the brain.
- Meninges.

SIGNS & SYMPTOMS—The following symptoms usually develop within 1 to 96 hours after a head injury:
- Unconsciousness for a short period of time, followed by a headache that steadily worsens.
- Drowsiness or unconsciousness.
- Nausea or vomiting.
- Inability to move the arms and legs.
- Change in the size of the eye pupils.

CAUSES—Head injury with a skull fracture that tears the middle meningeal artery.

RISK INCREASES WITH
- Contact sports such as boxing, football or hockey.
- Activities with a risk of falling.
- Auto, motorcycle or bike racing.
- During surgery, surgical risk increases with smoking and use of drugs, including anticoagulants, muscle relaxants, tranquilizers, sleep inducers, insulin, sedatives, beta-adrenergic blockers, corticosteroids or mind-altering drugs.

HOW TO PREVENT—Wear a protective helmet for any activity with risk of head injury.

 WHAT TO EXPECT

APPROPRIATE HEALTH CARE
- Doctor's diagnosis.
- Immediate surgery to remove the clot causing pressure on the brain.
- Physical therapy for rehabilitation if there is any residual paralysis or other disability.

DIAGNOSTIC MEASURES
- Your own observation of symptoms.
- Medical history and physical exam by a doctor.

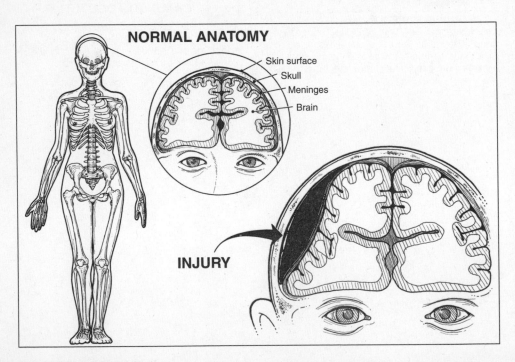

NORMAL ANATOMY

Skin surface
Skull
Meninges
Brain

INJURY

- Laboratory studies of blood and cerebrospinal fluid.
- Diagnostic tests such as x-rays, arteriography, radioactive uptake studies and a CT scan or MRI (see Glossary for all).

POSSIBLE COMPLICATIONS
- Death or permanent brain damage, including partial or complete paralysis, behavioral and personality changes and speech problems.
- Convulsions following surgery.

PROBABLE OUTCOME—The degree of recovery depends upon one's general health, age, severity of the injury, rapidity of the treatment and extensiveness of the bleeding or clot. After the clot is removed, brain tissue that has been compressed usually expands slowly to fill its original space. If speech or muscle control has been damaged, physical therapy or speech therapy may be necessary. The outlook for complete recovery is good with quick diagnosis and prompt surgery.

 HOW TO TREAT

NOTE—Follow your doctor's instructions. These instructions are supplemental.

FIRST AID—After any head injury:
- If the victim is wearing headgear with a face guard, cut the face guard off, *but don't remove the headgear or move the head or neck for any reason.* Brain injury is frequently associated with neck injury.
- If the victim vomits, support the head and neck completely and carefully while rotating the entire body to the side and clearing the airway to prevent aspiration.
- Splint the head and neck, and transport the person to the nearest well-equipped emergency facility.
- Elevate the head of the stretcher slightly. Do not use pillows.

- Watch closely for vomiting, convulsions, changes in consciousness, paralysis or impaired breathing. Be ready to render CPR if needed.

CONTINUING CARE—Surgery is the only treatment for an extradural hemorrhage and hematoma. With the patient under local or light general anesthesia, small holes are bored through the skull. The blood clot (which looks like currant jelly) is removed manually or by suction. After surgery, symptoms usually improve rapidly.

MEDICATION—Your doctor may prescribe:
- Corticosteroid drugs to reduce swelling inside the skull.
- Anticonvulsant medication.
- Antibiotics to fight infection.

ACTIVITY—After surgery, stay as active as your strength allows. Work and exercise moderately, and rest often. Once you have had an extradural hemorrhage, don't participate in contact sports.

DIET—During recovery, balance the amount of food you eat with any change in your level of physical activity. Eat a variety of foods to get the energy, protein, vitamins, minerals and fiber you need for good health and healing.

REHABILITATION—Consult your doctor or a physical therapist.

 CALL YOUR DOCTOR IF

- You observe signs of an extradural hemorrhage in someone following a head injury. Call immediately. This is an emergency!
- The following occur after surgery:
  Temperature rises to 101°F (38.3°C) or higher.
  Surgical wound becomes red, swollen or tender.
  Headache worsens.

HEAD INJURY, INTRACEREBRAL HEMATOMA

 GENERAL INFORMATION

DEFINITION—Bleeding (hemorrhage) that causes blood to collect and partially clot (hematoma) inside the brain. The collection of blood can produce pressure on the otherwise uninjured surrounding brain tissues and progressively worsen brain function. CT scans (see Glossary) have shown that this condition occurs more frequently than doctors previously thought.

BODY PARTS INVOLVED
- Brain.
- Blood vessels to the brain.

SIGNS & SYMPTOMS—The following symptoms develop within 1 to 96 hours (occasionally longer) after a head injury:
- Unconsciousness for a short period of time, followed by a headache that steadily worsens.
- Drowsiness or unconsciousness.
- Nausea or vomiting.
- Inability to move the arms and legs.
- Change in the size of the eye pupils.

CAUSES—Severe blow to the head.

RISK INCREASES WITH
- Contact sports such as boxing, football or hockey.
- Activities with a risk of falling.
- Auto, motorcycle or bike racing.
- During surgery, surgical risk increases with smoking and use of drugs, including anticoagulants, muscle relaxants, tranquilizers, sleep inducers, insulin, sedatives, beta-adrenergic blockers, corticosteroids or mind-altering drugs.

HOW TO PREVENT—Wear a protective helmet for any activity with risk of head injury.

 WHAT TO EXPECT

APPROPRIATE HEALTH CARE
- Surgery to remove the clot causing pressure on the brain.
- Physical therapy for rehabilitation if there is any residual paralysis or other disability.

DIAGNOSTIC MEASURES
- Your own observation of symptoms.
- Medical history and physical exam by a doctor.
- Laboratory studies of blood and cerebrospinal fluid.

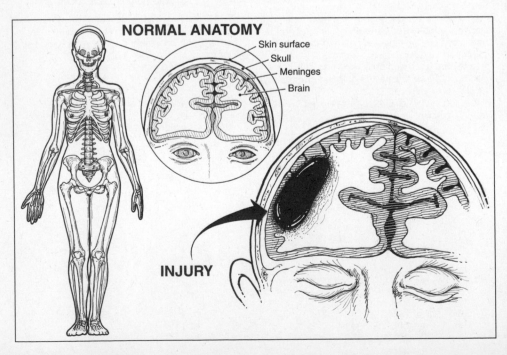

NORMAL ANATOMY

Skin surface
Skull
Meninges
Brain

INJURY

- Diagnostic tests such as x-rays, arteriography, radioactive uptake studies and a CT scan or MRI (see Glossary for all).

POSSIBLE COMPLICATIONS
- Death or permanent brain damage, including partial or complete paralysis, behavioral and personality changes and speech problems.
- Convulsions following surgery.

PROBABLE OUTCOME—The degree of recovery depends upon one's general health, age, severity of the injury, rapidity of the treatment and extensiveness of the bleeding or clot. After the clot is removed, brain tissue that has been compressed usually expands slowly to fill its original space. If speech or muscle control has been damaged, physical therapy or speech therapy may be necessary. The outlook for complete recovery is good with quick diagnosis and prompt surgery.

 HOW TO TREAT

NOTE—Follow your doctor's instructions. These instructions are supplemental.

FIRST AID—After any head injury:
- If the victim is wearing headgear with a face guard, cut the face guard off, *but don't remove the headgear or move the head or neck for any reason.* Brain injury is frequently associated with neck injury.
- If the victim vomits, support the head and neck completely and carefully while rotating the entire body to the side and clearing the airway to prevent aspiration.
- Splint the head and neck, and transport the person to the nearest well-equipped emergency facility.
- Elevate the head of the stretcher slightly. Do not use pillows.
- Watch closely for vomiting, convulsions, changes in consciousness, paralysis or impaired breathing. Be ready to render CPR if needed.

CONTINUING CARE—Surgery s the only treatment for an intracerebral hemorrhage and hematoma. With the patient under local or light general anesthesia, small holes are bored through the skull. The blood clot (which looks like currant jelly) is removed manually or by suction. After surgery, symptoms usually improve rapidly.

MEDICATION—Your doctor may prescribe:
- Corticosteroid drugs to reduce swelling inside the skull.
- Anticonvulsant medication.
- Antibiotics to fight infection.

ACTIVITY—After surgery, stay as active as your strength allows. Work and exercise moderately, and rest often. Once you have had an intracerebral hemorrhage, don't participate in contact sports.

DIET—During recovery, balance the amount of food you eat with any change in your level of physical activity. Eat a variety of foods to get the energy, protein, vitamins, minerals and fiber you need for good health and healing.

REHABILITATION—Consult your doctor or a physical therapist.

 CALL YOUR DOCTOR IF

- You observe signs of an intracerebral hemorrhage in someone following a head injury. Call immediately. This is an emergency!
- The following occur after surgery:
  Temperature rises to 101°F (35.3°C) or higher.
  Surgical wound becomes red, swollen or tender.
  Headache worsens.

HEAD INJURY, SKULL FRACTURE

GENERAL INFORMATION

DEFINITION—Skull fractures may be of two types:
• A closed or simple break in the bone without breaking the skin or bone covering (periosteum).
• An open or compound break that breaks the skin and periosteum.

BODY PARTS INVOLVED
• Skull.
• Periosteum (fibrous covering of bone).
• Soft tissues adjacent to the skull, including skin and underlying tissues, muscles, nerves and tendons.
• Brain (sometimes) if bone fragments are depressed into the brain.

SIGNS & SYMPTOMS
Signs of skull fracture only:
• Pain and swelling over the skull fracture.
• Bruising over the fracture and around the eyes and nose.
• Profuse bleeding from the scalp if the skin is broken.
• Leakage of clear fluid (cerebrospinal fluid) into the ear or nose.
Additional signs if brain damage accompanies the skull fracture:
• Drowsiness or confusion.
• Vomiting and nausea.
• Blurred vision.

• Loss of consciousness—either temporarily or for long periods.
• Amnesia or memory lapses.
• Irritability.
• Headache.

CAUSES—Direct blow to the head.

RISK INCREASES WITH
• Contact sports, especially if the head is not protected adequately.
• Sports that involve heavy equipment such as baseball bats or golf clubs.
• Sports such as basketball, gymnastics, diving or cycling in which falling on the head is possible.
• Poor nutrition, especially calcium deficiency.

HOW TO PREVENT—Wear a protective helmet or other appropriate headgear during athletic activity in which head injury is possible.

WHAT TO EXPECT

APPROPRIATE HEALTH CARE
• Doctor's diagnosis and care.
• Hospitalization (serious skull fractures).
• Home care if hospitalization is not necessary.

DIAGNOSTIC MEASURES
• Your own observation of symptoms.
• Medical history and physical exam by a doctor. Total extent of the injury may not be apparent for 48 to 72 hours following injury.

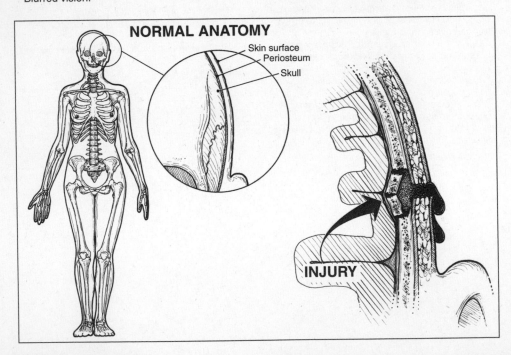

NORMAL ANATOMY

Skin surface
Periosteum
Skull

INJURY

- X-rays of the head and neck to assess total injury to soft tissues.
- CT scan or MRI (see Glossary for both) of the head.
- Laboratory studies of blood and cerebrospinal fluid.

POSSIBLE COMPLICATIONS
- Hematoma (a collection of blood) that creates pressure on the brain. This can cause permanent brain damage or death, depending on the extent of injury.
- Prolonged healing time if activity is resumed too soon.
- Infection if skin over the skull fracture is broken.

PROBABLE OUTCOME—Most skull fractures without complications heal within 4 to 6 weeks. Prompt medical evaluation and treatment are essential to prevent or treat complications. These can be life-threatening or cause permanent brain damage.

HOW TO TREAT

NOTE—Follow your doctor's instructions. These instructions are supplemental.

FIRST AID—After any head injury:
- If the victim is wearing headgear with a face guard, cut the face guard off, *but don't remove the headgear or move the head or neck for any reason*. Brain injury is frequently associated with neck injury.
- If the victim vomits, support the head and neck completely and carefully while rotating the entire body to the side and clearing the airway to prevent aspiration.
- Splint the head and neck, and transport the person to the nearest well-equipped emergency facility.
- Elevate the head of the stretcher slightly. Do not use pillows.
- Watch closely for vomiting, convulsions, changes in consciousness, paralysis or impaired breathing. Be ready to render CPR if needed.

CONTINUING CARE—The extent of injury can be determined only with careful examination and observation. After a doctor's examination, the injured person may be sent home—but a responsible person must stay with the person and watch for serious symptoms. The first 24 hours after injury are critical, although serious aftereffects can appear later. If you are watching the patient, awaken him or her every hour for 24 hours. Report to the doctor immediately if you can't awaken or arouse the person. Also report any of the following:
- Vomiting.
- Inability to move arms and legs equally well on both sides.
- Temperature above 100°F (37.8°C).
- Stiff neck.
- Pupils of unequal sizes or shapes.
- Convulsions.
- Noticeable restlessness.
- Severe headache that persists longer than 4 hours after injury.
- Confusion.

MEDICATION—Don't give any medicine except nonprescription acetaminophen until the extent of injury is certain.

ACTIVITY—The patient should rest in bed until the doctor determines that the danger of complications—especially hematomas—is over. Normal activity may then be resumed as symptoms improve.

DIET—Follow a full liquid diet for 24 to 48 hours until the danger of complications passes.

REHABILITATION—Depends on whether brain damage occurs. Consult your doctor.

CALL YOUR DOCTOR IF

- You have signs and symptoms of a skull fracture after a blow to the head or you observe signs of a head injury in someone else.
- After returning home, any signs or symptoms appear that are listed under Continuing Care.

HEAD INJURY, SUBDURAL HEMORRHAGE & HEMATOMA

 GENERAL INFORMATION

DEFINITION—Bleeding (hemorrhage) that causes blood to collect and clot (hematoma) beneath the membranes (meninges) that cover the brain. There are 2 types of subdural hematomas:
• An acute subdural hematoma occurs soon after a severe head injury. It is the most frequent cause of death from injury in contact sports.
• A chronic subdural hematoma may develop weeks after a head injury. The injury may have been so minor that the patient does not remember it.

BODY PARTS INVOLVED
• Brain.
• Meninges.
• Blood vessels to the brain.

SIGNS & SYMPTOMS
• Recurrent, worsening headaches.
• Fluctuating drowsiness, dizziness, mental changes or confusion.
• Weakness or numbness on one side of the body.
• Vision disturbances.
• Vomiting without nausea.
• Pupils of different sizes (sometimes).

CAUSES
• Acute hematoma—Severe blow to the head that bruises and tears the brain and its blood vessels.
• Chronic hematoma—Minor (even forgotten) head injury. Blood in the enclosed space in the brain forms a hematoma that gradually increases with further bleeding.

RISK INCREASES WITH
• Contact sports such as boxing, football or hockey.
• Auto, motorcycle or bike racing.
• During surgery, surgical risk increases with smoking and use of drugs, including anticoagulants, muscle relaxants, tranquilizers, sleep inducers, insulin, sedatives, beta-adrenergic blockers, corticosteroids or mind-altering drugs.

HOW TO PREVENT—Wear a protective helmet for any activity with risk of head injury.

 WHAT TO EXPECT

APPROPRIATE HEALTH CARE
• Doctor's diagnosis.
• Surgery to remove the clot causing pressure on the brain.
• Physical therapy for rehabilitation if there is any residual paralysis or other disability.

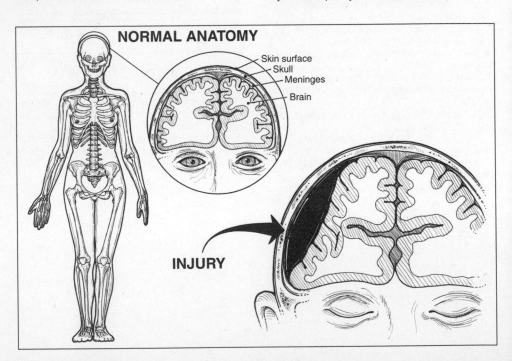

NORMAL ANATOMY

Skin surface
Skull
Meninges
Brain

INJURY

DIAGNOSTIC MEASURES
- Your own observation of symptoms.
- Medical history and physical exam by a doctor.
- Laboratory studies of blood and cerebrospinal fluid.
- Diagnostic tests such as x-rays, arteriography, radioactive uptake studies and a CT scan or MRI (see Glossary for all).

POSSIBLE COMPLICATIONS
- Death or permanent brain damage, including partial or complete paralysis, behavioral and personality changes and speech problems.
- Convulsions following surgery.

PROBABLE OUTCOME—The degree of recovery depends upon one's general health, age, severity of the injury, rapidity of the treatment and extensiveness of the bleeding or clot. After the clot is removed, brain tissue that has been compressed usually expands slowly to fill its original space. If speech or muscle control has been damaged, physical therapy or speech therapy may be necessary. The outlook for complete recovery is good with quick diagnosis and prompt surgery.

 HOW TO TREAT

NOTE—Follow your doctor's instructions. These instructions are supplemental.

FIRST AID—After any head injury:
- If the victim is wearing headgear with a face guard, cut the face guard off, but don't remove the headgear or move the head or neck for any reason. Brain injury is frequently associated with neck injury.
- If the victim vomits, support the head and neck completely and carefully while rotating the entire body to the side and clearing the airway to prevent aspiration.
- Splint the head and neck, and transport the person to the nearest well-equipped emergency facility.

- Elevate the head of the stretcher slightly. Do not use pillows.
- Watch closely for vomiting, convulsion, changes in consciousness, paralysis or impaired breathing. Be ready to render CPR if needed.

CONTINUING CARE—Surgery is the only treatment for a subdural hemorrhage and hematoma. With the patient under local or light general anesthesia, small holes are bored through the skull. The blood clot (which looks like currant jelly) is removed manually or by suction. After surgery, symptoms usually improve rapidly.

MEDICATION—Your doctor may prescribe:
- Corticosteroid drugs to reduce swelling inside the skull.
- Anticonvulsant medication.
- Antibiotics to fight infection.

ACTIVITY—After surgery, stay as active as your strength allows. Work and exercise moderately, and rest often. Once you have had a subdural hemorrhage, don't participate in contact sports.

DIET—During recovery, balance the amount of food you eat with any change in your level of physical activity. Eat a variety of foods to get the energy, protein, vitamins, minerals and fiber you need for good health and healing.

REHABILITATION—Consult your doctor or a physical therapist.

 CALL YOUR DOCTOR IF

- You have had a head injury—even if it seems minor—and you develop any symptoms of a subdural hemorrhage. This is an emergency!
- The following occur during or after surgery:
  Temperature rises to 101°F (38.3°C) or higher.
  Surgical wound becomes red, swollen or tender.
  Headache worsens.

HIP BURSITIS

GENERAL INFORMATION

DEFINITION—Inflammation of the bursa surrounding either of the big knobs of bone (trochanters) at the top of the femur (thigh bone). Bursitis may vary in degree from mild irritation to an abscess formation that causes excruciating pain. Hip bursitis is associated with snapping hip syndrome.

BODY PARTS INVOLVED
- One of two bursas in the hip joint where the trochanters fit into their socket. A bursa is a soft sac filled with lubricating fluid that facilitates motion in the hip and protects it from injury.
- Soft tissues surrounding the hip joint, including nerves, tendons, ligaments, blood vessels (both large vessels and capillaries), periosteum (the outside lining of bone) and muscles.

SIGNS & SYMPTOMS
- Pain in the hip.
- A "crackling" feeling when moving the hip.
- Tenderness.
- Swelling.
- Redness (sometimes) over the effected bursa.
- A "snapping" noise with stepping or other hip motion.
- Fever if infection is present.
- Limitation of motion in the hip.

CAUSES
- Injury to the hip.
- Acute or chronic infection.
- Arthritis.
- Gout.
- Unknown (frequently).

RISK INCREASES WITH
- Participating in competitive athletics, particularly contact sports.
- Running and bouncing activities.
- Previous history of bursitis in any joint.
- Exposure to cold weather.
- Poor conditioning and inadequate warmup.
- Inadequate protective equipment in contact sports.

HOW TO PREVENT
- Use protective gear such as hip pads for contact sports.
- Warm up adequately before athletic practice or competition.
- Wear warm clothing in cold weather.
- To prevent recurrence, continue to wear extra protection over the hips until healing is complete.

? WHAT TO EXPECT

APPROPRIATE HEALTH CARE
- Doctor's diagnosis and treatment.
- Surgery (sometimes), particularly for recurrent severe bursitis.

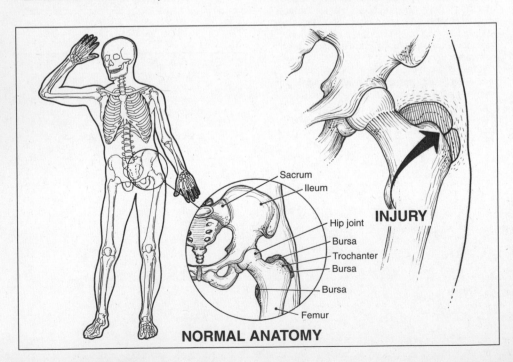

Sacrum
Ileum
Hip joint
Bursa
Trochanter
Bursa
Bursa
Femur

INJURY

NORMAL ANATOMY

DIAGNOSTIC MEASURES
- Your own observation of symptoms.
- Medical history and physical exam by a doctor.
- X-rays of the hips.

POSSIBLE COMPLICATIONS
- Permanent limitation of the hip's normal mobility.
- Prolonged healing time if activity is resumed too soon.
- Proneness to repeated flare-ups.
- Spontaneous rupture of bursa if severe infection is present.

PROBABLE OUTCOME—Hip bursitis is a common—but not a serious—problem. Painful symptoms usually subside in 3 to 4 weeks with treatment, but they frequently recur.

 ## HOW TO TREAT

NOTE—Follow your doctor's instructions. These instructions are supplemental.

FIRST AID—None. This problem develops slowly.

CONTINUING CARE
- Use frequent ice massage. Fill a large styrofoam cup with water and freeze. Tear a small amount of foam from the top so ice protrudes. Massage firmly over the injured area in a circle about the size of a softball. Do this for 15 minutes at a time 3 or 4 times a day, and also before workouts or competition.
- After 72 hours, apply heat instead of ice if it feels better. Use heat lamps, hot soaks, hot showers, heating pads or heat liniments and ointments.
- Take whirlpool treatments, if available.
- Use crutches to prevent weight-bearing on the hip joint, if needed. See Appendix 3 (Safe Use of Crutches).

- Elevate the hips above the level of the heart to reduce swelling and prevent accumulation of fluid. Use pillows for propping.
- Gentle massage will frequently provide comfort and decrease swelling.

MEDICATION—Your doctor may prescribe:
- Nonsteroidal anti-inflammatory drugs.
- Antibiotics if the bursa is infected.
- Prescription pain relievers for severe pain. Use nonprescription aspirin, acetaminophen or ibuprofen for mild pain.
- Injections with a long-lasting local anesthetic mixed with a corticosteroid drug, such as triamcinolone.

ACTIVITY—Rest the inflamed area as much as possible. If you must resume normal activity immediately, use crutches until the pain becomes more bearable. Begin normal, slow joint movement as soon as possible.

DIET—During recovery, balance the amount of food you eat with any change in your level of physical activity. Eat a variety of foods to get the energy, protein, vitamins, minerals and fiber you need for good health and healing. Your doctor may suggest vitamin and mineral supplements to promote healing.

REHABILITATION—See Rehabilitation section for hip and pelvis exercises.

 ## CALL YOUR DOCTOR IF

- You have symptoms of hip bursitis.
- Pain increases despite treatment.
- You develop signs of infection (headache, muscle aches, dizziness or a general ill feeling and fever).
- New, unexplained symptoms develop. Drugs used in treatment may produce side effects.

HIP DISLOCATION

GENERAL INFORMATION

DEFINITION—A serious hip injury in which adjoining bones in the hip are displaced so they no longer touch each other. Dislocations are frequently accompanied by bone fractures, torn ligaments and torn tendons. Temporary or permanent damage to bone or to the sciatic nerve may also occur. This injury is considered an urgent surgical emergency. The hip must be manipulated to reposition it.

BODY PARTS INVOLVED
- Femur (thigh bone) and pelvis.
- Strong ligaments that hold the hip in place.
- Sciatic nerve.
- Soft tissues surrounding the dislocated hip, including periosteum (covering of bone), other nerves, tendons, blood vessels and connective tissues.

SIGNS & SYMPTOMS
- Severe pain in the hip at the time of injury and when trying to move hip.
- Loss of hip function.
- Visible deformity if the dislocated bones have locked in the dislocated positions. The leg may appear shortened and turned in or fixed in flexion. Bones may spontaneously reposition themselves and leave no deformity, but damage is the same.
- Tenderness over the dislocation.
- Swelling and bruising at the injury site.
- Numbness or paralysis below the dislocation from pressure, pinching or cutting of blood vessels or nerves.

CAUSES
- Direct or indirect blow to a flexed knee and hip.
- End result of a severe hip sprain.
- Congenital abnormality, such as shallow or malformed joint surfaces.

RISK INCREASES WITH
- Contact sports, especially football and hockey.
- Previous hip dislocation or sprain.
- Repeated hip injury of any type.
- Poor muscle conditioning.

HOW TO PREVENT
- Participate in a strengthening, flexibility and conditioning program appropriate for your sport.
- Warm up adequately before physical activity.
- After healing, protect vulnerable joints with special hip pads.
- Consider avoiding contact sports if treatment is unsuccessful in restoring a strong, stable hip.

WHAT TO EXPECT

APPROPRIATE HEALTH CARE
- Doctor's treatment.
- Manipulation and sometimes surgery to restore the joint to its normal position and repair torn ligaments and tendons. Acute or recurring dislocations may require surgical reconstruction or replacement of the joint.
- Self-care during rehabilitation.

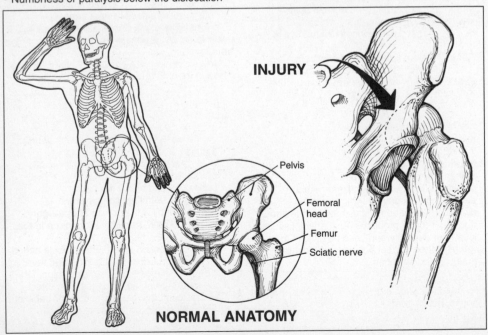

INJURY

Pelvis

Femoral head

Femur

Sciatic nerve

NORMAL ANATOMY

DIAGNOSTIC MEASURES
- Your own observation of symptoms.
- Medical history and exam by a doctor.
- X-rays of the hip, pelvis and knee.

POSSIBLE COMPLICATIONS
At the time of injury:
- Shock.
- Pressure on or injury to nearby nerves, ligaments, tendons, muscles, blood vessels and connective tissues.

After treatment or surgery:
- Excessive internal bleeding.
- Impaired blood supply to the dislocated area.
- Avascular necrosis (death of bone cells due to interruption of the blood supply), which may lead to collapse of the femoral head and arthritis of the joint.
- Infection introduced during surgical treatment.
- Prolonged healing if activity is resumed too soon.
- Repeated hip dislocations.
- Unstable or arthritic hip after repeated injury.
- Loose bodies within the hip joint, causing locking or catching.

PROBABLE OUTCOME—After the dislocation has been corrected, the joint may require immobilization for 4 to 6 weeks in a body cast or brace that encloses the hip. Complete healing of injured ligaments requires a minimum of 6 weeks. Allow at least 3 months of healing before resuming active participation in sports.

 HOW TO TREAT

NOTE—Follow your doctor's instructions. These instructions are supplemental.

FIRST AID
- Keep the person warm with blankets to decrease the possibility of shock.
- Follow instructions for R.I.C.E., the first letters of *rest ice, compression* and *elevation.* See Appendix 1 for details.
- Support the injured area with pillows during movement for transportation.
- The doctor will manipulate the hip bones to return them to their normal position. Manipulation should be done as soon as possible after injury. Shortly after a hip dislocation, bleeding in the hip area and displacement of body fluids may lead to shock and other major problems. Also, many tissues lose their elasticity and become difficult to return to their normal positions within 4 to 6 hours after dislocation.

CONTINUING CARE—At home:
- Apply heat frequently. Use heat lamps, hot soaks, hot showers or heating pads.

- Take whirlpool treatments, if available.
- Massage gently and often to provide comfort and decrease swelling.

MEDICATION—Your doctor may prescribe:
- General anesthesia or muscle relaxants to make joint manipulation possible.
- Acetaminophen to relieve moderate pain.
- Stronger pain relievers for severe pain.
- Stool softeners to prevent constipation due to decreased activity.
- Antibiotics to fight infection.

ACTIVITY
- Walk only with crutches until after the cast is removed and you can safely bear weight. See Appendix 3 (Safe Use of Crutches).
- Begin weight-bearing and reconditioning of the hip and leg after clearance from your doctor.
- If surgery is necessary, resume normal activities and reconditioning gradually.

DIET
- Do not eat or drink before manipulation or surgery to correct the dislocation. Fluid or solid food in your stomach makes vomiting while under general anesthesia more hazardous.
- Balance the amount of food you eat with any change in your level of physical activity.

REHABILITATION
- Begin daily rehabilitation exercises when pain subsides.
- Use ice massage for 10 minutes before and after workouts. Fill a large styrofoam cup with water and freeze. Tear a small amount of foam from the top so ice protrudes. Massage firmly in a circle over the injured area.
- See Rehabilitation section for hip and pelvis exercises.

 CALL YOUR DOCTOR IF

- You have symptoms of a hip dislocation. Call immediately if the leg becomes numb, pale or cold after injury. This is an emergency!
- Any of the following occurs after treatment:
  Swelling above or below the cast.
  Blue or gray skin color beyond the cast, particularly under the toenails.
  Loss of feeling below the hip.
  Nausea or vomiting; constipation.
- Any of the following occurs after surgery:
  Increased pain, swelling or drainage in the surgical area.
  Signs of infection (headache, muscle aches, dizziness or a general ill feeling and fever).
- New, unexplained symptoms develop. Drugs used in treatment may produce side effects.
- Hip dislocations that you can "pop" back into normal position occur repeatedly.

HIP FRACTURE

GENERAL INFORMATION

DEFINITION—A complete or incomplete break in the head of the femur, the major bone in the hip joint.

BODY PARTS INVOLVED
- Femur (the large bone extending from the knee to the hip).
- Acetabulum (hip socket in bony pelvis).
- Hip joint.
- Soft tissues around the fracture site, including muscles, nerves, tendons, ligaments, periosteum (covering of bone), blood vessels and connective tissues.

SIGNS & SYMPTOMS
- Severe pain in the hip.
- Inability to stand or bear weight on the leg.
- Swelling and bruising around the fracture.
- Visible deformity and leg rotation if the fracture is complete and the bone fragments separate enough to distort normal body contours.
- Tenderness to the touch.
- Numbness or coldness in the leg and foot if blood supply is impaired or nerves are injured.

CAUSES—Direct blow or indirect stress to the hip joint. Indirect stress may be caused by twisting or a violent muscle contraction.

RISK INCREASES WITH
- Age over 60.
- Contact sports.
- Cycling.
- History of bone or joint disease, especially osteoporosis.
- Obesity.
- Poor nutrition, especially insufficient calcium and protein.
- If surgery is needed, surgical risk increases with smoking and use of drugs, including mind-altering drugs, muscle relaxants, antihypertensives, tranquilizers, sleep inducers, insulin, sedatives, beta-adrenergic blockers or corticosteroids.

HOW TO PREVENT
- Build your strength with a good conditioning program before beginning regular athletic practice or competition. Increased muscle mass helps protect bones and underlying tissues.
- Use appropriate protective equipment, such as hip pads, when competing in contact sports.
- Ensure an adequate calcium intake (1000 mg to l500 mg a day) with milk and milk products or calcium supplements.

WHAT TO EXPECT

APPROPRIATE HEALTH CARE
- Doctor's treatment.
- Anesthesia and surgery to set the broken hip fragments, usually by surgically pinning them together, but sometimes by replacing the joint.
- Physical therapy and rehabilitation.

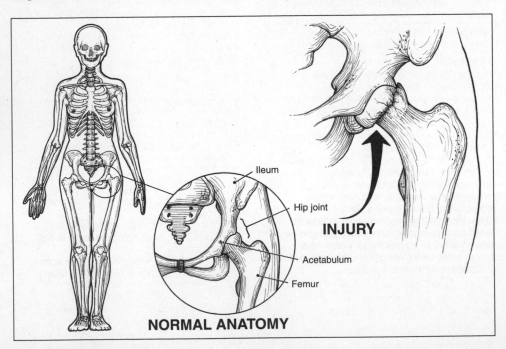

Ileum

Hip joint

INJURY

Acetabulum

Femur

NORMAL ANATOMY

DIAGNOSTIC MEASURES
- Your own observation of symptoms.
- Medical history and exam by a doctor.
- X-rays of the hip, femur and pelvis.

POSSIBLE COMPLICATIONS
At the time of fracture:
- Shock.
- Pressure on or injury to nearby nerves, ligaments, tendons, blood vessels or connective tissues.

After treatment, including surgery:
- Excessive bleeding.
- Impaired blood supply to the healing bone.
- Avascular necrosis (death of bone cells due to interruption of the blood supply), which may lead to collapse of the femoral head and arthritis of the joint.
- Problems arising from plaster casts, splints or other immobilizing materials. See Appendix 2 (Care of Casts).
- Shortening or deformity of the fractured bone.
- Poor healing (nonunion) of the fracture.
- Arrest of bone growth in young people.
- Infection introduced during surgical treatment.
- Unstable or arthritic hip joint following repeated injury.

PROBABLE OUTCOME—The average healing time for this fracture is 8 to 12 weeks. Healing is considered complete when there is no pain or motion at the fracture site and when x-rays show complete bone union.

 HOW TO TREAT

NOTE—Follow your doctor's instructions. These instructions are supplemental.

FIRST AID
- Cut away clothing, if possible, but don't move the injured area to do so.
- Use a padded splint or backboard to immobilize the hip joint before transporting the injured person to an emergency facility.
- Apply ice packs to the injury site to decrease swelling and pain.
- Elevate the foot of the backboard or splint so the pelvis is above the level of the heart. This reduces swelling and fluid accumulation.
- Keep the person warm with blankets to decrease the possibility of shock.
- The doctor will manipulate and set broken bones during surgery. Manipulation should be done as soon as possible after injury. Also, many tissues lose elasticity and become difficult to return to their normal positions.

CONTINUING CARE
- Immobilization will be necessary. In hip fractures, the fractured bone is usually fixed and held with surgical steel pins or screws. A cast is then necessary, although sometimes bracing may be used in recovery period.
- Use frequent ice massage after the cast is removed. Fill a large styrofoam cup with water and freeze. Tear a small amount of foam from the top so ice protrudes. Massage firmly over the injured area in a circle about the size of a softball. Do this for 15 minutes at a time 3 or 4 times a day.
- Apply heat instead of ice if it feels better. Use heat lamps, hot soaks, hot showers, heating pads or heat liniments and ointments.
- Take whirlpool treatments, if available.
- Massage gently and often to provide comfort and decrease swelling.

MEDICATION—Your doctor may prescribe:
- General anesthesia to make joint manipulation possible.
- Stronger pain relievers for severe pain.
- Stool softeners to prevent constipation.
- Acetaminophen for mild pain.
- Antibiotics to fight infection following surgery.

ACTIVITY
- Begin reconditioning and rehabilitation after clearance from your doctor.
- Resume normal daily activities gradually.

DIET
- Do not eat or drink before manipulation or surgery to treat the fracture. Fluid or solid food in your stomach makes vomiting while under anesthesia more hazardous.
- Balance the amount of food you eat with any change in your level of physical activity.

REHABILITATION—Begin daily rehabilitation exercises when movement is comfortable. Use ice massage for 10 minutes prior to exercise. See Rehabilitation section for hip and pelvis exercises.

 CALL YOUR DOCTOR IF

- You have signs or symptoms of a hip fracture. Call immediately if you have numbness or loss of feeling below the fracture site. This is an emergency!
- Any of the following occurs after surgery:
  Increased pain, swelling or drainage in the surgical area.
  Signs of infection (headache, muscle aches, dizziness or a general ill feeling and fever).
  Nausea or vomiting; constipation.
  Swelling above or below the cast.
  Blue or gray skin color beyond the cast, especially under the toenails.

HIP STRAIN

GENERAL INFORMATION

DEFINITION—Injury to the muscles and tendons attached to the trochanter, the large end of the femur (thigh bone) that forms part of the hip joint. Muscles, tendons and their attached bones comprise contractile units. These units stabilize the hip joint and allow its motion. A strain occurs at the weakest part of a unit. Strains are of 3 types:
● Mild (Grade I)—Slightly pulled muscle without tearing of muscle or tendon fibers. There is no loss of strength.
● Moderate (Grade II)—Tearing of fibers in a muscle or tendon or at the attachment to bone. Strength is diminished.
● Severe (Grade III)—Rupture of the muscle-tendon-bone attachment, with separation of fibers. A severe strain may require surgical repair. Chronic strains are caused by overuse. Acute strains are caused by direct injury or overstress.

BODY PARTS INVOLVED
● Trochanter of the femur.
● Muscles or tendons that attach to the trochanter.
● Soft tissues surrounding the strain, including nerves, periosteum (covering of bone), blood vessels and lymph vessels.

SIGNS & SYMPTOMS
● Pain when moving, stretching or twisting.
● Muscle spasm in the hip area.
● Swelling around the injury.
● Limping.
● Loss of strength (moderate or severe strain).
● Crepitation ("crackling" feeling and sound when the injured area is pressed with fingers).
● Calcification of muscles or tendons (visible with x-ray).

CAUSES
● Prolonged overuse of muscle-tendon units in the buttock area or around the hip joint.
● Single violent injury or force applied to the muscle-tendon units in the region of the buttock and hip joint.

RISK INCREASES WITH
● Contact sports, such as football, hockey or soccer.
● Sports that require quick starts, such as running races.
● Medical history of any bleeding disorder.
● Obesity.
● Poor nutrition.
● Previous buttock or hip injury.
● Poor muscle conditioning.

HOW TO PREVENT
● Participate in a strengthening, flexibility and conditioning program appropriate for your sport.
● Warm up before practice or competition.
● Wear proper protective equipment, such as hip pads, for contact sports.

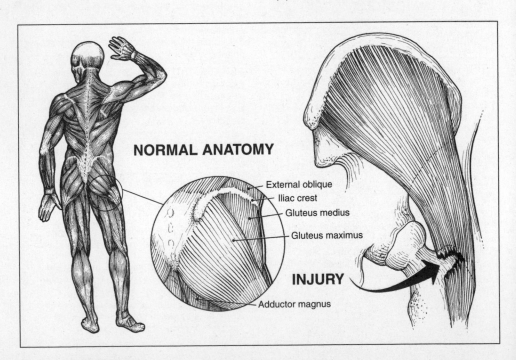

NORMAL ANATOMY

External oblique
Iliac crest
Gluteus medius
Gluteus maximus

INJURY

Adductor magnus

? WHAT TO EXPECT

APPROPRIATE HEALTH CARE
- Doctor's diagnosis.
- Self-care during rehabilitation.
- Physical therapy (moderate or severe strain).
- Surgery (severe strain).

DIAGNOSTIC MEASURES
- Your own observation of symptoms.
- Medical history and exam by a doctor.
- X-rays of the hip area to rule out fractures

POSSIBLE COMPLICATIONS
- Prolonged healing time if activity is resumed too soon.
- Proneness to repeated injury.
- Inflammation at the attachment to bone (periostitis).
- Prolonged disability (sometimes).

PROBABLE OUTCOME—If this is a first-time injury, proper care and sufficient healing time before resuming activity should prevent permanent disability. Torn ligaments and tendons require as long to heal as fractured bones. Average healing times are:
- Mild strain—2 to 10 days.
- Moderate strain—10 days to 6 weeks.
- Severe strain—6 to 10 weeks. If this is a repeat injury, complications listed above are more likely to occur.

HOW TO TREAT

NOTE—Follow your doctor's instructions. These instructions are supplemental.

FIRST AID—Use instructions for R.I.C.E., the first letters of *rest, ice, compression* and *elevation* (if possible). See Appendix 1 for details.

CONTINUING CARE
- Use ice massage 3 or 4 times a day for 15 minutes at a time. Fill a large styrofoam cup with water and freeze. Tear a small amount of foam from the top so ice protrudes. Massage firmly over the injured area in a circle about the size of a softball.

- After the first 72 hours, apply heat instead of ice if it feels better. Use heat lamps, hot soaks, hot showers, heating pads or heat liniments and ointments.
- Take whirlpool treatments, if available.
- Massage gently and often to provide comfort and decrease swelling.

MEDICATION
- For minor discomfort, you may use:
  Aspirin, acetaminophen or ibuprofen.
  Topical liniments and ointments.
- Your doctor may prescribe:
  Stronger pain relievers.
  Injection of a long-acting local anesthetic to reduce pain.
  Injections of corticosteroids, such as triamcinolone, to reduce inflammation.

ACTIVITY
- For a moderate or severe strain, walk with crutches for at least 72 hours—longer with a cast or splints. See Appendix 3 (Safe Use of Crutches).
- Resume your normal activities gradually.
- Pad the injured area if you participate in contact sports.

DIET—During recovery, balance the amount of food you eat with any change in your level of physical activity. Eat a variety of foods to get the energy, protein, vitamins, minerals and fiber you need for good health and healing.

REHABILITATION—Begin daily rehabilitation exercises when pain subsides. See Rehabilitation section for hip and pelvis exercises.

CALL YOUR DOCTOR IF

- You have symptoms of a moderate or severe hip strain or a mild strain persists longer than 10 days.
- Pain or swelling worsens despite treatment.

HIP SYNOVITIS

GENERAL INFORMATION

DEFINITION—Inflammation of the synovium, the smooth, lubricated lining of the hip joint. The synovium's lubricating fluid allows the hip to move freely and prevents bone surfaces from rubbing against each other. Synovitis is often a complication of an injury, such as a fracture, or of rheumatologic diseases, such as gout or rheumatoid arthritis.

BODY PARTS INVOLVED
• Lining of the hip joint
• Bones of the hip, including the thigh bone and pelvis.

SIGNS & SYMPTOMS
• Pain in the hip joint with movement.
• Swelling in the hip.
• Limping.
• Tenderness and redness in the hip area if inflammation is caused by infection or a disease rather than by an athletic injury.

CAUSES
• Any direct blow to the hip or other hip injury that damages the synovium of the hip joint. Most hip synovitis can be traced back to an injury, even though the athlete cannot always remember the injury.

• Bacterial infection in the hip.
• A complication of an open hip fracture.
• Inflammatory joint disease, such as gout or rheumatoid arthritis.

RISK INCREASES WITH
• Contact sports, such as football or soccer.
• Previous hip injury or childhood hip problems.
• Vitamin or mineral deficiency, which makes complications following injury more likely.
• Congenital abnormalities, such as shallow or malformed joint surfaces.

HOW TO PREVENT
• Engage in a muscle strengthening, flexibility and conditioning program prior to beginning regular participation in sports. Overall strength and muscle tone make injury less likely. Also, warm up adequately before competition or workouts.
• When appropriate, wear hip pads to protect the hip area during participation in contact sports.

WHAT TO EXPECT

APPROPRIATE HEALTH CARE
• Doctor's care.
• Self-care during rehabilitation.
• Physical therapy.

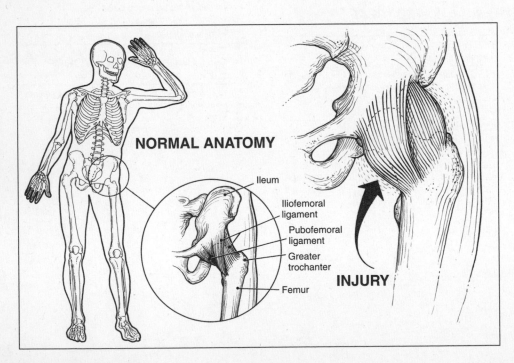

NORMAL ANATOMY

Ileum
Iliofemoral ligament
Pubofemoral ligament
Greater trochanter
Femur

INJURY

DIAGNOSTIC MEASURES
- Your own observation of symptoms.
- Medial history and physical exam by a doctor.
- X-rays of the hip joint.
- Laboratory examination of any fluid removed.

POSSIBLE COMPLICATIONS
- Prolonged healing time if activity is resumed too soon.
- Proneness to repeated hip injury.
- Unstable or arthritic hip following repeated bouts of synovitis.
- Chronic synovitis that may prevent athletic participation.

PROBABLE OUTCOME—Hip synovitis can usually be cured completely in 3 to 5 weeks with rest, heat and corticosteroid injections. However, recurrences are common following minor hip injuries.

 ## HOW TO TREAT

NOTE—Follow your doctor's instructions. These instructions are supplemental.

FIRST AID—None. This condition develops gradually.

CONTINUING CARE
- Follow your doctor's instructions for treatment of any underlying condition.
- Apply heat frequently. Use heat lamps, hot soaks, hot showers, heating pads or heat liniments and ointments.
- Take whirlpool treatments, if available.
- Massage gently and often to provide comfort and decrease swelling.

MEDICATION
- Your doctor may prescribe:
  Antibiotics if infection is present.
  Nonsteroidal anti-inflammatory drugs or antigout medicine.
  Injection of a long-acting local anesthetic mixed with a corticosteroid to help reduce pain and inflammation.
- You may take aspirin or ibuprofen for minor discomfort.

ACTIVITY—Use crutches to limit weight-bearing until pain subsides. See Appendix 3 (Safe Use of Crutches). Resume normal activity gradually.

DIET—During recovery, balance the amount of food you eat with any change in your level of physical activity. Eat a variety of foods to get the energy, protein, vitamins, minerals and fiber you need for good health and healing.

REHABILITATION
- Begin daily rehabilitation exercises when pain subsides after clearance from your doctor.
- Use ice massage for 10 minutes before and after exercise. Fill a large styrofoam cup with water and freeze. Tear a small amount of foam from the top so ice protrudes. Massage firmly over the injured area in a circle about the size of a softball.
- See Rehabilitation section for hip and pelvis exercises.

 ## CALL YOUR DOCTOR IF

- Your hip becomes red, hot, tender and painful.
- You develop signs of infection (headache, fever, muscle aches, dizziness or a general ill feeling) after injection of the hip.

JAW DISLOCATION, TEMPOROMANDIBULAR JOINT

 GENERAL INFORMATION

DEFINITION—Injury and displacement of the end of the lower jaw from its normal niche in a small depression at the base of the skull.

BODY PARTS INVOLVED
- Skull.
- Lower jaw (mandible).
- Soft tissues surrounding the dislocation, including nerves, tendons, ligaments, muscles and blood vessels.

SIGNS & SYMPTOMS
- Inability to close the mouth.
- Excruciating pain in the jaw at the time of injury.
- Visible deformity if dislocated bones lock in the dislocated positions. If they spontaneously reposition themselves, no deformity will be apparent, but damage will be the same.
- Tenderness over the dislocation.
- Swelling and bruising around the jaw.
- Numbness or paralysis in muscles of the face, jaw and neck from pressure, pinching or cutting of blood vessels or nerves

CAUSES
- Direct blow to the jaw.
- Any action that forces the mandible open wider than its normal range on either side.

Muscle spasm follows immediately. This can occur with yawning, yelling or taking a very large bite.
- End result of a severe jaw sprain.

RISK INCREASES WITH
- Contact sports such as boxing.
- Previous jaw dislocation or sprain.
- Repeated injury to the temporomandibular joint.

HOW TO PREVENT—For participation in contact sports, wear protective equipment, including a mouthpiece and helmet.

 WHAT TO EXPECT

APPROPRIATE HEALTH CARE
- Doctor's treatment. This may include manipulating the joint to reposition the bones.
- Surgery (sometimes) to restore the joint to its normal position. Acute or recurring dislocations may require surgical reconstruction or replacement of the joint.
- Self-care during rehabilitation.

DIAGNOSTIC MEASURES
- Your own observation of symptoms.
- Medical history and exam by a doctor.
- X-rays of the jaw.

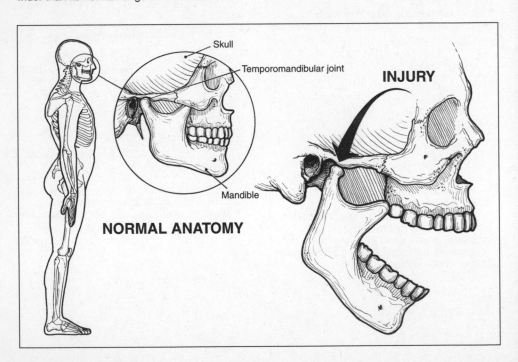

Skull

Temporomandibular joint

INJURY

Mandible

NORMAL ANATOMY

POSSIBLE COMPLICATIONS
- Temporary or permanent damage to nearby nerves or major blood vessels, causing numbness and impaired circulation.
- Shock or loss of consciousness.
- Obstruction of the airway and inhalation of mucus and blood into the lungs, leading to pneumonia. This occurs most often with dislocation and fracture.
- Excessive internal bleeding around the dislocation site.
- Proneness to recurrent jaw dislocations, particularly if a previous dislocation has not healed completely.

PROBABLE OUTCOME—After the dislocation has been corrected, the joint may require immobilization for 2 to 8 weeks with a special device fitted by your doctor or dentist. Complete healing of injured ligaments requires a minimum of 6 weeks.

HOW TO TREAT

NOTE—Follow your doctor's instructions. These instructions are supplemental.

FIRST AID
- Don't panic—try to stay calm. You will not be able to talk. Write messages on paper.
- Don't push or force your mouth or try to make it close. Your mouth cannot close in a normal way until the dislocation is corrected.
- Keep warm with blankets to decrease the possibility of shock.
- Ice helps stop internal bleeding. Prepare an ice pack of ice cubes or chips wrapped in plastic or placed in a container. Place a towel over the injured area to prevent skin damage. Apply ice for 20 minutes, then rest 10 minutes until you obtain medical treatment.
- Go to the nearest dental office or hospital emergency room for help.

CONTINUING CARE
- Continue ice massage 3 or 4 times a day for 15 minutes at a time. Fill a large styrofoam cup with water and freeze. Tear a small amount of foam from the top so ice protrudes. Massage firmly over the injured area in a circle about the size of a softball.
- After 48 hours, application of localized heat promotes healing by increasing blood circulation in the injured area. Use hot compresses, hot lamps, heating pads or heat ointments and liniments.

- If you have recurrent jaw dislocations, you can learn to reposition the jaw. Ask your doctor or dentist for instructions. Use the following points as reminders:

  Place your index finger on your back lower teeth (or the gums in this area, if you have no teeth).

  At the same time, place both thumbs under the center of your chin.

  Push the fingers down while simultaneously raising upward with the thumbs. The proper motion is more of a rotating movement than a straight one. It should be gentle—not fast or jerking. Note: It is probably easier for someone else to perform the relocation than for you to do it.

MEDICATION—Your doctor may prescribe:
- General anesthesia or muscle relaxants to make jaw manipulation easier.
- Acetaminophen or aspirin to relieve moderate pain.
- Narcotic pain relievers for severe pain.

ACTIVITY—No restrictions except those imposed by a mouth appliance. Resume your normal activities gradually over several days. After the dislocation has been corrected, use caution when opening your mouth. Be careful when you yawn, take large bites, yell or scream during excitement, call someone loudly or sing.

DIET—If a mouth appliance is necessary, drink a full liquid diet until the appliance can be removed. If no appliance is necessary, eat a soft diet for a few days until discomfort decreases. Avoid chewy foods that require big bites for a while. Balance the amount of food you eat with any change in your level of physical activity.

REHABILITATION—Rehabilitation exercises must be individualized. Follow your doctor's or surgeon's directions.

CALL YOUR DOCTOR IF

- You have difficulty moving your jaw after injury.
- Any part of the face becomes numb, pale or cold after injury. This is an emergency!
- Jaw dislocations that you can "pop" back into normal position occur repeatedly.

JAW (MANDIBLE) FRACTURE

GENERAL INFORMATION

DEFINITION—A complete or incomplete break in the lower jaw bone (mandible). The temporomandibular joints (TMJs) are located just in front of the ears. These joints connect the lower jaw with the skull end are used to open and close the mouth. A fracture usually occurs at the condyle, or head of the mandible.

BODY PARTS INVOLVED
- Lower jawbone (mandible).
- Temporomandibular joint.
- Soft tissues surrounding the fracture site, including nerves, muscles, tendons, ligaments and blood vessels.

SIGNS & SYMPTOMS
- Severe pain at the fracture site.
- Swelling of soft tissues surrounding the fracture.
- Blood at the base of the teeth near the fracture site.
- Visible deformity if the fracture is complete and bone fragments separate enough to distort normal facial contours.
- Tenderness to the touch.
- Numbness around the fracture site (sometimes).

CAUSES—Direct blow (usually) or indirect stress to the bone. Indirect stress may be caused by violent muscle contraction.

RISK INCREASES WITH
- Contact sports, especially boxing.
- History of bone or joint disease, especially osteoporosis.
- Poor nutrition, especially calcium deficiency.
- If surgery and anesthesia are needed, surgical risk increases with smoking and use of drugs, including mind-altering drugs, muscle relaxants, antihypertensives, tranquilizers, sleep inducers, insulin, sedatives, beta-adrenergic blockers or corticosteroids.

HOW TO PREVENT—Use appropriate protective equipment, such as a face mask or mouthpiece, when participating in contact sports.

WHAT TO EXPECT

APPROPRIATE HEALTH CARE
- Doctor's or dentist's treatment to manipulate and set the broken bone.
- Anesthesia and surgery to set the fracture and wire the jaw or insert screws, plates or pins.
- X-rays of injured area.

DIAGNOSTIC MEASURES
- Your own observation of symptoms.
- Medical history and physical exam by a doctor.
- X-rays of injured areas.

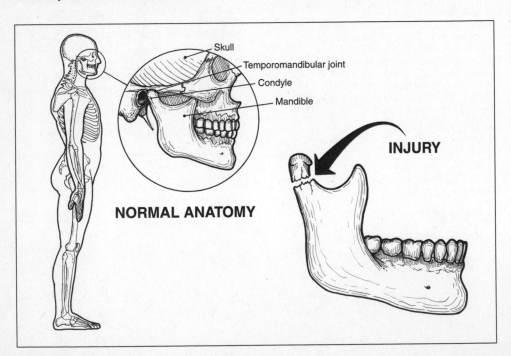

Skull
Temporomandibular joint
Condyle
Mandible

NORMAL ANATOMY

INJURY

POSSIBLE COMPLICATIONS

At the time of injury:
- Shock.
- Pressure on or injury to nearby nerves, ligaments, tendons, muscles, blood vessels and connective tissues.

After treatment or surgery:
- Delayed union or nonunion of the fracture (rare).
- Impaired blood supply to the fracture site.
- Infection in open fracture (skin broken over fracture site), or at the incision if surgical setting was necessary.
- Malocclusion (teeth do not meet correctly with bite).
- Proneness to repeated jaw injury.
- Unstable or arthritic jaw following repeated injury.
- Prolonged healing if activity is resumed too soon.
- Nutritional problems arising because the jaw is wired closed.

PROBABLE OUTCOME—It is impossible to predict exactly how long it will take for any fracture to heal. Variable factors include age, sex and previous state of health and conditioning. The average healing time for this fracture is 6 to 8 weeks. Healing is considered complete when there is no motion at the fracture site and when x-rays show complete bone union.

 HOW TO TREAT

NOTE—Follow your doctor's instructions. These instructions are supplemental.

FIRST AID
- Keep the person warm with blankets to decrease the possibility of shock.
- Use instructions for R.I.C.E., the first letters of *rest, ice, compression* and *elevation*. See Appendix 1 for details.
- The doctor will realign and set the broken bones either with surgery or, if possible, without. Manipulation should be done as soon as possible after injury. Also, many tissues lose their elasticity and become difficult to return to their normal positions.

CONTINUING CARE
- Immobilization will be necessary. Mandible fractures usually require wiring the jaw together.
- Use an ice pack 3 or 4 times a day. Wrap ice chips or cubes in a plastic bag, and wrap the bag in a moist towel. Place it over the injured area for 20 minutes at a time.
- After 72 hours, apply heat instead of ice if it feels better. Use heat lamps, hot soaks, hot showers or a heating pad.
- Learn how to "quick-release" your wired teeth for any emergency, such as severe coughing or vomiting.

MEDICATION—Your doctor may prescribe:
- General anesthesia, local anesthesia or muscle relaxants to make bone manipulation and fixation of bone fragments possible.
- Pain relievers in liquid form for severe pain.
- Stool softeners in liquid form to prevent constipation due to a liquid diet.
- Liquid acetaminophen (available without prescription) for mild pain after initial treatment.

ACTIVITY—Rest quietly for two days, then resume normal activities gradually. Don't exercise to the point that you pant for breath, because breathing may be difficult for a while.

DIET—A normal diet may be difficult, especially if the jaw is wired or bandaged. If so, eat soft or liquid foods until a regular diet is possible.

REHABILITATION—No special rehabilitation program. Begin using jaw muscles carefully after the fracture heals.

 CALL YOUR DOCTOR IF

- You have signs or symptoms of a jaw fracture.
- Any of the following occurs after surgery or their treatment:
  Increased pain, swelling or drainage in the surgical area.
  Signs of infection (headache, muscle aches, dizziness or a general ill feeling and fever).
  Nausea or vomiting.
  Numbness or complete loss of feeling around the jaw.
  Constipation.

JAW SPRAIN, TEMPOROMANDIBULAR JOINT

GENERAL INFORMATION

DEFINITION—Violent overstretching of one or more ligaments in the temporomandibular joint. Sprains involving two or more ligaments cause considerably more disability than single-ligament sprains. When the ligament is overstretched, it becomes tense and gives way at its weakest point, either where it attaches to bone or within the ligament itself. If the ligament pulls loose a fragment of bone, it is called an avulsion fracture. There are 3 types of sprains:
- Mild (Grade I)—Tearing of some ligament fibers. There is no loss of function.
- Moderate (Grade II)—Rupture of a portion of the ligament, resulting in some loss of function.
- Severe (Grade III)—Complete rupture of the ligament or complete separation of ligament from bone. There is total loss of function. A severe sprain may require surgical repair.

BODY PARTS INVOLVED
- Ligaments of the temporomandibular joint of the jaw.
- Tissues surrounding the sprain, including blood vessels, tendons, bone, periosteum (covering of bone) and muscles.

SIGNS & SYMPTOMS
- Severe pain at the time of injury.
- A feeling of popping or tearing inside the jaw.
- Difficulty opening and closing the mouth.
- Tenderness at the injury site.
- Swelling around the jaw.
- Bruising that appears soon after injury.

CAUSES—Stress that forces the jaw through a wider range of motion than ligaments normally permit.

RISK INCREASES WITH
- Contact sports, especially boxing.
- Previous temporomandibular joint injury or disorder.
- Inadequate protection from equipment

HOW TO PREVENT—Wear protective equipment, such as a face mask and mouthpiece, when appropriate.

WHAT TO EXPECT

APPROPRIATE HEALTH CARE
- Doctor's diagnosis.
- Bandaging or wiring of the jaw (sometimes).
- Biofeedback training (see Glossary) during the healing phase.
- Physical therapy (moderate or severe sprain).
- Surgery (severe sprain).

DIAGNOSTIC MEASURES
- Your own observation of symptoms.
- Medical history and exam by a doctor.
- X-rays of the jaw to rule out fractures or dislocations.

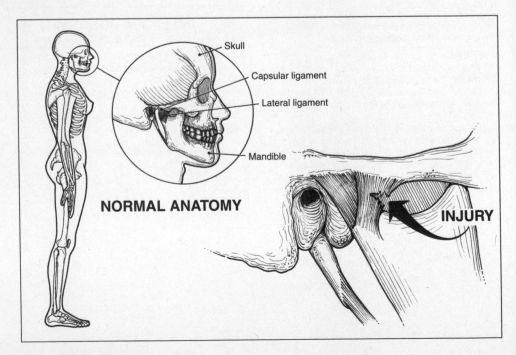

Skull

Capsular ligament

Lateral ligament

Mandible

NORMAL ANATOMY

INJURY

POSSIBLE COMPLICATIONS
- Proneness to repeated jaw injury.
- Inflammation at the ligament attachment to bone (periostitis).

PROBABLE OUTCOME—Jaw sprains usually cause no permanent problems if allowed to heal sufficiently. Ligaments have a poor blood supply, and torn ligaments require as much healing time as fractures. Average healing times are:
- Mild sprains—2 to 6 weeks.
- Moderate sprains—6 to 8 weeks.
- Severe sprains—8 to 10 weeks.

 ## HOW TO TREAT

NOTE—Follow your doctor's instructions. These instructions are supplemental.

FIRST AID—Use instructions for R.I.C.E., the first letters of *rest, ice, compression* and *elevation*. See Appendix 1 for details.

CONTINUING CARE
- Continue using an ice pack 3 or 4 times a day. Place ice chips or cubes in a plastic bag. Wrap the bag in a moist towel, and place it over the jaw. Use for 20 minutes at a time.
- After 72 hours, apply heat instead of ice if it feels better. Use heat lamps, hot soaks, hot showers, heating pads or heat liniments and ointments.
- Massage gently and often to provide comfort and decrease swelling.

MEDICATION
- For minor discomfort, you may use aspirin, acetaminophen or ibuprofen.
- Your doctor may prescribe:
  Stronger pain relievers.
  Injection of a long-acting local anesthetic to reduce pain.
  Injections of a corticosteroid, such as triamcinolone, to reduce inflammation.
  Stool softeners if constipation results from a liquid or soft diet.

ACTIVITY—Resume your normal activities gradually after clearance from your doctor.

DIET—A normal diet may be difficult, especially if the jaw is wired or bandaged. If so, eat soft or liquid foods until a regular diet is possible.

REHABILITATION—Consult your doctor or oral surgeon for rehabilitation exercises.

 ## CALL YOUR DOCTOR IF

- You have symptoms of a moderate or severe temporomandibular sprain or a mild sprain persists longer than 2 weeks.
- Pain, swelling or bruising worsens despite treatment.
- You feel numbness or coldness around the injury.
- Any of the following occurs after surgery:
  Increased pain, swelling, redness, drainage or bleeding in the surgical area.
  Signs of infection (headache, muscle aches, dizziness or a general ill feeling with fever).
- New, unexplained symptoms develop. Drugs used in treatment may produce side effects.

KIDNEY INJURY

GENERAL INFORMATION

DEFINITION—Bruising or tearing of the kidney or ureter. The kidneys filter waste material from the bloodstream and produce urine. The ureters are the tubes that carry urine from the kidneys to the bladder. The most common injury to the kidney is contusion. In contact sports, this may result from a blow from a knee or helmet, with the shock penetrating the flank muscles and reaching the kidney.

BODY PARTS INVOLVED
- Kidney.
- Ureter (tube that carries urine from the kidney to the bladder).
- Muscles of the abdominal wall.
- Subcutaneous tissues, nerves, blood vessels and connective tissues.
- Urethra (tube that carries urine from the bladder out of the body).

SIGNS & SYMPTOMS
- Pain and tenderness in the flank or back, just below the ribs on the injured side.
- Fever to 101°F (38.3°C).
- Blood in the urine. There may be enough to make the urine look "smoky" or bloody. Lesser bleeding can only be determined by studying the urine under a microscope.

- If infection of the injured kidney complicates the injury, sudden onset of:
  Fever and shaking chills.
  Burning, frequent urination.
  Cloudy urine or blood in the urine.
  Aching (sometimes severe) in one or both sides of the lower back.
  Abdominal pain.
  Marked fatigue.

CAUSES
- A blow or penetrating wound to the kidney, located at the side of the body under the ribs.
- Urinary tract infection caused by kidney damage that leads to decreased rate of urine flow. Decreased urine flow allows bacteria to grow and infect the parts of the urinary tract— the kidneys, ureters, bladder and urethra.

RISK INCREASES WITH
- Contact sports.
- Any underlying abnormality of the kidney or genitourinary tract, such as polycystic kidneys.
- Poor muscle conditioning.
- Medical history of any bleeding disorder.
- Congenital or abnormal shape or position of the kidney.

HOW TO PREVENT
- Use adequate protective equipment for contact sports.
- Develop good muscle conditioning in the flank area. Increased muscle mass helps protect underlying organs and other tissues.

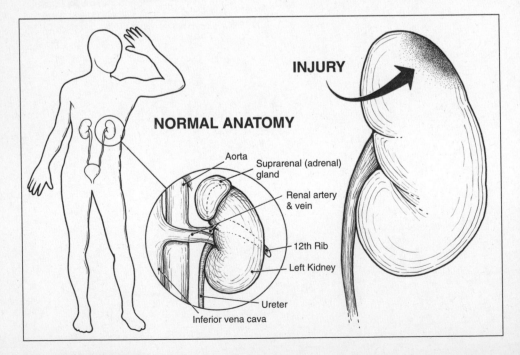

INJURY

NORMAL ANATOMY

Aorta

Suprarenal (adrenal) gland

Renal artery & vein

12th Rib

Left Kidney

Ureter

Inferior vena cava

WHAT TO EXPECT

APPROPRIATE HEALTH CARE
• Doctor's treatment.
• Hospitalization for shock or internal bleeding.
• Surgery to repair the ureter or remove the kidney if other treatment fails.

DIAGNOSTIC MEASURES
• Your own observation of symptoms.
• Medical history and physical exam by a doctor.
• Laboratory urine studies.
• X-rays of the urinary tract.

POSSIBLE COMPLICATIONS
• Internal bleeding.
• Shock (sweating; faintness; nausea; panting; rapid pulse; pale, cold, moist skin).
• Urine leakage into the abdomen, causing abdominal inflammation or infection.
• Scarring and narrowing of the injured ureter.

PROBABLE OUTCOME—Usually heals with time, bed rest, protection against infection and surgery (sometimes). Surgery to remove an injured kidney (if it does not heal with other measures) may be necessary. After recovery, you can lead a normal life with one kidney, but you must avoid contact sports. Allow about 4 weeks for recovery from surgery.

HOW TO TREAT

NOTE—Follow your doctor's instructions. These instructions are supplemental.

FIRST AID—Use instructions for R.I.C.E., the first letters of *rest ice, compression* and *elevation*. See Appendix 1 for details.

CONTINUING CARE—No special instructions except those under other headings. If surgery is required, your surgeon will supply postoperative instructions.

MEDICATION—Your doctor may prescribe:
• Pain relievers.
• Antibiotics to treat or protect against infection.

ACTIVITY—You may need bed rest for 1 to 2 weeks after the injury. After recovery, resume normal activities gradually.

DIET
• Drink 6 to 8 glasses of fluid daily.
• Don't drink alcohol.
• During recovery, balance the amount of food you eat with any change in your level of physical activity. Eat a variety of foods to get the energy, protein, vitamins, minerals and fiber you need for good health and healing.

REHABILITATION—Rehabilitation exercises must be individualized. Follow your doctor's or surgeon's directions.

CALL YOUR DOCTOR IF

• You have any symptoms of kidney or ureter injury.
• Symptoms recur after treatment, especially blood in the urine.
• You have symptoms of a kidney infection.
• Symptoms and fever persist after 48 hours of antibiotic treatment. Occasionally a different antibiotic is needed.
• Symptoms return (especially if accompanied by fever) after antibiotic treatment.
• New, unexplained symptoms develop. Drugs used in treatment may produce side effects.

KNEE BURSITIS

GENERAL INFORMATION

DEFINITION—Inflammation of a bursa in the knee. Bursitis may vary in degree from mild irritation to an abscess formation that causes excruciating pain. There are many bursas in the knee:
- In front of the kneecap.
- On both sides of the knee, just below the jointline.
- Behind the patellar tendon.
- Behind the hamstring tendons.

BODY PARTS INVOLVED
- Knee bursas—soft sacs in the knee area filled with lubricating fluid that facilitate motion in the knee.
- Soft tissues surrounding the knee, including nerves, tendons, ligaments, blood vessels (both large vessels and capillaries), periosteum (the outside lining of bone) and muscles.

SIGNS & SYMPTOMS
- Pain, especially when moving the knee.
- Tenderness.
- Swelling.
- Redness (sometimes) over the affected bursa.
- Fever if infection is present.
- Limitation of motion in the knee.

CAUSES
- Injury to the knee, especially falling on a bent knee.
- Acute or chronic infection in the knee.
- Arthritis.
- Gout.
- Unknown (frequently).

RISK INCREASES WITH
- Participation in competitive athletics, particularly contact sports such as football.
- Previous history of bursitis in any joint.
- Exposure to cold weather.
- Poor conditioning and inadequate warmup.
- Inadequate protective equipment in contact sports.

HOW TO PREVENT
- Warm up adequately before athletic practice or competition.
- Wear warm clothing in cold weather.
- To prevent recurrence, continue to wear extra knee pads until healing is complete.

WHAT TO EXPECT

APPROPRIATE HEALTH CARE
- Doctor's exam for precise diagnosis and treatment.
- Surgery (sometimes), particularly for a frozen knee.

DIAGNOSTIC MEASURES
- Your own observation of symptoms.
- Medical history and physical exam by a doctor.
- X-rays of the knee.

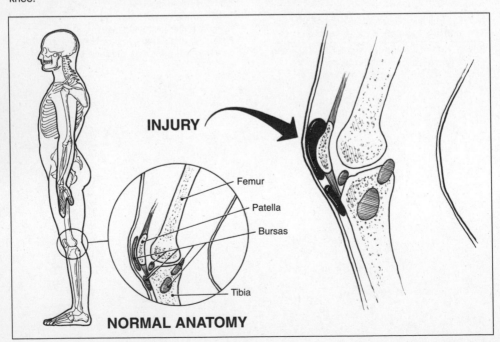

INJURY

Femur

Patella

Bursas

Tibia

NORMAL ANATOMY

POSSIBLE COMPLICATIONS
● Infection from wound or caused by injections or surgery.
● Prolonged healing time if activity or weight-bearing is resumed too soon.
● Proneness to repeated flare-ups.

PROBABLE OUTCOME—Knee bursitis is commonly a chronic problem. Symptoms may subside with treatment, but recurrent flare-ups are common. If surgery becomes necessary, allow 6 to 8 weeks for healing.

 ## HOW TO TREAT

NOTE—Follow your doctor's instructions. These instructions are supplemental.

FIRST AID—None. This problem develops slowly.

CONTINUING CARE
● Use frequent ice massage. Fill a large styrofoam cup with water and freeze. Tear a small amount of foam from the top so ice protrudes. Massage firmly over the injured area in a circle about the size of a softball. Do this for 15 minutes at a time 3 or 4 times a day, and also before workouts or competition.
● After 72 hours, apply heat instead of ice if it feels better. Use heat lamps, hot soaks, hot showers, heating pads or heat liniments and ointments.
● Take whirlpool treatments, if available.
● Use crutches to prevent weight-bearing on the knee, if needed.
● Whenever possible, elevate the knee above the level of the heart to reduce swelling and prevent accumulation of fluid. Use pillows for propping, or elevate the foot of the bed.
● Gentle massage will frequently provide comfort and decrease swelling.

MEDICATION—Your doctor may prescribe:
● Nonsteroidal anti-inflammatory drugs.
● Antibiotics if the bursa is infected.
● Prescription pain relievers for severe pain. Use nonprescription aspirin, acetaminophen or ibuprofen for mild pain.
● Injection with a long-lasting local anesthetic mixed with a corticosteroid drug, such as triamcinolone.
● Steroid creams applied by ultrasound (phonophoresis) (see Glossary).

ACTIVITY—Rest the knee as much as possible. If you must resume normal activity, use crutches until the pain becomes more bearable. Begin normal, slow knee movement as soon as possible.

DIET—During recovery, balance the amount of food you eat with any change in your level of physical activity. Eat a variety of foods to get the energy, protein, vitamins, minerals and fiber you need for good health and healing. Your doctor may suggest vitamin and mineral supplements to promote healing.

REHABILITATION—See Rehabilitation section for knee exercises.

 ## CALL YOUR DOCTOR IF

● You have symptoms of knee bursitis.
● Pain increases despite treatment.
● Pain, swelling, tenderness, drainage or bleeding increases in the surgical area.
● You develop signs of infection (headache, muscle aches, dizziness or a general ill feeling and fever).
● New, unexplained symptoms develop. Drugs used in treatment may produce side effects.

KNEE CARTILAGE (MENISCUS) INJURY

GENERAL INFORMATION

DEFINITION—Damage to cartilage in the knee at the top of the lower leg bone (tibia). Knee cartilage injuries frequently accompany ligament sprains in the knee. This is sometimes a vaguely diagnosed knee injury that resists conservative treatment.

BODY PARTS INVOLVED
- Cartilage at the top of the tibia that normally cushions force applied to the knee.
- Knee joint.
- Ligaments that lend stability to the knee.
- Soft tissues that include nerves, synovial membranes, periosteum (covering of bone), blood vessels, lymph vessels and synovium (lining) of the knee joint.

SIGNS & SYMPTOMS
- Pain and tenderness in the knee, especially when bearing weight.
- Locking of the knee joint.
- "Giving way" of the knee.
- "Water" on the knee (effusion).

CAUSES
- Prolonged overuse of an injured knee.
- Twisting injury to the knee or violent muscle contraction.
- Landing on a very flexed knee; kneeling or squatting.

RISK INCREASES WITH
- Contact sports, especially football.
- Obesity.
- Poor nutrition.
- Previous knee injury, with residual ligament looseness in the knee.
- Poor muscle conditioning.

HOW TO PREVENT
- Participate in a strengthening, flexibility and conditioning program appropriate for your sport.
- Avoid concrete or asphalt surfaces and other rigid surfaces for continuous conditioning exercises.
- Warm up adequately before practice or competition.
- Tape the knee before practice or competition if you have had a previous knee injury.

WHAT TO EXPECT

APPROPRIATE HEALTH CARE
- Doctor's care.
- Arthroscopic surgery to remove the damaged meniscus or repair the meniscus tear. Arthroscopy is visual examination of a joint using an arthroscope, a fiberoptic instrument with a lighted tip.
- Self-care during recovery following surgery.
- Physical therapy and rehabilitation after surgery.

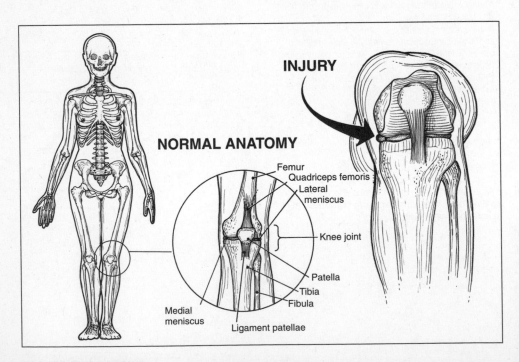

INJURY

NORMAL ANATOMY

Femur
Quadriceps femoris
Lateral meniscus
Knee joint
Patella
Tibia
Fibula
Medial meniscus
Ligament patellae

DIAGNOSTIC MEASURES
- Your own observation of symptoms.
- Medical history and physical exam by a doctor.
- X-rays of the knee to rule out fracture.
- MRI (see Glossary) to establish or confirm diagnosis.
- Arthroscopy to diagnose knee injuries that have some, but not all, signs of cartilage injury. This technique is also used for surgery on the knee.

POSSIBLE COMPLICATIONS
- Prolonged disability, knee instability and pain without surgery.
- Arthritic changes in later years whether surgery was performed or not.
- Proneness to repeated knee injury.
- Postoperative complications, including bleeding into the knee joint, surgical wound infection and slow healing.

PROBABLE OUTCOME—Surgery is the only definitive treatment for knee cartilage injuries. With surgery, expect complete healing if no complications occur. Allow 3 to 6 weeks for full recovery from surgery.

 ## HOW TO TREAT

NOTE—Follow your doctor's instructions. These instructions are supplemental.

FIRST AID
- Use instructions for R.I.C.E., the first letters of *rest, ice, compression* and *elevation*. See Appendix 1 for details.
- Keep the person warm with blankets to decrease the possibility of shock.
- Cut away clothing, if possible. Don't move the injured knee to remove clothing.
- Use a padded splint to immobilize the knee, hip and ankle before transporting the injured person to the doctor's office or emergency facility.

CONTINUING CARE—During the postoperative phase:
- Walk on crutches until your doctor instructs otherwise.
- After the dressing is removed, use an electric heating pad, heat lamp or warm compress to relieve incisional pain.

- Take whirlpool treatments, if available.
- Wrap the injured knee with an elasticized bandage between treatments.
- Massage gently and often to provide comfort and decrease swelling.
- On follow-up visits, your surgeon may aspirate fluid that has accumulated in the knee joint.

MEDICATION
- For minor discomfort, you may use non-prescription medicines such as aspirin, acetaminophen or ibuprofen.
- Your doctor may prescribe stronger medicine for pain, if needed.

ACTIVITY—Return gradually to previous level of activity. You may return to full activity when the range of motion and strength in the injured leg is equal to that in the normal leg.

DIET—During recovery, balance the amount of food you eat with any change in your level of physical activity. Eat a variety of foods to get the energy, protein, vitamins, minerals and fiber you need for good health and healing.

REHABILITATION
- Begin non-weight-bearing rehabilitation exercises the first day after surgery.
- Begin daily rehabilitation exercises when movement is comfortable.
- Use ice massage for 10 minutes before and after exercise. Fill a large styrofoam cup with water and freeze. Tear a small amount of foam from the top so ice protrudes. Massage firmly over the injured area in a circle about the size of a softball.
- See Rehabilitation section for knee exercises.

 ## CALL YOUR DOCTOR IF

- You have symptoms of a knee cartilage injury.
- Any of the following occurs after surgery:
  Increased pain, swelling, redness, drainage or bleeding in the surgical area.
  Signs of infection (headache, muscle aches, dizziness or a general ill feeling and fever).
  Nausea or vomiting.

KNEE CONTUSION

GENERAL INFORMATION

DEFINITION—Bruising of the skin and underlying tissues of the knee due to a direct blow. Contusions cause bleeding from ruptured small capillaries that allow blood to infiltrate muscles, tendons or other soft tissues. The knee is highly vulnerable to contusions.

BODY PARTS INVOLVED—Knee, including blood vessels, muscles, tendons, nerves, covering of bone (periosteum) and connective tissues.

SIGNS & SYMPTOMS
- Swelling—either superficial or deep.
- Pain and tenderness over the knee.
- Feeling of firmness when pressure is exerted on the knee.
- Discoloration under the skin, beginning with redness and progressing to the characteristic "black-and-blue" bruise.
- Restricted knee activity proportional to the extent of injury.
- Break in skin over the contusion (frequent in knee injury).

CAUSES—Direct blow to the front or side of the knee.

RISK INCREASES WITH
- Contact, running or riding sports, especially if the knees are not adequately protected.
- Medical history of any bleeding disorder.
- Poor nutrition, including vitamin deficiency.
- Use of anticoagulants or aspirin.

HOW TO PREVENT—Wear protective knee pads during competition or other athletic activity if there is risk of a knee contusion.

WHAT TO EXPECT

APPROPRIATE HEALTH CARE
- Doctor's care unless the injury is quite small.
- Self-care for minor contusions and for serious contusions during rehabilitation.
- Physical therapy for serious contusions.

DIAGNOSTIC MEASURES
- Your own observation of symptoms.
- Medical history and physical exam by a doctor for all except minor injuries.
- X-rays of the knee to assess total injury to soft tissues and to rule out the possibility of underlying fractures. The total extent of injury may not be apparent for 48 to 72 hours.

POSSIBLE COMPLICATIONS
- Excessive bleeding, leading to disability. Infiltrative-type bleeding can sometimes lead to calcification and impaired function of injured muscles, ligaments or tendons.
- Prolonged healing time if usual activities are resumed too soon.
- Infection if skin over the contusion is broken.

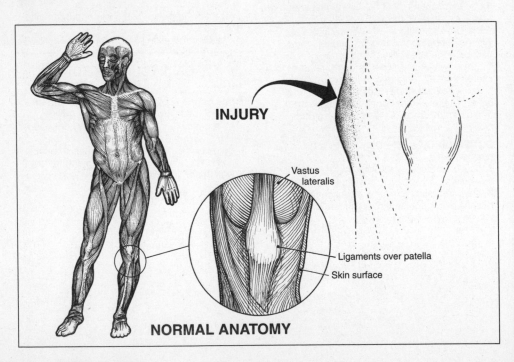

INJURY

Vastus lateralis

Ligaments over patella

Skin surface

NORMAL ANATOMY

PROBABLE OUTCOME—Healing time varies from 3 to 10 days, depending on the extent of injury.

HOW TO TREAT

NOTE—Follow your doctor's instructions. These instructions are supplemental.

FIRST AID—Use instructions for R.I.C.E., the first letters of *rest, ice, compression* and *elevation*. See Appendix 1 for details.

CONTINUING CARE
• Wrap an elasticized bandage over a felt pad on the knee. Keep the area compressed for about 72 hours.
• Use an ice pack 3 or 4 times a day. Wrap ice chips or cubes in a plastic bag, and wrap the bag in a moist towel. Place it over the injured area for 20 minutes at a time.
• After 72 hours, apply heat instead of ice if it feels better. Use heat lamps, hot soaks, hot showers, heating pads, heat liniments and ointments or whirlpool treatments.
• Massage gently and often to provide comfort and decrease swelling.
• Return to activity with protective knee pad to prevent a repeat injury from a direct blow.

MEDICATION
• For minor discomfort, you may use:
  Acetaminophen or ibuprofen.
  Topical liniments and ointments.
• Your doctor may prescribe stronger medicine for pain.

ACTIVITY—Begin activities slowly, and stop exercise as soon as pain begins. Increase activity as healing progresses.

DIET—During recovery, balance the amount of food you eat with any change in your level of physical activity. Eat a variety of foods to get the energy, protein, vitamins, minerals and fiber you need for good health and healing.

REHABILITATION
• Begin daily rehabilitation exercises when supportive wrapping is no longer needed.
• Use ice massage for 10 minutes before and after workouts. Fill a large styrofoam cup with water and freeze. Tear a small amount of foam from the top so ice protrudes. Massage firmly over the injured area in a circle about the size of a softball.
• See Rehabilitation section for knee exercises.

CALL YOUR DOCTOR IF

• You have a knee contusion that doesn't improve in 1 or 2 days.
• Skin is broken and signs of infection (drainage, increasing pain, fever, headache, muscle aches, dizziness or a general ill feeling) occur.

KNEE DISLOCATION, TIBIA-FEMUR

GENERAL INFORMATION

DEFINITION—Injury to the knee joint in which the upper and lower leg bones are displaced and no longer touch each other. Knee dislocations always include torn or ruptured ligaments in the knee.

BODY PARTS INVOLVED
- Tibia (large lower leg bone), femur (thigh bone) and patella (kneecap).
- Ligaments of the knee joint.
- Meniscus (cartilage) of the knee joint.
- Soft tissues surrounding the dislocated knee, including periosteum (covering of bone), nerves, tendons, blood vessels and connective tissues.

SIGNS & SYMPTOMS
- Severe knee pain at the time of injury.
- Loss of function of the knee and severe pain when attempting to move it.
- Visible deformity if the dislocated bones have locked in the dislocated positions. Bones may spontaneously reposition themselves and leave no deformity, but damage is the same.
- Tenderness over the dislocation.
- Swelling and bruising around the knee.
- Numbness or paralysis below the dislocation.

CAUSES
- Overextension of the knee.
- Direct blow to the tibia.

- Direct blow to the thigh, driving the knee to either side.
- End result of a severe knee sprain.
- Congenital knee abnormality, such as shallow or malformed joint surfaces.

RISK INCREASES WITH
- Contact sports, especially football, hockey or rugby.
- Previous knee sprain or dislocation.
- Repeated knee injury of any sort.
- Poor muscle conditioning.

HOW TO PREVENT
- Participate in a strengthening, flexibility and conditioning program appropriate for your sport.
- Warm up adequately before physical activity.
- After healing, wear protective equipment such as special knee pads and knee braces during participation in contact sports.

WHAT TO EXPECT

APPROPRIATE HEALTH CARE
- Doctor's treatment.
- Manipulation and frequently surgery to restore the knee to its normal position and repair torn ligaments and tendons. Acute or recurring dislocation may require reconstruction of the knee ligaments. At times, cast immobilization may be used instead of surgery.

DIAGNOSTIC MEASURES
- You own observation of symptoms.

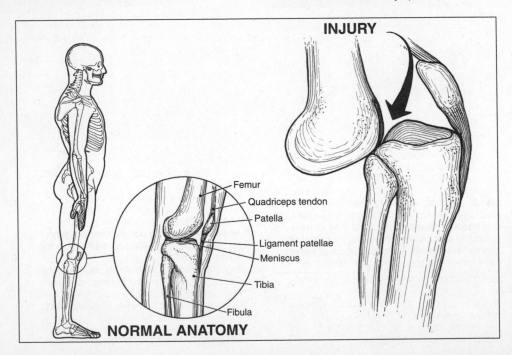

INJURY

Femur
Quadriceps tendon
Patella
Ligament patellae
Meniscus
Tibia
Fibula

NORMAL ANATOMY

- Medical history and exam by a doctor.
- X-rays of the knee, hip and ankle.
- Arteriogram to rule out artery injury.

POSSIBLE COMPLICATIONS
At the time of injury:
- Shock.
- Injury to the major artery and nerves to the foot and ankle. These may require urgent surgery or chronic brace use due to foot drop.
- Cartilage surface fractures that may lead to development of arthritis.

After treatment or surgery:
- Excessive internal bleeding around the knee.
- Impaired blood supply to the knee.
- Death of bone cells from interruption of the blood supply (avascular necrosis).
- Infection introduced during surgical treatment.
- Excessive looseness and giving way of the knee.
- Prolonged healing if activity is resumed too soon.
- Permanently stiff or arthritic knee joint.

PROBABLE OUTCOME—After the dislocation has been corrected, the knee may require immobilization with a cast or splint for 6 to 8 weeks. Complete healing of injured ligaments requires a minimum of 6 weeks. Avoid contact sports if all treatments are unsuccessful in restoring a strong, stable knee.

HOW TO TREAT

NOTE—Follow your doctor's instructions. These instructions are supplemental.

FIRST AID
- This is a medical emergency. Get help as soon as possible.
- Follow instructions for R.I.C.E., the first letters of *rest, ice, compression* and *elevation*. See Appendix 1 for details.
- Cut away clothing if possible. Don't move the injured leg to do so.
- Immobilize the knee, hip and ankle joints with padded splints.
- The doctor will repair torn ligaments and tendons and manipulate the dislocated knee to return it to its normal position. Manipulation should be done within 6 hours after injury or bleeding and displacement of body fluids may lead to shock. Also, many tissues lose elasticity and become difficult to return to their normal positions. Manipulation may require spinal or general anesthesia. If blood vessels or nerves have major damage, surgery is mandatory.

CONTINUING CARE—After removal of the cast or splint:
- Use an ice pack 3 or 4 times a day. Place ice chips or cubes in a plastic bag, and wrap the bag in a moist towel. Place it over the injured area for 20 minutes at a time.

- Apply heat instead of ice if it feels better. Use heat lamps, hot soaks, hot showers, heating pads or whirlpool treatments.
- Wrap the injured knee with an elasticized bandage between treatments.
- Massage gently and often to provide comfort and decrease swelling.

MEDICATION—Your doctor may prescribe:
- General anesthesia, spinal anesthesia or muscle relaxants prior to joint manipulation.
- Acetaminophen to relieve moderate pain.
- Narcotic pain relievers for severe pain.
- Stool softeners to prevent constipation.
- Antibiotics to fight infection if surgery is necessary.

ACTIVITY
- Walk with crutches while the cast is in place. See Appendix 3 (Safe Use of Crutches). Begin weight-bearing and reconditioning of the knee after clearance from your doctor.
- If surgery is necessary, resume activity gradually.

DIET
- Do not eat or drink before manipulation or surgery to correct the dislocation. Fluid or solid food in your stomach makes vomiting while under general anesthesia more hazardous.
- During recovery, eat a well-balanced diet.

REHABILITATION
- Begin daily rehabilitation exercises after clearance from your doctor.
- Use ice massage for 10 minutes before and after workouts. Fill a large styrofoam cup with water and freeze. Tear a small amount of foam from the top so ice protrudes. Massage firmly in a circle over the injured area. See the Rehabilitation section for knee exercises.

CALL YOUR DOCTOR IF

- You have symptoms of a dislocated knee, even if the knee goes back into position. Call immediately if the leg becomes numb, pale, or cold. This is an emergency!
- Any of the following occurs after treatment:
  Nausea or vomiting.
  Swelling above or below the cast.
  Blue or gray skin color below the cast, particularly under the toenails.
- Any of the following occurs after surgery:
  Increasing pain, swelling or drainage in the surgical area.
  Signs of infection (headache, muscle aches, dizziness or a general ill feeling and fever).
- New, unexplained symptoms develop. Drugs used in treatment may produce side effects.
- Knee dislocations that you can "pop" back into normal position occur repeatedly.

KNEE DISLOCATION, TIBIA-FIBULA

GENERAL INFORMATION

DEFINITION—Injury and displacement of the bones of the lower leg so they no longer touch each other. This is less common than dislocation of the kneecap. It often occurs with fracture of the tibia.

BODY PARTS INVOLVED
- Knee joint.
- Lower leg bones (tibia and fibula) where they join the knee joint.
- Soft tissues surrounding the dislocation, including nerves, periosteum (covering of bone), tendons, ligaments, muscles and blood vessels.
- Ligaments supporting the outside of the knee and attached fibula.

SIGNS & SYMPTOMS
- A feeling of "giving way" of the knee.
- Excruciating pain at the time of injury.
- Locking of the dislocated bones in the abnormal position or spontaneous reposition, leaving no apparent deformity.
- Tenderness over the dislocation.
- Swelling and discoloration of the knee.
- Numbness or paralysis in the lower leg and foot from pressure, pinching or cutting of blood vessels or nerves.

CAUSES
- Direct blow to the knee.
- End result of a severe sprain caused by a twisting injury.

- Powerful muscle contractions related to quick changes of direction while running.

RISK INCREASES WITH
- Contact and running sports.
- A wide pelvis and "knock knees."
- Previous knee sprains.
- Repeated knee injury.
- Poor muscle conditioning.
- Congenital abnormalities of the knee joint.

HOW TO PREVENT
- Participate in a strengthening, flexibility and conditioning program appropriate for your sport.
- Warm up adequately before physical activity.
- After recovery, protect the knee during contact or running sports by wearing wrapped elastic bandages, tape wraps, knee pads or special support stockings.

WHAT TO EXPECT

APPROPRIATE HEALTH CARE
- Doctor's treatment. This may include manipulation of the knee to reposition the bones.
- Surgery (sometimes) to restore the knee to normal function.
- Self-care during rehabilitation.

DIAGNOSTIC MEASURES
- Your own observation of symptoms.
- Medical history and exam by a doctor.
- X-rays of the knee joint and adjacent bones.

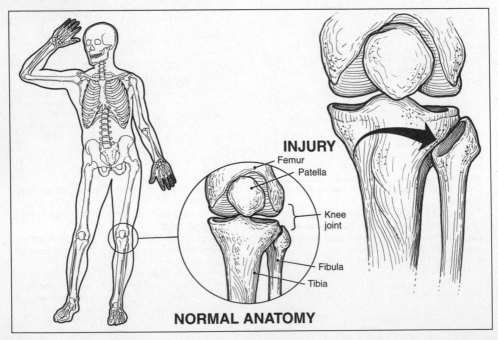

INJURY

Femur
Patella
Knee joint
Fibula
Tibia

NORMAL ANATOMY

POSSIBLE COMPLICATIONS

At the time of injury:
- Shock.
- Pressure on or injury to nearby nerves, ligaments, tendons, muscles, blood vessels and connective tissues. This causes numbness, coldness and paleness in the leg or foot.

After treatment or surgery:
- Impaired blood supply to the dislocated area.
- Infection introduced during surgical treatment.
- Excessive internal bleeding around the knee.
- Recurrent dislocations, particularly if the previous dislocation has not healed completely.
- Loss of muscle strength.
- Unstable or arthritic knee following repeated injury.

PROBABLE OUTCOME—After the dislocation has been corrected and the knee has been surgically repaired, the knee may require immobilization in a long leg cast for 3 weeks. Complete healing of injured ligaments requires a minimum of 6 weeks. Avoid contact sports if all treatments are unsuccessful in restoring a strong, stable knee.

 HOW TO TREAT

NOTE—Follow your doctor's instructions. These instructions are supplemental.

FIRST AID
- Keep the person warm with blankets to decrease the possibility of shock.
- Cut away clothing if possible. Don't move the injured area to remove clothing.
- Immobilize the knee, hip and ankle joints with padded splints.
- Follow instructions for R.I.C.E., the first letters of *rest, ice, compression* and *elevation*. See Appendix 1 for details.
- The doctor will realign the dislocated bones with surgery or, if possible, without. This should be done as soon as possible after injury. Within 6 hours after the dislocation, bleeding and displacement of body fluids may lead to shock. Also, many tissues lose their elasticity and become difficult to return to their normal positions.

CONTINUING CARE—After removal of the cast:
- Use an ice pack 3 or 4 times a day. Wrap ice chips or cubes in a plastic bag, and wrap the bag in a moist towel. Place it over the injured area for 20 minutes at a time.
- You may try heat instead of ice if it feels better. Use heat lamps, hot soaks, hot showers, healing pads or heat liniments and ointments.
- Take whirlpool treatments, if available.
- Massage gently and often to provide comfort and decrease swelling.

MEDICATION—Your doctor may prescribe:
- General anesthesia or muscle relaxants to make joint manipulation possible.
- Acetaminophen or aspirin to relieve moderate pain.
- Pain relievers for severe pain.
- Stool softeners to prevent constipation due to decreased activity.
- Antibiotics to fight infection following surgery.

ACTIVITY
- Walk on crutches while the cast is in place.
- Resume usual activities gradually after surgery.
- Begin weight-bearing and reconditioning at the knee after clearance from your doctor.

DIET
- Do not eat or drink before manipulation or surgery to correct the dislocation. Fluid or solid food in your stomach makes vomiting while under general anesthesia more hazardous.
- During recovery, balance the amount of food you eat with any change in your level of physical activity. Eat a variety of foods to get the energy, protein, vitamins, minerals and fiber you need for good health and healing.

REHABILITATION
- Begin daily rehabilitation exercises after clearance from your doctor.
- Use ice massage for 10 minutes before and after workouts. Fill a large styrofoam cup with water and freeze. Tear a small amount of foam from the top so ice protrudes. Massage firmly over the injured area in a circle about the size of a softball.
- See Rehabilitation section for knee exercises.

 CALL YOUR DOCTOR IF

- Your have symptoms of a dislocated knee, even if it repositions itself. Call immediately if the leg becomes numb, pale, or cold. This is an emergency!
- Any of the following occurs after treatment or surgery:
   Nausea or vomiting.
   Swelling above or below the cast.
   Blue or gray skin color below the cast, particularly under the toenails.
   Numbness or complete loss of feeling below the knee.
   Increasing pain, swelling or drainage in the surgical area.
   Signs of infection (headache, muscle aches, dizziness or a general ill feeling and fever).
   Constipation.
- New, unexplained symptoms develop. Drugs used in treatment may produce side effects.
- Knee dislocations that you can "pop" back into normal position occur repeatedly.

KNEE SPRAIN

GENERAL INFORMATION

DEFINITION—Violent overstretching of one or more ligaments in the knee. Sprains involving two or more ligaments cause considerably more disability than single-ligament sprains. When the ligament is overstretched, it becomes tense and gives way at its weakest point, either where it attaches to bone or within the ligament itself. If the ligament pulls loose a fragment of bone, it is called an avulsion fracture. There are 3 types of sprains:
- Mild (Grade I)—Tearing of some ligament fibers. There is no loss of function.
- Moderate (Grade II)—Rupture of a portion of the ligament, resulting in some loss of function.
- Severe (Grade III)—Complete rupture of the ligament or complete separation of ligament from bone. There is total loss of function. A severe sprain may require surgical repair.

BODY PARTS INVOLVED
- Any of the many ligaments in the knee: ACL (anterior cruciate ligament), PCL (posterior cruciate ligament), and MCL (medial collateral ligament).
- Tissues surrounding the sprain, including blood vessels, tendons, bone, periosteum (covering of bone) and muscles.

SIGNS & SYMPTOMS
- Severe pain at the time of injury.
- A feeling of popping or tearing inside the knee.
- Tenderness at the injury site.
- Giving way of the weakened knee joint.
- Swelling in the knee (effusion).
- Bruising that appears soon after injury.

CAUSES—Stress on a ligament that temporarily forces or pries the knee out of its normal location. Sprains occur frequently in runners, walkers and those who jump in such sports as basketball, soccer, volleyball, skiing and distance or high jumping. These athletes often accidentally land on the side of the foot.

RISK INCREASES WITH.
- Contact, running and jumping sports.
- Previous knee injury.
- Obesity.
- Poor muscle conditioning.
- Inadequate protection from equipment.

HOW TO PREVENT
- Participate in a strengthening, flexibility and conditioning program appropriate for your sport.
- Warm up before practice or competition.
- Tape vulnerable joints before practice or competition.
- Wear proper protective shoes. A twist or injury to the foot can affect the knee.

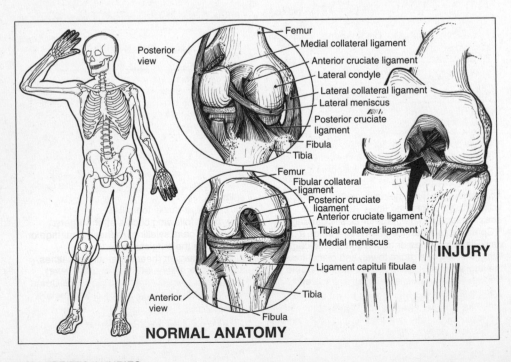

Posterior view

Femur
Medial collateral ligament
Anterior cruciate ligament
Lateral condyle
Lateral collateral ligament
Lateral meniscus
Posterior cruciate ligament
Fibula
Tibia

Femur
Fibular collateral ligament
Posterior cruciate ligament
Anterior cruciate ligament
Tibial collateral ligament
Medial meniscus
Ligament capituli fibulae
Tibia

Anterior view

Fibula

NORMAL ANATOMY

INJURY

WHAT TO EXPECT

APPROPRIATE HEALTH CARE
- Doctor's diagnosis.
- Application of tape, cast or elastic bandage.
- Self-care during rehabilitation.
- Physical therapy (moderate or severe sprain).
- Surgery (severe sprain).

DIAGNOSTIC MEASURES
- Your own observation of symptoms.
- Medical history and exam by a doctor.
- X-rays of the knee, hip and ankle to rule out fractures.
- MRI (see Glossary) to identify meniscal cartilage tear.

POSSIBLE COMPLICATIONS
- Prolonged healing time if usual activities are resumed too soon.
- Proneness to repeated injury.
- Inflammation at the ligament attachment to bone (periostitis).
- Prolonged disability (sometimes).
- Unstable or arthritic knee following repeated injury.
- Meniscal cartilage injuries.

PROBABLE OUTCOME—If this is a first-time injury, proper care and sufficient healing time before resuming activity should prevent permanent disability. Ligaments have a poor blood supply, and torn ligaments require as much healing time as fractures. Average healing times are:
- Mild sprains—2 to 6 weeks.
- Moderate sprains—6 to 8 weeks.
- Severe sprains—8 weeks to 10 months.

HOW TO TREAT

NOTE—Follow your doctor's instructions. These instructions are supplemental.

FIRST AID—Use instructions for R.I.C.E., the first letters of *rest, ice, compression* and *elevation*. See Appendix 1 for details.

CONTINUING CARE—The doctor usually applies a splint from the ankle to the groin to immobilize the sprained knee. If the doctor does not apply a cast, tape or elastic bandage:
- Continue using an ice pack 3 or 4 times a day. Place ice chips or cubes in a plastic bag. Wrap the bag in a moist towel, and place it over the injured knee. Use for 20 minutes at a time.
- Wrap the injured knee with an elasticized bandage.

- After 72 hours, apply heat instead of ice if it feels better. Use heat lamps, hot soaks, hot showers, heating pads or heat liniments and ointments.
- Take whirlpool treatments, if available.
- Massage gently and often to provide comfort and decrease swelling.

MEDICATION
- For minor discomfort, you may use:
  Aspirin, acetaminophen or ibuprofen.
  Topical liniments and ointments.
- Your doctor may prescribe:
  Stronger pain relievers.
  Injection of a long-acting local anesthetic to reduce pain.
  General anesthetic for surgery or arthroscopy (see Glossary) of the knee joint.

ACTIVITY—Resume your normal activities gradually after clearance from your doctor.

DIET—During recovery, balance the amount of food you eat with any change in your level of physical activity. Eat a variety of foods to get the energy, protein, vitamins, minerals and fiber you need for good health and healing.

REHABILITATION
- Begin daily rehabilitation exercises when the cast or supportive wrapping is no longer necessary.
- Use ice massage for 10 minutes before and after exercise. Fill a large styrofoam cup with water and freeze. Tear a small amount of foam from the top so ice protrudes. Massage firmly over the injured area in a circle about the size of a softball.
- See Rehabilitation section for knee exercises.

CALL YOUR DOCTOR IF

- You have symptoms of a moderate or severe knee sprain or a mild sprain persists longer than 2 weeks.
- Pain, swelling or bruising worsens despite treatment.
- Any of the following occurs after casting or splinting:
  Pain, numbness or coldness below the cast or splint.
  Blue, gray or dusky toenails.
- Any of the following occurs after surgery:
  Increased pain, swelling, redness, drainage or bleeding in the surgical area.
  Signs of infection (headache, muscle aches, dizziness or a general ill feeling with fever).
- New, unexplained symptoms develop. Drugs used in treatment may produce side effects.

KNEE STRAIN

GENERAL INFORMATION

DEFINITION—Injury to the muscles or tendons that attach to bones in the knee. Muscles, tendons and their attached bones comprise contractile units. These units stabilize the knee joint and allow its motion. A strain occurs at a unit's weakest part. Strains are of 3 types:
• Mild (Grade I)—Slightly pulled muscle without tearing of muscle or tendon fibers. There is no loss of strength.
• Moderate (Grade II)—Tearing of fibers in a muscle or tendon or at the attachment to bone. Strength is diminished.
• Severe (Grade III)—Rupture of the muscle-tendon-bone attachment, with separation of fibers. A severe strain may require surgical repair. Chronic strains are caused by overuse. Acute strains are caused by direct injury or overstress.

BODY PARTS INVOLVED
• Tendons and muscles in the knee region, especially the quadriceps and the hamstrings.
• Bones in the knee area, including the femur, patella, tibia and fibula.
• Soft tissues surrounding the strain, including nerves, periosteum (covering of bone), blood vessels and lymph vessels.

SIGNS & SYMPTOMS
• Pain when moving or stretching the knee.
• Muscle spasm in the knee area.
• Swelling over the injury.
• Loss of strength (moderate or severe strain).
• Crepitation ("crackling" feeling and sound when the injured area is pressed with fingers).
• Calcification of the muscle or tendon (visible with x-rays).
• Inflammation of the tendon sheath.

CAUSES
• Prolonged overuse of muscle-tendon units in the knee.
• Single violent blow or force applied to the knee.

RISK INCREASES WITH
• Contact sports.
• Sports that require quick starts, such as running races.
• Overly "tight" hamstrings or quadriceps muscles or poor muscle conditioning.
• Medical history of any bleeding disorder.
• Obesity.
• Poor nutrition.
• Previous knee injury.

HOW TO PREVENT
• Participate in a strengthening, flexibility and conditioning program appropriate for your sport.
• Warm up before practice or competition.
• Tape the knee area before practice or competition.

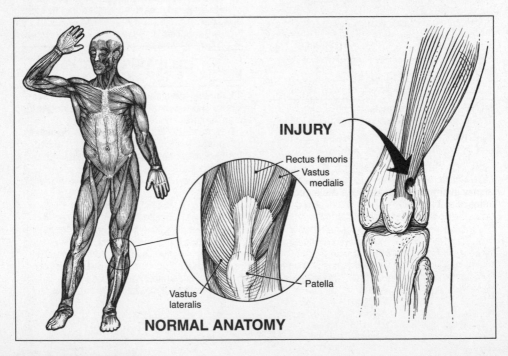

INJURY

Rectus femoris
Vastus medialis

Patella

Vastus lateralis

NORMAL ANATOMY

WHAT TO EXPECT

APPROPRIATE HEALTH CARE
- Doctor's diagnosis.
- Application of tape or of plaster splints or casts (sometimes).
- Self-care during rehabilitation.
- Physical therapy (moderate or severe strain).
- Surgery (severe strain).

DIAGNOSTIC MEASURES
- Your own observation of symptoms.
- Medical history and exam by a doctor.
- X-rays of the knee to rule out fractures.

POSSIBLE COMPLICATIONS
- Prolonged healing time if activity is resumed too soon.
- Proneness to repeated injury.
- Inflammation at the attachment to bone (periostitis).
- Prolonged disability (weakness).

PROBABLE OUTCOME—If this is a first-time injury, proper care and sufficient healing time before resuming activity should prevent permanent disability. Torn ligaments and tendons require as long to heal as fractured bones. Average healing times are:
- Mild strain—2 to 10 days.
- Moderate strain—10 days to 6 weeks.
- Severe strain—6 to 10 weeks.

If this is a repeat injury, complications listed above are more likely to occur.

HOW TO TREAT

NOTE—Follow your doctor's instructions. These instructions are supplemental.

FIRST AID—Use instructions for R.I.C.E., the first letters of *rest, ice, compression* and *elevation*. See Appendix 1 for details.

CONTINUING CARE
- Use ice massage 3 or 4 times a day for 15 minutes at a time. Fill a large styrofoam cup with water and freeze. Tear a small amount of foam from the top so ice protrudes. Massage firmly over the injured area in a circle about the size of a softball.

- After the first 72 hours, apply heat instead of ice if it feels better. Use heat lamps, hot soaks, hot showers, heating pads or heat liniments and ointments.
- Take whirlpool treatments, if available.
- Wrap the injured knee with an elasticized bandage between treatments.
- Massage gently and often to provide comfort and decrease swelling.

MEDICATION
- For minor discomfort, you may use:
  Aspirin, acetaminophen or ibuprofen.
  Topical liniments and ointments.
- Your doctor may prescribe:
  Stronger pain relievers.
  Injection of a long-acting local anesthetic to reduce pain.

ACTIVITY
- For a moderate or severe strain, walk with crutches for at least 72 hours—longer with a cast or splints. See Appendix 3 (Safe Use of Crutches).
- Do frequent, gentle stretching exercises during the healing phase.
- Resume your normal activities gradually.

DIET—During recovery, balance the amount of food you eat with any change in your level of physical activity. Eat a variety of foods to get the energy, protein, vitamins, minerals and fiber you need for good health and healing.

REHABILITATION—Begin daily rehabilitation exercises when supportive wrapping is no longer needed. Use ice massage for 10 minutes prior to exercise. See Rehabilitation section for knee exercises.

CALL YOUR DOCTOR IF

- You have symptoms of a moderate or severe knee strain or a mild strain persists longer than 10 days.
- Pain or swelling worsens despite treatment.
- The following occur with a cast or splints:
  Pain, numbness or coldness below the injury.
  Dusky, blue or gray toenails.

KNEE SYNOVITIS WITH EFFUSION
("Water on the Knee")

GENERAL INFORMATION

DEFINITION—Inflammation of the synovium, the smooth, lubricated lining of the knee. The synovium's lubricating fluid helps the knee move freely and prevents bone surfaces from rubbing against each other. Inflammation triggers an excess of fluid production and accumulation in the knee (effusion). Synovitis with effusion is often a complication of a knee injury or of rheumatologic diseases such as gout or rheumatoid arthritis.

BODY PARTS INVOLVED
- Synovium of the knee.
- Bones of the knee joint, including the patella (kneecap), femur (thigh bone), and tibia and fibula (lower leg bones).
- Ligaments and soft tissues of the knee joint, including the meniscus (cartilage of the knee).

SIGNS & SYMPTOMS
- Pain in the knee (sometimes).
- Swelling above the kneecap.
- Generalized swelling and redness if the inflammation is caused by infection or joint disease, such as gout, rather than by athletic injury.

CAUSES
- Single injury or repeated injury that damages any part of the knee.
- Bacterial infection, such as gonorrhea.
- Metabolic disturbance, such as an acute attack of gout or rheumatoid arthritis.
- Meniscal injury or internal derangement.

RISK INCREASES WITH
- Participation in contact sports such as football, baseball, soccer or rugby.
- Repeated knee injury.
- Poor muscle strength or conditioning, which makes knee injury more likely.
- Medical history of gout, rheumatoid arthritis, or other inflammatory joint diseases.
- Infection in another joint.
- Vitamin or mineral deficiency, which makes complications following injury more likely.

HOW TO PREVENT
- Participate in a strengthening, flexibility and conditioning program appropriate for your sport.
- Warm up adequately before workouts or competition.
- Wear protective knee pads during participation in contact sports.

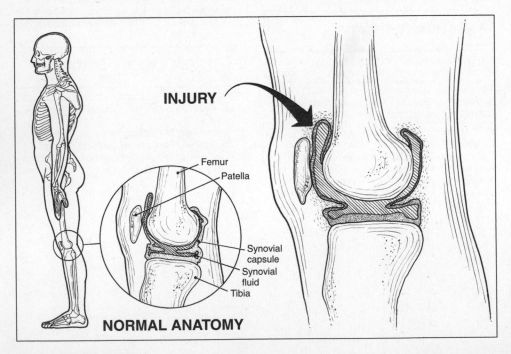

INJURY

Femur
Patella
Synovial capsule
Synovial fluid
Tibia

NORMAL ANATOMY

WHAT TO EXPECT

APPROPRIATE HEALTH CARE
- Doctor's care, including aspiration of fluid from the knee. Because most knee synovitis with effusion is caused by injury to some part of the knee, treating the underlying injury is as important as treating the effusion.
- Self-care during rehabilitation.
- Physical therapy.

DIAGNOSTIC MEASURES
- Your own observation of symptoms.
- Medical history and physical exam by a doctor.
- X-ray of the knee joint.
- Laboratory examination of fluid removed from the knee.
- MRI (see Glossary) to identify meniscal cartilage or ligament tear.

POSSIBLE COMPLICATIONS
- Prolonged healing time if activity is resumed too soon.
- Proneness to repeated knee injury.
- Unstable or arthritic knee following repeated bouts of synovitis.
- Chronic synovitis that may prevent athletic participation.

PROBABLE OUTCOME—Knee synovitis with effusion can usually be cured completely in 2 to 4 weeks with treatment. However, recurrences are common following minor knee injuries.

HOW TO TREAT

NOTE—Follow your doctor's instructions. These instructions are supplemental.

FIRST AID—None. This condition develops gradually.

CONTINUING CARE
- Follow doctor's instructions for treatment of the underlying condition.
- Use an elastic bandage to compress the knee after fluid has been removed and between physical therapy sessions.
- Apply heat frequently. Use heat lamps, hot soaks, hot showers, heating pads or heat liniments and ointments.
- Take whirlpool treatments, if available.
- Massage gently and often to provide comfort and decrease swelling.

MEDICATION
- Your doctor may prescribe:
  Antibiotics if infection is present.
  Nonsteroidal anti-inflammatory drugs or antigout medicine.
  Injection of a long-acting local anesthetic mixed with a corticosteroid to help reduce pain and inflammation.
- You may take aspirin or ibuprofen for minor discomfort.

ACTIVITY—Continue your usual activities during treatment if there in no pain, but protect the knee with tape and an elastic bandage during competitive sports. If you have pain, reduce activities until pain subsides.

DIET—During recovery, balance the amount of food you eat with any change in your level of physical activity. Eat a variety of foods to get the energy, protein, vitamins, minerals and fiber you need for good health and healing.

REHABILITATION
- Begin daily rehabilitation exercises when pain subsides.
- Use ice massage for 10 minutes before and after exercise. Fill a large styrofoam cup with water and freeze. Tear a small amount of foam from the top so ice protrudes. Massage firmly over the injured area in a circle about the size of a softball.
- See Rehabilitation section for knee exercises.

CALL YOUR DOCTOR IF

- Your knee becomes red, hot, swollen or painful.
- After aspiration of fluid from the knee you develop signs of infection (headache, fever, muscle aches, dizziness or a general ill feeling).

KNEECAP (PATELLA) DISLOCATION

GENERAL INFORMATION

DEFINITION—A displacement of the patella (kneecap) so it no longer touches adjoining bones. Adolescents and young adults are most prone to injury.

BODY PARTS INVOLVED
- Knee joint and patella.
- Femur and tibia, the bones of the lower leg.
- Soft tissues surrounding the dislocation, including nerves, periosteum (covering of bone), tendons, ligaments, muscles and blood vessels.

SIGNS & SYMPTOMS
- A feeling of the knee "giving way."
- Excruciating pain in the knee at the time of injury.
- Loss of function of the knee and severe pain when attempting to move it.
- Visible deformity if the dislocated bones have locked in the dislocated positions. Bones may spontaneously reposition themselves and leave no deformity, but damage is the same.
- Tenderness over the dislocation.
- Swelling and bruising around the knee.
- Numbness or paralysis below the dislocation from pressure, pinching or cutting of blood vessels or nerves.

CAUSES
- Direct blow to the knee.
- Congenital abnormal shape of the patella or femur, leading to poor tracking and making dislocation easier.
- End result of a severe knee sprain.
- Powerful muscle contraction.
- "Cutting" moves (movements in which an athlete changes direction suddenly, causing bones in the knee joint to rotate and dislocate the patella).

RISK INCREASES WITH
- A wide pelvis and "knock knees."
- Contact sports such as football or soccer.
- Running sports; jumping sports such as gymnastics and basketball.
- Previous knee sprains.
- Repeated knee injury of any sort.
- Poor muscle conditioning.
- Congenital abnormalities of the knee joint.

HOW TO PREVENT
- Participate in a strengthening, flexibility and conditioning program appropriate for your sport. Include special exercises for the knee.
- Warm up adequately before physical activity.
- After injury, protect the knee from reinjury by wearing wrapped elastic bandages, tape wraps, knee pads or special support sleeves.

[?] WHAT TO EXPECT

APPROPRIATE HEALTH CARE
- Doctor's treatment. This will include manipulation of the joint to reposition the bones, and aspirate the fluid from the knee joint.

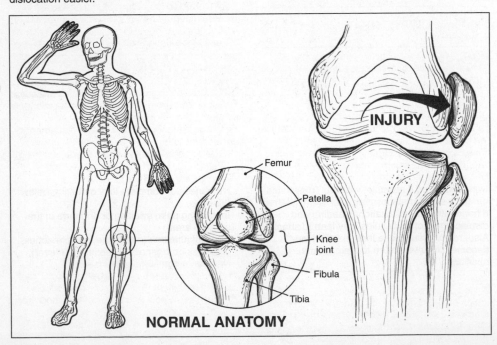

INJURY

Femur

Patella

Knee joint

Fibula

Tibia

NORMAL ANATOMY

- Surgery (usually) to restore normal knee joint function and stability.

DIAGNOSTIC MEASURES
- Your own observation of symptoms.
- Medical history and exam by a doctor.
- X-rays of the knee joint and adjacent bones.

POSSIBLE COMPLICATIONS
At the time of injury:
- Shock.
- Pressure on or injury to nearby nerves, ligaments, tendons, muscles, blood vessels or connective tissues, causing numbness, coldness and paleness in the leg or foot.
- Excessive internal bleeding around the kneecap.
- Fracture from the cartilage surfaces of the patella or femur. This may lead to loose bodies or arthritis.
After surgery:
- Impaired blood supply to the dislocated area.
- Infection introduced during surgical treatment.
- Recurrent dislocations, particularly if the previous dislocation has not healed completely.
- Unstable or arthritic knee joint following repeated injury.

PROBABLE OUTCOME—After treatment or surgery to correct the dislocation, the joint may be immobilized with a cast for 6 to 8 weeks. Complete healing of injured ligaments requires a minimum of 6 weeks.

 HOW TO TREAT

NOTE—Follow your doctor's instructions. These instructions are supplemental.

FIRST AID
- Keep the person warm with blankets to decrease the possibility of shock.
- Cut away clothing if possible. Don't move the injured area to remove clothing.
- Immobilize the knee, hip and ankle joints with padded splints.
- Follow instructions for R.I.C.E., the first letters of *rest, ice, compression* and *elevation*. See Appendix 1 for details.
- The doctor will realign the dislocated bones with surgery or, if possible, without. This should be done as soon as possible after injury. Within 6 hours after the dislocation, bleeding and displacement of body fluids may lead to shock. Also, many tissues lose their elasticity and become difficult to return to their normal positions.

CONTINUING CARE—After cast removal:
- Use an ice pack 3 or 4 times a day. Wrap ice chips or cubes in a plastic bag, and wrap the bag in a moist towel. Place it over the injured area for 20 minutes at a time.

- You may try heat instead of ice if it feels better. Use heat lamps, hot soaks, hot showers, heating pads, or heat liniments and ointments.
- Take whirlpool treatments, if available.
- Massage gently and often to provide comfort and decrease swelling.

MEDICATION—Your doctor may prescribe:
- General anesthesia or muscle relaxants to make joint manipulation possible or for surgery.
- Acetaminophen to relieve moderate pain.
- Narcotic pain relievers for severe pain.
- Stool softeners to prevent constipation due to decreased activity.
- Antibiotics to fight infection.

ACTIVITY
- Walk on crutches while the cast is in place.
- Resume usual activities gradually after surgery.
- Begin weight-bearing and reconditioning of the knee after clearance from your doctor.

DIET
- Do not eat or drink before manipulation or surgery to correct the dislocation. Fluid or solid food in your stomach makes vomiting while under general anesthesia more hazardous.
- Balance the amount of food you eat with any change in your level of physical activity.

REHABILITATION
- Begin daily rehabilitation exercises when supportive wrapping is no longer needed.
- Use ice massage for 10 minutes before and after workouts. Fill a large styrofoam cup with water and freeze. Tear a small amount of foam from the top so ice protrudes. Massage firmly in a circle over the injured area.
- See Rehabilitation section for knee exercises.

 CALL YOUR DOCTOR IF

- You have symptoms of a dislocated kneecap. Call immediately if the leg becomes numb, pale or cold. This is an emergency!
- Any of the following occurs after treatment or surgery:
  Swelling above or below the cast.
  Blue or gray skin color below the cast, particularly under the toenails.
  Numbness or complete loss of feeling below the knee.
  Increasing pain, swelling or drainage in the surgical area.
  Signs of infection (headache, muscle aches, dizziness or a general ill feeling and fever).
  Nausea or vomiting; constipation.
- New, unexplained symptoms develop. Drugs used in treatment may produce side effects.
- Kneecap dislocations that you can "pop" back into normal position occur repeatedly.

KNEECAP (PATELLA) FRACTURE

GENERAL INFORMATION

DEFINITION—A complete or incomplete break in the upper or lower portion of the patella (kneecap). Most fractures of the patella are accompanied by sprain or rupture of ligaments or tendons attached to the patella. Usually there is disruption of the quadriceps contractile unit and inability to straighten the knee against resistance.

BODY PARTS INVOLVED
- Patella and knee joint.
- Soft tissues surrounding the fracture site, including nerves, tendons, ligaments and blood vessels.

SIGNS & SYMPTOMS
- Severe pain at the fracture site.
- Pain when moving the knee forward or backward.
- Swelling around the fracture.
- Visible deformity if the fracture is complete and bone fragments separate enough to distort normal knee contours.
- "Catching" or locking of the knee.
- Tenderness when pressing the kneecap against underlying bones.
- Numbness and coldness beyond the fracture site if the blood supply is impaired.

CAUSES—Direct blow or indirect stress to the kneecap. Indirect stress may be caused by twisting or violent muscle contraction.

RISK INCREASES WITH
- Contact sports, especially football.
- History of bone or joint disease, especially osteoporosis.
- Obesity.
- Poor nutrition, especially calcium deficiency.
- If surgery or anesthesia is needed, surgical risk increases with smoking and use of drugs, including mind-altering drugs, muscle relaxants, antihypertensives, tranquilizers, sleep inducers, insulin, sedatives, beta-adrenergic blockers or corticosteroids.

HOW TO PREVENT
- Participate in a strengthening, flexibility and conditioning program appropriate for your sport. Increased muscle mass helps protect bones and underlying tissues.
- Use appropriate protective equipment, such as knee pads, when participating in contact sports.

WHAT TO EXPECT

APPROPRIATE HEALTH CARE
- Doctor's treatment to manipulate and set the broken bones.
- Hospitalization (sometimes) for anesthesia and surgery to remove the fractured pieces of bone, repair the damaged soft tissues or repair broken patella pieces with wires and screws.
- Whirlpool, ultrasound or massage after healing (to displace fluid from the injured joint space).

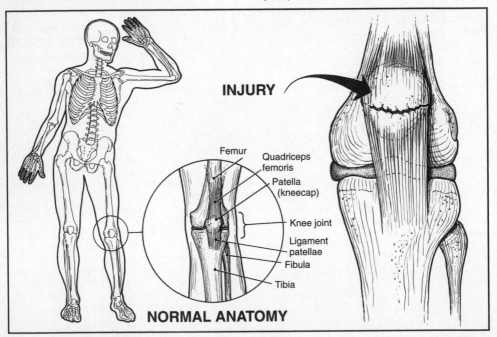

INJURY

Femur
Quadriceps femoris
Patella (kneecap)
Knee joint
Ligament patellae
Fibula
Tibia

NORMAL ANATOMY

DIAGNOSTIC MEASURES
- Your own observation of symptoms.
- Medical history and exam by a doctor.
- X-rays of the knee joint.

POSSIBLE COMPLICATIONS
At the time of injury:
- Shock.
- Pressure on or injury to nearby nerves, ligaments, tendons, muscles, blood vessels or connective tissues.
- Loss of smooth cartilage surface beneath the kneecap.

After treatment or surgery:
- Delayed union or nonunion of the fracture.
- Impaired blood supply to the fracture site.
- Avascular necrosis (death of bone cells due to interruption of the blood supply).
- Arrest of normal bone growth in children.
- Infection in open fractures (skin broken over fracture site) or at the incision if surgical setting was necessary.
- Proneness to repeated knee problems. After healing, the fracture often leaves a roughened contact surface in the kneecap.
- Unstable or arthritic knee following repeated injury.
- Problems caused by casts. See Appendix 2 (Care of Casts).

PROBABLE OUTCOME—The average healing time for this fracture is 6 to 8 weeks. Healing is considered complete when there is no motion at the fracture site and when x-rays show complete bone union.

HOW TO TREAT

NOTE—Follow your doctor's instructions. These instructions are supplemental.

FIRST AID
- Keep the person warm with blankets to decrease the possibility of shock.
- Cut away clothing, if possible. Don't move the injured knee to remove clothing.
- Use a padded splint to immobilize the hip joint and the ankle joint before transporting the injured person to the doctor's office or emergency facility.
- Follow instructions for R.I.C.E., the first letters of *rest, ice, compression* and *elevation.* See Appendix 1 for details.
- The doctor will realign and set the broken bones with surgery or, if possible, without. Manipulation should be done as soon as possible after injury. Also, many tissues lose their elasticity and become difficult to return to a normal position.

CONTINUING CARE
- Immobilization will be necessary. A rigid cast will be used from the upper leg to the ankle.
- After the cast is removed, use frequent ice massage. Fill a large styrofoam cup with water and freeze. Tear a small amount of foam from the top so ice protrudes. Massage firmly over the injured area in a circle about the size of a softball. Do this for 15 minutes at a time 3 or 4 times a day, and also before workouts or competition.
- Apply heat instead of ice if it feels better. Use heat lamps, hot soaks, hot showers, heating pads or heat liniments and ointments.
- Take whirlpool treatments, if available.

MEDICATION—Your doctor may prescribe:
- General anesthesia or local anesthesia for surgery to remove or repair the fractured patella fragments.
- Pain relievers for severe pain.
- Stool softeners to prevent constipation.
- Acetaminophen (available without prescription).

ACTIVITY
- Actively exercise all muscle groups not immobilized. The resulting muscle contractions promote fracture alignment and hasten healing.
- Resume normal activities gradually after treatment.

DIET
- Do not eat or drink before manipulation or surgery to treat the fracture. Fluid or solid food in your stomach makes vomiting while under anesthesia more hazardous.
- During recovery, balance the amount of food you eat with any change in your level of physical activity.

REHABILITATION—Begin reconditioning the injured knee after clearance from your doctor. See Rehabilitation section for knee exercises.

CALL YOUR DOCTOR IF

- You have signs or symptoms of a kneecap fracture.
- Any of the following occurs after surgery or other treatment:
  Increased pain, swelling or drainage in the surgical area.
  Signs of infection (headache, muscle aches, dizziness or a general ill feeling and fever).
  Nausea or vomiting; constipation.
  Swelling above or below the cast.
  Blue or gray skin color beyond the cast, particularly under the toenails.
  Numbness or complete loss of feeling below the fracture site.
  Constipation.

LEG CONTUSION, LOWER LEG

GENERAL INFORMATION

DEFINITION—Bruising of the skin and underlying tissues of the lower leg due to a direct blow. Contusions cause bleeding from ruptured small capillaries that allow blood to infiltrate muscles, tendons or other soft tissues. The lower leg is particularly susceptible to contusions because it is frequently exposed to direct blows. If the blow is over the tibia (shin bone) it is much more likely to be severe.

BODY PARTS INVOLVED
• Lower leg tissues, including blood vessels, muscles, tendons, nerves, covering of bone (periosteum) and connective tissues.
• The peroneal nerve where it wraps around the upper portion of the fibula. Injury to the nerve can lead to painful neuritis or temporary paralysis and a dropped foot.

SIGNS & SYMPTOMS
• Swelling—either superficial or deep.
• Pain at the contusion site.
• Feeling of firmness when pressure is exerted on the injury.
• Tenderness.
• Discoloration under the skin, beginning with redness and progressing to the characteristic "black-and-blue" bruise.
• Restricted leg function proportional to the extent of injury.

• Feeling an "electrical shock" followed by temporary muscle paralysis, causing the foot to drop.

CAUSES—Direct blow to the leg, usually from a blunt object.

RISK INCREASES WITH
• Violent contact sports—especially when lower legs are not adequately protected.
• Medical history of any bleeding disorder.
• Poor nutrition, including vitamin deficiency.
• Use of anticoagulants or aspirin.

HOW TO PREVENT—Wear appropriate protective devices, such as shin guards over felt or sponge rubber, if there is risk of a lower leg contusion during athletic activity.

WHAT TO EXPECT

APPROPRIATE HEALTH CARE
• Doctor's care unless the contusion is quite small.
• Self-care for minor contusions and for serious contusions during rehabilitation.
• Physical therapy for serious contusions.

DIAGNOSTIC MEASURES
• Your own observation of symptoms.
• Medical history and physical exam by a doctor for all except minor injuries.

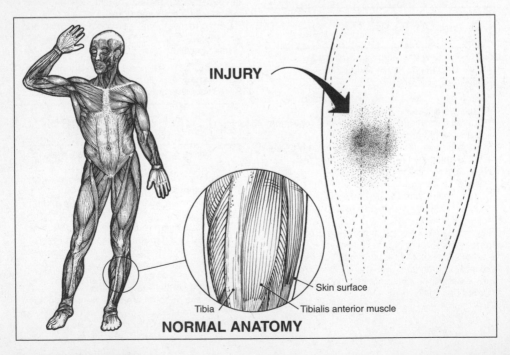

INJURY

Tibia

Skin surface

Tibialis anterior muscle

NORMAL ANATOMY

- X-rays of the lower leg, ankle and knee to assess total injury to soft tissues and to rule out the possibility of underlying fractures. The total extent of injury may not be apparent for 48 to 72 hours.

POSSIBLE COMPLICATIONS
- Excessive bleeding, leading to disability. Infiltrative-type bleeding can sometimes lead to calcification and impaired function of the injured muscle.
- Prolonged healing time if usual activities are resumed too soon.
- Infection if skin over the contusion is broken.
- Foot drop from blow to peroneal nerve.

PROBABLE OUTCOME—Healing time varies with the extent of injury, but average healing time for a lower leg contusion is 1 to 2 weeks. If foot drop has occurred, return of strength may require 2 months or more.

 # HOW TO TREAT

NOTE—Follow your doctor's instructions. These instructions are supplemental.

FIRST AID—Use instructions for R.I.C.E., the first letters of *rest, ice, compression* and *elevation.* See Appendix 1 for details.

CONTINUING CARE
- Wrap an elasticized bandage over a sponge rubber donut on the injured area. Keep the area compressed for about 72 hours.
- Continue ice massage. Fill a large styrofoam cup with water and freeze. Tear a small amount of foam from the top so ice protrudes. Massage gently over the injured area in a circle about the size of a softball. Do this for 15 minutes at a time 3 or 4 times a day, and also before workouts or competition.

- After 72 hours, apply heat instead of ice if it feels better. Use heat lamps, hot soaks, hot showers, heating pads, heat liniments and ointments or whirlpool treatments.
- Massage gently and often to provide comfort and decrease swelling.

MEDICATION
- For minor discomfort, you may use: Acetaminophen or ibuprofen. Topical liniments and ointments.
- Your doctor may prescribe stronger medicine for pain.

ACTIVITY—Begin activities slowly, and stop exercise as soon as pain begins. Increase activity as healing progresses.

DIET—During recovery, balance the amount of food you eat with any change in your level of physical activity. Eat a variety of foods to get the energy, protein, vitamins, minerals and fiber you need for good health and healing.

REHABILITATION—Begin daily rehabilitation exercises when supportive wrapping is no longer needed. See Rehabilitation section for knee exercises and ankle and foot exercises.

 # CALL YOUR DOCTOR IF

- You have a lower leg contusion that doesn't improve in 1 or 2 days.
- Skin is broken and signs of infection (increasing pain, fever, headache, muscle aches, dizziness or a general ill feeling) occur.
- Signs of peroneal nerve injury appear (paralysis, dropped foot or loss of sensation in the foot).

LEG EXOSTOSIS

GENERAL INFORMATION

DEFINITION—An overgrowth of bone in the tibia (the larger bone in the lower leg). It extends out from the bone like a spur and is visible on x-rays. An exostosis occurs at the site of repeated injury, usually from direct blows. This benign overgrowth of bone can be mistaken for a bone tumor.

BODY PARTS INVOLVED
- Tibia.
- Knee joint (sometimes).
- Ankle joint (sometimes).
- Soft tissues surrounding the exostosis, including nerves, lymph vessels, blood vessels and periosteum (covering of bone).

SIGNS & SYMPTOMS
- No symptoms for mild cases.
- Pain and tenderness in the lower leg at the site of the exostosis.
- Extreme sensitivity to pressure or even minor injury.
- Change in contour of the tibia, ranging from a slight lump to the appearance of a large calcified spur (1 cm or more in length). In the worst cases, the exostosis may break away and feel like a distinct mass. An x-ray will show it to be loose in the tissues of the lower leg.
- Snapping or locking of the lower leg if a tendon catches on the exostosis during exercise.

CAUSES
- Repeated injury (contusions, sprains or strains) that involve the periosteum—the covering of the large bone (tibia) in the lower leg.
- Chronic irritation to an already damaged area.
- Congenital abnormality at the edge of the growth plate.

RISK INCREASES WITH
- Participation in contact sports such as football, basketball or soccer or in throwing sports such as softball.
- History of bone or joint disease, such as osteomyelitis, osteomalacia or osteoporosis.
- Vitamin or mineral deficiency.
- Poor muscle strength or conditioning, which makes injury more likely.
- If surgery or anesthesia is needed, risk increases with smoking, use of mind-altering drugs, muscle relaxants, tranquilizers, sleep inducers, insulin, sedatives, beta-adrenergic blockers or corticosteroids.

HOW TO PREVENT
- Participate in a strengthening, flexibility and conditioning program appropriate for your sport.
- Warm up adequately before competition or workouts to decrease the risk of injury.
- Allow adequate recovery time for any leg, ankle or knee injury.
- Wear protective equipment, such as shin guards and knee pads, for participation in contact sports.
- Practice and learn the proper moves and techniques for your sport to decrease injury risk.

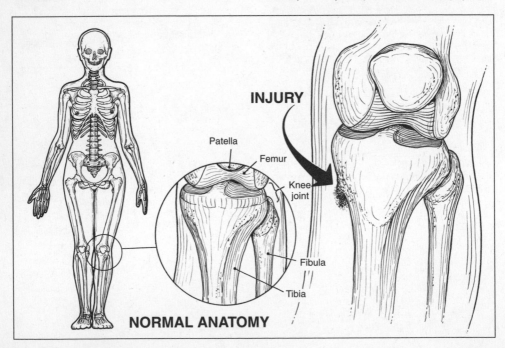

INJURY

Patella

Femur

Knee joint

Fibula

Tibia

NORMAL ANATOMY

WHAT TO EXPECT

APPROPRIATE HEALTH CARE
- Doctor's care.
- Surgery (sometimes) to remove the exostosis.
- Self-care during rehabilitation.
- Physical therapy.

DIAGNOSTIC MEASURES
- Your own observation of signs and symptoms.
- Medical history and physical exam by a doctor.
- X-rays of the lower leg, ankle and knee.

POSSIBLE COMPLICATIONS
- Overlooking a mild exostosis that produces no symptoms, despite signs of diminished performance. Athletes and coaches frequently assume that decreased performance is due to loss of competitive drive or emotional causes rather than due to the physical disability that actually exists.
- Proneness to repeated injury.
- Unstable or arthritic knee or ankle following repeated injury.
- Pressure on or injury to nearby nerves, ligaments, tendons, blood vessels or connective tissues.
- Impaired blood supply to the injured area.
- Tendinitis from direct irritation.

PROBABLE OUTCOME—Lower leg exostosis usually causes no disability if it is treated properly. Treatment usually involves resting the injured leg for 2 to 4 weeks, heat treatments, corticosteroid injections and protection against additional injury. In a few cases, surgery is necessary to remove the exostosis.

 HOW TO TREAT

NOTE—Follow your doctor's instructions. These instructions are supplemental.

FIRST AID—None. This condition develops gradually.

CONTINUING CARE
- Rest the injured area. Use splints or crutches if needed.

- Apply heat frequently. Use heat lamps, hot soaks, hot showers, heating pads or heat liniments and ointments.
- Take whirlpool treatments, if available.
- Follow instructions under How to Prevent to avoid a recurrence of the injury.

MEDICATION
- Medication usually is not necessary for this disorder. For minor pain, you may use non-prescription drugs such as aspirin.
- If surgery is necessary, your doctor may prescribe:
  Nonsteroidal anti-inflammatory drugs to help control swelling or adjacent tendinitis.
  Stronger pain relievers.
  Antibiotics to fight infection.

ACTIVITY—Decrease activity for 2 to 4 weeks. If surgery is necessary, resume normal activity gradually.

DIET—During recovery, balance the amount of food you eat with any change in your level of physical activity. Eat a variety of foods to get the energy, protein, vitamins, minerals and fiber you need for good health and healing. Your doctor may suggest vitamin and mineral supplements to promote healing.

REHABILITATION
- Begin daily rehabilitation exercises when movement is comfortable.
- Use ice massage for 10 minutes before and after exercise. Fill a large styrofoam cup with water and freeze. Tear a small amount of foam from the top so ice protrudes. Massage firmly over the injured area in a circle about the size of a softball.
- See Rehabilitation section for knee exercises and ankle and foot exercises.

 CALL YOUR DOCTOR IF

- You have symptoms of lower leg exostosis.
- Any of the following occurs after surgery:
  Increased pain, swelling, redness, drainage, or bleeding in the surgical area.
  Signs of infection (headache, muscle aches, dizziness or a general ill feeling and fever).
  New, unexplained symptoms. Drugs used in treatment may cause side effects.

LEG FRACTURE, FIBULA

GENERAL INFORMATION

DEFINITION—A complete or incomplete break in the fibula, the smaller of the two bones of the lower leg. Fractures of the fibula are not uncommon, and displacement is seldom severe. They sometimes accompany severe ankle sprains.

BODY PARTS INVOLVED
- Fibula.
- Soft tissues surrounding the fracture site, including nerves, tendons, ligaments and blood vessels.

SIGNS & SYMPTOMS
- Severe pain at the fracture site.
- Swelling of soft tissues surrounding the fracture.
- Visible deformity if the fracture is complete and bone fragments separate enough to distort normal leg contours.
- Tenderness to the touch.
- Numbness or coldness in the foot if the blood supply is impaired.

CAUSES—Direct blow or indirect stress to the bone. Indirect stress may be caused by twisting, turning quickly or violent muscle contraction. These fractures may occur with severe ankle or leg sprains or dislocations. In these cases, treatment is determined by the type of ankle or leg injury.

RISK INCREASES WITH
- Contact sports such as football, soccer or hockey.
- History of bone or joint disease, especially osteoporosis.
- Obesity.
- Poor nutrition, especially calcium deficiency.

HOW TO PREVENT—Participate in a strengthening, flexibility and conditioning program appropriate for your sport. Increased muscle mass helps protect bones and underlying tissues.

WHAT TO EXPECT

APPROPRIATE HEALTH CARE
- Doctor's diagnosis. Setting of the fracture is usually not necessary.
- Self-care during rehabilitation.

DIAGNOSTIC MEASURES
- Your own observation of symptoms.
- Medical history and physical exam by a doctor.
- X-rays of injured areas, including the knee and ankle.

POSSIBLE COMPLICATIONS
- Pressure on or injury to nearby nerves, ligaments, tendons, muscles, blood vessels or connective tissues.
- Delayed union or nonunion of the fracture (rare).

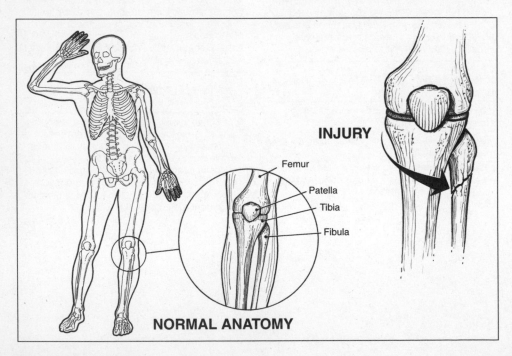

INJURY

Femur
Patella
Tibia
Fibula

NORMAL ANATOMY

- Impaired blood supply to the fracture site.
- Arrest of normal bone growth in children.
- Shortening of the injured bones.
- Prolonged healing time if activity is resumed too soon.
- Proneness to repeated injury.

PROBABLE OUTCOME—It is impossible to predict exactly how long it will take for any fracture to heal. Variable factors include age, sex and previous state of health and conditioning. The average healing time for this fracture is 4 to 6 weeks. Healing is considered complete when there is no motion at the fracture site and when x-rays show complete bone union.

 # HOW TO TREAT

NOTE—Follow your doctor's instructions. These instructions are supplemental.

FIRST AID
- Keep the person warm with blankets to decrease the possibility of shock.
- Cut away clothing, if possible. Don't move the injured area to remove clothing.
- Follow instructions for R.I.C.E., the first letters of *rest, Ice, compression* and *elevation*. See Appendix 1 for details.

CONTINUING CARE
- Setting the broken bone for a fibula fracture is usually not necessary. The tibia (the big bone adjacent to the fibula) provides immobilization and supports weight-bearing.
- A fibula fracture usually requires only a snug, toe-to-knee cotton elastic bandage. If pain is severe, a walking cast or removable boot below the knee may be necessary for about 5 weeks.
- After the bandage or cast is removed, use frequent ice massage. Fill a large styrofoam cup with water and freeze. Tear a small amount of foam from the top so ice protrudes. Massage firmly over the injured area in a circle about the size of a softball. Do this for 15 minutes at a time 3 or 4 times a day.
- Apply heat instead of ice if it feels better. Use heat lamps, hot soaks, hot showers, heating pads or heat liniments and ointments.
- Take whirlpool treatments, if available.

MEDICATION—Your doctor may prescribe:
- Pain relievers for severe pain.
- Stool softeners to prevent constipation due to inactivity.
- Acetaminophen (available without prescription) for mild pain after initial treatment.

ACTIVITY
- Actively exercise all muscle groups not immobilized. Muscle contractions promote fracture alignment and hasten healing.
- Begin walking and light running when there is no pain or tenderness.
- Resume normal activities gradually after treatment.

DIET—During recovery, balance the amount of food you eat with any change in your level of physical activity. Eat a variety of foods to get the energy, protein, vitamins, minerals and fiber you need for good health and healing.

REHABILITATION
- Begin reconditioning the injured area after clearance form your doctor. Use ice massage for 10 minutes before and after workouts.
- See Rehabilitation section for knee exercises and ankle and foot exercises.

 # CALL YOUR DOCTOR IF

- You have signs or symptoms of a leg fracture.
- Any of the following occurs after surgery or other treatment:

  Signs of infection (headache, muscle aches, dizziness or a general ill feeling and fever).
  Swelling above or below the bandage or cast.
  Change in skin color to blue or gray beyond the cast, particularly under the toenails.
  Numbness or complete loss of feeling below the fracture site.
  Nausea or vomiting.
  Constipation.

LEG FRACTURE, TIBIA

GENERAL INFORMATION

DEFINITION—A complete or incomplete break of the tibia, one of the two large bones of the leg between the knee and the ankle.

BODY PARTS INVOLVED
- Tibia.
- Knee or ankle joint.
- Soft tissues around the fracture site, including nerves, tendons, ligaments and blood vessels.

SIGNS & SYMPTOMS
- Severe leg pain at the time of injury.
- Swelling of soft tissues around the fracture.
- Visible deformity if the fracture is complete and the bone fragments separate enough to distort normal leg contours.
- Tenderness to the touch.
- Numbness and coldness in the leg and foot beyond the fracture site if the blood supply is impaired.

CAUSES
- Direct blow to the leg.
- Weakening of the bone from repeated stress, resulting in a stress fracture that progresses to a complete fracture. This is especially common in joggers, marathon runners and walkers.
- Indirect stress caused by twisting or violent muscle contractions.

RISK INCREASES WITH
- Contact sports and cycling activities.
- History of bone or joint disease.
- Obesity.
- Poor nutrition, especially calcium deficiency.
- If surgery or anesthesia is needed, risk increases with smoking and use of drugs, including mind-altering drugs, muscle relaxants, antihypertensives, tranquilizers, sleep inducers, insulin, sedatives, beta-adrenergic blockers or corticosteroids.

HOW TO PREVENT
- Build your strength with a good conditioning program before beginning regular athletic practice or competition. Increased muscle mass helps protect bones and underlying tissues.
- Use appropriate protective equipment, including good running shoes for running and shin guards for participation in contact sports.

? WHAT TO EXPECT

APPROPRIATE HEALTH CARE
- Doctor's treatment.
- Anesthesia and surgery to set the fracture.
- Whirlpool, ultrasound or massage after healing (to displace excess fluid from the knee and ankle).

DIAGNOSTIC MEASURES
- Your own observation of symptoms.
- Medical history and exam by a doctor.
- X-rays of the injured area, including the knee joint above and the ankle joint below.

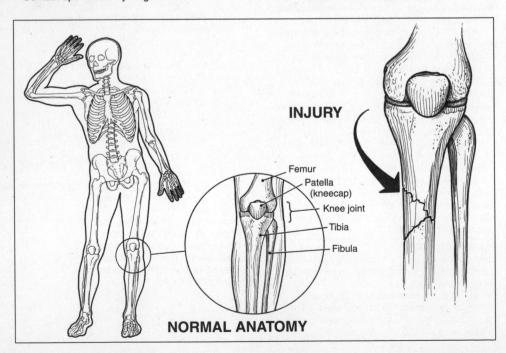

INJURY

Femur
Patella (kneecap)
Knee joint
Tibia
Fibula

NORMAL ANATOMY

POSSIBLE COMPLICATIONS

At the time of injury:
- Shock.
- Pressure on or injury to nearby nerves, ligaments, tendons, muscles, blood vessels or connective tissues.

After treatment or surgery:
- Delayed union or nonunion of the fracture.
- Impaired blood supply to the fracture site.
- Avascular necrosis (death of bone cells due to interruption of the blood supply).
- Shortening of the injured bones.
- Arrest of normal bone growth in children.
- Compartment syndrome (see Glossary), requiring emergency compartment release.
- Infection in open fractures (skin broken over fracture site) or at the incision if surgical setting was necessary.
- Unstable or arthritic ankle or knee joint if the fracture is close to either.
- Prolonged healing time if activity is resumed too soon.
- Proneness to repeated leg injury.
- Problems caused by casts. See Appendix 2 (Care of Casts).

PROBABLE OUTCOME—The average healing time for this fracture is 12 to 20 weeks. Healing is considered complete when there is no motion at the fracture site and when x-rays show complete bone union.

HOW TO TREAT

NOTE—Follow your doctor's instructions. These instructions are supplemental.

FIRST AID
- Keep the person warm with blankets to decrease the possibility of shock.
- Cut away clothing, if possible, but don't move the injured leg to do so.
- Follow instructions for R.I.C.E., the first letters of *rest, ice, compression* and *elevation*. See Appendix 1 for details.
- The doctor will set (realign) the broken bones with surgery or, if possible, without. In tibia fractures, the segments are sometimes fixed together with screws, metal plates or rods. Realignment should be done as soon as possible after injury. Also, many tissues lose their elasticity and become difficult to return to their normal positions.

CONTINUING CARE
- Immobilization will be necessary. A rigid cast is placed around the injured leg to immobilize the knee and ankle.
- After 96 hours, localized heat promotes healing by increasing blood circulation in the injured area. Use a heat lamp or heating pads so heat can penetrate the casts.
- After the cast is removed, use frequent ice massage. Fill a large styrofoam cup with water and freeze. Tear a small amount of foam from the top so ice protrudes. Massage firmly in a circle over the injured area.

MEDICATION—Your doctor may prescribe:
- General anesthesia, local anesthesia or muscle relaxants to make bone manipulation and fixation of bone fragments possible.
- Strong pain relievers for severe pain.
- Stool softeners to prevent constipation due to inactivity.
- Acetaminophen for mild pain.

ACTIVITY
- Learn to walk with crutches. See Appendix 3 (Safe Use of Crutches).
- Actively exercise all muscle groups not immobilized. These muscle contractions promote fracture alignment and hasten healing.
- Begin reconditioning the injured leg after clearance from your doctor.
- Resume normal activities gradually after treatment.

DIET
- Do not eat or drink before manipulation or surgery to treat the fracture. Fluid or solid food in your stomach makes vomiting while under anesthesia more hazardous.
- During recovery, balance the amount of food you eat with any change in your level of physical activity.

REHABILITATION—Begin daily rehabilitation exercises when supportive wrapping is no longer needed. Use ice massage for 10 minutes prior to exercise. See Rehabilitation section for knee exercises and ankle and foot exercises.

CALL YOUR DOCTOR IF

- You have signs or symptoms of a tibia fracture.
- Any of the following occurs after surgery or other treatment:
  Increased pain, swelling or drainage in the surgical area.
  Signs of infection (headache, muscle aches, dizziness or a general ill feeling and fever).
  Swelling above or below the cast.
  Blue or gray skin color beyond the cast, especially under the toenails.
  Loss of feeling below the fracture site.
  Nausea or vomiting; constipation.
  Marked pain in the leg with passive movement of toes.

LEG HEMATOMA, LOWER LEG

GENERAL INFORMATION

DEFINITION—A collection of pooled blood in a small area of the lower leg. Hematomas in the lower leg can be quite disabling. A large hematoma in the enclosed space over the tibia (the "shin bone") can be a surgical emergency if it causes compartment syndrome (see Glossary).

BODY PARTS INVOLVED
- Lower leg.
- Soft tissues surrounding the hematoma, including nerves, tendons, ligaments, muscles and blood vessels.

SIGNS & SYMPTOMS
- Swelling over the injury site.
- Fluctuance (feeling of tenseness to the touch, like pushing on an overinflated balloon).
- Tenderness.
- Redness that progresses through several color changes—purple, green-yellow, yellow—before it completely heals.

CAUSES—Direct injury, usually with a blunt object. Bleeding into tissues causes the surrounding tissues to be pushed away.

RISK INCREASES WITH
- Contact sports, especially if the lower leg is not adequately protected.
- Medical history of any bleeding disorder.
- Poor nutrition, including vitamin deficiency.
- Use of anticoagulants or aspirin.

HOW TO PREVENT—Wear appropriate protective gear and equipment, such as shin pads, during competition or other athletic activity if there is risk of a lower leg injury.

WHAT TO EXPECT

APPROPRIATE HEALTH CARE
- Doctor's care unless the hematoma is very small.
- Needle aspiration of blood from the hematoma if the hematoma is accessible. At the same time hyaluronidase (an enzyme) can be injected into the hematoma space. Hyaluronidase may hasten absorption of blood.
- Self-care for minor hematomas or for serious hematomas during the rehabilitation phase.
- Physical therapy following serious hematomas.

DIAGNOSTIC MEASURES
- Your own observation of symptoms.
- Physical exam and medical history by a doctor for all except minor injuries.
- X-rays of the injured area to assess total injury to the lower leg and to rule out the possibility of underlying bone fractures. Total extent of the injury may not be apparent for 48 to 72 hours.

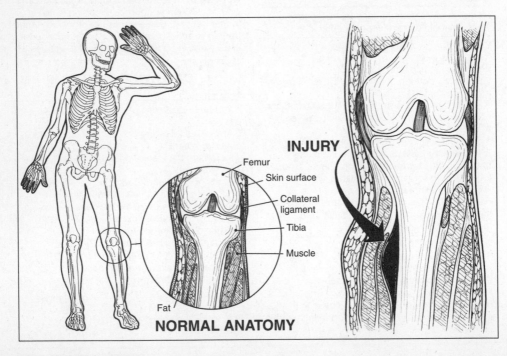

INJURY

Femur
Skin surface
Collateral ligament
Tibia
Muscle
Fat

NORMAL ANATOMY

POSSIBLE COMPLICATIONS
- Hematoma formation about the tibia may place excess pressure on muscles in the leg, leading to loss of their blood supply. This is called acute compartment syndrome and requires emergency treatment.
- Permanent damage to muscles and nerves, causing muscle atrophy and a weak foot, if treatment is delayed.
- Infection introduced through a break in the skin at the time of injury or during aspiration of the hematoma by a doctor.
- Prolonged healing time if activity is resumed too soon.
- Calcification of the blood remaining in the hematoma if the blood is not completely removed or absorbed.

PROBABLE OUTCOME—Average healing time is 2 weeks to 2 months unless blood is removed with aspiration. Healing time is much less with this treatment.

 ## HOW TO TREAT

NOTE—Follow your doctor's instructions. These instructions are supplemental.

FIRST AID—Use instructions for R.I.C.E., the first letters of *rest, ice, compression* and *elevation*. See Appendix 1 for details.

CONTINUING CARE
- Use an ice pack 3 or 4 times a day. Wrap ice chips or cubes in a plastic bag, and wrap the bag in a moist towel. Place it over the injured area for 20 minutes at a time.
- After 48 hours, application of localized heat promotes healing by increasing blood circulation in the injured area. Use hot baths, showers, compresses, heat lamps, healing pads, heat ointments and liniments or whirlpools.
- Don't massage the leg. You may trigger bleeding again.

MEDICATION
- For minor discomfort, you may use: Nonprescription medicines such as acetaminophen or ibuprofen. Topical liniments and ointments.
- Your doctor may prescribe stronger medicine for pain if needed.

ACTIVITY—Begin activities slowly, and stop exercise as soon as pain begins. Increase activity as healing progresses. To prevent healing delay, protect the hematoma area against excessive motion soon after injury. Motion breaks down the clot and causes irritation throughout the lower leg, leading to possible scar formation, calcification and restricted movement after healing.

DIET—During recovery, balance the amount of food you eat with any change in your level of physical activity. Eat a variety of foods to get the energy, protein, vitamins, minerals and fiber you need for good health and healing.

REHABILITATION
- Begin daily rehabilitation exercises when supportive wrapping is no longer needed.
- Use gentle ice massage for 10 minutes before and after workouts. Fill a large styrofoam cup with water and freeze. Tear a small amount of foam from the top so ice protrudes. Massage firmly over the injured area in a circle about the size of a softball.
- See Rehabilitation section for knee exercises and ankle and foot exercises.

 ## CALL YOUR DOCTOR IF

- You have signs or symptoms of a lower leg hematoma that doesn't begin to improve in 1 or 2 days.
- Skin is broken and signs of infection (drainage, increasing pain, fever, headache, muscle aches, dizziness or a general ill feeling) occur.
- There is marked pain in the leg with passive motion of the toes or marked tense swelling in the leg. These are symptoms of compartment syndrome.

LEG SPRAIN
(Syndesmotic Ankle Sprain; High Ankle Sprain)

GENERAL INFORMATION

DEFINITION—Violent overstretching of the ligaments between the tibia and the fibula in the lower leg. Sprains involving two or more ligaments cause considerably more disability than single-ligament sprains. When the ligament is overstretched, it becomes tense and gives way at its weakest point, either where it attaches to bone or within the ligament itself. If the ligament pulls loose a fragment of bone, it is called an avulsion fracture. There are 3 types of sprains:
- Mild (Grade I)—Tearing of some ligament fibers. There is no loss of function.
- Moderate (Grade II)—Rupture of a portion of the ligament, resulting in some loss of function.
- Severe (Grade III)—Complete rupture of the ligament or complete separation of ligament from bone. There is total loss of function. A severe sprain usually require s surgical repair.

BODY PARTS INVOLVED
- Ligaments between the tibia and the fibula.
- Tissues surrounding the sprain, including blood vessels, tendons, bone, periosteum (covering of bone) and muscles.
- The fibula may be fractured with this injury (well above the ankle joint).

SIGNS & SYMPTOMS
- Severe pain at the time of injury.
- A feeling of popping or tearing inside the lower leg.
- Tenderness at the injury site.
- Swelling in the lower leg.
- Bruising that appears soon after injury.

CAUSES—Stress on a ligament that temporarily forces or pries the tibia and fibula apart. Sprains occur frequently in runners, walkers and those who jump in such sports as basketball, soccer, skiing and distance and high jumping. These athletes often accidentally land on the side of the foot.

RISK INCREASES WITH
- Contact, running and jumping sports.
- Previous lower leg injury.
- Obesity.
- Poor muscle conditioning.
- Inadequate protection from equipment.

HOW TO PREVENT
- Build your strength with a conditioning program appropriate for your sport.
- Warm up before practice or competition.
- Tape vulnerable joints before practice or competition.
- Wear proper protective shoes.

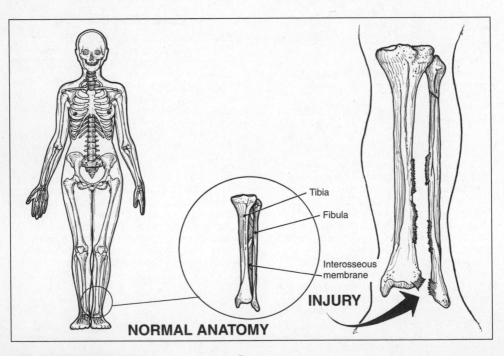

Tibia

Fibula

Interosseous membrane

INJURY

NORMAL ANATOMY

APPROPRIATE HEALTH CARE
- Doctor's diagnosis.
- Application of tape, cast or elastic bandage.
- Self-care during rehabilitation.
- Physical therapy (moderate or severe sprain).
- Surgery (severe sprain) to place a screw from the fibula to the tibia to temporarily hold them together and allow ligaments to heal.

DIAGNOSTIC MEASURES
- Your own observation of symptoms.
- Medical history and exam by a doctor.
- X-rays of the lower leg, knee, hip and ankle to rule out fractures.

POSSIBLE COMPLICATIONS
- Prolonged healing time if usual activities are resumed too soon.
- Proneness to repeated injury.
- Inflammation at the ligament attachment to bone (periostitis).
- Calcification in torn ligaments.
- Prolonged disability (sometimes).
- Associated fibula fracture.

PROBABLE OUTCOME—If this is a first-time injury, proper care and sufficient healing time before resuming activity should prevent permanent disability. Ligaments have a poor blood supply, and torn ligaments require as much healing time as fractures. Average healing times are:
- Mild sprains—2 to 6 weeks.
- Moderate sprains—6 to 10 weeks.
- Severe sprains—10 to 16 weeks.

 HOW TO TREAT

NOTE—Follow your doctor's instructions. These instructions are supplemental.

FIRST AID—Use instructions for R.I.C.E., the first letters of *rest, ice, compression* and *elevation*. See Appendix 1 for details.

CONTINUING CARE—The doctor usually applies a cast from the toes to the knee to immobilize the severely sprained leg. If the doctor does not apply a cast, tape or elastic bandage:
- Use an ice pack 3 or 4 times a day. Put ice chips or cubes in a plastic bag. Wrap the bag in a moist towel, and place it over the injured area. Use for 20 minutes at a time.
- Wrap the injured leg with an elasticized bandage between ice treatments.
- After 72 hours, apply heat instead of ice if it feels better. Use heat lamps, hot soaks, hot showers, heating pads or heat liniments and ointments.

- Take whirlpool treatments, if available.
- Massage the leg gently and often to provide comfort and decrease swelling.

MEDICATION
- For minor discomfort, you may use:
Aspirin, acetaminophen or ibuprofen.
Topical liniments and ointments.
- Your doctor may prescribe:
General anesthesia for surgery.
Stronger pain relievers.
Injection of a long-acting local anesthetic to reduce pain.
Injection of a corticosteroid, such as triamcinolone, to reduce inflammation.

ACTIVITY—Resume your normal activities gradually after clearance from your doctor.

DIET—During recovery, balance the amount of food you eat with any change in your level of physical activity. Eat a variety of foods to get the energy, protein, vitamins, minerals and fiber you need for good health and healing.

REHABILITATION
- Begin daily rehabilitation exercise when the cast or supportive wrapping is no longer necessary.
- Use ice massage for 10 minutes before and after exercise. Fill a large styrofoam cup with water and freeze. Tear a small amount of foam from the top so ice protrudes. Massage firmly over the injured area in a circle about the size of a softball.
- See Rehabilitation section for knee exercises and ankle and foot exercises.

 CALL YOUR DOCTOR IF

- You have symptoms of a moderate or severe lower leg sprain or a mild sprain persists longer than 2 weeks.
- Pain, swelling or bruising worsens despite treatment.
- Any of the following occurs after casting or splinting:
Pain, numbness or coldness below the cast or splint.
Blue, gray or dusky toenails.
- Any of the following occurs after surgery:
Increased pain, swelling, redness, drainage or bleeding in the surgical area.
Signs of infection (headache, muscle aches, dizziness or a general ill feeling with fever).
New, unexplained symptoms. Drugs used in treatment may produce side effects.

LEG STRAIN, CALF
(Lower Leg Strain)

GENERAL INFORMATION

DEFINITION—Injury to muscles and tendons in the lower leg (calf). Muscles, tendons and their attached bones comprise contractile units. These units stabilize the knee and allow its motion. A strain occurs at the weakest part of a unit. Strains are of 3 types:
● Mild (Grade I)—Slightly pulled muscle without tearing of muscle or tendon fibers. There is no loss of strength.
● Moderate (Grade II)—Tearing of fibers in a muscle or tendon or at the attachment to bone. Strength is diminished.
● Severe (Grade III)—Rupture of the muscle-tendon-bone attachment, with separation of fibers. A severe strain occasionally requires surgical repair. Chronic strains are caused by overuse. Acute strains are caused by direct injury or overstress.

BODY PARTS INVOLVED
● Tendons and muscles of the calf and lower leg.
● Leg bones (femur, tibia and fibula).
● Soft tissues surrounding the strain, including nerves, periosteum (covering of bone), blood vessels and lymph vessels.

SIGNS & SYMPTOMS
● Pain when moving or stretching the foot or ankle.
● Sudden loss of foot arch.
● Limping.
● Muscle spasm in the calf.
● Swelling over the injury.
● Loss of strength (moderate or severe strain).
● Crepitation ("crackling" feeling and sound when the injured area is pressed with fingers).
● Calcification of the muscle or the tendon (visible with x-rays).
● Inflammation of tendon sheath.

CAUSES
● Prolonged overuse of muscle-tendon units in the calf.
● Single violent injury or force applied to the calf.

RISK INCREASES WITH
● Contact sports such as football, soccer or hockey.
● Sports that require quick starts, such as running races.
● Medical history of any bleeding disorder.
● Obesity.
● Poor nutrition.
● Previous lower leg injury.
● Poor muscle conditioning.

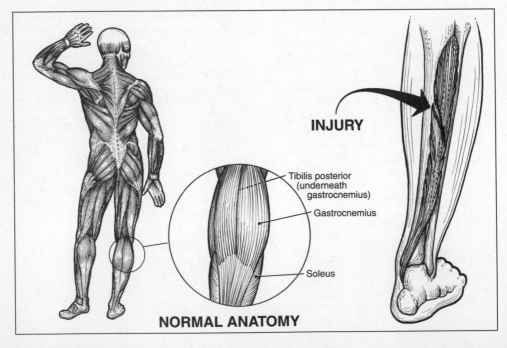

INJURY

Tibilis posterior (underneath gastrocnemius)

Gastrocnemius

Soleus

NORMAL ANATOMY

HOW TO PREVENT
- Participate in a strengthening, flexibility and conditioning program appropriate for your sport.
- Warm up before practice or competition.

? WHAT TO EXPECT

APPROPRIATE HEALTH CARE
- Doctor's care.
- Self-care during rehabilitation.
- Physical therapy (for moderate and severe strains).
- Orthotics (shoe inserts) to help correct foot misalignment and support fallen arch.
- Surgery (severe strain).

DIAGNOSTIC MEASURES
- Your own observation of symptoms.
- Medical history and exam by a doctor.
- X-rays of the leg, ankle, knee and foot to rule out fractures.

POSSIBLE COMPLICATIONS
- Prolonged healing time if activity is resumed too soon.
- Proneness to repeated injury.
- Unstable or arthritic knee following repeated injury.
- Inflammation at the attachment to bone (periostitis).
- Prolonged disability (sometimes).

PROBABLE OUTCOME—If this is a first-time injury, proper care and sufficient healing time before resuming activity should prevent permanent disability. Torn ligaments and tendons require as long to heal as fractured bones. Average healing times are:
- Mild strain—2 to 10 days.
- Moderate strain—10 days to 6 weeks.
- Severe strain—6 to 10 weeks.

✎ HOW TO TREAT

NOTE—Follow your doctor's instructions. These instructions are supplemental.

FIRST AID—Use instructions for R.I.C.E., the first letters of *rest, ice, compression* and *elevation.* See Appendix 1 for details.

CONTINUING CARE—If a cast or splints are necessary, keep toes free and exercise them frequently. If a cast or splints are not necessary:
- Use ice massage 3 or 4 times a day for 15 minutes at a time. Fill a large styrofoam cup with water and freeze. Tear a small amount of foam from the top so ice protrudes. Massage firmly over the injured area in a circle about the size of a softball.

- Apply heat instead of ice if it feels better. Use heat lamps, hot soaks, hot showers, heating pads or heat liniments and ointments.
- Take whirlpool treatments, if available.
- Wrap the injured leg with an elasticized bandage between treatments.
- Massage gently and often to provide comfort and decrease swelling.
- Elevate the heels of your shoes to relax the calf. Use half of heel pad in each shoe.

MEDICATION
- For minor discomfort, you may use:
  Aspirin, acetaminophen or ibuprofen.
  Topical liniments and ointments.
- Your doctor may prescribe:
  Stronger pain relievers.
  Injection of a long-acting local anesthetic to reduce pain (rare).
  Injections of a corticosteroid, such as triamcinolone, to reduce inflammation (rare).

ACTIVITY
- For a moderate or severe strain, walk with crutches for at least 72 hours—longer with a cast or splints. See Appendix 3 (Safe Use of Crutches).
- Resume your normal activities gradually as pain subsides and participate in a stretching routine.

DIET—During recovery, balance the amount of food you eat with any change in your level of physical activity. Eat a variety of foods to get the energy, protein, vitamins, minerals and fiber you need for good health and healing.

REHABILITATION—Begin daily rehabilitation exercises when supportive wrapping is no longer needed. Use ice massage for 10 minutes prior to exercise. See Rehabilitation section for knee exercises and ankle and foot exercises.

☎ CALL YOUR DOCTOR IF

- You have symptoms of a moderate or severe calf strain or a mild strain persists longer than 10 days.
- Pain or swelling worsens despite treatment.
- The following occurs with a cast or splints:
  Pain, numbness or coldness below the injury.
  Dusky, blue or gray toenails.

LEG STRESS FRACTURE, FIBULA
(Fatigue Fracture of the Fibula)

 GENERAL INFORMATION

DEFINITION—A hairline fracture of the fibula that develops after repeated stress, such as from prolonged standing, marching, running, jogging or hiking.

BODY PARTS INVOLVED
- Fibula (smaller bone in the lower leg).
- Soft tissues around the fracture site, including muscles, joints, nerves, tendons, ligaments, periosteum (covering of bone), blood vessels and connective tissues.

SIGNS & SYMPTOMS
- Pain at the fracture site that lessens or disappears when the load is taken off the legs.
- Tenderness to the touch.
- Warmth over the site of the fractured fibula.

CAUSES—Fatigue of the fibula caused by repeated overload.

RISK INCREASES WITH
- Hiking, jumping, running, jogging or standing for long periods, especially with rapid increases in activity or weight carried.
- History of bone or joint disease, especially osteoporosis.
- Obesity.
- Oligomenorrhea or amenorrhea (lessened or absent menstrual periods) due to marked decrease of body fat seen in women with eating disorders and habitual exercisers.
- Poor nutrition, especially calcium deficiency.

HOW TO PREVENT
- Heed early warnings of an impending fracture, such as leg pain during or after extended hiking, walking or running. Reduce activities before a fracture occurs.
- Avoid rapid increases in training regimen.
- Ensure adequate calcium intake (1000 mg to 1500 mg a day) with milk and milk products or calcium supplements.

 WHAT TO EXPECT

APPROPRIATE HEALTH CARE
- Doctor's diagnosis and care.
- Self-care during rehabilitation.

DIAGNOSTIC MEASURES
- Your own observation of symptoms.
- Medical history and physical exam by a doctor.
- X-rays of the lower leg. X-rays are often normal for 10 to 24 days after symptoms begin before changes appear.

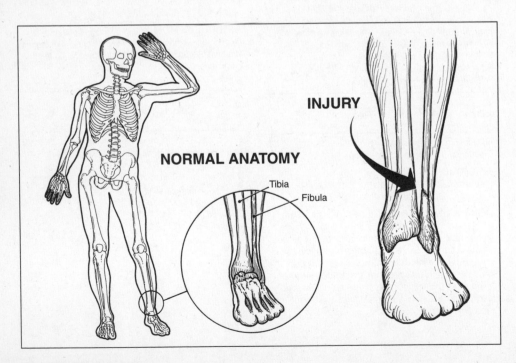

NORMAL ANATOMY

Tibia

Fibula

INJURY

• Radioactive technetium 99 scan (see Glossary) if symptoms are typical but x-rays are negative.

POSSIBLE COMPLICATIONS
• Complete fibula fracture with possible dislocation of broken fragments if overuse of the leg continues after symptoms begin.
• Pressure on or injury to nearby nerves, ligaments, tendons, blood vessels or connective tissues.

PROBABLE OUTCOME—It is impossible to predict exactly how long it will take for any fracture to heal. Variable factors include age, sex and previous state of health and conditioning. The average healing time for this fracture is 6 to 8 weeks with adequate treatment. Healing is considered complete when there is no pain at the fracture site and when x-rays show complete bone union.

 HOW TO TREAT

NOTE—Follow your doctor's instructions. These instructions are supplemental.

FIRST AID—None. This injury develops gradually.

CONTINUING CARE
• This fracture does not require setting (realignment), because the fractured bone is not displaced.
• Use frequent ice massage. Fill a large styrofoam cup with water and freeze. Tear a small amount of foam from the top so ice protrudes. Massage firmly over the injured area in a circle about the size of a softball. Do this for 15 minutes at a time 3 or 4 times a day, and also before workouts or competition.
• Apply heat instead of ice if it feels better. Use heat lamps, hot soaks, hot showers, heating pads or heat liniments and ointments.
• Take whirlpool treatments, if available.

• Treatment often requires elimination of repetitive weight-bearing exercise for 4 to 6 weeks and then a gradual progressive return to activity with care to avoid abrupt additions to training regimen.
• Massage gently and often to provide comfort and decrease swelling.

MEDICATION—Your doctor may prescribe:
• Pain relievers for severe pain.
• Stool softeners to prevent constipation due to inactivity.
• Acetaminophen or ibuprofen (available without prescription) for mild pain after initial treatment.

ACTIVITY
• Don't bear weight on the injured leg. Learn to walk with crutches (see Appendix 3, Safe Use of Crutches), and prop your leg up whenever possible. Immobilization in a cast is not usually necessary.
• Begin reconditioning and rehabilitation after clearance from your doctor.
• Resume normal daily activities gradually after treatment.

DIET—During recovery, balance the amount of food you eat with any change in your level of physical activity. Eat a variety of foods to get the energy, protein, vitamins, minerals and fiber you need for good health and healing.

REHABILITATION—Begin daily rehabilitation exercises when movement is comfortable. Use ice massage for 10 minutes prior to exercise. See Rehabilitation section for knee exercises and ankle and foot exercises.

 CALL YOUR DOCTOR IF

• You have symptoms of a fibula stress fracture.
• After diagnosis, pain worsens despite treatment.

LEG STRESS FRACTURE, TIBIA
(Fatigue Fracture of the Tibia)

 GENERAL INFORMATION

DEFINITION—A hairline fracture of the tibia (the larger bone in the lower leg) that develops after repeated stress, such as prolonged hiking, marching, running or jogging.

BODY PARTS INVOLVED
- Tibia.
- Soft tissues around the fracture site, including muscles, joints, nerves, tendons, ligaments, periosteum (covering of bone), blood vessels and connective tissues.

SIGNS & SYMPTOMS
- Pain at the fracture site that lessens or disappears when the load is taken off the legs.
- Tenderness to the touch.
- Warmth over the site of the fractured tibia.

CAUSES—Fatigue of the tibia caused by repeated overload.

RISK INCREASES WITH
- Hiking, running, jogging or jumping for long periods, especially with rapid increases in activity level or weight carried.
- History of bone or joint disease, especially osteoporosis.
- Obesity.

- Oligomenorrhea or amenorrhea (lessened or absent menstrual periods) due to marked decrease of body fat seen in women with eating disorders and habitual exercisers.
- Poor nutrition, especially calcium deficiency.

HOW TO PREVENT
- Heed early warnings of an impending fracture, such as leg pain during or after extended hiking, walking or running. Reduce activities before a fracture occurs.
- Avoid rapid increases in training regimen.
- Ensure an adequate calcium intake (1000 mg to 1500 mg a day) with milk and milk products or calcium supplements.

 WHAT TO EXPECT

APPROPRIATE HEALTH CARE
- Doctor's diagnosis end care.
- Self-care during rehabilitation.

DIAGNOSTIC MEASURES
- Your own observation of symptoms.
- Medical history and physical exam by a doctor.
- X-rays of the lower leg. X-rays are often normal for 10 to 24 days after symptoms begin before bone changes appear.

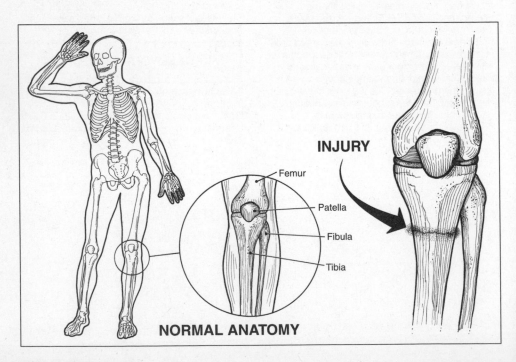

Femur

Patella

Fibula

Tibia

INJURY

NORMAL ANATOMY

• Radioactive technetium 99 scan (see Glossary), if symptoms are typical but x-rays are negative.

POSSIBLE COMPLICATIONS
• Complete fracture with possible dislocation of broken bone fragments if overuse of leg continues after symptoms begin.
• Pressure on or injury to nearby nerves, ligaments, tendons, blood vessels or connective tissues.
• Problems arising from plaster casts, splints or other immobilizing materials. See Appendix 2 (Care of Casts).

PROBABLE OUTCOME—It is impossible to predict exactly how long it will take for any fracture to heal. Variable factors include age, sex and previous state of health and conditioning. The average healing time for this fracture is 6 to 8 weeks with adequate rest and treatment. Healing is considered complete when there is no pain at the fracture site and when x-rays show complete bone union.

 ## HOW TO TREAT

NOTE—Follow your doctor's instructions. These instructions are supplemental.

FIRST AID—None. This injury develops gradually.

CONTINUING CARE
• This fracture does not require setting (realignment), because the fractured bone is not displaced.
• Immobilization is sometimes required. If so, a rigid walking cast or removable boot is placed around the lower leg.
• After cast removal, use frequent ice massage. Fill a large styrofoam cup with water and freeze. Tear a small amount of foam from the top so ice protrudes. Massage firmly over the injured area in a circle about the size of a baseball. Do this for 15 minutes at a time 3 or 4 times a day, and also before workouts or competition.

• Apply heat instead of ice if it feels better. Use heat lamps, hot soaks, hot showers, heating pads or heat liniments and ointments.
• Take whirlpool treatments, if available.
• Massage gently and often to provide comfort and decrease swelling.
• Treatment often requires elimination of repetitive weight-bearing exercise for 4 to 6 weeks and then a gradual progressive return to activity with care to avoid abrupt additions to the training regimen.

MEDICATION—Your doctor may prescribe:
• Strong pain relievers for severe pain.
• Stool softeners to prevent constipation due to inactivity.
• Acetaminophen or ibuprofen (available without prescription) for mild pain after initial treatment.

ACTIVITY
• Don't bear weight on the injured leg. Learn to walk with crutches, and prop your leg up whenever possible. See Appendix 3 (Safe Use of Crutches).
• Begin reconditioning and rehabilitation after clearance from your doctor.
• Resume normal daily activities gradually as symptoms disappear.

DIET—During recovery, balance the amount of food you eat with any change in your level of physical activity. Eat a variety of foods to get the energy, protein, vitamins, minerals and fiber you need for good health and healing.

REHABILITATION—Begin daily rehabilitation exercises when movement is comfortable. Use ice massage for 10 minutes prior to exercise. See Rehabilitation section for knee exercises and ankle and foot exercises.

 ## CALL YOUR DOCTOR IF

• You have symptoms of a tibia stress fracture.
• Your toes become dark, blue, cold or numb while the cast is on.

LIVER INJURY

GENERAL INFORMATION

DEFINITION—Laceration, contusion or rupture of the liver. A severe liver injury is an emergency!

BODY PARTS INVOLVED
- Liver.
- Muscles of the abdominal wall.
- Peritoneum (membranous covering of the intestines).
- Ribs (sometimes) if they are fractured at the same time the liver is injured.

SIGNS & SYMPTOMS
- Vomiting.
- Pain in the abdomen.
- Abdominal tenderness and rigidity.
- Pain in the right shoulder or right side of the neck.
- Rapid heart rate.
- Low blood pressure.
- Signs of shock: pale, moist and sweaty skin; anxiety with a feeling of impending doom; shortness of breath and rapid breathing; disorientation and confusion.

CAUSES—Direct blow to the liver, located in the upper right abdomen or the right side of the chest.

RISK INCREASES WITH
- Contact sports.

- Recent injury to the right side of the abdomen or flank (side or back between the ribs and hip).
- Rib fracture.
- Medical history of any bleeding disorder.
- Any illness that causes enlargement of the liver, such as cirrhosis.
- If surgery is necessary, surgical risk increases with smoking, use of mind-altering drugs, muscle relaxants, tranquilizers, sleep inducers, insulin, sedatives, beta-adrenergic blockers or corticosteroids.

HOW TO PREVENT—Avoid causes and risk factors when possible.

WHAT TO EXPECT

APPROPRIATE HEALTH CARE
- Doctor's treatment.
- Hospitalization for intravenous fluids or transfusions to treat shock.
- Surgery under general anesthesia to clamp off bleeding blood vessels and repair the injured liver.

DIAGNOSTIC MEASURES
Before surgery:
- Blood and urine studies.
- X-rays of the abdomen and chest.
After surgery:
- Examination of all tissues removed.
- Additional blood studies.

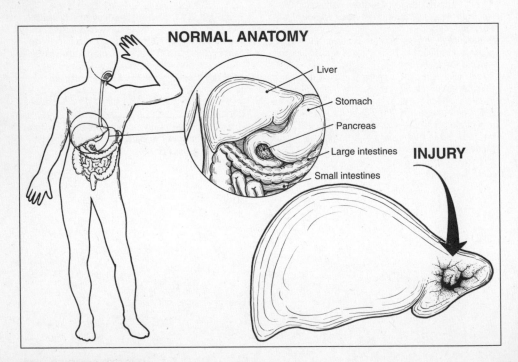

NORMAL ANATOMY

Liver
Stomach
Pancreas
Large intestines
Small intestines

INJURY

POSSIBLE COMPLICATIONS

At the time of injury:
- Rapid deterioration due to internal bleeding, possibly leading to death.

After surgery:
- Excessive bleeding.
- Infection.
- Incisional hernia.
- Lung collapse.
- Inflammation of the pancreas.
- Deep vein blood clots.
- Pneumonia.

PROBABLE OUTCOME—Expect complete healing if no complications occur. Allow about 4 weeks for recovery from surgery.

 HOW TO TREAT

NOTE—Follow your doctor's instructions. These instructions are supplemental.

FIRST AID
- Cover the victim with a blanket to combat shock.
- Carry the injured person to the nearest emergency facility.
- Don't give the person water or food. If surgery is necessary, food or water in the stomach makes vomiting while under general anesthesia more dangerous.
- Don't give the person pain relievers. They may mask symptoms and hinder diagnosis.

CONTINUING CARE—No specific instructions except those under other headings. If surgery is required, your surgeon will supply postoperative instructions.

MEDICATION
- Your doctor may prescribe:
  Pain relievers. Don't take prescription pain medication longer than 4 to 7 days. Use only as much as you need.
  Antibiotics to fight infection.
  Stool softeners to prevent constipation.
  Pneumonia vaccinations.
- You may use nonprescription drugs such as acetaminophen for minor pain.

ACTIVITY—Return to work, play and normal activity as soon as possible. This reduces postoperative depression, which is common. Avoid vigorous exercise for 6 weeks after surgery.

DIET
- Do not eat or drink before surgery.
- Following surgery, a clear liquid diet will be necessary until the gastrointestinal tract functions again.
- During recovery, balance the amount of food you eat with any change in your level of physical activity. Eat a variety of foods to get the energy, protein, vitamins, minerals and fiber you need for good health and healing.

REHABILITATION—Rehabilitation exercises must be individualized. Follow your doctor's or surgeon's directions.

 CALL YOUR DOCTOR IF

- You receive an abdominal injury and the symptoms last longer than a few minutes or the symptoms diminish and recur within hours or days. This may be an emergency!
- Any of the following occurs after surgery:
  You develop signs of infection (headache, muscle aches, dizziness or a general ill feeling and fever).
  Pain, swelling, redness, drainage or bleeding increases in the surgical area.
  New, unexplained symptoms develop. Drugs used in treatment may produce side effects.
- Symptoms return after recovery.

MEDIAL TIBIA STRESS SYNDROME (MTSS)
(Shin Splints)

GENERAL INFORMATION

DEFINITION
• Pain in the lower leg brought on by exercise or athletic activity. Shin splints is a common term that has been used to describe a variety of different leg injuries and it is generally being replaced by more specific diagnostic terms. The most common shin pain an athlete experiences is caused by medial tibia stress syndrome (MTSS). It is an overuse condition that can be caused by several factors. This shin problem usually develops gradually over weeks to months or could occur after a single excessive or intense training session.
• Other shin disorders that may be causing the symptoms include muscle strain, tendinopathy (microtears in the tendon), tibial stress fracture, or compartment syndrome (caused by lack of blood and oxygen to the leg muscles during exercise).

BODY PARTS INVOLVED—The tibia (shin bone) is the larger of the two bones between the knee and the ankle. Medial refers to the inside part of the tibia (the most common site for MTSS). Leg muscles, tendons and the bone covering are also involved.

SIGNS & SYMPTOMS
• Pain, dull ache, or tenderness, and some-times swelling, redness and warmth, in the inner side (medial), back side (posterior), or outer side (anterior) of the lower leg.
• Pain may come and go as activity continues.

CAUSES—The problem is exercise-induced, but the specific cause of the pain is difficult to pinpoint. It may be periostitis (inflammation of the outer layer of the bone), myositis (muscle inflammation), tendinitis (inflammation of the muscle-tendon complex) or a combination of two of these. Faulty foot mechanics contribute to the injury.

RISK INCREASES WITH
• Sports involving extensive amounts of running (e.g., runners and sprinters; football, basketball, soccer and rugby players); jumping activities such as gymnastics or figure skating.
• A beginning runner or training that is being done too quickly, too hard and too long.
• Training that involves switching from one type of sport to another (e.g., a triathlon).
• High impact aerobics or aerobic dancing.
• Poorly fitting or worn out running shoes.
• Foot arches that are flat (pronated) or high (supinated) or muscle imbalance in leg muscles.

HOW TO PREVENT
• Stretch and strengthen the muscles in the lower leg. Stretch before and after running.
• Avoid hard and uneven surfaces—use soft surfaces such as dirt or grass for jogging, running and walking.

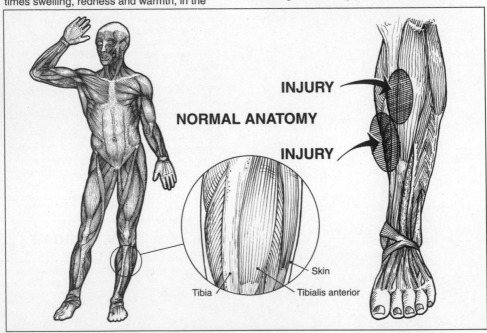

INJURY

NORMAL ANATOMY

INJURY

Skin

Tibia

Tibialis anterior

- Warm up adequately before the activity.
- Wear well-fitting shoes with good arch support during physical activities.
- Avoid overtraining.
- Consider sports activities such as swimming or biking that have less impact on the shins.

 WHAT TO EXPECT

APPROPRIATE HEALTH CARE
- Self care for minor pain or discomfort.
- Doctor's treatment if pain is more severe or when pain and other symptoms persist.

DIAGNOSTIC MEASURES
- Your own observation of symptoms.
- Medical history and physical by a doctor.
- The diagnosis may include an evaluation of your training schedule, competition schedule, your running shoes and a biomechanical study to check your running style.
- A bone scan, MRI or x-ray may be done to help rule out stress fracture.

POSSIBLE COMPLICATIONS
- Prolonged healing time if activity is resumed too soon.
- May progress to stress fracture.
- Proneness to recurrence.
- Rarely, surgery may be recommended.

PROBABLE OUTCOME—Complete cure usually requires rest and slow rehabilitation. Total time may range from a few days to 2 weeks to 2 months. The activity that brought on the pain should be avoided until you can exercise regularly without pain.

 HOW TO TREAT

NOTE—Follow your doctor's instructions. These instructions are supplemental.

FIRST AID—Follow instructions for R.I.C.E., the first letters of *rest, ice, compression* and *elevation.* See Appendix 1 for details.

CONTINUING CARE
- Use ice massage. Fill a large styrofoam cup with water and freeze. Tear a small amount of foam from the top so ice protrudes. Massage firmly over the painful area in a circle about the size of a softball. Do this for 15 minutes at a time 3 or 4 times a day, and also before workouts or competition.
- After a few days, apply heat instead of ice if it feels better. Use heat lamps, hot soaks, hot showers, heating pads or heat liniments and ointments.
- Take whirlpool treatments, if available.
- Massage gently and often to provide comfort and decrease swelling. This also helps increase circulation to the area. Apply lubricating oil to skin over the painful area during massage.

MEDICATION
- For minor discomfort, you may use non-prescription anti-inflammatory drugs such as aspirin or ibuprofen.
- Your doctor may prescribe other nonsteroidal anti-inflammatory medicines.

ACTIVITY
- Stop participating in the sport or activity until the pain is gone. Return to pre-injury activity level slowly.
- In some cases, severe pain may require the use of crutches for a short period of time.
- If foot mechanics are a problem, such as excessive pronation, your doctor may prescribe special shoes, heal lifts, or orthotics (inserts for the shoes). Orthotics can be over-the-counter products or in some cases, custom-made orthotics may be prescribed.
- Try alternate exercising (cross-training) such as swimming, bicycle riding, walking or walking or running in water.
- After treatment, when ready to resume your normal athletic activity:
  Cut back on your training schedule.
  Ice the legs 5 to 10 minutes before warmup and after running.

DIET—During recovery, balance the amount of food you eat with any change in your level of physical activity. Eat a variety of foods to get the energy, protein, vitamins, minerals and fiber you need for good health and healing. Your doctor may suggest vitamin and mineral supplements to promote healing.

REHABILITATION
- Stretching routines and strengthening exercises can be started after the pain and inflammation have been resolved. Calf raises and toe raises are often recommended. Stop if too much discomfort or pain occurs. The stretching routines can be repeated several times a day (approximately every 2 hours).
- See Rehabilitation section of the book for knee exercises and ankle and foot exercises.
- Physical therapy may be necessary for patients whose pain is not relieved in 2-3 weeks.
- Electrical stimulation and ultrasound may be used to treat the affected area.

 CALL YOUR DOCTOR IF

- You have symptoms of medial tibial stress syndrome that continue after self care routine.
- Numbness or tingling occurs in the foot or ankle, or there is an increase in swelling.
- Pain does not improve after resting.
- Symptoms persist or intensify after treatment.

METATARSALGIA

GENERAL INFORMATION

DEFINITION—Metatarsalgia is a general term for pain over the bottom front (forefoot) of one or both feet. The area is also referred to as the ball of the foot. Metatarsalgia is a common occurrence and can be very painful. The onset is usually gradual, but may happen suddenly, or it can be a recurrent problem.

BODY PARTS INVOLVED
• Juncture of the big toe or other toes with the rest of the foot.
• Bones and joints at the ball-of-the-foot. The metatarsal bones are the long bones of the feet. They are located between the bones that form the ankle (tarsal bones) and the bones of the toes (phalanges).

SIGNS & SYMPTOMS
• Pain, dull ache or burning sensation in the area of the ball of the forefoot. Occasionally, pain is felt throughout the sole of the foot or may feel sharp or shooting pains in the toes.
• Pain worsens when walking barefoot and may lessen when walking in shoes with good forefoot cushioning.
• Feels like "have a stone in my shoe" or "walking on pebbles," are frequent complaints.
• Swelling may be present.

CAUSES—There is no one specific cause of metatarsalgia. It most often occurs as a result of faulty distribution of weight on the forefoot.

This could come from doing too much of a weight-bearing activity such as running, jumping, or walking. The metatarsal heads become painful and/or inflamed. It may happen suddenly if there is trauma to the area. Sometimes no cause is found. Metatarsalgia is often referred to as a symptom, rather than as a specific disease.

RISK INCREASES WITH
• High-impact sports involving running or jumping.
• Wearing shoes that do not fit properly, are poorly designed or are worn-out.
• For women, wearing high heels and shoes that are too tight across the ball of the foot.
• Certain foot shapes (such as high arches) or deformities may be at risk for metatarsalgia.
• With aging, the fat pad in the foot tends to thin out which causes the foot to be more susceptible to pain.
• Medical problems that may be a risk factor for metatarsalgia include obesity, gout, inflammatory arthritis, other inflammatory joint disorders, bunions, nerve problems, poor circulation and diabetes.

HOW TO PREVENT
• Wear good shoes that fit well and are appropriate for the activity involved.
• Weight loss may be helpful if overweight.
• See your doctor for evaluation if you have a medical problem that could lead to metatarsalgia.

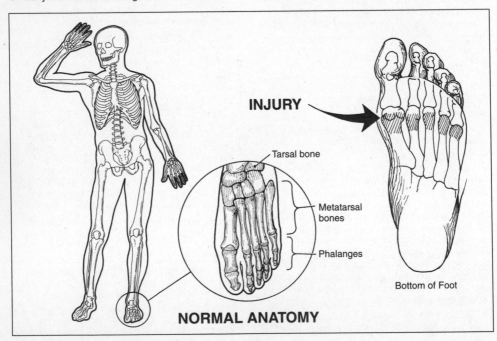

INJURY

Tarsal bone

Metatarsal bones

Phalanges

Bottom of Foot

NORMAL ANATOMY

WHAT TO EXPECT

APPROPRIATE HEALTH CARE
- Doctor's care for moderate to severe symptoms.
- Self-care for milder symptoms.

DIAGNOSTIC MEASURES
- Your own observation of symptoms.
- Medical history and physical exam by a doctor.
- X-rays of injured area to see if a foot bone is fractured. If you have metatarsalgia, the x-ray will show no break. Bone scan may also be done if a stress fracture is suspected.

POSSIBLE COMPLICATIONS
- Joint instability or toe dislocation.
- A loss of flexibility which could lead to some loss in range of motion, or chronic stiffness.
- Prolonged healing time or worsening of metatarsalgia if activities are resumed too soon.

PROBABLE OUTCOME
- A good outcome is expected in uncomplicated cases caused by shoes or training problems. Appropriate treatment can usually relieve symptoms in 10 to 14 days.
- In some cases, recovery may depend on treatment of any underlying medical disorder.

HOW TO TREAT

NOTE—Follow your doctor's instructions. These instructions are supplemental.

FIRST AID—If the problem occurs suddenly, use instructions for R.I.C.E., the first letters of *rest, ice, compression* and *elevation*. See Appendix 1 for details.

CONTINUING CARE
- Rest with your feet elevated after periods of activity.
- Fill a large styrofoam cup with water and freeze. Tear a small amount of foam from the top so ice protrudes. Massage firmly over the painful area for about 15 minutes at a time with the foot elevated. Switch to moist heat after 72 hours if it feels better.
- For some, pain relief occurs by wearing adhesive felt, gel or foam padding around the painful area. Cushioned insoles, metatarsal pads or arch supports may also help.
- Orthotics (for inserting into shoes) may be prescribed by your doctor to relieve pressure and redistribute weight from the painful area to more tolerant areas. Orthotics may be custom-made to fit the anatomy of the foot.

- Chronic symptoms may be treated with a metatarsal bar that can be added to the running or athletic shoe.
- Wear shoes that are roomier with a wide toe-box, have thick soles, or have energy-absorbing soles.
- Surgery may be recommended if there is a correctable problem such as bunions, hammertoes, or pinched nerves.

MEDICATION—For minor discomfort, you may use nonsteroidal anti-inflammatory drugs, such as ibuprofen.

ACTIVITY
- Your activities may need to be limited until the symptoms go away. Workouts should be less lengthy and intense. If metatarsalgia is severe, training may have to stop until symptoms subside.
- Try swimming or bicycling instead of running or walking.
- Return to your regular sports or fitness activity on a gradual basis. You should have full range of motion and full strength of the injured foot, and be able to walk or run without pain.

DIET—During recovery, balance the amount of food you eat with any change in your level of physical activity. Eat a variety of foods to get the energy, protein, vitamins, minerals and fiber you need for good health and healing.

REHABILITATION
- Usually, there is no specific physical therapy needed.
- Your doctor may recommend foot and ankle exercises for range of motion, flexibility, and strength building.
- See Rehabilitation section for foot and ankle exercises.

CALL YOUR DOCTOR IF

- You have tried self treatment measures and the symptoms continue or interfere with normal activities.
- You have symptoms of moderate or severe forefoot pain that persists longer than 2 weeks. Metatarsalgia is similar to other problems of the foot which may require different treatment.
- Pain or discomfort worsens despite treatment.

NECK (CERVICAL SPINE) DISLOCATION
(Cervical Spine Facet Dislocation)

 GENERAL INFORMATION

DEFINITION—A displacement of spinal vertebrae in the neck so that adjoining bones no longer touch each other. Subluxation is a minor dislocation; the joint surfaces still touch, but not in normal relation to each other. Neck subluxation followed by spontaneous reposition can occur in athletes. A neck dislocation is a serious injury that can lead to spinal cord damage and paralysis of all four extremities, and it sometimes leads to death.

BODY PARTS INVOLVED
• Vertebrae of the spine in the cervical (neck) region and ligaments that hold the vertebrae in proper alignment.
• Cartilage between the vertebrae that cushions the bones.
• Spinal cord and nerve roots (sometimes).

SIGNS & SYMPTOMS
• Excruciating pain at the time of injury.
• Loss of function in the neck and severe pain when attempting to move it.
• Visible deformity if the dislocated bones have locked in the dislocated positions. Bones may spontaneously reposition themselves and leave no deformity, but damage is the same.
• Tenderness over the dislocation.
• Swelling and bruising in the neck.

• Numbness or paralysis below the neck dislocation site from pressure, pinching or cutting of blood vessels or nerves.

CAUSES
• Forceful flexing, extension or rotation of the neck; direct blow to or violent force exerted on the neck or head.
• End result of a severe neck sprain.

RISK INCREASES WITH
• Contact and collision sports such as football, hockey or basketball.
• Gymnastics or diving.
• Previous neck dislocation or sprain.
• Repeated neck injury of any sport.
• Poor muscle conditioning.

HOW TO PREVENT
• Participate in a strengthening, flexibility and conditioning program appropriate for your sport.
• Warm up adequately before physical activity.
• After healing, wear protective devices (such as a soft or rigid neck collar) to decrease the likelihood of reinjury during participation in any sports. Avoid all contact or collision sports.

 WHAT TO EXPECT

APPROPRIATE HEALTH CARE
• Surgery to restore the cervical vertebrae and torn ligaments to their normal positions. This

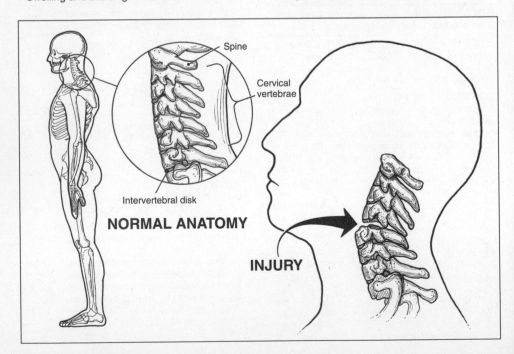

Spine

Cervical vertebrae

Intervertebral disk

NORMAL ANATOMY

INJURY

requires fusion of one or more vertebrae and use of a halo vest for immobilization of the head and neck.
• Self care during rehabilitation.

DIAGNOSTIC MEASURES
• Your own observation of symptoms.
• Medical history and exam by a doctor.
• X-rays of the neck and skull.
• CT scan (see Glossary) of the neck to identify fracture; MRI (see Glossary) of the neck to identify disk injuries.

POSSIBLE COMPLICATIONS
At time of injury:
• Shock.
• Serious injury to neck cartilage, the spinal cord and roots of the spinal nerves as they emerge from between the vertebrae to serve other parts of the body. Neck dislocation can lead to paralysis from the neck down.
• Pressure on or damage to other nearby smaller nerves, tendons, muscles, blood vessels and connective tissues.
• Trouble swallowing or clearing secretions.
After treatment of surgery:
• Excessive internal bleeding in the neck area.
• Impaired blood supply to the dislocated area.
• Death of bone cells due to interruption of the blood supply (avascular necrosis).
• Infection introduced during surgical treatment.
• Prolonged healing if activity is resumed too soon.
• Unstable or arthritic neck joint following repeated injury.

PROBABLE OUTCOME—After the dislocation has been corrected, the neck may require immobilization with a soft or rigid collar for 8 weeks or more. Complete healing of injured ligaments requires a minimum of 6 weeks.

 # HOW TO TREAT

NOTE—Follow your doctor's instructions. These instructions are supplemental.

FIRST AID
• *Don't move anyone with a neck injury* except on sturdy boards and with the neck immobilized. Don't remove the victim's headgear, but do remove the face mask.
• Transport the victim immediately to an emergency facility.
• Ice helps stop internal bleeding. Prepare an ice pack of ice cubes or chips wrapped in plastic or placed in a container. Place a towel over the injured area to prevent skin damage. Apply ice for 20 minutes, then rest 10 minutes until medical help is available. Compress the area with a loose-fitting elastic wrap to hold ice in place. Don't wrap too tightly. This can cause further damage.

• The doctor will manipulate the dislocated bones or apply traction for 12 to 24 hours to return the bones to their normal positions. Manipulation should be done as soon as possible after injury. Delays may lead to compression of the spinal cord—a surgical emergency. Also, many tissues lose their elasticity and become difficult to return to their normal functional positions.

CONTINUING CARE—At home:
• Apply heat frequently. Use heat lamps, hot soaks, hot showers or heating pads.
• Massage gently and often to provide comfort and decrease swelling.

MEDICATION—Your doctor may prescribe:
• General anesthesia or muscle relaxants prior to joint manipulation or application of traction.
• Acetaminophen, aspirin or nonsteroidal anti-inflammatory drugs for mild pain.
• Narcotic pain relievers for severe pain.
• Stool softeners to prevent constipation due to decreased activity.
• Antibiotics to fight infection.
• Special corticosteroids, such as dexamethasone, to reduce swelling and minimize spinal cord damage.

ACTIVITY—Resume activities gradually after surgery. Follow your doctor's instructions.

DIET
• Do not eat or drink before manipulation or surgery to correct the dislocation. Fluid or solid food in your stomach makes vomiting while under general anesthesia more hazardous.
• During recovery, eat a well-balanced diet.

REHABILITATION—Your doctor will advise you when and how to begin your rehabilitation.

 # CALL YOUR DOCTOR IF

• You have any neck injury—especially if any part of your body becomes numb, pale or cold after injury. This is an emergency!
• Any of the following occurs after treatment:
  Loss of feeling below the dislocation site.
  Blue or gray skin color, particularly under the fingernails or toenails.
  Swelling above or below the neck collar.
  Nausea or vomiting; constipation.
• Any of the following occurs after surgery:
  Increased pain, swelling or drainage in the surgical area.
  Signs of infection (headache, muscle aches, dizziness or a general ill feeling and fever).
• New, unexplained symptoms develop. Drugs used in treatment may produce side effects.
• Neck dislocations that you can "pop" back into normal position occur repeatedly.

NECK (CERVICAL SPINE) FRACTURE

GENERAL INFORMATION

DEFINITION—A complete or incomplete break in a bone in the neck (cervical spine). Injuries to this region of the spine are frequently a combination of sprain, dislocation and fracture. The most serious can injure the spinal cord, leading to paralysis or death.

BODY PARTS INVOLVED
- Bones in the neck (cervical spine).
- Joints in the cervical spine.
- Spinal cord (sometimes).
- Soft tissues surrounding the fracture site, including muscles, nerves, tendons, ligaments, periosteum (covering of bone), blood vessels and connective tissues.

SIGNS & SYMPTOMS
- Severe pain in the neck at the fracture site.
- Swelling of soft tissues around the fracture.
- Tenderness to the touch.
- Numbness below the fracture site (sometimes).
- Weakness in the hands or feet.

CAUSES—Direct blow or indirect stress to the neck. Indirect stress may be caused by twisting.

RISK INCREASES WITH
- Diving; contact sports, particularly football.
- Gymnastics (tumbling or trampoline activities).
- History of bone or joint disease, especially osteoporosis.
- Obesity.
- Poor nutrition, especially insufficient calcium.
- If surgery or anesthesia is necessary, risk increases with smoking and use of drugs, including mind-altering drugs, muscle relaxants, antihypertensives, tranquilizers, sleep inducers, insulin, sedatives, beta-adrenergic blockers or corticosteroids.

HOW TO PREVENT
- Build your strength with a good conditioning program before beginning regular athletic practice or competition. Increased muscle mass provides additional protection to your bones.
- Use a "spotter" (helper) when attempting difficult moves in gymnastics or similar activities.
- Use appropriate protective equipment, such as padded collars and shoulder pads, when competing in contact sports.
- Ensure an adequate calcium intake (l000 mg to 1500 mg a day) with milk and milk products or calcium supplements.

WHAT TO EXPECT

APPROPRIATE HEALTH CARE
- Doctor's treatment.
- Hospitalization for traction to the skull so the fracture can become properly aligned.
- Whirlpool, ultrasound or massage to displace excess fluid from the injured joint space.
- Surgery to reposition bone fragments and fuse vertebrae. Use of a halo vest to immobilize the head and neck.

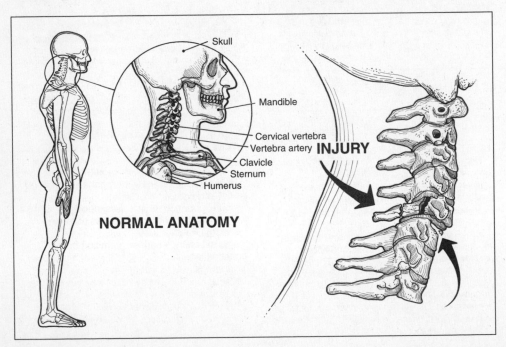

Skull

Mandible

Cervical vertebra
Vertebra artery **INJURY**
Clavicle
Sternum
Humerus

NORMAL ANATOMY

DIAGNOSTIC MEASURES
- Your own observation of symptoms.
- Medical history and exam by a doctor.
- X-rays of the skull and neck.
- CT scan (see Glossary) of the neck.

POSSIBLE COMPLICATIONS
At the time of injury:
- Shock.
- Pressure on or injury to the spinal cord and nearby nerves, ligaments, tendons, muscles, blood vessels or connective tissues.
- Paralysis—temporary or permanent, partial or complete—below the neck.

After treatment:
- Delayed union or nonunion of the fracture.
- Impaired blood supply to the fracture site.
- Infection in open fractures (skin broken over the fracture site) or at the incision if surgical setting was necessary.
- Prolonged healing time if activity is resumed too soon.
- Proneness to repeated neck injury.
- Unstable or arthritic neck joint following repeated injury.

PROBABLE OUTCOME—The average healing time for this fracture is 3 to 7 days in traction, followed by 3 to 4 months in a halo brace. Healing is complete when there is no pain or motion at the fracture site and when x-rays show complete bone union.

 ## HOW TO TREAT

NOTE—Follow your doctor's instructions. These instructions are supplemental.

FIRST AID
- Keep the person warm with blankets to decrease the possibility of shock.
- *Don't move the injured area.* Don't try to remove a helmet or other headgear.
- Use a stretcher or spine board with sandbags or a cervical collar to immobilize the neck while transporting the injured person to an emergency facility. Do this only if you are trained in emergency medical assistance or if no help is available.
- The doctor will apply traction to manipulate the broken bones slowly back to their original positions. Traction lines up and holds the broken neck bones as close to their normal positions as possible. Manipulation should be done as soon as possible after injury. Also, many tissues lose their elasticity and become difficult to return to their normal positions.
- Immobilization will be necessary. The best method must be determined by your doctor based on your age, sex and the possibility of spinal cord injury.

CONTINUING CARE—Treatment after manipulation and healing:
- Take whirlpool treatments, if available.
- Massage gently and often to provide comfort and decrease swelling.

MEDICATION—Your doctor may prescribe:
- Strong pain relievers for severe pain.
- Special corticosteroids, such as dexamethasone, to reduce swelling and minimize spinal cord damage.
- Stool softeners to prevent constipation due to inactivity.
- Acetaminophen for mild pain.
- Antibiotics to fight infection if skin is broken or surgery is needed.

ACTIVITY
- Actively exercise all muscle groups not immobilized. Muscle contractions promote fracture alignment and hasten healing.
- Resume normal daily activities gradually after treatment.

DIET
- Do not eat or drink before manipulation or surgery to treat the fracture. Fluid or solid food in your stomach makes vomiting while under anesthesia more hazardous.
- During recovery, balance the amount of food you eat with any change in your level of physical activity. Eat a variety of foods to get the energy, protein, vitamins, minerals and fiber you need for good health and healing.

REHABILITATION
- Begin reconditioning and rehabilitation after clearance from your doctor.
- Use ice massage for 10 minutes before and after workouts. Fill a large styrofoam cup with water and freeze. Tear a small amount of foam from the top so ice protrudes. Massage firmly over the injured area in a circle about the size of a softball.
- See Rehabilitation section for neck exercises.

 ## CALL YOUR DOCTOR IF

- You have any serious neck injury.
- You develop signs of infection (headache, muscle aches, dizziness or a general ill feeling and fever) while in traction.
- You experience muscle weakness, numbness normal position, or complete loss of feeling below the fracture site.
- You experience nausea, vomiting or constipation.

NECK (CERVICAL SPINE) SPRAIN

GENERAL INFORMATION

DEFINITION—Violent overstretching of one or more ligaments in the cervical (neck) region of the vertebral column. Sprains involving two or more ligaments cause considerably more disability than single-ligament sprains. When the ligament is overstretched, it becomes tense and gives way at its weakest point, either where it attaches to bone or within the ligament itself. If the ligament pulls loose a fragment of bone, it is called an avulsion fracture. There are 3 types of sprains:
- Mild (Grade I)—Tearing of some ligament fibers. There is no loss of function.
- Moderate (Grade II)—Rupture of a portion of the ligament, resulting in some loss of function.
- Severe (Grade III)—Complete rupture of the ligament or complete separation of ligament from bone. There is total loss of function. A severe sprain may require surgical repair.

BODY PARTS INVOLVED
- Any ligament in the neck.
- Tissues surrounding the sprain, including blood vessels, tendons, bone, periosteum (covering of bone) and muscle.

SIGNS & SYMPTOMS.
- Severe pain at the time of injury.
- A feeling of popping or tearing inside the neck.
- Muscle spasm with soreness and stiffness in the neck.
- Tenderness at the injury site.
- Swelling in the neck.
- Bruising that appears soon after injury.

CAUSES—Stress on a ligament that temporarily forces the joints in the neck out of their normal locations. Neck sprains occur frequently in contact sports and auto accidents.

RISK INCREASES WITH
- Contact sports, especially football and wrestling.
- Diving or gymnastics.
- Auto racing.
- Previous neck injury.
- Obesity.
- Poor muscle conditioning.
- Inadequate protection from equipment.

HOW TO PREVENT
- Use appropriate equipment and precautions.
- Build your strength with a conditioning program appropriate for your sport.
- Warm up before practice or competition.
- Wear protective equipment, such as padded soft collars, for participation in contact sports.

WHAT TO EXPECT

APPROPRIATE HEALTH CARE
- Doctor's diagnosis.
- Traction (sometimes).
- Self-care during rehabilitation.
- Physical therapy (moderate or severe sprain).
- Surgery (severe sprain).

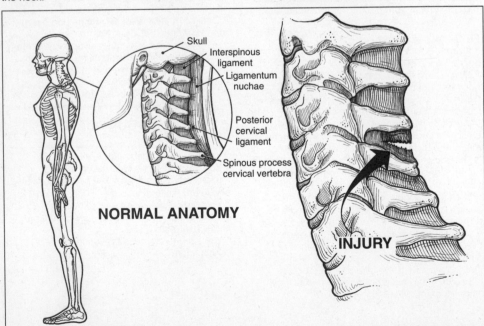

Skull
Interspinous ligament
Ligamentum nuchae
Posterior cervical ligament
Spinous process cervical vertebra

NORMAL ANATOMY

INJURY

DIAGNOSTIC MEASURES
- Your own observation of symptoms.
- Medical history and exam by a doctor.
- X-rays of the neck to rule out fractures.

POSSIBLE COMPLICATIONS
- Prolonged healing time if usual activities are resumed too soon.
- Proneness to repeated injury.
- Inflammation at the ligament attachment to bone (periostitis).
- Prolonged disability (sometimes).

PROBABLE OUTCOME—If this is a first-time injury, proper care and sufficient healing time before resuming activity should prevent permanent disability. Ligaments have a poor blood supply, and torn ligaments require as much healing time as fractures. Average healing times are:
- Mild sprains—2 to 6 weeks.
- Moderate sprains—6 to 8 weeks.
- Severe sprains—8 to 10 weeks.

 ## HOW TO TREAT

NOTE—Follow your doctor's instructions. These instructions are supplemental.

FIRST AID—Use Instructions for R.I.C.E., the first letters of *rest, ice, compression* and *elevation*. See Appendix 1 for details.

CONTINUING CARE
- Your doctor may suggest an adjustable cervical brace, a plastic cervical collar or a cloth collar to immobilize the neck while it heals.
- Continue using an ice pack 3 or 4 times a day. Wrap ice chips or cubes in a plastic bag. Wrap the bag in a moist towel, and place it over the injured area. Use for 20 minutes at a time.
- After 72 hours, apply heat instead of ice if it feels better. Use heat lamps, hot soaks, hot showers, heating pads or heat liniments and ointments.
- Take whirlpool treatments, if available.
- Massage gently and often to provide comfort and decrease swelling.
- Cervical traction devices that can be rented or purchased may provide pain relief. Follow your doctor's instructions or instructions supplied with the product.

MEDICATION
- For minor discomfort, you may use: Aspirin, acetaminophen or ibuprofen. Topical liniments and ointments.
- Your doctor may prescribe: Stronger pain relievers. Injection of a long-acting local anesthetic to reduce pain. Injection of a corticosteroid, such as triamcinolone, to reduce inflammation.

ACTIVITY—Resume your normal activities gradually after clearance from your doctor.

DIET—During recovery, balance the amount of food you eat with any change in your level of physical activity. Eat a variety of foods to get the energy, protein, vitamins, minerals and fiber you need for good health and healing.

REHABILITATION
- Begin daily rehabilitation exercises when the supportive collar is no longer necessary.
- Use ice massage for 10 minutes before and after exercise. Fill a large styrofoam cup with water and freeze. Tear a small amount of foam from the top so ice protrudes. Massage firmly over the injured area in a circle about the size of a softball.
- See Rehabilitation section for neck exercises.

 ## CALL YOUR DOCTOR IF

- You have symptoms of a moderate or severe neck sprain or a mild sprain persists longer than 2 weeks.
- Pain, swelling or bruising worsens despite treatment.
- Numbness or weakness occurs in muscles of the face, shoulder, arm or hand.
- Any of the following occurs after surgery: Increased pain, swelling, redness, drainage or bleeding in the surgical area. Signs of infection (headache, muscle aches, dizziness or a general ill feeling with fever). New unexplained symptoms. Drugs used in treatment may produce side effects.

NECK (CERVICAL SPINE) STRAIN

GENERAL INFORMATION

DEFINITION—Injury to the muscles or tendons that attach to the vertebral column in the neck, to the skull and to the trunk. Muscles, tendons and their attached bones comprise contractile units. These units stabilize the neck and head and allow their motion. A strain occurs at the unit's weakest part. Strains are of 3 types:
• Mild (Grade I)—Slightly pulled muscle without tearing of muscle or tendon fibers. There is no loss of strength.
• Moderate (Grade II)—Tearing of fibers in a muscle or tendon or at the attachment to bone. Strength is diminished.
• Severe (Grade III)—Rupture of the muscle-tendon-bone attachment, with separation of fibers. Severe strains may require surgical repair. Chronic strains are caused by overuse. Acute strains are caused by direct injury or overstress.

BODY PARTS INVOLVED
• Tendons and muscles with multiple attachments to bones in the neck, skull and shoulder.
• Bones in the neck, shoulder and skull.
• Soft tissues surrounding the strain, including nerves, periosteum (covering of bone), blood vessels and lymph vessels.

SIGNS & SYMPTOMS
• Pain when moving or stretching the neck.
• Muscle spasm in the neck.
• Swelling in the neck area.
• Loss of strength (moderate or severe strain).
• Crepitation ("cracking" feeling and sound when the injured area is pressed with fingers).
• Calcification (visible with x-ray) of the injured muscle or tendon.

CAUSES
• Prolonged overuse of muscle-tendon units in the neck.
• Single violent injury or force applied to the muscle-tendon units in the neck.

RISK INCREASES WITH
• Contact sports, especially wrestling and football.
• Medical history of any bleeding disorder.
• Obesity.
• Poor nutrition.
• Previous neck strain.
• Poor muscle conditioning.

HOW TO PREVENT
• Participate in a strengthening, flexibility and conditioning program appropriate for your sport.
• Warm up before practice or competition.
• Wear proper protective equipment, such as neck rolls.

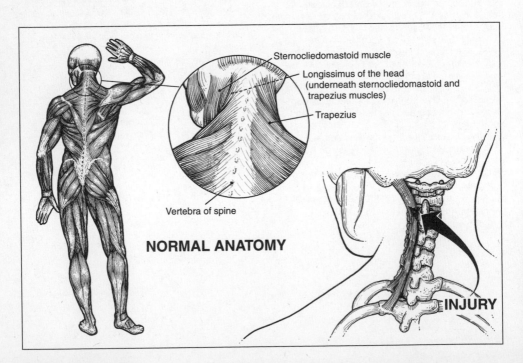

Sternocliedomastoid muscle

Longissimus of the head (underneath sternocliedomastoid and trapezius muscles)

Trapezius

Vertebra of spine

NORMAL ANATOMY

INJURY

WHAT TO EXPECT

APPROPRIATE HEALTH CARE
- Doctor's diagnosis.
- Self-care during rehabilitation.
- Physical therapy (moderate or severe strain).
- Surgery (severe strain).

DIAGNOSTIC MEASURES
- Your own observation of symptoms.
- Medical history and exam by a doctor.
- X-rays of the neck to rule out fractures.

POSSIBLE COMPLICATIONS
- Prolonged healing time if activity is resumed too soon.
- Proneness to repeated injury.
- Headaches from muscle spasm.
- Inflammation at the attachment to bone (periostitis).
- Prolonged disability (sometimes).

PROBABLE OUTCOME—If this is a first-time injury, proper care and sufficient healing time before resuming activity should prevent permanent disability. Torn ligaments and tendons require as long to heal as fractured bones. Average healing times are:
- Mild strain—2 to 10 days.
- Moderate strain—10 days to 6 weeks.
- Severe strain—6 to 10 weeks.
If this is a repeat injury, complications listed above are more likely to occur.

HOW TO TREAT

NOTE—Follow your doctor's instructions. These instructions are supplemental.

FIRST AID—Use instructions for R.I.C.E., the first letters of *rest, ice, compression* and *elevation.* See Appendix 1 for details.

CONTINUING CARE
- Rest in bed with traction on the neck if your doctor advises you to do so.
- Use ice massage 3 or 4 times a day for 15 minutes at a time. Fill a large styrofoam cup with water and freeze. Tear a small amount of foam from the top so ice protrudes. Massage firmly over the injured area in a circle about the size of a softball.

- After the first 24 hours, apply heat instead of ice if it feels better. Use heat lamps, hot soaks, hot showers, heating pads or heat liniments and ointments.
- Use a support collar to reduce movement and support the neck during healing.
- Massage gently and often to provide comfort and decrease swelling.

MEDICATION
- For minor discomfort, you may use:
  Aspirin, acetaminophen or ibuprofen.
  Topical liniments and ointments.
- Your doctor may prescribe:
  Stronger pain relievers.
  Muscle relaxants.
  Injection of a long-acting local anesthetic to reduce pain (rare).
  Injections of a corticosteroid, such as triamcinolone, to reduce inflammation (rare).

ACTIVITY—Resume your normal activities gradually after pain subsides.

DIET—During recovery, balance the amount of food you eat with any change in your level of physical activity. Eat a variety of foods to get the energy, protein, vitamins, minerals and fiber you need for good health and healing.

REHABILITATION
- Begin daily rehabilitation exercises when support collar is no longer needed. Use ice massage for 10 minutes prior to exercise.
- See Rehabilitation section for neck exercises.

CALL YOUR DOCTOR IF

- You have symptoms of a moderate or severe neck strain or a mild strain persists longer than 5 days.
- Pain or swelling worsens despite treatment.
- Symptoms of neck strain recur after treatment.

NOSE INJURY

GENERAL INFORMATION

DEFINITION—Nose injuries include:
- Fractures of the nasal bones.
- Dislocations of nasal bones and cartilage.
- Contusions of the nose.
- Nosebleeds.

BODY PARTS INVOLVED
- Nasal bones and cartilage.
- Sinuses and eustachian tubes (indirectly sometimes).
- Soft tissues surrounding the injury, including eyes, periosteum (covering of bone), nerves, blood vessels, mucous membrane lining the inside of the nose and connective tissues.

SIGNS & SYMPTOMS
- Pain or tenderness in the nose.
- Swollen, bruised nose.
- Inability to breathe through the nose.
- Crooked or misshapen nose (sometimes).
- Brisk bleeding or blood oozing from a nostril. If the nosebleed is close to the nostril, the blood is bright red. If the nosebleed is deeper in the nose, the blood may be bright or dark.
- Lightheadedness from blood loss.
- Rapid heartbeat, shortness of breath and pallor (with significant blood loss only).

CAUSES—Direct blow to the nose.

RISK INCREASES WITH
- Contact sports, particularly boxing and wrestling. The nose is fairly well protected by a face guard in football.
- Previous nose injury.
- Medical history of any bleeding disorder.
- Use of certain drugs, such as anticoagulants or aspirin, or prolonged use of nose drops.
- Exposure to irritating chemicals.
- High altitude or dry climate.

HOW TO PREVENT—Protect your nose from injury whenever possible. Wear protective headgear for contact sports or when riding motorcycles or bicycles. Wear auto seat belts.

WHAT TO EXPECT

APPROPRIATE HEALTH CARE
- Self-care (see Continuing Care).
- Doctor's treatment or emergency room treatment if self-care is unsuccessful.
- Surgery (for severe bleeding only) to tie off the artery feeding the bleeding area.
- Surgery if the nose is crooked or breathing is impaired.

DIAGNOSTIC MEASURES
- Your own observation of symptoms.
- Medical history and physical exam by a doctor.
- Laboratory blood tests if bleeding is heavy.
- X-rays of the nose.

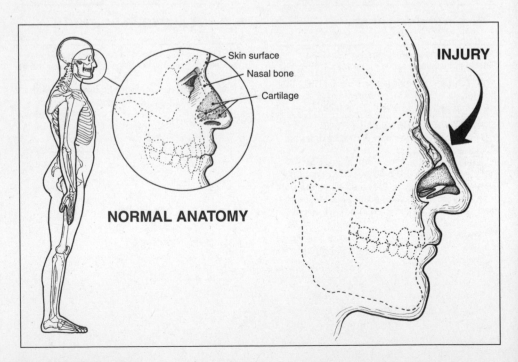

Skin surface
Nasal bone
Cartilage

NORMAL ANATOMY

INJURY

POSSIBLE COMPLICATIONS
- Infection of the nose and sinuses.
- Shock from loss of blood (rare).
- Bleeding severe enough to require a transfusion.
- Permanent breathing difficulty.
- Permanent change in appearance.

PROBABLE OUTCOME
- Minor fractures and contusions with no deformity usually heal in 4 weeks.
- Major fractures can be repaired with surgery. If surgery is necessary, it should be done within 2 weeks or not until 6 months after injury.
- Most bleeding can be controlled with home treatment. Severe bleeding requires emergency care and packing of nose by a doctor.

 ## HOW TO TREAT

NOTE—Follow your doctor's instructions. These instructions are supplemental.

FIRST AID
- Apply ice packs to the nose immediately after injury to minimize swelling and decrease bleeding.
- If the nose is deformed or if a nosebleed is heavy or cannot be stopped, obtain emergency medical treatment. Gauze packing may be inserted to absorb blood, stop dripping and exert pressure on ruptured blood vessels. Continued bleeding may require cauterization (see Glossary).

CONTINUING CARE
For a nosebleed with fracture:
- If surgery is required to set a broken nose or insert a nasal pack, your doctor will give you postoperative instructions.

For a nosebleed without fracture:
- Sit up with your head bent forward.
- Clamp your nose closed with your fingers for 5 uninterrupted minutes. During this time, breathe through your mouth.
- If bleeding stops and recurs, repeat—but pinch your nose firmly on both sides for 8 to 10 minutes. Holding your nose tightly closed allows the blood to clot and seal the damaged blood vessels.
- You may apply cold compresses at the same time.
- Don't blow your nose for 12 hours after bleeding stops to avoid dislodging the blood clot.
- Don't swallow blood. It may upset your stomach or make you gag, causing you to inhale blood.
- Don't talk (also to avoid gagging).

MEDICATION
- For minor discomfort, you may use non-prescription drugs such as acetaminophen. Aspirin should not be used because it makes bleeding more likely.
- Your doctor may prescribe:
  Stronger pain relievers, if needed.
  Antibiotics if infection develops.
  Drugs to treat any underlying serious disorder.

ACTIVITY—Resume your normal activities as soon as bleeding stops or other symptoms improve.

DIET—During recovery, balance the amount of food you eat with any change in your level of physical activity. Eat a variety of foods to get the energy, protein, vitamins, minerals and fiber you need for good health and healing.

REHABILITATION—Rehabilitation exercises must be individualized. Follow your doctor's directions.

 ## CALL YOUR DOCTOR IF

- You have a nosebleed that won't stop with the self-care described above.
- After the nosebleed, you become nauseous or vomit.
- After the nose has been packed, your temperature rises to 101°F (38.3°C) or higher.

PELVIS STRAIN, HIP-TRUNK

GENERAL INFORMATION

DEFINITION—Injury to the muscles or tendons in the region of the hip and trunk where these parts attach to the upper pelvis. Tendons, muscles and their attached bones comprise contractile units. These units stabilize the pelvis and allow its motion. A strain occurs at the weakest part of a unit. Strains are of 3 types:
- Mild (Grade I)—Slightly pulled muscle without tearing of muscle or tendon fibers. There is no loss of strength.
- Moderate (Grade II)—Tearing of fibers in a muscle or tendon or at the attachment to bone. Strength is diminished.
- Severe (Grade III)—Rupture of the muscle-tendon-bone attachment, with separation of fibers. A severe strain may require surgical repair. Chronic strains are caused by overuse. Acute strains are caused by direct injury or overstress.

BODY PARTS INVOLVED
- Muscles and tendons of the trunk and hip.
- Iliac crest bone.
- Soft tissues surrounding the strain, including nerves, periosteum (covering of bone), blood vessels and lymph vessels.

SIGNS & SYMPTOMS
- Pain when moving or stretching the leg or trunk.
- Muscle spasm at the injury site.
- Swelling at the injury site.
- Weakened trunk and thigh muscles (moderate or severe strain).
- Crepitation ("crackling" feeling and sound in when the injured area is pressed with fingers).
- Calcification of the muscle or tendon (visible with x-rays).
- Inflammation of the tendon sheath.

CAUSES
- Prolonged overuse of muscle-tendon units in the region of the iliac crest.
- Single violent injury or force applied to the muscle-tendon units in the upper pelvic area.

RISK INCREASES WITH
- Contact sports such as football, soccer or hockey.
- Sports that require quick starts, such as running races.
- Medical history of any bleeding disorder.
- Obesity.
- Poor nutrition.
- Previous pelvic injury.
- Poor muscle conditioning.

HOW TO PREVENT
- Participate in a strengthening, flexibility and conditioning program appropriate for your sport.
- Warm up before practice or competition.
- Wear proper protective equipment for contact sports.

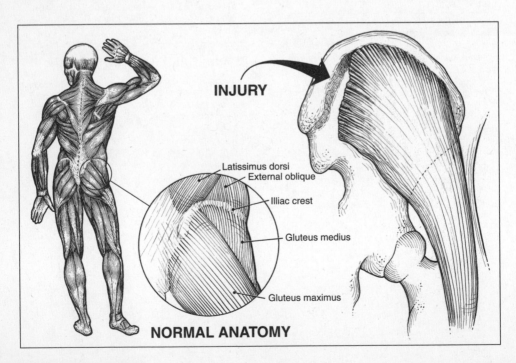

INJURY

Latissimus dorsi
External oblique
Iliac crest
Gluteus medius
Gluteus maximus

NORMAL ANATOMY

WHAT TO EXPECT

APPROPRIATE HEALTH CARE
- Doctor's diagnosis.
- Self-care during rehabilitation.
- Physical therapy (moderate or severe strain).
- Surgery (severe strain).

DIAGNOSTIC MEASURES
- Your own observation of symptoms.
- Medical history and exam by a doctor.
- X-rays of the hip, thigh and pelvis to rule out fractures.

POSSIBLE COMPLICATIONS
- Prolonged healing time if activity is resumed too soon.
- Proneness to repeated injury.
- Inflammation at the attachment to bone (periostitis).
- Prolonged disability (sometimes).

PROBABLE OUTCOME—If this is at first-time injury, proper care and sufficient healing time before resuming activity should prevent permanent disability. Torn ligaments and tendons require as long to heal as fractured bones do. Average healing times are:
- Mild strain—2 to 10 days.
- Moderate strain—10 days to 6 weeks.
- Severe strain—6 to 10 weeks.

If this is a repeat injury, complications listed above are more likely to occur.

HOW TO TREAT

NOTE—Follow your doctor's instructions. These instructions are supplemental.

FIRST AID—Use instructions for R.I.C.E., the first letters of *rest, ice, compression* and *elevation* (if possible). See Appendix 1 for details.

CONTINUING CARE
- Use ice massage 3 or 4 times a day for 15 minutes at a time. Fill a large styrofoam cup with water and freeze. Tear a small amount of foam from the top so ice protrudes. Massage firmly over the injured area in a circle about the size of a softball.

- After the first 72 hours, apply heat instead of ice if it feels better. Use heat lamps, hot soaks, hot showers, heating pads or heat liniments and ointments.
- Take whirlpool treatments, if available.
- Massage gently and often to provide comfort and decrease swelling.

MEDICATION
- For minor discomfort, you may use:
  Aspirin, acetaminophen or ibuprofen or other nonsteroidal anti-inflammatories.
  Topical liniments and ointments.
- Your doctor may prescribe:
  Stronger pain relievers.
  Injection of a long-acting local anesthetic to reduce pain.
  Injections of corticosteroids, such as triamcinolone, to reduce inflammation.

ACTIVITY
- For a moderate or severe strain, walk with crutches for at least 72 hours. See Appendix 3 (Safe Use of Crutches).
- Resume your normal activities gradually.

DIET—During recovery, balance the amount of food you eat with any change in your level of physical activity. Eat a variety of foods to get the energy, protein, vitamins, minerals and fiber you need for good health and healing.

REHABILITATION
- Begin daily rehabilitation exercises when pain subsides. Use ice massage for 10 minutes prior to exercise.
- See Rehabilitation section for hip and pelvis exercises.

CALL YOUR DOCTOR IF

- You have symptoms of a moderate or severe hip-trunk pelvic strain or a mild strain persists longer than 10 days.
- Pain or swelling worsens despite treatment.

PELVIS STRAIN, ISCHIUM

GENERAL INFORMATION

DEFINITION—Injury to the muscles or tendons of the lower pelvis (ischium) or injury at places where muscles attach to pelvic bones. Tendons, muscles and their attached bones comprise contractile units. These units stabilize the pelvis and allow its motion. A strain occurs at the weakest part of a unit. Strains are of 3 types:
- Mild (Grade I)—Slightly pulled muscle without tearing of muscle or tendon fibers. There is no loss of strength.
- Moderate (Grade II)—Tearing of fibers in a muscle or tendon or at the attachment to bone. Strength is diminished.
- Severe (Grade III)—Rupture of the muscle-tendon-bone attachment, with separation of fibers. A severe strain may require surgical repair. Chronic strains are caused by overuse. Acute strains are caused by direct injury or overstress.

SIGNS & SYMPTOMS
- Pain when moving or stretching the thigh.
- Spasm in muscles that attach to the pelvis.
- Swelling in the lower pelvic area.
- Loss of strength (moderate or severe strain).
- Crepitation ("crackling" feeling and sound when the injured area is pressed with fingers).
- Calcification of the muscle or tendon (visible with x-rays).
- Inflammation of the tendon sheath.

CAUSES
- Prolonged overuse of muscle-tendon units in the pelvis.
- Single violent injury or force applied to the muscle-tendon units in the lower pelvis. Strains of pelvic muscles are common in sports in which the hip is bent and the knee is straight, as with a hurdler's leading leg. Forceful straight leg-raising exercises also lead to pelvic strain.

RISK INCREASES WITH
- Hurdling, high jumping, vaulting or long jumping.
- Sports that require quick starts.
- Contact sports (e.g., football).
- Medical history of any bleeding disorder.
- Obesity.
- Poor nutrition.
- Previous pelvic injury.
- Poor muscle conditioning.

HOW TO PREVENT
- Participation in a strengthening, flexibility and conditioning program appropriate for your sport.
- Warm up before practice or competition.

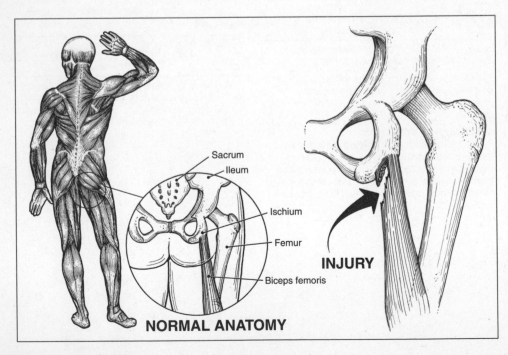

Sacrum
Ileum
Ischium
Femur
Biceps femoris

NORMAL ANATOMY

INJURY

WHAT TO EXPECT

APPROPRIATE HEALTH CARE
- Doctor's diagnosis.
- Self-care during rehabilitation.
- Physical therapy (moderate or severe strain).
- Surgery (severe strain).

DIAGNOSTIC MEASURES
- Your own observation of symptoms.
- Medical history and exam by a doctor.
- X-rays of pelvic bones to rule out fractures.

POSSIBLE COMPLICATIONS
- Prolonged healing time if activity is resumed too soon.
- Proneness to repeated injury.
- Inflammation at the attachment to bone (periostitis).
- Prolonged disability, especially weakness.

PROBABLE OUTCOME—If this is a first-time injury, proper care and sufficient healing time before resuming activity should prevent permanent disability. Torn ligaments and tendons require as long to heal as fractured bones do. Average healing times are:
- Mild strain—2 to 10 days.
- Moderate strain—10 days to 6 weeks.
- Severe strain—6 to 10 weeks.

If this is a repeat injury, complications listed above are more likely to occur.

HOW TO TREAT

NOTE—Follow your doctor's instructions. These instructions are supplemental.

FIRST AID—Use instructions for R.I.C.E., the first letters of *rest, ice, compression* and *elevation* (if possible). See Appendix 1 for details.

CONTINUING CARE
- Use ice massage 3 or 4 times a day for 15 minutes at a time. Fill a large styrofoam cup with water and freeze. Tear a small amount of foam from the top so ice protrudes. Massage firmly over the injured area in a circle about the size of a softball.

- After the first 72 hours, apply heat instead of ice if it feels better. Use heat lamps, hot soaks, hot showers, heating pads or heat liniments and ointments.
- Take whirlpool treatments, if available.
- Wrap the injured pelvic muscles loosely with an elasticized bandage or wear a corset between treatments.
- Massage gently and often to provide comfort and decrease swelling.

MEDICATION
- For minor discomfort, you may use:
  Aspirin, acetaminophen or ibuprofen.
  Topical liniments and ointments.
- Your doctor may prescribe:
  Stronger pain relievers.
  Injection of a long-acting local anesthetic to reduce pain (rare).
  Injections of a corticosteroid, such as triamcinolone, to reduce inflammation (rare).

ACTIVITY
- For a moderate or severe strain, walk with crutches for at least 72 hours. See Appendix 3 (Safe Use of Crutches).
- Resume your normal activities gradually.

DIET—During recovery, balance the amount of food you eat with any change in your level of physical activity. Eat a variety of foods to get the energy, protein, vitamins, minerals and fiber you need for good health and healing.

REHABILITATION
- Begin daily rehabilitation exercises when supportive wrapping is no longer needed. Use ice massage for 10 minutes prior to exercise.
- See Rehabilitation section for hip and pelvis exercises.

CALL YOUR DOCTOR IF

- You have symptoms of a moderate or severe lower pelvic strain or a mild strain persists longer than 10 days.
- Pain or swelling worsens despite treatment.

PERINEUM CONTUSION

GENERAL INFORMATION

DEFINITION—A direct blow to the floor of the pelvis and associated structures, including the genitals, causing bruising of skin and underlying tissues. Contusions cause bleeding from ruptured small capillaries that allow blood to infiltrate muscles, tendons, nerves or other soft tissues. See also Genital Contusion.

BODY PARTS INVOLVED
- The perineum.
- Vaginal labia (lips), mons pubis (pubic mound), vagina, anus, penis, scrotum, testicles.
- Skin, subcutaneous tissues, tendons, ligaments, blood vessels (both large vessels and capillaries), periosteum (the outside lining of bone), muscles and connective tissues.

SIGNS & SYMPTOMS
- Swelling in the perineal area—either superficial or deep.
- Pain in the perineum.
- Feeling of firmness when pressure is exerted from outside.
- Tenderness.
- Discoloration under the skin, beginning with redness and progressing to the characteristic "black-and-blue" discoloration.

CAUSES
- Direct blow to the perineum, usually by a blunt object or because of a fall.

- Damage to tiny blood vessels, causing bleeding that infiltrates into muscle and other surrounding tissues.

RISK INCREASES WITH
- Ice skating.
- Gymnastics.
- Cycling.
- Horseback riding.
- Medical history of any bleeding disorder.
- Poor nutrition.
- Inadequate protection of exposed areas during sports.
- Obesity.

HOW TO PREVENT—Usually cannot be prevented.

WHAT TO EXPECT

APPROPRIATE HEALTH CARE
- Doctor's care unless the injury is quite small.
- Self-care for minor contusions.

DIAGNOSTIC MEASURES
- Your own observation of symptoms.
- Physical exam and medical history by a doctor for all except minor injuries. The total extent of injury may not be apparent for 48 to 72 hours.
- X-rays of the pelvis to assess total injury to perineal soft tissues and to rule out the possibility of underlying fracture.

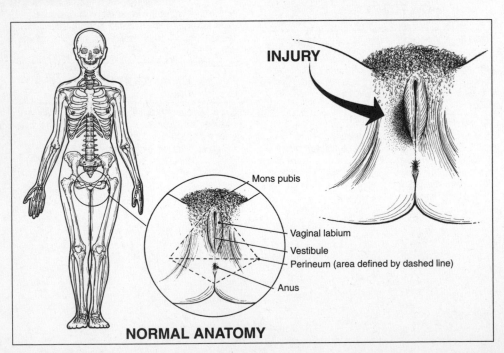

INJURY

Mons pubis

Vaginal labium

Vestibule

Perineum (area defined by dashed line)

Anus

NORMAL ANATOMY

POSSIBLE COMPLICATIONS
- Excessive bleeding, leading to disability. Infiltrative-type bleeding can (rarely) lead to calcification and impaired function of injured muscle.
- Repeated injury with prolonged healing time if usual activities are resumed too soon.
- Infection if skin over the injury site was broken.
- Scarring and narrowing of the birth canal in women (rare).

PROBABLE OUTCOME—Healing is usually complete in 1 to 4 weeks, depending on the extent of injury.

 HOW TO TREAT

NOTE—Follow your doctor's instructions. These instructions are supplemental.

FIRST AID—Use instructions for R.I.C.E., the first letters of *rest, ice, compression* and *elevation* (if possible). See Appendix 1 for details.

CONTINUING CARE
- Use an ice pack 3 or 4 times a day. Wrap ice chips or cubes in a plastic bag, and wrap the bag in a moist towel. Place it over the injured area for 20 minutes at a time.
- After 72 hours, apply heat instead of ice if it feels better. Use heat lamps, hot soaks, hot showers, heating pads or heat liniments and ointments.
- Take whirlpool treatments, if available.
- Protect the injured area with pads between treatments.

MEDICATIONS
- For minor discomfort, you may use non-prescription medicines such as acetaminophen or ibuprofen. Do not use aspirin for injuries involving bleeding.
- Your doctor may prescribe stronger medicine for pain if needed.

ACTIVITY
- Begin activities slowly, and stop exercise as soon as pain begins. Increase activity as healing progresses.
- Delay sexual activity unit healing is complete.

DIET—During recovery, balance the amount of food you eat with any change in your level of physical activity. Eat a variety of foods to get the energy, protein, vitamins, minerals and fiber you need for good health and healing.

REHABILITATION—None.

 CALL YOUR DOCTOR IF

- The injured perineum doesn't improve within a day or two.
- Signs of infection (drainage from skin, headache, muscle aches, dizziness, fever or a general ill feeling) occur if skin was broken.
- You have discomfort with sexual intercourse after healing.

RIB DISLOCATION
(Costochondral Separation)

 GENERAL INFORMATION

DEFINITION—Injury and displacement of a rib where it joins the sternum (breastbone) or spinal column. Dislocation means the rib and adjoining bones no longer touch each other. Subluxation is a minor dislocation in which the joint surfaces still touch, but not in normal relation to each other.

BODY PARTS INVOLVED
• Rib and sternum or spinal column.
• Ligaments attaching ribs to the sternum or spinal column.
• Soft tissues surrounding the site, including periosteum (covering of bone), nerves, tendons, blood vessels and connective tissues.

SIGNS & SYMPTOMS
• Excruciating pain at the time of injury.
• Loss of function of the injured rib, causing breathing difficulty.
• Severe pain when moving.
• Visible deformity (lump) if the dislocated bones have locked in the dislocated positions. Bones may spontaneously reposition themselves and leave no deformity, but damage is the same.
• Tenderness over the dislocation.
• Swelling and bruising over the rib.
• Pain when taking a deep breath, coughing or laughing.

• Numbness or paralysis of other ribs below the dislocation or subluxation from pressure, pinching or cutting of blood vessels or nerves.

CAUSES
• Direct blow to the ribs.
• End result of a severe rib sprain.

RISK INCREASES WITH
• Contact sports, especially football, boxing, wrestling, basketball or hockey.
• Previous rib dislocation or sprain.
• Repeated chest injury.
• Poor muscle conditioning.

HOW TO PREVENT
• Build your overall strength and muscle tone with a long-term conditioning program appropriate for your sport.
• Warm up adequately before physical activity.
• After healing, wear protective devices, such as wrapped elastic bandages or a special rib vest, to prevent reinjury during participation in contact sports.
• Consider avoiding contact sports if treatment is unsuccessful in restoring strong normal rib connections.

 WHAT TO EXPECT

APPROPRIATE HEALTH CARE
• Doctor's treatment.

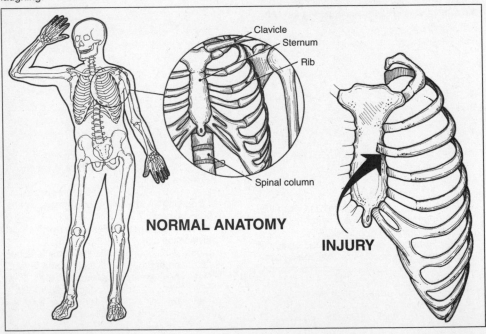

Clavicle
Sternum
Rib
Spinal column

NORMAL ANATOMY

INJURY

- Surgery (rare) to restore the rib to its normal position and repair torn ligaments and tendons.

DIAGNOSTIC MEASURES
- Your own observation of symptoms.
- Medical history and exam by a doctor.
- X-rays of the chest and spine.

POSSIBLE COMPLICATIONS
At the time of injury:
- Shock.
- Pressure or damage to nearby nerves, ligaments, tendons, muscles, blood vessels or connective tissues.
- Injury to the underlying lung.

After treatment or surgery:
- Excessive internal bleeding.
- Impaired blood supply to the dislocated area.
- Death of bone cells due to interruption of the blood supply (avascular necrosis).
- Infection introduced during surgical treatment.
- Continuing dislocations, often with progressively less provocation.
- Prolonged healing if activity is resumed too soon.
- Unstable or arthritic rib joints following repeated injury or permanent prominence at the injury site.

PROBABLE OUTCOME—After the dislocation has been corrected, the chest may require an elasticized bandage. Injured ligaments require a minimum of 6 weeks to heal.

 ## HOW TO TREAT

NOTE—Follow your doctor's instructions. These instructions are supplemental.

FIRST AID
- Use instructions for R.I.C.E., the first letters of *rest, ice, compression* and *elevation*. See Appendix 1 for details.
- The doctor may manipulate the dislocated rib to return it to its normal position. Manipulation should be done within 6 hours, if possible. After that time, internal bleeding and displacement of body fluids may lead to shock. Also, many tissues lose their elasticity and become difficult to return to their normal positions.

CONTINUING CARE—At home:
- Use an ice pack 3 or 4 times a day. Wrap ice chips or cubes in a plastic bag, and wrap the bag in a moist towel. Place it over the injured area for 20 minutes at a time.
- After 72 hours, apply heat instead of ice if it feels better. Use heat lamps, hot soaks, hot showers, heating pads or heat liniments and ointments.
- Take whirlpool treatments, if available.
- If directed, wrap the injured chest with an elasticized bandage between treatments.

- Massage gently and often to provide comfort and decrease swelling.

MEDICATION—Your doctor may prescribe:
- General anesthesia or muscle relaxants to make joint manipulation possible.
- Acetaminophen to relieve moderate pain.
- Stronger pain relievers for severe pain.
- Stool softeners after manipulation to prevent constipation due to decreased activity.
- Antibiotics to fight infection if surgery is necessary.

ACTIVITY
- Begin reconditioning the chest area after clearance from your doctor.
- If surgery is necessary, resume normal activities and reconditioning gradually after surgery.

DIET
- Do not eat or drink before manipulation or surgery to correct the dislocation. Fluid or solid food in your stomach makes vomiting while under general anesthesia more hazardous.
- During recovery, balance the amount of food you eat with any change in your level of physical activity. Eat a variety of foods to get the energy, protein, vitamins, minerals and fiber you need for good health and healing. Your doctor may suggest vitamin and mineral supplements to promote healing.

REHABILITATION
- Begin daily rehabilitation exercises when supportive wrapping is no longer needed.
- Use ice massage for 10 minutes before and after workouts. Fill a large styrofoam cup with water and freeze. Tear a small amount of foam from the top so ice protrudes. Massage firmly in a circle over the injured area.
- See Rehabilitation section for upper back exercises.

 ## CALL YOUR DOCTOR IF

- Any of the following occurs after chest injury: The skin of the chest wall becomes numb, pale or cold.
  You experience nausea or vomiting.
  You feel very short of breath or have an extreme hunger for air.
- Any of the following occurs after surgery: Increasing pain, swelling or drainage in the surgical area.
  Numbness or loss of feeling below the dislocation site.
  Signs of infection (headache, muscle aches, dizziness or a general ill feeling and fever).
- New, unexplained symptoms develop. Drugs used in treatment may produce side effects.
- Rib dislocations that you can "pop" back into normal position occur repeatedly.

RIB FRACTURE

GENERAL INFORMATION

DEFINITION—A complete or incomplete fracture of any of the 12 ribs on either side. Most rib fractures are accompanied by sprain or rupture of muscles, tendons or ligaments between the ribs (intercostal structures). Rib fractures are relatively common injuries in athletes, particularly those who compete in contact sports.

BODY PARTS INVOLVED
- Any one or several of the 12 ribs.
- Soft tissues surrounding the fracture site, including nerves, tendons, ligaments, cartilage and blood vessels.

SIGNS & SYMPTOMS
- Severe pain at the fracture site.
- Tenderness to the touch.
- A feeling that the "wind has been knocked out" of you (sometimes).
- Abdominal pain if the fractured ribs are below the diaphragm (the 11th and 12th ribs).
- Severe chest pain when coughing, sneezing or breathing deeply.
- A feeling of small air pockets under the skin of the chest or neck it the lung has been injured and leaked air.
- Swelling and bruising over the fracture site.

CAUSES
- Direct blow to the chest from a blunt object, such as an arm or elbow.
- Compression of the chest, as when a player falls on his side with a ball or helmet between him and the ground or when a player is crushed in a pile-up.

RISK INCREASES WITH
- Contact sports (especially football, hockey, boxing, wrestling or rugby) and weightlifting.
- History of bone or joint disease.
- Poor nutrition, especially calcium deficiency.
- If surgery is needed to remove air or blood from the chest, surgical risk increases with smoking and use of drugs, including mind-altering drugs, muscle relaxants, antihypertensives, tranquilizers, sleep inducers, insulin, sedatives, beta-adrenergic blockers or corticosteroids.

HOW TO PREVENT—No specific preventive measures. The chance of reinjury can be minimized by using a chest support or binder that has a rigid pad in it to prevent a direct blow to the injured area.

WHAT TO EXPECT

APPROPRIATE HEALTH CARE
- Doctor's diagnosis.

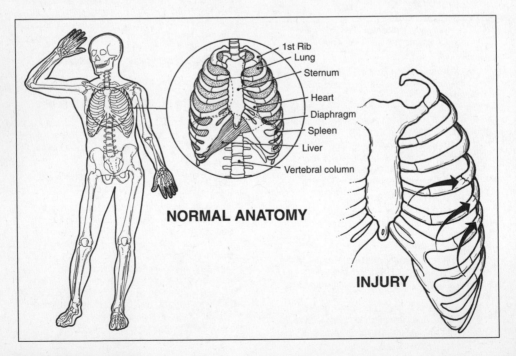

1st Rib
Lung
Sternum
Heart
Diaphragm
Spleen
Liver
Vertebral column

NORMAL ANATOMY

INJURY

- Application of a wide elastic wrap or chest binder to decrease movement of the chest muscles and reduce pain with breathing. The binder should be applied around the lower chest beneath the breasts, even if the rib fracture is in the upper chest.
- Hospitalization if symptoms of injury to the lung, spleen or liver appear. Blood or air in the chest may need to be removed if the lung is punctured by the raw edge of a fractured rib. A lacerated liver may need to be surgically repaired. A ruptured spleen frequently requires surgical removal.

DIAGNOSTIC MEASURES
- Your own observation of symptoms.
- Medical history and exam by a doctor.
- X-rays of the ribs and vertebral column. Early x-rays may not show fractures if they are not dislocated, but repeat x-rays taken 4 or more days later usually reveal them. The early treatment for an uncomplicated rib fracture is the same as for bruised ribs, so a delay in diagnosis does not hinder treatment.

POSSIBLE COMPLICATIONS
- Rupture of the lung, with bleeding or escape of air into the chest wall or under the skin in the neck.
- Pneumonia (pain with rib motion prevents deep breathing and coughing, so secretions may build up and lead to pneumonia).
- Injury to the liver if the right 11th and 12th ribs are fractured and have jagged edges.
- Injury or rupture of the spleen if the 11th and 12th ribs on the left are fractured and have jagged edges.
- Prolonged pain and slow healing.

PROBABLE OUTCOME—If this is a first-time chest injury and there are no complications of internal injury, proper care and sufficient healing time before resuming contact sports should prevent later complications. Healing is usually complete in 4 to 6 weeks.

 HOW TO TREAT

NOTE—Follow your doctor's instructions. These instructions are supplemental.

FIRST AID—With uncomplicated rib fractures, no first aid is necessary. If injury to the lung, liver or spleen is suspected, seek emergency medical help.

CONTINUING CARE
- Use the binder or wrap as long as needed for pain and support—usually 4 to 6 weeks.
- Use an ice pack 3 or 4 times a day. Place ice chips in a plastic bag. Wrap the bag in a moist towel, and place over the injured area. Use for 20 minutes at a time.
- After 2 or 3 days, if heat is more soothing than ice, use heat lamps, hot soaks, hot showers or heating pads.
- Attempt deep breathing and light coughing to help clear secretions.

MEDICATION
- For minor discomfort, you may use:
  Aspirin, acetaminophen or ibuprofen.
  Topical liniments and ointments.
- Your doctor may prescribe:
  Stronger pain relievers.
  Injection of a long-acting local anesthesia into the fracture site to reduce pain and allow normal breathing and coughing.

ACTIVITY—Resume your normal activities gradually after clearance from your doctor.

DIET—During recovery, balance the amount of food you eat with any change in your level of physical activity. Eat a variety of foods to get the energy, protein, vitamins, minerals and fiber you need for good health and healing.

REHABILITATION—None. Continue exercising uninjured parts during recovery.

 CALL YOUR DOCTOR IF

- You have symptoms of a fractured rib.
- Any of the following occurs after diagnosis:
  Shortness of breath.
  Uncontrollable chest pain.
  Sudden or severe abdominal pain.
  Nausea or vomiting.
  Swelling of the abdomen.
  New, unexplained symptoms. Drugs used in treatment may produce side effects.

RIB SPRAIN
(Costochondral Sprain; Costal-Vertebral Sprain)

 GENERAL INFORMATION

DEFINITION—Violent overstretching of one or more ligaments where ribs attach to the vertebral column in the back or the breastbone (sternum) in the front. Sprains involving two or more ligaments cause considerably more disability than single-ligament sprains. When the ligament is overstretched, it becomes tense and gives way at its weakest point, either where it attaches to bone or within the ligament itself. If the ligament pulls loose a fragment of bone, it is called an avulsion fracture. There are 3 types at sprains:
- Mild (Grade I)—Tearing of some ligament fibers. There is no loss of function.
- Moderate (Grade II)—Rupture of a portion of the ligament, resulting in some loss of function.
- Severe (Grade III)—Complete rupture of the ligament or complete separation of ligament from bone. There is total loss of function. A severe sprain may require surgical repair.

BODY PARTS INVOLVED
- Ligaments attaching ribs to the vertebral column or to cartilage of the breastbone.
- Tissues surrounding the sprain, including blood vessels, tendons, bone, periosteum (covering of bone) and muscles.

SIGNS & SYMPTOMS
- Severe pain at the time of injury.
- A feeling of popping or tearing at the injury site.
- Swelling and tenderness over the injury.
- Bruising that appears soon after injury.
- Pain when rotating the body, coughing, sneezing or breathing deeply.

CAUSES—Stress on a ligament, temporarily forcing or prying ligaments attached to ribs out of their normal location (usually caused by a direct blow to the chest wall with a blunt instrument).

RISK INCREASES WITH
- Contact sports.
- Gymnastics.
- Skiing.
- Crewing.
- Previous back or chest injury.
- Obesity.
- Poor muscle conditioning.
- Inadequate protection from equipment, especially shoulder pads.

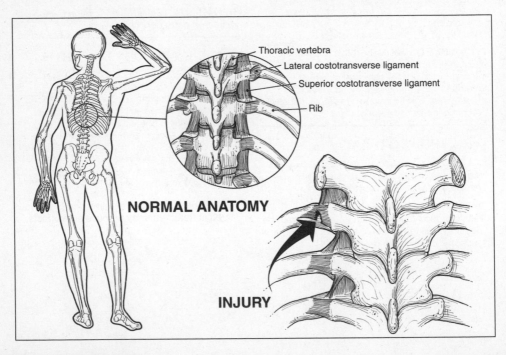

Thoracic vertebra
Lateral costotransverse ligament
Superior costotransverse ligament
Rib

NORMAL ANATOMY

INJURY

HOW TO PREVENT
- Participate in a strengthening, flexibility and conditioning program appropriate for your sport.
- Warm up before practice or competition.
- Wear protective equipment appropriate for your sport.

 WHAT TO EXPECT

APPROPRIATE HEALTH CARE
- Doctor's diagnosis.
- Application of an elastic bandage or rib belt.
- Self-care during rehabilitation.
- Physical therapy (moderate or severe sprain).

DIAGNOSTIC MEASURES
- Your own observation of symptoms.
- Medical history and exam by a doctor.
- X-rays of the ribs and injury site to rule out fractures.

POSSIBLE COMPLICATIONS
- Prolonged healing time if usual activities are resumed too soon.
- Proneness to repeated injury.
- Inflammation at the ligament attachment to bone (periostitis).
- Prolonged disability (sometimes).
- Unstable or arthritic rib attachment to the sternum or vertebra following repeated injury.

PROBABLE OUTCOME—If this is a first-time injury, proper care and sufficient healing time before resuming activity should prevent permanent disability. Ligaments have a poor blood supply, and torn ligaments require as much healing time as fractures. Average healing times are:
- Mild sprains—2 to 6 weeks.
- Moderate sprains—6 to 8 weeks.
- Severe sprains—8 to 10 weeks.

 HOW TO TREAT

NOTE—Follow your doctor's instructions. These instructions are supplemental.

FIRST AID—Use instructions for R.I.C.E., the first letters of *rest, ice, compression* and *elevation*. See Appendix 1 for details.

CONTINUING CARE
- If your doctor fits you with an elastic wrap, rib belt or rib binder, continue to use it for pain and support—usually 4 to 6 weeks.

- Use an ice pack 3 or 4 times a day. Wrap ice chips or cubes in a plastic bag. Wrap the bag in a moist towel, and place it over the injured area. Use for 20 minutes at a time.
- After 72 hours, apply heat instead at ice if it feels better. Use heat lamps, hot soaks, hot showers, heating pads or heat liniments and ointments.
- Take whirlpool treatments, if available.
- Massage gently and often to provide comfort and decrease swelling.

MEDICATION
- For minor discomfort, you may use:
  Aspirin, acetaminophen or ibuprofen.
  Topical liniments and ointments.
- Your doctor may prescribe:
  Stronger pain relievers.
  Injection of a long-acting local anesthetic to reduce pain.
  Injections of a corticosteroid, such as triamcinolone, to reduce inflammation.

ACTIVITY—Resume your normal activities gradually after clearance from your doctor.

DIET—During recovery, balance the amount of food you eat with any change in your level of physical activity. Eat a variety of foods to get the energy, protein, vitamins, minerals and fiber you need for good health and healing.

REHABILITATION
- Begin daily rehabilitation exercises when supportive wrapping is no longer necessary.
- Use ice massage for 10 minutes before and after exercise. Fill a large styrofoam cup with water and freeze. Tear a small amount of foam from the top so ice protrudes. Massage firmly over the injured area in a circle about the size of a softball.
- See Rehabilitation section for upper back exercises.

 CALL YOUR DOCTOR IF

- You have symptoms of a moderate or severe rib sprain or a mild sprain persists longer than 2 weeks.
- Pain, swelling or bruising worsens despite treatment.
- New, unexplained symptoms develop. Drugs used in treatment may produce side effects.

RIB STRAIN
(Intercostal Muscle Strain)

GENERAL INFORMATION

DEFINITION—Injury to any of the muscles or tendons that attach to the ribs. Muscles, tendons and their attached ribs comprise contractile units. The units stabilize the chest, breastbone and upper spine and allow their motion. A strain occurs at the weakest part of a unit. Strains are of 3 types:
- Mild (Grade I)—Slightly pulled muscle without tearing of muscle or tendon fibers. There is no loss of strength.
- Moderate (Grade II)—Tearing of fibers in a muscle or tendon or at the attachment to a rib. Strength is diminished.
- Severe (Grade III)—Rupture of the muscle-tendon-rib attachment, with separation of fibers. A severe strain may require surgical repair. Chronic strains are caused by overuse. Acute strains are caused by direct injury or overstress.

BODY PARTS INVOLVED
- Tendons and muscles of the chest, back and abdomen that attach to any of the ribs.
- Ribs.
- Soft tissues surrounding the strain, including nerves, periosteum (covering of bone), blood vessels and lymph vessels.

SIGNS & SYMPTOMS
- Pain with motion, breathing, coughing or stretching.
- Muscle spasm.
- Tenderness to the touch.
- Swelling.
- Crepitation ("crackling" feeling and sound when the injured area is pressed with fingers).
- Calcification of the muscle or tendon (visible with x-rays).
- Loss of strength (moderate or severe strain).

CAUSES
- Prolonged overuse of muscle-tendon units that attach to the ribs.
- Single violent injury or force applied to the muscle-tendon units in the chest.

RISK INCREASES WITH
- Contact sports such as wrestling.
- Weightlifting.
- Any cardiovascular medical problem that results in decreased circulation.
- Medical history of any bleeding disorder.
- Obesity.
- Poor nutrition.
- Previous rib injury.
- Poor muscle conditioning.

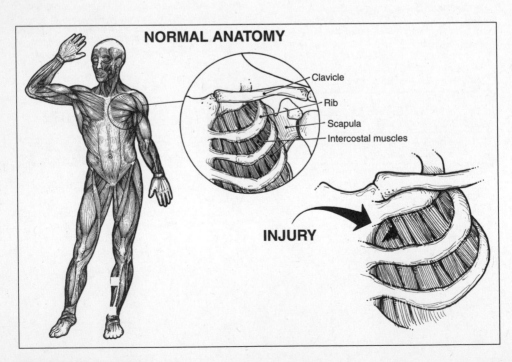

NORMAL ANATOMY

Clavicle
Rib
Scapula
Intercostal muscles

INJURY

HOW TO PREVENT
• Participate in a strengthening and conditioning program appropriate for your sport.
• Warm up before practice or competition.
• To prevent a recurrence, tape the rib area before practice or competition.

 # WHAT TO EXPECT

APPROPRIATE HEALTH CARE
• Doctor's diagnosis.
• Application of tape or elastic wrap (sometimes).
• Self-care during rehabilitation.
• Physical therapy (moderate or severe strain).
• Surgery (rare).

DIAGNOSTIC MEASURES
• Your own observation of symptoms.
• Medical history and exam by a doctor.
• X-rays of the chest to rule out fractures.

POSSIBLE COMPLICATIONS
• Prolonged healing time if activity is resumed too soon.
• Proneness to repeated injury.
• Inflammation at the attachment to the rib (periostitis).

PROBABLE OUTCOME—Most rib strains are more painful than disabling. If this is a first-time injury, proper care and sufficient healing time before resuming activity should prevent permanent disability. Average healing times are:
• Mild strain—2 to 10 days.
• Moderate strain—10 days to 6 weeks.
• Severe strain—6 to 10 weeks.

 # HOW TO TREAT

NOTE—Follow your doctor's instructions. These instructions are supplemental.

FIRST AID—Use instructions for R.I.C.E., the first letters of *rest, ice, compression* and *elevation* (if possible). See Appendix 1 for details.

CONTINUING CARE
• Continue ice massage 3 or 4 times a day for 15 minutes at a time. Fill a large styrofoam cup with water and freeze. Tear a small amount of foam from the top so ice protrudes. Massage firmly over the injured area in a circle about the size of a softball.
• After the first 24 hours, apply heat instead of ice if it feels better. Use heat lamps, hot soaks, hot showers, heating pads or heat liniments and ointments.
• Take whirlpool treatments, if available.
• Wrap the injured chest cage with an elasticized bandage or rib belt between treatments.
• Massage gently and often to provide comfort and decrease swelling.

MEDICATION
• For minor discomfort, you may use:
Aspirin, acetaminophen or ibuprofen.
Topical liniments and ointments.
• Your doctor may prescribe:
Stronger pain relievers.
Injection of a long-acting local anesthetic to reduce pain (rare).
Injections of corticosteroids, such as triamcinolone, to reduce inflammation (rare).

ACTIVITY—Resume your normal activities gradually after treatment.

DIET—During recovery, balance the amount of food you eat with any change in your level of physical activity. Eat a variety of foods to get the energy, protein, vitamins, minerals and fiber you need for good health and healing.

REHABILITATION—Begin daily rehabilitation exercises when supportive wrapping is no longer needed. Use ice massage for 10 minutes prior to exercises. See Rehabilitation section for upper back exercises.

 # CALL YOUR DOCTOR IF

• You have symptoms of a moderate or severe rib strain or a mild strain persists longer than 10 days.
• Pain or swelling worsens despite treatment.

SHOULDER BLADE (SCAPULA) BURSITIS

GENERAL INFORMATION

DEFINITION—Inflammation of any of the bursas of the scapula (shoulder blade). Bursitis may vary in degree from mild irritation to an abscess formation that causes excruciating pain. There are several bursas around the body of the scapula. Scapula bursitis develops most frequently in the bursa between the body of the scapula and the muscles of the chest wall.

BODY PARTS INVOLVED
● Scapula bursas (soft sacs filled with lubricating fluid that facilitate motion in the scapula area).
● Soft tissues surrounding the scapula, including nerves, tendons, ligaments, large blood vessels, capillaries, periosteum (the outside lining of bone) and muscles.

SIGNS & SYMPTOMS
● Pain around or under the scapula.
● Tenderness.
● Swelling.
● Redness (sometimes) over the affected bursa.
● Fever if infection is present.
● Limitation of motion in the scapula area, including the shoulder.

CAUSES
● Injury to the scapula.
● Acute or chronic infection.
● Arthritis.
● Gout.
● Unknown (frequently).

RISK INCREASES WITH
● Participation in competitive athletics, particularly contact sports such as football.
● Previous history of bursitis in any joint.
● Exposure to cold weather.
● Poor conditioning and inadequate warmup.
● Inadequate protective equipment in contact sports.

HOW TO PREVENT
● Use protective gear for contact sports.
● Warm up adequately before athletic practice or competition.
● Wear warm clothing in cold weather.
● To prevent recurrence, continue to wear extra protection over the scapula until healing is complete.

WHAT TO EXPECT

APPROPRIATE HEALTH CARE
● Doctor's diagnosis and treatment.
● Surgery (sometimes), particularly for a frozen joint.

DIAGNOSTIC MEASURES
● Your own observation of symptoms.
● Medical history and physical exam by a doctor.
● Acute or chronic infection.
● X-rays of the shoulder and scapula.

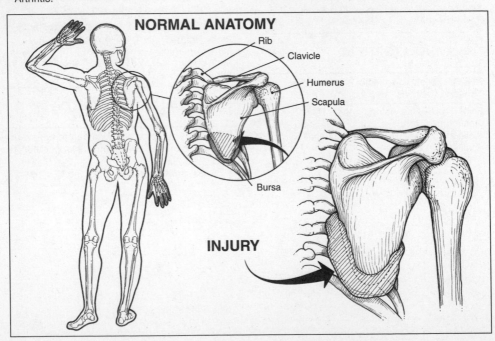

NORMAL ANATOMY

Rib

Clavicle

Humerus

Scapula

Bursa

INJURY

POSSIBLE COMPLICATIONS
• Frozen scapula, with temporary or permanent limitation of the normal mobility of both scapula and shoulder.
• Prolonged healing time if activity is resumed too soon.
• Proneness to repeated flare-ups.
• Spontaneous rupture of the bursa if severe infection is present.

PROBABLE OUTCOME—Scapula bursitis is a common problem. Symptoms usually subside in 7 to 14 days with treatment. Chronic bursitis may require 6 to 8 months to heal.

 ## HOW TO TREAT

NOTE—Follow your doctor's instructions. These instructions are supplemental.

FIRST AID—None. This problem develops slowly.

CONTINUING CARE
• Use ice massage. Fill a large styrofoam cup with water and freeze. Tear a small amount of foam from the top so ice protrudes. Massage firmly over the injured area in a circle about the size of a softball. Do this for 15 minutes at a time 3 or 4 times a day, and also before workouts or competition.
• After 72 hours of ice treatment, apply heat if it feels better. Use heat lamps, hot soaks, hot showers, heating pads or heat liniments and ointments.
• Use a sling to support the shoulder and scapula if needed.
• Elevate the inflamed scapula and shoulder above the level of the heart to reduce swelling and prevent accumulation of fluid. Use pillows for propping.
• Gentle massage will frequently provide comfort and decrease swelling.

MEDICATION—Your doctor may prescribe:
• Nonsteroidal anti-inflammatory drugs.
• Prescription pain relievers for severe pain. Use nonprescription aspirin, acetaminophen or ibuprofen (available under many trade names) for mild pain.
• Injections into the inflamed bursa of a long-lasting local anesthetic mixed with a corticosteroid drug such as triamcinolone.

ACTIVITY—Rest the inflamed area as much as possible. If you must resume normal activity immediately, use a sling to immobilize the shoulder and scapula and help reduce pain. To prevent a frozen shoulder, begin normal, slow joint movement as soon as possible.

DIET—During recovery, balance the amount of food you eat with any change in your level of physical activity. Eat a variety of foods to get the energy, protein, vitamins, minerals and fiber you need for good health and healing. Your doctor may suggest vitamin and mineral supplements to promote healing.

REHABILITATION—See Rehabilitation section for shoulder exercises.

 ## CALL YOUR DOCTOR IF

• You have symptoms of scapula bursitis.
• Pain increases despite treatment.
• Pain, swelling, tenderness, drainage or bleeding increases in the surgical area.
• You develop signs of infection (headache, muscle aches, dizziness or a general ill feeling and fever).
• New, unexplained symptoms develop. Drugs used in treatment may produce side effects.

SHOULDER BLADE (SCAPULA) CONTUSION

GENERAL INFORMATION

DEFINITION—Bruising of skin and underlying tissues caused by a direct blow to the scapula (shoulder blade). Contusions cause bleeding from ruptured small capillaries that allow blood to infiltrate muscles, tendons or other soft tissues.

BODY PARTS INVOLVED—Tissues surrounding the scapula, including blood vessels, tendons, nerves, covering of the bone (periosteum) and connective tissues between the scapula and the skin.

SIGNS & SYMPTOMS
- Local swelling—either superficial or deep.
- Pain and tenderness over the injury.
- Feeling of firmness when pressure is exerted on the injured area.
- Discoloration under the skin, beginning with redness and progressing to the characteristic "black-and-blue" bruise.
- Restricted shoulder blade motion proportional to the extent of injury.

CAUSES—Direct blow to the skin, usually from a blunt object.

RISK INCREASES WITH
- Contact sports, especially when the shoulder area is not adequately protected.
- Medical history of any bleeding disorder.
- Poor nutrition, including vitamin deficiency.
- Use of anticoagulants or aspirin.

HOW TO PREVENT—Wear appropriate protective gear and equipment, such as shoulder pads, during competition or other athletic activity if there is risk of a scapula contusion.

WHAT TO EXPECT

APPROPRIATE HEALTH CARE
- Doctor's care unless the contusion is quite small.
- Self-care for minor contusions and for serious contusions during the rehabilitation phase.
- Physical therapy following serious contusions.

DIAGNOSTIC MEASURES
- Your own observation of symptoms.
- Medical history and physical exam by a doctor for all except minor injuries.
- X-rays of the clavicle, shoulder and scapula to assess total injury to soft tissues and to rule out the possibility of underlying fractures. The total extent of injury may not be apparent for 48 to 72 hours.

POSSIBLE COMPLICATIONS
- Excessive bleeding, leading to disability. Infiltrative-type bleeding can (rarely) lead to calcification and impaired function of injured muscle.

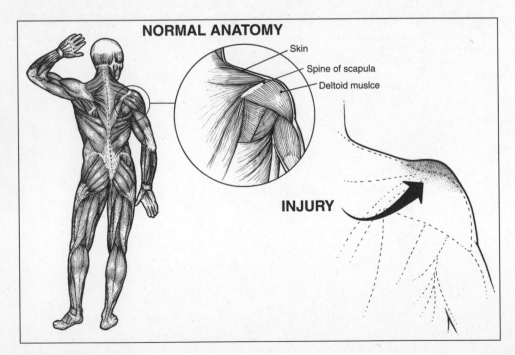

NORMAL ANATOMY

Skin

Spine of scapula

Deltoid muslce

INJURY

- Prolonged healing time if usual activities are resumed too soon.
- Infection if skin is broken over the contusion.

PROBABLE OUTCOME—Healing time varies with the extent of injury, but all but the most serious contusions should heal in 6 to 10 days.

 ## HOW TO TREAT

NOTE—Follow your doctor's instructions. These instructions are supplemental.

FIRST AID—Use instructions for R.I.C.E., the first letters of *rest, ice, compression* and *elevation*. See Appendix 1 for details.

CONTINUING CARE
- Use an ice pack 3 or 4 times a day. Wrap ice chips or cubes in a plastic bag, and wrap the bag in a moist towel. Place over the injured area for 20 minutes at a time.
- After 72 hours, apply heat instead of ice if it feels better. Use heat lamps, hot soaks, hot showers, heating pads, heat liniments and ointments or whirlpool treatments.
- Massage gently and often to provide comfort and decrease swelling.

MEDICATION
- For minor discomfort, you may use:
  Aspirin, acetaminophen or ibuprofen.
  Topical liniments and ointments.
- Your doctor may prescribe stronger medicine for pain.

ACTIVITY—Begin activities slowly, and stop exercise as soon as pain begins. Increase activity as healing progresses.

DIET—During recovery, balance the amount of food you eat with any change in your level of physical activity. Eat a variety of foods to get the energy, protein, vitamins, minerals and fiber you need for good health and healing.

REHABILITATION
- Begin daily rehabilitation exercises when pain subsides.
- Use ice massage for 10 minutes before and after workouts. Fill a large styrofoam cup with water and freeze. Tear a small amount of foam from the top so ice protrudes. Massage firmly over the injured area in a circle about the size of a softball.
- See Rehabilitation section for shoulder exercises.

 ## CALL YOUR DOCTOR IF

- You have a contusion that doesn't improve in 1 or 2 days.
- Skin is broken and signs of infection (drainage, increasing pain, fever, headache, muscle aches, dizziness or a general ill feeling) occur.

SHOULDER BLADE (SCAPULA) FRACTURE, ACROMION

GENERAL INFORMATION

DEFINITION—A complete or incomplete break of the acromion (the part of the shoulder blade that projects over the shoulder joint and forms the highest point of the shoulder).

BODY PARTS INVOLVED
- Acromion.
- Shoulder joint.
- Soft tissues around the fracture site, including nerves, tendons, ligaments and blood vessels.
- Broken ribs frequently accompany any scapula fracture.

SIGNS & SYMPTOMS
- Severe pain at the fracture site.
- Swelling of soft tissues around the fracture.
- Visible deformity if the fracture is complete and bone fragments separate enough to distort normal body contours.
- Tenderness to the touch.
- Numbness and coldness in the arm if the blood supply is impaired.

CAUSES
- Direct injury caused by an upward blow occurring at the same time as a shoulder dislocation. This can result in a major injury requiring surgery for repair.
- Indirect stress caused by twisting or by a violent muscle contraction.

RISK INCREASES WITH
- Contact sports such as football, soccer and hockey.
- A history of bone or joint disease.
- Obesity.
- Poor nutrition, especially calcium deficiency.
- If surgery or anesthesia is needed, risk increases with smoking and use of drugs, including mind-altering drugs, muscle relaxants, antihypertensives, tranquilizers, sleep inducers, insulin, sedatives, beta-adrenergic blockers or corticosteroids.

HOW TO PREVENT
- Participate in a strengthening, flexibility and conditioning program appropriate for your sport, especially a shoulder-strengthening and -conditioning program, prior to throwing sports.
- Use appropriate protective equipment, such as shoulder pads, for contact sports.

WHAT TO EXPECT

APPROPRIATE HEALTH CARE
- Doctor's treatment to manipulate and set the broken bones.
- Hospitalization (sometimes) for anesthesia and surgery to set the fracture.
- Self-care during rehabilitation.
- Whirlpool, ultrasound or massage (to displace excess fluid from the injured joint space).

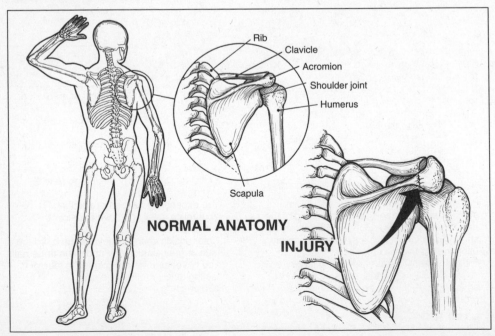

Rib
Clavicle
Acromion
Shoulder joint
Humerus
Scapula

NORMAL ANATOMY

INJURY

DIAGNOSTIC MEASURES
- Your own observation of symptoms.
- Medical history and physical exam by a doctor.
- X-rays of injured areas.

POSSIBLE COMPLICATIONS
At the time of injury:
- Shock.
- Pressure on or injury to nearby nerves, ligaments, tendons, muscles, blood vessels or connective tissues.

After treatment or surgery:
- Delayed union or nonunion of the fracture.
- Impaired blood supply to the fracture site.
- Arrest of normal bone growth in children.
- Infection in open fractures (skin broken over fracture site) or at the incision if surgical setting was necessary.
- Shortening of the injured bones.
- Unstable or arthritic joint following repeated injury.
- Prolonged healing time if activity is resumed too soon.
- Proneness to repeated injury.

PROBABLE OUTCOME—The average healing time for this fracture is 6 to 8 weeks. Healing is considered complete when there is no motion at the fracture site and when x-rays show complete bone union.

 ## HOW TO TREAT

NOTE—Follow your doctor's instructions. These instructions are supplemental.

FIRST AID
- Keep the person warm with blankets to decrease the possibility of shock.
- Cut away clothing, if possible, but don't move the injured area to do so.
- Follow instructions for R.I.C.E., the first letters of *rest, ice, compression* and *elevation*. See Appendix 1 for details.
- The doctor will set the broken bones with surgery or, if possible, without. Manipulation should be done as soon as possible after injury. Many tissues lose their elasticity and become difficult to return to their normal positions.

CONTINUING CARE
- Immobilization will be necessary. A firm compression bandage plus suspension of the arm in a sling usually supplies satisfactory support and immobilization. Casts are rarely used for this injury.
- Use frequent ice massage. Fill a large styrofoam cup with water and freeze. Tear a small amount of foam from the top so ice protrudes. Massage firmly over the injured area in a circle about the size of a baseball. Do this for 15 minutes at a time 3 or 4 times a day, and also before workouts or competition.
- After 48 hours, application of localized heat promotes healing by increasing blood circulation in the injured area. Use hot baths, showers, compresses, heat lamps, heating pads, heat ointments and liniments or whirlpools.

MEDICATION—Your doctor may prescribe:
- General anesthesia, local anesthesia or muscle relaxants to make bone manipulation and fixation of bone fragments possible.
- Strong pain relievers for severe pain.
- Stool softeners to prevent constipation due to inactivity.
- Acetaminophen (available without prescription) for mild pain after initial treatment.

ACTIVITY
- Actively exercise all muscle groups not immobilized. Muscle contractions promote fracture alignment and hasten healing.
- Resume normal activities gradually after treatment.
- Begin reconditioning the injured area after clearance from your doctor.

DIET—During recovery, balance the amount of food you eat with any change in your level of physical activity. Eat a variety of foods to get the energy, protein, vitamins, minerals and fiber you need for good health and healing.

REHABILITATION—Begin daily rehabilitation exercises when movement is comfortable. Use ice massage for 10 minutes prior to exercise. See Rehabilitation section for shoulder exercises.

 ## CALL YOUR DOCTOR IF

- You have signs or symptoms of a shoulder blade injury.
- Any of the following occurs after surgery or treatment:
  Pain, swelling or drainage increases in the surgical area.
  You develop signs of infection (headache, muscle aches, dizziness or a general ill feeling and fever).
  You experience nausea or vomiting.
  You notice swelling above or below the bandage.
  Color of skin changes beyond the bandage to blue or gray, particularly under the fingernails.
  You have numbness or complete loss of feeling below the fracture site.
  You become constipated.

SHOULDER BLADE (SCAPULA) FRACTURE, CORACOID PROCESS

GENERAL INFORMATION

DEFINITION—A compete or incomplete break in the coracoid process of the scapula (shoulder blade).

BODY PARTS INVOLVED
- Scapula.
- Shoulder joint.
- Soft tissues around the fracture site, including nerves, tendons, ligaments and blood vessels.

SIGNS & SYMPTOMS
- Severe pain at the fracture site.
- Swelling of soft tissues around the fracture.
- Tenderness to the touch.

CAUSES—Direct blow or indirect stress to the bone. Indirect stress may be caused by twisting ligaments, tendons, muscles, blood vessels or violent muscle contraction.

RISK INCREASES WITH
- Contact sports such as football, soccer or hockey.
- History of bone or joint disease, especially osteoporosis.
- Poor nutrition, especially calcium deficiency.

HOW TO PREVENT
- Build your strength with a good conditioning program before beginning regular athletic practice or competition. Increased muscle mass helps protect bones and underlying tissues.
- Use appropriate protective equipment.

WHAT TO EXPECT

APPROPRIATE HEALTH CARE
- Doctor's diagnosis.
- Self-care during rehabilitation.

DIAGNOSTIC MEASURES
- Your own observation of symptoms.
- Medical history and physical exam by a doctor.
- X-rays of injured areas.

POSSIBLE COMPLICATIONS
At the time of injury:
- Shock.
- Pressure on or injury to nearby nerves, ligaments, tendons, muscles, blood vessels or connective tissues.

After treatment or surgery:
- Delayed union or nonunion of the fracture.
- Impaired blood supply to the fracture site.
- Arrest of normal bone growth in children.
- Infection in open fractures (skin broken over fracture site) or at the incision if surgical setting was necessary.

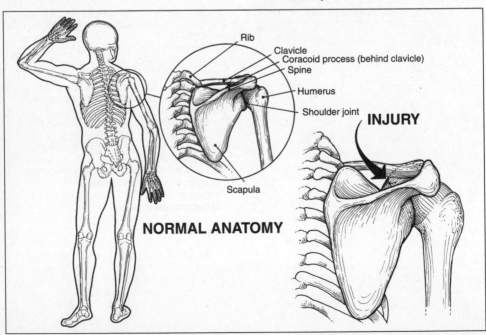

Rib
Clavicle
Coracoid process (behind clavicle)
Spine
Humerus
Shoulder joint
INJURY
Scapula
NORMAL ANATOMY

- Shortening of the injured bones.
- Unstable or arthritic joint following repeated injury
- Prolonged healing time if activity is resumed too soon.
- Proneness to repeated injury.

PROBABLE OUTCOME—It is impossible to predict exactly how long it will take for any fracture to heal. Variable factors include age, sex and previous state of health and conditioning. The average healing time for this fracture is 8 to 10 weeks. Healing is complete when there is no motion at the fracture site and when x-rays show complete bone union.

 ## HOW TO TREAT

NOTE—Follow your doctor's instructions. These instructions are supplemental.

FIRST AID
- Keep the person warm with blankets to decrease the possibility of shock.
- Cut away clothing, if possible. Don't move the injured area to do so.
- Follow instructions for R.I.C.E., the first letters of *rest, ice, compression* and *elevation.* See Appendix 1 for details.

CONTINUING CARE
After injury:
- If bone fragments are displaced, the doctor will set the broken bones with surgery or, if possible, without. The bones should be set as soon as possible after injury. Many tissues lose their elasticity and become difficult to return to their normal positions.
- If bone fragments are not displaced, these fractures require only simple treatment and heal relatively quickly. The strong muscles that attach to and surround the scapula usually prevent the displacement of the fractured parts.
- Immobilization with a compression bandage and sling will be necessary for 14 days.
- After 45 hours, application of localized heat promotes healing by increasing blood circulation in the injured area. Use hot baths, showers, compresses, heat lamps, heating pads or heat ointments and liniments.

After immobilization:
- Use ice massage. Fill a large styrofoam cup with water and freeze. Tear a small amount of foam from the top so ice protrudes. Massage firmly over the injured area in a circle about the size of a baseball. Do this for 15 minutes at a time 3 or 4 times a day, and also before workouts or competition.

MEDICATION—Your doctor may prescribe:
- Strong pain relievers for severe pain.
- Stool softeners to prevent constipation due to inactivity.
- Acetaminophen (available without prescription) for mild pain after initial treatment.

ACTIVITY
- Actively exercise all muscle groups not immobilized. Muscle contractions promote fracture alignment and hasten healing.
- Resume normal activities gradually after treatment.
- Begin reconditioning the injured area after clearance from your doctor.

DIET—During recovery, balance the amount of food you eat with any change in your level of physical activity. Eat a variety of foods to get the energy, protein, vitamins, minerals and fiber you need for good health and healing.

REHABILITATION—Use ice massage for 10 minutes prior to exercise. See Rehabilitation section for shoulder exercises.

 ## CALL YOUR DOCTOR IF

- You have signs or symptoms of a shoulder blade fracture.
- Any of the following occurs after surgery or treatment:
  Pain, swelling or drainage increases in the surgical area.
  You develop signs of infection (headache, muscle aches, dizziness or a general ill feeling and fever).
  You experience nausea or vomiting.
  You notice swelling above or below the compression bandage.
  You have numbness or complete loss of feeling below the fracture site.
  Pain continues for more than 6 weeks.
  You become constipated.

SHOULDER BLADE (SCAPULA) FRACTURE, GLENOID FOSSA

GENERAL INFORMATION

DEFINITION—A complete or incomplete break in the glenoid fossa of the scapula (shoulder blade). The glenoid fossa functions as a receptacle—like a socket—for the upper end of the humerus (the large bone between the elbow and the shoulder). The glenoid fossa, along with bones, tendons, joint capsules and other soft tissues, forms the shoulder.

BODY PARTS INVOLVED
- Glenoid fossa of the scapula.
- Shoulder joint.
- Soft tissues around the fracture site, including nerves, tendons, ligaments, joint membranes and capsules and blood vessels.

SIGNS & SYMPTOMS
- Severe pain at the fracture site.
- Swelling of soft tissues around the fracture.
- Visible deformity if the fracture is complete and the bone fragments separate enough to distort normal body contours.
- Tenderness to the touch.
- Numbness in the arm and hand (sometimes).
- 1

CAUSES
- Direct injury—A direct blow to the side of the shoulder produces a star-shaped minor fracture of the glenoid fossa.
- Indirect injury—Falling on a bent elbow can fracture the glenoid fossa.

RISK INCREASES WITH
- Participation in contact sports such as football, soccer or hockey.
- History of bone or joint disease, especially osteoporosis.
- Obesity.
- Poor nutrition, especially calcium deficiency.
- If surgery or anesthesia is needed, risk increases with smoking and use of drugs, including mind-altering drugs, muscle relaxants, antihypertensives, tranquilizers, sleep inducers, insulin, sedatives, beta-adrenergic blockers or corticosteroids.

HOW TO PREVENT
- Build your strength with a good conditioning program before beginning regular athletic practice or competition. Increased muscle mass helps protect bones and underlying tissues.
- Try to avoid falling on a bent elbow.
- Use appropriate protective equipment, such as shoulder pads, for contact sports.

WHAT TO EXPECT

APPROPRIATE HEALTH CARE
- Doctor's treatment to manipulate and set the broken bones.

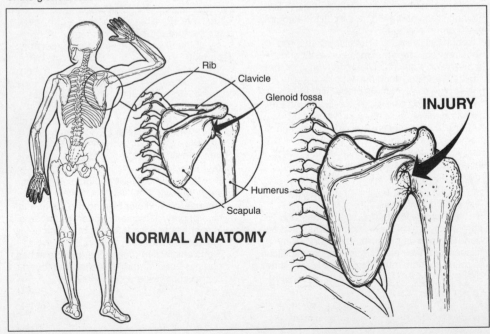

Rib
Clavicle
Glenoid fossa
Humerus
Scapula

NORMAL ANATOMY

INJURY

- Anesthesia and surgery to set bones for all except minimal fractures without displacement.
- Self-care during rehabilitation.
- Ultrasound or massage (to displace excess fluid from the injured joint space).

DIAGNOSTIC MEASURES
- Your own observation of symptoms.
- Medical history and physical exam by a doctor.
- X-rays of injured areas.

POSSIBLE COMPLICATIONS
At the time of injury:
- Shock.
- Pressure on or injury to nearby nerves, ligaments, tendons, muscles, blood vessels or connective tissues.

After treatment or surgery:
- Delayed union or nonunion of the fracture.
- Impaired blood supply to the fracture site.
- Arrest of normal bone growth in children.
- Infection in open fractures (skin broken over fracture site) or at the incision if surgical setting was necessary.
- Shortening of the injured bones.
- Unstable or arthritic joint due to extension of fracture into the cartilage surface of the joint.
- Prolonged healing time if activity is resumed too soon.
- Proneness to repeated injury.

PROBABLE OUTCOME—It is impossible to predict exactly how long it will take for any fracture to heal. Variable factors include age, sex and previous state of health and conditioning. The average healing time for this fracture is 8 to 10 weeks. Healing is complete when there is no motion at the fracture site and when x-rays show complete bone union.

 # HOW TO TREAT

NOTE—Follow your doctor's instructions. These instructions are supplemental.

FIRST AID
- Keep the person warm with blankets to decrease the possibility of shock.
- Cut away clothing, if possible, but don't move the injured area to do so.
- Follow instructions for R.I.C.E., the first letters of *rest ice, compression* and *elevation*. See Appendix 1 for details.
- The doctor will set the broken bones with surgery or, if possible, without. This should be done as soon as possible after injury. Many tissues lose their elasticity and become difficult to return to their normal positions. Most injuries to the glenoid fossa require surgical treatment.

CONTINUING CARE
- Immobilization will be necessary. Wearing a triangular sling for 3 to 4 weeks is usually sufficient.

- Use frequent ice massage. Fill a large styrofoam cup with water and freeze. Tear a small amount of foam from the top so ice protrudes. Massage firmly over the injured area in a circle about the size of a baseball. Do this for 15 minutes at a time 3 or 4 times a day, and also before workouts or competition.
- After 72 hours, application of localized heat promotes healing by increasing blood circulation in the injured area. Use hot baths, showers, compresses, heat lamps, heating pads or heat ointments and liniments.

MEDICATION—Your doctor may prescribe:
- General anesthesia, local anesthesia or muscle relaxants to make bone manipulation and fixation of bone fragments possible.
- Narcotic or synthetic narcotic pain relievers for severe pain.
- Stool softeners to prevent constipation due to inactivity.
- Acetaminophen (available without prescription) for mild pain after initial treatment.

ACTIVITY
- Actively exercise all muscle groups not immobilized. Muscle contractions promote fracture alignment and hasten healing.
- Resume normal activities gradually after treatment.
- Begin reconditioning the injured area after clearance from your doctor.

DIET—During recovery, balance the amount of food you eat with any change in your level of physical activity. Eat a variety of foods to get the energy, protein, vitamins, minerals and fiber you need for good health and healing.

REHABILITATION—Start shoulder exercises 2 weeks after injury. Use ice massage for 10 minutes prior to exercise. See Rehabilitation section for shoulder exercises.

 # CALL YOUR DOCTOR IF

- You have signs or symptoms of a shoulder blade fracture.
- Any of the following occurs after surgery or other treatment:
  Increased pain, swelling or drainage in the surgical area.
  Change in skin color beyond the fracture to blue or gray, particularly under the fingernails.
  Numbness or complete loss of feeling below the fracture site.
  Signs of infection (headache, muscle aches, dizziness or a general ill feeling and fever).
  Nausea or vomiting; constipation.

SHOULDER BLADE (SCAPULA) FRACTURE, NECK

GENERAL INFORMATION

DEFINITION—A complete or incomplete break in the neck of the scapula (shoulder blade). This injury results in marked displacement of the broken bone.

BODY PARTS INVOLVED
- Scapula; shoulder joint.
- Soft tissues around the fracture site, including nerves, tendons, ligaments, joint membranes and blood vessels.

SIGNS & SYMPTOMS
- Severe pain at the fracture site.
- Swelling of soft tissues around the fracture.
- Visible deformity if the fracture is complete and bone fragments separate enough to distort normal body contours.
- Tenderness to the touch.
- Numbness in the arm and hand (sometimes).
- Cold arm and hand if the blood supply is impaired.

CAUSES—Direct blow to or indirect stress on the bone. Indirect stress may be caused by twisting or violent muscle contraction.

RISK INCREASES WITH
- Contact sports such as football.
- History of bone or joint disease, especially osteoporosis.
- Poor nutrition, especially calcium deficiency.
- Obesity.
- If surgery or anesthesia is needed, risk increases with smoking and use of certain drugs.

HOW TO PREVENT
- Build your strength with a good conditioning program before beginning regular athletic practice or competition. Increased muscle mass helps protect bones and underlying tissues.
- Use appropriate protective equipment, such as shoulder pads, for contact sports.

WHAT TO EXPECT

APPROPRIATE HEALTH CARE
- Doctor's treatment to manipulate and set the broken bones.
- Hospitalization (sometimes) for anesthesia and surgery to set the fracture.
- Hospitalization for traction (sometimes).
- Self-care during rehabilitation.
- Ultrasound or massage after healing (to displace excess fluid from the injured joint space).

DIAGNOSTIC MEASURES
- Your own observation of symptoms.
- Medical history and exam by a doctor.
- X-rays of injured areas.

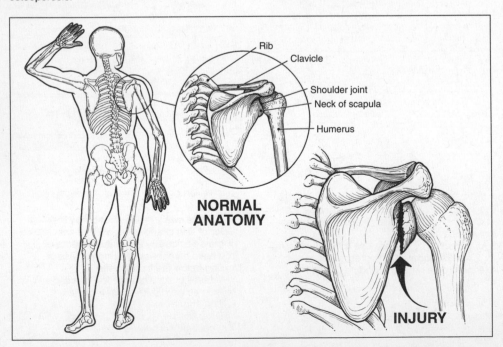

Rib
Clavicle
Shoulder joint
Neck of scapula
Humerus

NORMAL ANATOMY

INJURY

POSSIBLE COMPLICATIONS

At the time of injury:
- Shock.
- Pressure on or injury to nearby nerves, ligaments, tendons, muscles, blood vessels or connective tissues.

After treatment or surgery:
- Delayed union or nonunion of the fracture.
- Impaired blood supply to the fracture site.
- Arrest of normal bone growth in children.
- Infection in open fractures (skin broken over fracture site) or at the incision if surgical setting was necessary.
- Shortening of the injured bones.
- Unstable or arthritic joint if fracture also extends into the cartilage-lined joint surface of the glenoid.
- Prolonged healing time if activity is resumed too soon.
- Proneness to repeated injury.

PROBABLE OUTCOME—It is impossible to predict exactly how long it will take for any fracture to heal. Variable factors include age, sex and previous state of health and conditioning. The average healing time for this fracture is 6 to 8 weeks. Healing is complete when there is no motion at the fracture site and when x-rays show complete bone union.

HOW TO TREAT

NOTE—Follow your doctor's instructions. These instructions are supplemental.

FIRST AID
- Keep the person warm with blankets to decrease the possibility of shock.
- Cut away clothing, if possible, but don't move the injured area to do so.
- Use instructions for R.I.C.E., the first letters of *rest, ice, compression* and *elevation*. See Appendix 1 for details.

CONTINUING CARE
- The doctor will set the broken bones with surgery or, if possible, without. Manipulation should be done as soon as possible after injury. Many tissues lose their elasticity and become difficult to return to their normal positions.
- Immobilization will be necessary. A rigid cast or sling placed around the injured area is the most common technique. Skeletal traction is sometimes necessary.
- After traction or surgery, use a triangular sling for 2 weeks, and begin progressive shoulder exercises on a regular schedule (5 to 10 minutes every waking hour).

- After immobilization, use frequent ice massage. Fill a large styrofoam cup with water and freeze. Tear a small amount of foam from the top so ice protrudes. Massage firmly over the injured area in a circle about the size of a baseball. Do this for 15 minutes at a time 3 or 4 times a day, and also before workouts or competition.
- Apply heat instead of ice if it feels better. Use heat lamps, hot soaks, hot showers, heating pads or heat liniments and ointments.

MEDICATION—Your doctor may prescribe:
- General anesthesia, local anesthesia or muscle relaxants to make bone manipulation and fixation of bone fragments possible.
- Narcotic or synthetic narcotic pain relievers for severe pain.
- Stool softeners to prevent constipation due to inactivity.
- Acetaminophen (available without prescription) for mild pain after initial treatment.

ACTIVITY
- Actively exercise all muscle groups not immobilized. Muscle contractions promote fracture alignment and hasten healing.
- Resume normal activities gradually after treatment.
- Begin reconditioning the injured area after clearance from your doctor.

DIET—During recovery, balance the amount of food you eat with any change in your level of physical activity. Eat a variety of foods to get the energy, protein, vitamins, minerals and fiber you need for good health and healing.

REHABILITATION—Begin daily rehabilitation exercises when movement is comfortable. Use ice massage for 10 minutes prior to exercise. See Rehabilitation section for shoulder exercises.

CALL YOUR DOCTOR IF

- You have signs or symptoms of a shoulder blade fracture.
- Any of the following occurs after surgery or treatment:
  Pain, swelling or drainage increases in the surgical area.
  You notice swelling above or below the cast.
  Color of skin changes beyond the cast to blue or gray, particularly under the fingernails.
  You have numbness or complete loss of feeling below the fracture site.
  You develop signs of infection (headache, muscle aches, dizziness or a general ill feeling and fever).
  You experience nausea or vomiting.
  You become constipated.

SHOULDER BLADE (SCAPULA) STRAIN

GENERAL INFORMATION

DEFINITION—Injury to muscles or tendons that attach to bone in the area of the scapula (shoulder blade). Muscles, tendons and their attached bones comprise contractile units. These units stabilize the shoulder and allow its motion. A strain occurs at a unit's weakest part. Strains are of 3 types:
* Mild (Grade I)—Slightly pulled muscle without tearing of muscle or tendon fibers. There is no loss of strength.
* Moderate (Grade II)—Tearing of fibers in a muscle or tendon or at the attachment to bone. Strength is diminished.
* Severe (Grade III)—Rupture of the muscle-tendon-bone attachment, with separation of fibers. A severe strain may require surgical repair. Chronic strains are caused by overuse. Acute strains are caused by direct injury or overstress.

BODY PARTS INVOLVED
* Tendons and muscles that attach the shoulder blade to the arm and chest wall.
* Shoulder blade, collarbone (clavicle), upper arm bone (humerus) or spinal column.
* Soft tissues surrounding the strain, including nerves, periosteum (covering of bone), blood vessels and lymph vessels.

SIGNS & SYMPTOMS
* Pain when moving or stretching muscles of the shoulder blade.
* Muscle spasm in the shoulder blade area.
* Swelling in the shoulder blade area.
* Loss of strength (moderate or severe strain).
* Crepitation ("crackling" feeling and sound when the injured area is pressed with fingers).
* Calcification of the muscle or its tendon (visible with x-ray).
* Inflammation of sheath covering the tendon.

CAUSES
* Prolonged overuse of muscle-tendon units of the shoulder blade.
* Single violent injury or force applied to the muscle-tendon unit of the shoulder blade.

RISK INCREASES WITH
* Any throwing sport or exercise, such as baseball, basketball, tennis, shotput or javelin.
* Contact sports.
* Any cardiovascular medical problem that results in decreased circulation.
* Medical history of any bleeding disorder.
* Obesity.
* Poor nutrition.
* Previous shoulder or shoulder blade injury.

HOW TO PREVENT
* Participate in a strengthening, flexibility and conditioning program appropriate for your sport.
* Warm up before practice or competition.
* Wear proper protective equipment, such as shoulder pads, for contact sports.

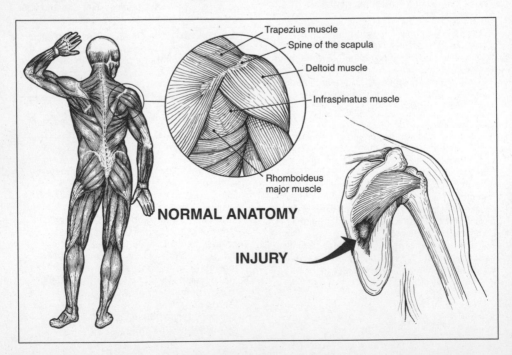

Trapezius muscle
Spine of the scapula
Deltoid muscle
Infraspinatus muscle
Rhomboideus major muscle

NORMAL ANATOMY

INJURY

WHAT TO EXPECT

APPROPRIATE HEALTH CARE
- Doctor's diagnosis.
- Self-care during rehabilitation.
- Physical therapy (moderate or severe strain).
- Surgery (rare).

DIAGNOSTIC MEASURES
- Your own observation of symptoms.
- Medical history and exam by a doctor.
- X-rays of the chest and shoulder to rule out fractures.

POSSIBLE COMPLICATIONS
- Prolonged healing time if activity is resumed too soon.
- Proneness to repeated injury.
- Unstable or arthritic shoulder and spine following repeated injury.
- Inflammation at the attachment to bone (periostitis).
- Prolonged disability (sometimes).

PROBABLE OUTCOME—If this is a first-time injury, proper care and sufficient healing time before resuming activity should prevent permanent disability. Torn ligaments and tendons require as long to heal as fractured bones do. Average healing times are:
- Mild strain—2 to 10 days.
- Moderate strain—10 days to 3 weeks.
- Severe strain—3 to 6 weeks.

If this is a repeat injury, complications listed above are more likely to occur.

 # HOW TO TREAT

NOTE—Follow your doctor's instructions. These instructions are supplemental.

FIRST AID—Use instructions for R.I.C.E., the first letters of *rest, ice, compression* and *elevation*. See Appendix 1 for details.

CONTINUING CARE
- Use ice massage 3 or 4 times a day for 15 minutes at a time. Fill a large styrofoam cup with water and freeze. Tear a small amount of foam from the top so ice protrudes. Massage firmly over the injured area in a circle about the size of a softball.

- After the first 72 hours, apply heat instead of ice if it feels better. Use heat lamps, hot soaks, hot showers, heating pads or heat liniments and ointments.
- Take whirlpool treatments, if available.
- Wrap the injured chest and shoulder blade with an elasticized bandage between treatments.
- Massage gently and often to provide comfort and decrease swelling.

MEDICATION
- For minor discomfort, you may use:
  Aspirin, acetaminophen or ibuprofen.
  Topical liniments and ointments.
- Your doctor may prescribe:
  Stronger pain relievers.
  Injection of a long-acting local anesthetic to reduce pain.
  Injections of corticosteroids, such as triamcinolone, to reduce inflammation.

ACTIVITY
- For a moderate or severe strain, use a sling for at least 72 hours—longer if it lessens discomfort.
- Resume your normal activities gradually.

DIET—During recovery, balance the amount of food you eat with any change in your level of physical activity. Eat a variety of foods to get the energy, protein, vitamins, minerals and fiber you need for good health and healing.

REHABILITATION—Begin daily rehabilitation exercises when supportive wrapping is no longer needed. See Rehabilitation section for shoulder exercises.

 # CALL YOUR DOCTOR IF

- You have symptoms of a moderate or severe shoulder blade strain or a mild strain persists longer than 10 days.
- Pain or swelling worsens despite treatment.

SHOULDER BURSITIS, SUBACROMIAL (Subdeltoid Bursitis; Subacromial Impingement Syndrome)

GENERAL INFORMATION

DEFINITION—Inflammation of the subdeltoid bursa (also known as the subacromial bursa), one of the important bursas of the shoulder. Bursitis may vary in degree from mild irritation to an abscess formation that causes excruciating pain.

BODY PARTS INVOLVED
- Subacromial bursa (a soft sac filled with lubricating fluid that facilitates motion in the shoulder).
- Soft tissues surrounding the shoulder, including nerves, tendons, ligaments, blood vessels (both large vessels and capillaries), periosteum (the outside lining of bone) and muscles.

SIGNS & SYMPTOMS
- Pain in the shoulder area.
- Tenderness.
- Swelling.
- Redness (sometimes) over the affected bursa.
- Fever if infection is present.
- Limitation of motion in the shoulder.

CAUSES
- Injury to the shoulder.
- Acute or chronic infection.
- Arthritis.
- Gout.
- Calcific tendinitis.
- Unknown (frequently).

RISK INCREASES WITH
- Participation in competitive athletics, particularly contact sports such as football and throwing sports.
- Previous history of bursitis in any joint.
- Previous shoulder injury involving the rotator cuff (see Glossary).
- Exposure to cold weather.
- Poor conditioning and inadequate warmup.
- Inadequate protective equipment in contact sports.

HOW TO PREVENT
- Participate in a strengthening, flexibility and conditioning program appropriate for your sport, especially a shoulder-strengthening and conditioning program prior to throwing sports.
- Use protective gear for contact sports.
- Warm up adequately before athletic practice or competition.
- Wear warm clothing in cold weather.

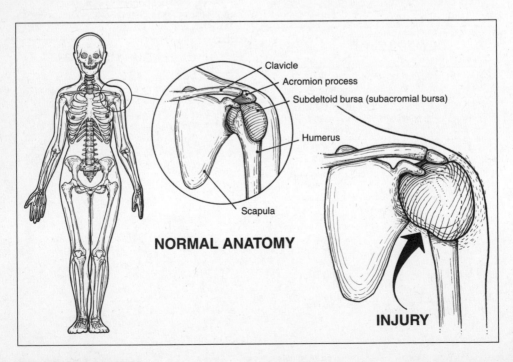

Clavicle
Acromion process
Subdeltoid bursa (subacromial bursa)
Humerus
Scapula

NORMAL ANATOMY

INJURY

- To prevent recurrence, continue to wear extra protection over the shoulder until healing is complete.

 ## WHAT TO EXPECT

APPROPRIATE HEALTH CARE
- Doctor's diagnosis and treatment.
- Surgery (sometimes) in worst cases, particularly for a frozen shoulder.

DIAGNOSTIC MEASURES
- Your own observation of symptoms.
- Medical history and physical exam by a doctor.
- X-rays of the shoulder.
- Diagnostic ultrasound or MRI (see Glossary for both) to look for rotator cuff tears.

POSSIBLE COMPLICATIONS
- Frozen shoulder, with temporary or permanent limitation of the shoulder's normal mobility.
- Prolonged healing time if activity is resumed too soon.
- Proneness to repeated flare-ups.
- Unstable or arthritic shoulder following repeated episodes of bursitis.
- Spontaneous rupture of the bursa if severe infection is present.

PROBABLE OUTCOME—Mild subdeltoid bursitis is a common—but not a serious—problem. Symptoms usually subside in 7 to 14 days with treatment. Chronic bursitis in any bursa of the shoulder can cause recurrent flare-ups.

 ## HOW TO TREAT

NOTE—Follow you doctor's instructions. These instructions are supplemental.

FIRST AID—None. This problem develops slowly.

CONTINUING CARE
- Use ice massage. Fill a large styrofoam cup with water and freeze. Tear a small amount of foam from the top so ice protrudes. Massage firmly over the injured area in a circle about the size of a softball. Do this for 15 minutes at a time 3 or 4 times a day, and also before workouts or competition.

- Apply heat instead of ice if it feels better. Use heat lamps, hot soaks, hot showers, heating pads or heat liniments and ointments. Sometimes heat makes the pain worse. If so, discontinue and use ice only.
- Use a sling to support the shoulder joint, if needed.
- Elevate the shoulder above the level of the heart to reduce swelling and prevent accumulation of fluid. Use pillows for propping.
- Gentle massage will frequently provide comfort and decrease swelling.

MEDICATION—Your doctor may prescribe:
- Nonsteroidal anti-inflammatory drugs.
- Prescription pain relievers for severe pain. Use nonprescription aspirin, acetaminophen or ibuprofen for mild pain.
- Injections into the inflamed bursa of a long-lasting local anesthetic mixed with a corticosteroid drug such as triamcinolone.

ACTIVITY—Rest the inflamed area as much as possible. If you must resume normal activity immediately, wear a sling until the pain becomes more bearable. To prevent a frozen shoulder, begin normal, slow joint movement as soon as possible.

DIET—During recovery, balance the amount of food you eat with any change in your level of physical activity. Eat a variety of foods to get the energy, protein, vitamins, minerals and fiber you need for good health and healing. Your doctor may suggest vitamin and mineral supplements to promote healing.

REHABILITATION—See Rehabilitation section for shoulder exercises.

 ## CALL YOUR DOCTOR IF

- You have symptoms of shoulder bursitis.
- Pain increases despite treatment.
- Pain, swelling, tenderness drainage or bleeding increases in the surgical area.
- You develop signs of infection (headache, muscle aches, dizziness or a general ill feeling and fever).
- New, unexplained symptoms develop. Drugs used in treatment may produce side effects.

SHOULDER CONTUSION

GENERAL INFORMATION

DEFINITION—Bruising of the skin and underlying tissues of the shoulder due to a direct blow. Contusions cause bleeding from ruptured small capillaries that allow blood to infiltrate muscles, tendons or other soft tissues.

BODY PARTS INVOLVED
* Shoulder, particularly the part over the acromion, the outer front end of the shoulder.
* Blood vessels, muscles, tendons, nerves, covering of bone (periosteum) and connective tissues.
* Injury to the axillary nerve, the most serious possible injury resulting from shoulder contusion.

SIGNS & SYMPTOMS
* Local swelling—either superficial or deep.
* Pain at the site of injury.
* Numbness and decreased function of the shoulder due to deltoid weakness if the axillary nerve is seriously injured.
* Feeling of firmness when pressure is exerted on the shoulder.
* Tenderness.
* Discoloration under the skin, beginning with redness and progressing to the characteristic "black-and-blue" bruise.
* Restricted activity of the shoulder directly proportional to the extent of injury.

CAUSES—Direct blow to the shoulder, usually from a blunt object.

RISK INCREASES WITH
* Contact sports, especially football, soccer, hockey, baseball or basketball.
* Medical history of any bleeding disorder.
* Poor nutrition, including vitamin deficiency.
* Inadequate protection of exposed areas during contact sports.
* Use of anticoagulants or aspirin.

HOW TO PREVENT—Wear appropriate protective gear and equipment, such as shoulder pads, during competition or other athletic activity if there is risk of a shoulder contusion.

WHAT TO EXPECT

APPROPRIATE HEALTH CARE
* Doctor's care unless the contusion is quite small.
* Self-care for minor contusions and during rehabilitation following serious contusions.
* Physical therapy for serious contusions.
* Possible surgery if the axillary nerve is damaged severely (rare).

DIAGNOSTIC MEASURES
* Your own observation of symptoms.
* Medical history and physical exam by a doctor, with particular attention to the possibility of axillary nerve damage, for all except minor injuries.

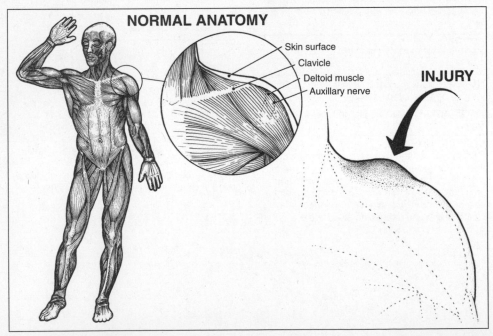

NORMAL ANATOMY

Skin surface
Clavicle
Deltoid muscle
Auxillary nerve

INJURY

- X-rays of the shoulder to assess total injury to soft tissues and to rule out the possibility of underlying fracture. The total extent of injury may not be apparent for 48 to 72 hours.

POSSIBLE COMPLICATIONS
- Excessive bleeding, leading to disability. Infiltrative-type bleeding can sometimes lead to calcification and impaired function of the injured muscle.
- Prolonged healing time if usual activities are resumed too soon.
- Infection if skin over the contusion is broken.
- Unstable or arthritic shoulder joint following repeated injury.

PROBABLE OUTCOME—Healing time varies from 2 to 6 weeks, depending on the site and the extent of injury.

 # HOW TO TREAT

NOTE—Follow your doctor's instructions. These instructions are supplemental.

FIRST AID—Use instructions for R.I.C.E., the first letters of *rest, ice, compression* and *elevation*. See Appendix 1 for details.

CONTINUING CARE
- Wrap an elasticized bandage over a felt pad on the injured area. Keep the area compressed for about 72 hours.
- Use an ice pack 3 or 4 times a day. Wrap ice chips or cubes in a plastic bag, and wrap the bag in a moist towel. Place it over the injured area for 20 minutes at a time.
- After 72 hours, apply heat instead of ice if it feels better. Use heat lamps, hot soaks, hot showers, heating pads, heat liniments and ointments or whirlpool treatments.
- Massage gently and often to provide comfort and decrease swelling.

MEDICATION
- For minor discomfort, you may use: Acetaminophen or ibuprofen. Topical liniments and ointments.
- Your doctor may prescribe stronger pain medicine if needed.

ACTIVITY—Begin activities slowly, and stop exercise as soon as pain begins. Increase activity as healing progresses.

DIET—During recovery, balance the amount of food you eat with any change in your level of physical activity. Eat a variety of foods to get the energy, protein, vitamins, minerals and fiber you need for good health and healing.

REHABILITATION
- Begin daily rehabilitation exercises when a sling is no longer needed.
- Use ice massage for 10 minutes before and after workouts. Fill a large styrofoam cup with water and freeze. Tear a small amount of foam from the top so ice protrudes. Massage firmly over the injured area in a circle about the size of a softball.
- See Rehabilitation section for shoulder exercises.

 # CALL YOUR DOCTOR IF

- You have a contusion that doesn't improve in 1 or 2 days.
- Skin is broken and signs of infection (drainage, increasing pain, fever, headache, muscle aches, dizziness or a general ill feeling) occur.
- Numbness or tingling in the arm begins. These may be signs of axillary nerve damage.

SHOULDER DISLOCATION
(Shoulder Subluxation)

GENERAL INFORMATION

DEFINITION—Displacement of the humerus (upper arm bone) from its socket in the shoulder joint. A forward displacement of the humerus is the most common type of shoulder dislocation. A temporary dislocation with immediate return to normal joint position is known as a subluxation.

BODY PARTS INVOLVED
- Shoulder joint; humerus.
- Soft tissues surrounding the dislocation, including nerves, tendons, ligaments, muscles and blood vessels. Injury to nerves in the axilla (armpit) is quite common, as is injury to the axillary nerve, which powers the deltoid muscle.

SIGNS & SYMPTOMS
- Excruciating pain at the time of injury.
- Loss of function of the dislocated shoulder joint and severe pain when attempting to move it.
- Visible deformity if dislocated bones lock in the dislocated positions. If they spontaneously reposition themselves, no deformity will be visible, but damage will be the same.
- Tenderness over the dislocation.
- Swelling and bruising at the injury site.
- Numbness or paralysis in the arm from pressure, pinching or cutting of blood vessels or nerves.

CAUSES
- Direct upward blow to the shoulder or backward force on an extended arm.
- End result of a severe shoulder sprain.
- Congenital abnormality, including shallow or malformed joint surfaces.
- Powerful muscle twisting or a violent muscle contraction (including contraction from seizures or electrocution). Some people can willfully produce a recurrent dislocation.

RISK INCREASES WITH
- Contact sports, especially football, wrestling or basketball.
- Any activity that involves forceful throwing, lifting, hitting or twisting.
- Shoulder fracture.
- Previous shoulder dislocation or sprain.
- Repeated shoulder injury of any sort.
- Arthritis of any type (rheumatoid, gout).
- Poor muscle conditioning.
- Increased ligamentous laxity.

HOW TO PREVENT
- Participate in a strengthening, flexibility and conditioning program appropriate for your sport, especially a shoulder-strengthening and conditioning program prior to throwing sports.
- Warm up adequately before physical activity.
- For participation in contact sports, protect shoulders with special equipment such as shoulder pads. After recovery, strapping or elastic wraps may protect against reinjury.

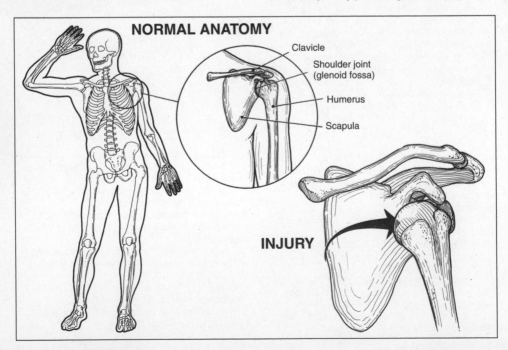

NORMAL ANATOMY

Clavicle

Shoulder joint (glenoid fossa)

Humerus

Scapula

INJURY

WHAT TO EXPECT

APPROPRIATE HEALTH CARE
• Doctor's treatment. This will include manipulation of the joint to reposition the bones.
• Surgery (sometimes) to restore the joint to its normal position. Acute or recurring dislocations may require surgical reconstruction to stabilize the joint.
• Self-care during rehabilitation.

DIAGNOSTIC MEASURES
• Your own observation of symptoms.
• Medical history and exam by a doctor.
• X-rays of the shoulder joint and adjacent bones.

POSSIBLE COMPLICATIONS
• Temporary or permanent damage to nearby nerves or major blood vessels, causing numbness, coldness and paleness.
• Excessive internal bleeding.
• Shock or loss of consciousness.
• Recurrent dislocations, particularly if the previous dislocation is not healed completely. Most recurrent dislocations are anterior (forward) dislocations caused by unhealed injuries to shoulder ligaments or congenital abnormalities of the glenohumeral joint.

PROBABLE OUTCOME—After the shoulder
dislocation has been corrected, it may require immobilization with a cast or sling for 2 to 8 weeks. Complete healing of injured ligaments requires a minimum of 6 weeks. If customary treatment does not prevent a recurrence, athletic activities should be modified until surgery can be done. Surgery should be followed by rehabilitation to prevent reinjury.

HOW TO TREAT

NOTE—Follow your doctor's instructions. These instructions are supplemental.

FIRST AID
• Keep the person warm with blankets to decrease the possibility of shock.
• Cut away clothing if possible, but don't move the injured area to remove clothing. Untrained persons should not attempt to reposition a dislocated shoulder.
• Immobilize the neck, dislocated shoulder and elbow with padded splints or a sling.
• Use instructions for R.I.C.E., the first letters of *rest, ice, compression* and *elevation*. See Appendix 1 for details.
• The doctor will manipulate the dislocated bones to return them to their normal positions. Manipulation should be done as soon as possible. Many tissues lose their elasticity and become difficult to return to their normal

positions. Relocating a dislocated shoulder may require general anesthesia.

CONTINUING CARE—At home:
• Use an ice pack 3 or 4 times a day. Wrap ice chips or cubes in a plastic bag, and wrap the bag in a moist towel. Place it over the injured area for 20 minutes at a time.
• After 72 hours, application of localized heat promotes healing by increasing blood circulation in the injured area. Use hot baths, showers, compresses, heat lamps, heating pads, heat ointments and liniments or whirlpools.
• Exercise all muscle groups not immobilized in a cast or sling. Muscle contractions promote alignment and hasten healing.
• Massage gently and often to provide comfort and decrease swelling.

MEDICATION—Your doctor may prescribe:
• General anesthesia or muscle relaxants to make joint manipulation possible.
• Acetaminophen to relieve moderate pain.
• Narcotic pain relievers for severe pain.
• Antibiotics to fight infection if surgery is necessary.

ACTIVITY—Resume your normal activities
gradually after treatment.

DIET—Do not eat or drink before manipulation
or surgery to correct the dislocation. Fluid or solid food in your stomach makes vomiting while under general anesthesia more hazardous. During recovery eat a well-balanced diet.

REHABILITATION
• Begin daily rehabilitation exercises when a supportive sling is no longer needed.
• Use ice massage for 10 minutes before and after workouts. Fill a large styrofoam cup with water and freeze. Tear a small amount of foam from the top so ice protrudes. Massage firmly in a circle over the injured area.
• See Rehabilitation section for shoulder exercises.

CALL YOUR DOCTOR IF

• You have difficulty moving your shoulder after dislocation.
• Your arm becomes numb, pale, or cold after a dislocation. This is an emergency!
• Any of the following occurs after surgery: Increased pain, swelling or drainage in the surgical area.
Signs of infection (headache, muscle aches, dizziness or a general ill feeling and fever). Constipation.
New, unexplained symptoms. Drugs used in treatment may produce side effects.
• Dislocations that you can "pop" back into normal position occur repeatedly.

SHOULDER SPRAIN, ACROMIOCLAVICULAR
(Shoulder Separation, Low-Grade)

GENERAL INFORMATION

DEFINITION—Violent overstretching of the acromioclavicular ligaments in the shoulder where it meets the collarbone (clavicle). Sprains involving two or more ligaments cause considerably more disability than single-ligament sprains. When the ligament is overstretched, it becomes tense and gives way at its weakest point, either where it attaches to bone or within the ligament itself. If the ligament pulls loose a fragment of bone, it is called an avulsion fracture. There are 3 types of sprains:
- Mild (Grade I)—Tearing of some ligament fibers. There is no loss of function.
- Moderate (Grade II)—Rupture of a portion of the ligament, resulting in some loss of function.
- Severe (Grade III)—Complete rupture of the ligament or complete separation of ligament from bone. There is total loss of function. A severe sprain may require surgical repair. The higher grades of shoulder separation (see Collarbone Dislocation at Shoulder Joint) show injury to the coracoclavicular ligaments as well as to the acromioclavicular ligaments.

BODY PARTS INVOLVED
- Acromioclavicular ligaments of the shoulder and collarbone.
- Tissues surrounding the sprain, including blood vessels, tendons, bone, periosteum (covering of bone) and muscles.

SIGNS & SYMPTOMS
- Severe pain at the time of injury.
- A feeling of popping or tearing inside the shoulder.
- Tenderness at the injury site.
- Swelling in the collarbone and shoulder.
- Bruising that appears soon after injury.

CAUSES
- Downward stress on the shoulder that temporarily forces the shoulder bones away from the collarbone.
- Falling on the point of the shoulder (acromion).
- Falling on outstretched hand or on the point of the elbow.

RISK INCREASES WITH
- Contact sports.
- Previous shoulder sprain or separation.
- Obesity.
- Poor muscle conditioning.
- Inadequate protection from equipment.

HOW TO PREVENT
- Participate in a strengthening, flexibility and conditioning program appropriate for your sport, especially a shoulder-strengthening and conditioning program, prior to throwing sports.

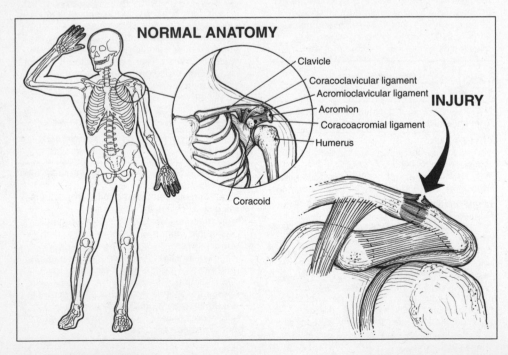

NORMAL ANATOMY

Clavicle
Coracoclavicular ligament
Acromioclavicular ligament
Acromion
Coracoacromial ligament
Humerus
Coracoid

INJURY

- Warm up before practice or competition.
- Wear protective equipment appropriate for your sport.
- To prevent reinjury, tape vulnerable joints before practice or competition.

 WHAT TO EXPECT

APPROPRIATE HEALTH CARE
- Doctor's diagnosis.
- Application of a sling, tape or elastic bandage.
- Self-care during rehabilitation.
- Physical therapy (moderate or severe sprain).

DIAGNOSTIC MEASURES
- Your own observation of symptoms.
- Medical history and exam by a doctor
- X-rays of the shoulder, elbow and collarbone to rule out fractures.

POSSIBLE COMPLICATIONS
- Prolonged healing time if usual activities are resumed too soon.
- Proneness to repeated injury.
- Inflammation at the ligament attachment to bone (periostitis).
- Prolonged disability (sometimes).
- Unstable or arthritic acromioclavicular joint following repeated injury.

PROBABLE OUTCOME—If this is a first-time injury, proper care and sufficient healing time before resuming activity should prevent permanent disability. Ligaments have a poor blood supply, and torn ligaments require as much healing time as fractures. Average healing times are:
- Mild sprains—2 to 3 weeks.
- Moderate sprains—3 to 6 weeks.
- Severe sprains—6 to 8 weeks.

 HOW TO TREAT

NOTE—Follow your doctor's instructions. These instructions are supplemental.

FIRST AID—Use instructions for R.I.C.E., the first letters of *rest, ice, compression* and *elevation.* See Appendix 1 for details.

CONTINUING CARE—If the doctor does not apply a sling, tape or elastic bandage:
- Continue using an ice pack 3 or 4 times a day. Place ice chips or cubes in a plastic bag. Wrap the bag in a moist towel, and place it over the injured area. Use for 20 minutes at a time.
- Wrap the injured shoulder with an elasticized bandage between treatments.

- After 72 hours, apply heat instead of ice if it feels better. Use heat lamps, hot soaks, hot showers, heating pads or heat liniments and ointments.
- Take whirlpool treatments, if available.
- Massage the shoulder and collarbone gently and often to provide comfort and decrease swelling.

MEDICATION
- For minor discomfort, you may use:
  Aspirin, acetaminophen or nonsteroidal anti-inflammatories.
  Topical liniments and ointments.
- Your doctor may prescribe:
  Stronger pain relievers.
  Injection of a long-acting local anesthetic to reduce pain.
  Injections of a corticosteroid, such as triamcinolone, to reduce inflammation.

ACTIVITY—Resume your normal activities gradually after clearance from your doctor.

DIET—During recovery, balance the amount of food you eat with any change in your level of physical activity. Eat a variety of foods to get the energy, protein, vitamins, minerals and fiber you need for good health and healing.

REHABILITATION
- Begin daily rehabilitation exercises when the cast or supportive wrapping is no longer necessary.
- Use ice massage for 10 minutes before and after exercise. Fill a large styrofoam cup with water and freeze. Tear a small amount of foam from the top so ice protrudes. Massage firmly over the injured area in a circle about the size of a softball.
- See Rehabilitation section for shoulder exercises.

 CALL YOUR DOCTOR IF

- You have symptoms of a moderate or severe shoulder sprain or a mild sprain persists longer than 2 weeks.
- Pain, swelling or bruising worsens despite treatment.
- You experience pain, numbness or coldness in the arm.
- Blue, gray or dusky color appears in the fingernails.
- Any of the following occurs after surgery:
  Increased pain, swelling, redness, drainage or bleeding in the surgical area.
  Signs of infection (headache, muscle aches, dizziness or a general ill feeling with fever).
- New, unexplained symptoms develop. Drugs used in treatment may produce side effects.

SHOULDER SPRAIN, GLENOHUMERAL

GENERAL INFORMATION

DEFINITION—Violent overstretching of one or more ligaments in the glenohumeral joint of the shoulder. Sprains involving two or more ligaments cause considerably more disability than single-ligament sprains. When the ligament is overstretched, it becomes tense and gives way at its weakest point, either where it attaches to bone or within the ligament itself. If the ligament pulls loose a fragment of bone, it is called an avulsion fracture. There are 3 types of sprains:
- Mild (Grade I)—Tearing of some ligament fibers. There is no loss of function.
- Moderate (Grade II)—Rupture of a portion of the ligament, resulting in some loss of function.
- Severe (Grade III)—Complete rupture of the ligament or complete separation of ligament from bone. There is total loss of function. A severe sprain may require surgical repair.

BODY PARTS INVOLVED
- Ligaments of the glenohumeral joint of the shoulder.
- Tissues surrounding the sprain, including blood vessels, tendons, bone, periosteum (covering of bone) and muscles.

SIGNS & SYMPTOMS
- Severe pain at the time of injury.
- A feeling of popping or tearing inside the shoulder.
- Tenderness at the injury site.
- Swelling in the shoulder.
- Bruising that appears soon after injury.

CAUSES—Backward and upward stress that temporarily forces or pries the ligaments and bones of the shoulder joint out of their normal locations.

RISK INCREASES WITH
- Contact sports such as boxing or wrestling.
- Throwing sports such as baseball, football and track events.
- Skiing.
- Previous shoulder injury.
- Obesity.
- Poor muscle conditioning.
- Inadequate protection from equipment.

HOW TO PREVENT
- Participate in a strengthening, flexibility and conditioning program appropriate for your sport, especially a shoulder-strengthening and conditioning program, prior to throwing sports.
- Warm up before practice or competition.
- Tape vulnerable joints before practice or competition.
- Wear protective equipment such as shoulder pads.

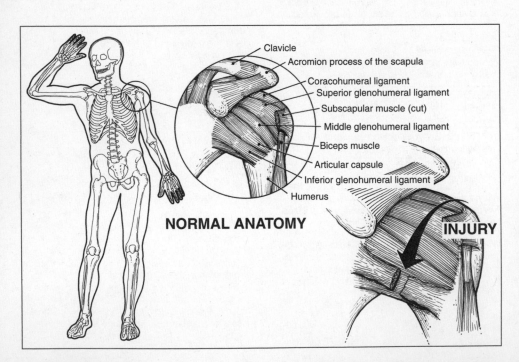

Clavicle
Acromion process of the scapula
Coracohumeral ligament
Superior glenohumeral ligament
Subscapular muscle (cut)
Middle glenohumeral ligament
Biceps muscle
Articular capsule
Inferior glenohumeral ligament
Humerus

NORMAL ANATOMY

INJURY

WHAT TO EXPECT

APPROPRIATE HEALTH CARE
- Doctor's diagnosis.
- Application of a sling, tape or elastic bandage.
- Self-care during rehabilitation.
- Physical therapy (moderate or severe sprain).

DIAGNOSTIC MEASURES
- Your own observation of symptoms.
- Medical history and exam by a doctor.
- X-rays of the shoulder joint to rule out fractures.

POSSIBLE COMPLICATIONS
- Prolonged healing time if usual activities are resumed too soon.
- Proneness to repeated injury.
- Inflammation at the ligament attachment to bone (periostitis).
- Prolonged disability (sometimes).
- Unstable or arthritic shoulder following repeated injury.

PROBABLE OUTCOME—If this is a first-time injury, proper care and sufficient healing time before resuming activity should prevent permanent disability. Ligaments have a poor blood supply, and torn ligaments require as much healing time as fractures. Average healing times are:
- Mild sprains—2 to 3 weeks.
- Moderate sprains—3 to 6 weeks.
- Severe sprains—6 to 8 weeks.

 HOW TO TREAT

NOTE—Follow your doctor's instructions. These instructions are supplemental.

FIRST AID—Use instructions for R.I.C.E., the first letters of *rest, ice, compression* and *elevation.* See Appendix 1 for details.

CONTINUING CARE—If the doctor does not apply a sling, tape or elastic bandage:
- Continue using an ice pack 3 or 4 times a day. Place ice chips or cubes in a plastic bag. Wrap the bag in a moist towel, and place it over the injured area. Use for 20 minutes at a time.
- Wrap the injured shoulder with an elasticized bandage between ice treatments.

- After 72 hours, apply heat instead of ice if it feels better. Use heat lamps, hot soaks, hot showers, heating pads or heat liniments and ointments.
- Take whirlpool treatments, if available.
- Massage the shoulder gently and often to provide comfort and decrease swelling.

MEDICATION
- For minor discomfort, you may use:
  Aspirin, acetaminophen or ibuprofen.
  Topical liniments and ointments.
- Your doctor may prescribe:
  Stronger pain relievers.
  Injection of a long-acting local anesthetic to reduce pain.
  Injections of a corticosteroid, such as triamcinolone, to reduce inflammation.

DIET—During recovery, balance the amount of food you eat with any change in your level of physical activity. Eat a variety of foods to get the energy, protein, vitamins, minerals and fiber you need for good health and healing.

REHABILITATION.
- Begin daily rehabilitation exercises when the supportive wrapping is no longer necessary.
- Use ice massage for 10 minutes before and after exercise. Fill a large styrofoam cup with water and freeze. Tear a small amount of foam from the top so ice protrudes. Massage firmly over the injured area in a circle about the size of a softball.
- See Rehabilitation section for shoulder exercises.

 CALL YOUR DOCTOR IF

- You have symptoms of a moderate or severe shoulder sprain or a mild sprain persists longer than 2 weeks.
- Pain, swelling or bruising worsens despite treatment.
- You experience pain, numbness or coldness in the arm or hand.
- Blue, gray or dusky color appears in the fingernails.
- New, unexplained symptoms develop. Drugs used in treatment may produce side effects.

SHOULDER STRAIN
(Rotator Cuff Strain, Partial or Complete Tear)

GENERAL INFORMATION

DEFINITION—Injury to muscles or tendons that attach to bones in the shoulder. Muscles, tendons and bones comprise contractile units. These units stabilize the shoulder and allow its motion. A strain occurs at a unit's weakest point. Strains are of 3 types:
* Mild (Grade I)—Slightly pulled muscle without tearing of muscle or tendon fibers. There is no loss of strength.
* Moderate (Grade II)—Tearing of fibers in a muscle or tendon or at the attachment to bone.
* Severe (Grade III)—Rupture of the muscle-tendon-bone attachment, with separation of fibers. A severe strain may require surgical repair. Chronic strains are caused by overuse. Acute strains are caused by direct injury or overstress.

BODY PARTS INVOLVED
* Muscles and tendons that attach to bones in the shoulder, including rotator cuff (see Glossary) muscles and tendons.
* Bones in the shoulder area, including the humerus, scapula and clavicle.

SIGNS & SYMPTOMS
* Soft tissues surrounding the strain, including nerves, periosteum (covering of bone), blood vessels and lymph vessels.
* Pain when moving or stretching the shoulder.
* Muscle spasm in the shoulder.
* Swelling over the injury.
* Loss of strength (moderate or severe strain).
* Crepitation ("crackling" feeling and sound when the injured area is pressed with finger).
* Calcification of the shoulder muscle or tendon (visible with x-rays).
* Inflammation of the tendon sheath.

CAUSES
* Prolonged overuse of muscle-tendon units in the shoulder.
* Single violent blow or force applied to the shoulder.

RISK INCREASES WITH
* Contact sports such as boxing, wrestling or rugby.
* Throwing sports such as baseball, football, basketball or tennis.
* Any cardiovascular medical problem that results in decreased circulation.
* Medical history of any bleeding disorder.
* Obesity.
* Poor nutrition.
* Previous shoulder injury.
* Poor muscle conditioning.

HOW TO PREVENT
* Participate in a strengthening, flexibility and conditioning program appropriate for your sport.

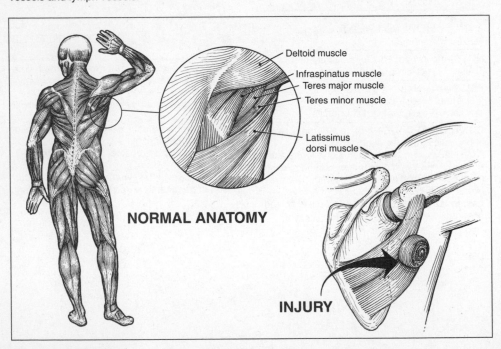

Deltoid muscle
Infraspinatus muscle
Teres major muscle
Teres minor muscle
Latissimus dorsi muscle

NORMAL ANATOMY

INJURY

- Warm up before practice or competition.
- Wear protective equipment, such as shoulder pads, for contact sports.
- Avoid overuse.
- To prevent a recurrence, tape the shoulder area before practice or competition.

 ## WHAT TO EXPECT

APPROPRIATE HEALTH CARE
- Doctor's diagnosis.
- Self-care during rehabilitation.
- Physical therapy (moderate or severe strain).
- Surgery (severe strain).

DIAGNOSTIC MEASURES
- Your own observation of symptoms.
- Medical history and exam by a doctor.
- X-rays of injured areas to rule out fractures.
- Diagnostic ultrasound or MRI (see Glossary for both) to confirm the diagnosis.

POSSIBLE COMPLICATIONS
- Prolonged healing time if activity is resumed too soon.
- Proneness to repeated injury.
- Unstable or arthritic shoulder following repeated injury.
- Inflammation at the attachment to bone (periostitis).
- Prolonged disability, usually weakness and pain, when using arm in the overhead position.

PROBABLE OUTCOME—If this is a first-time injury, proper care and sufficient healing time before resuming activity should prevent permanent disability. Torn ligaments and tendons require as long to heal as fractured bones do. Average healing times are:
- Mild strain—2 to 10 days.
- Moderate strain—10 days to 6 weeks.
- Severe strain—6 to 10 weeks.

If this is a repeat injury, complications listed above are more likely to occur.

 ## HOW TO TREAT

NOTE—Follow your doctor's instructions. These instructions are supplemental.

FIRST AID—Use instructions for R.I.C.E., the first letters of *rest, ice, compression* and *elevation*. See Appendix 1 for details.

CONTINUING CARE
- Use ice massage 3 or 4 times a day for 15 minutes at a time. Fill a large styrofoam cup with water and freeze. Tear a small amount of foam from the top so ice protrudes. Massage firmly over the injured area in a circle about the size of a softball.
- After the first 72 hours, apply heat instead of ice if it feels better. Use heat lamps, hot soaks, hot showers, heating pads or heat liniments and ointments.
- Take whirlpool treatments, if available.
- Wrap the injured shoulder with an elasticized bandage between treatments.
- Massage gently and often to provide comfort and decrease swelling.

MEDICATION
- For minor discomfort, you may use:
  Aspirin, acetaminophen or ibuprofen.
  Topical liniments and ointments.
- Your doctor may prescribe:
  Stronger pain relievers.
  Injection of a long-acting local anesthetic to reduce pain.
  Injections of corticosteroids, such as triamcinolone, to reduce inflammation.

ACTIVITY
- For a moderate or severe strain, use a sling for at least 72 hours.
- Resume your normal activities gradually.

DIET—During recovery, balance the amount of food you eat with any change in your level of physical activity. Eat a variety of foods to get the energy, protein, vitamins, minerals and fiber you need for good health and healing.

REHABILITATION—Begin daily rehabilitation exercises when supportive wrapping is no longer needed. Use ice massage for 10 minutes prior to exercise. See Rehabilitation section for shoulder exercises.

 ## CALL YOUR DOCTOR IF

- You have symptoms of a moderate or severe shoulder strain or a mild strain persists longer than 10 days.
- Pain or swelling worsens despite treatment.

SHOULDER SYNOVITIS, GLENOHUMERAL

GENERAL INFORMATION

DEFINITION—Inflammation of one of the bursas in the shoulder. Synovitis may vary in degree from mild irritation to an abscess formation that causes excruciating pain.

BODY PARTS INVOLVED
- Glenohumeral joint or other shoulder joint.
- Synovium (joint lining that produces lubricating fluid that facilitates motion in the shoulder).
- Soft tissues surrounding the shoulder, including nerves, tendons, ligaments, blood vessels (both large vessels and capillaries), periosteum (the outside lining of bone) and muscles.

SIGNS & SYMPTOMS
- Shoulder pain, especially when moving the shoulder.
- Tenderness.
- Swelling.
- Redness (sometimes) over the affected joint.
- Fever if infection is present.
- Limitation of shoulder motion.

CAUSES
- Injury to the shoulder.
- Acute or chronic infection.
- Arthritis.
- Gout.
- Unknown (frequently).

RISK INCREASES WITH
- Participation in competitive athletics, particularly contact sports such as football or soccer.
- Previous history of synovitis in any joint.
- Previous shoulder injury involving muscles of the rotator cuff (see Glossary).
- Exposure to cold weather.
- Poor conditioning and inadequate warmup.
- Inadequate protective equipment in contact.

HOW TO PREVENT
- Use protective gear for contact sports.
- Warm up adequately before athletic practice or competition.
- Wear warm clothing in cold weather.
- To prevent recurrence, continue to wear extra protection over the shoulder until healing is complete.

WHAT TO EXPECT

APPROPRIATE HEALTH CARE
- Doctor's diagnosis and treatment.
- Surgery (sometimes), particularly for a frozen shoulder.

DIAGNOSTIC MEASURES
- Your own observation of symptoms.
- Medical history and physical exam by a doctor.
- X-rays of the shoulder.
- Diagnostic ultrasound or MRI (see Glossary for both) to look for rotator cuff tear.

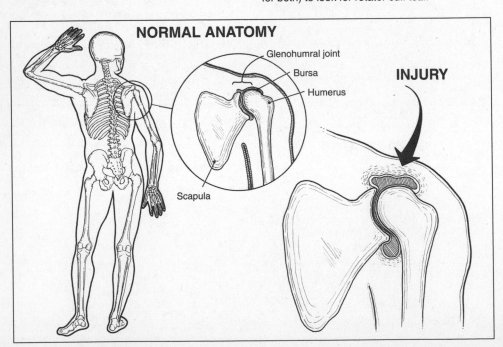

NORMAL ANATOMY

Glenohumral joint

Bursa

Humerus

Scapula

INJURY

POSSIBLE COMPLICATIONS
- Frozen shoulder (sustained marked stiffness of the shoulder joint), which may require 6 to 24 months to resolve.
- Permanent limitation of the shoulder's normal mobility.
- Prolonged healing time if activity is resumed too soon.
- Proneness to repeated flare-ups.
- Unstable or arthritic shoulder following repeated episodes of synovitis.

PROBABLE OUTCOME—Mild, acute shoulder synovitis is a common—but not serious—problem. Symptoms usually subside in 7 to 14 days with treatment. Chronic or recurrent synovitis, resulting from undertreatment of the acute form of synovitis, can lead to a frozen shoulder and years of discomfort.

 HOW TO TREAT

NOTE—Follow your doctor's instructions. These instructions are supplemental.

FIRST AID—None. This problem develops slowly.

CONTINUING CARE
- Use ice massage. Fill a large styrofoam cup with water and freeze. Tear a small amount of foam from the top so ice protrudes. Massage firmly over the injured area in a circle about the size of a softball. Do this for 15 minutes at a time 3 or 4 times a day, and also before workouts or competition.
- Apply heat instead of ice if it feels better. Use heat lamps, hot soaks, hot showers, heating pads or heat liniments and ointments. Sometimes heat makes the pain worse. If so, discontinue and use ice only.
- Use a sling to support the shoulder joint, if needed.
- Elevate the shoulder above the level of the heart to reduce swelling and prevent accumulation of fluid. Use pillows for propping.
- Gentle massage will frequently provide comfort and decrease swelling.

MEDICATION—Your doctor may prescribe:
- Nonsteroidal anti-inflammatory drugs.
- Prescription pain relievers for severe pain. Use nonprescription aspirin, acetaminophen or ibuprofen for mild pain.
- Your doctor may inject the inflamed joint with a long-lasting local anesthetic mixed with a corticosteroid drug such as triamcinolone.

ACTIVITY—Rest the inflamed area as much as possible. If you must resume normal activity immediately, wear a sling until the pain becomes more bearable. To prevent a frozen shoulder, begin normal, slow joint movement as soon as possible.

DIET—During recovery, balance the amount of food you eat with any change in your level of physical activity. Eat a variety of foods to get the energy, protein, vitamins, minerals and fiber you need for good health and healing. Your doctor may suggest vitamin and mineral supplements to promote healing.

REHABILITATION
- Begin stretching exercises of the shoulder (performed with pendulum motion, or use a broomstick, pulleys or a towel) daily to regain lost motion.
- See Rehabilitation section for additional shoulder exercises.

 CALL YOUR DOCTOR IF

- You have symptoms of shoulder synovitis.
- Pain increases despite treatment.
- Pain, swelling, tenderness drainage or bleeding increases in the surgical area.
- You develop signs of infection (headache, muscle aches, dizziness or a general ill feeling and fever).
- New, unexplained symptoms develop. Drugs used in treatment may produce side effects.

SHOULDER TENDINITIS & TENOSYNOVITIS

GENERAL INFORMATION

DEFINITION— Inflammation of the tendon (tendinitis) or the lining of the tendon sheath (tenosynovitis) in the shoulder. The lining secretes a fluid that lubricates the tendon. When the lining or the sheath becomes inflamed, the tendon cannot glide smoothly in its covering.

BODY PARTS INVOLVED
- Tendons of the shoulder muscles. These muscles include the teres minor, infraspinatus, supraspinatus, subscapularis, deltoid and biceps muscles. These muscles and tendons allow movement of the shoulder and hold the head of the humerus snugly against the glenoid cavity to stabilize the shoulder joint.
- Linings of the tendon sheaths (tough, fibrous tissues covering the tendons).
- Soft tissues in the surrounding area, including blood vessels, nerves, ligaments, periosteum (covering of bone) and connective tissues.

SIGNS & SYMPTOMS
- Constant pain or pain with motion of the shoulder.
- Limited motion of the shoulder.
- Crepitation (a "crackling" sound when the tendon moves or is touched).
- Weakness of the shoulder, especially when in an elevated position.
- Pain with elevation of the shoulder.
- Redness and tenderness over the injured tendon.

CAUSES
- Strain from unusual use or overuse of the shoulder.
- Direct blow or injury to muscles and tendons in the shoulder. Tenosynovitis becomes more likely with repeated injury.

RISK INCREASES WITH
- Contact sports, especially football and basketball.
- Throwing sports such as baseball.
- Racquet sports.
- Swimming or water polo.
- If surgery is needed, surgical risk increases with smoking, poor nutrition, alcoholism, drug abuse and recent or chronic illness.

HOW TO PREVENT
- Participate in a strengthening, flexibility and conditioning program appropriate for your sport, especially a shoulder-strengthening and conditioning program, prior to participation in throwing sports.
- Warm up adequately before practice or competition.
- Wear protective gear, such as shoulder pads, if they are appropriate for your sport.
- Learn proper moves and techniques for your sport.

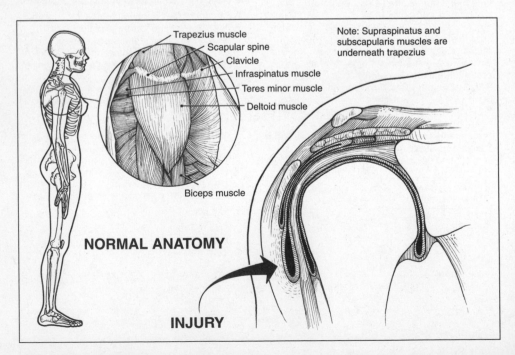

Trapezius muscle
Scapular spine
Clavicle
Infraspinatus muscle
Teres minor muscle
Deltoid muscle

Note: Supraspinatus and subscapularis muscles are underneath trapezius

Biceps muscle

NORMAL ANATOMY

INJURY

WHAT TO EXPECT

APPROPRIATE HEALTH CARE
- Doctor's examination and diagnosis.
- Surgery (sometimes) to enlarge the bony tunnel through which the tendon passes or to repair torn tendons. The surgical procedure is performed under general anesthesia in an outpatient surgical facility or hospital operating room.

DIAGNOSTIC MEASURES
- Your own observation of symptoms and signs.
- Medical history and physical examination by your doctor.
- X-rays of the shoulder and arm to rule out other abnormalities.
- Diagnostic ultrasound or MRI (see Glossary for both) to evaluate rotator cuff tendons for tears.

POSSIBLE COMPLICATIONS
- Prolonged healing time if activity is resumed too soon.
- Proneness to repeated shoulder injury.
- Adhesive tenosynovitis—The tendon and its covering become bound together. Loss of motion may be complete or partial. Surgery is necessary to remove the covering or transfer the tendon to a new area.
- Constrictive tenosynovitis—The walls of the covering thicken and narrow the opening, preventing the tendon from sliding through. Surgery is necessary to cut away part of the covering.
- Progression to rotator cuff tear.

PROBABLE OUTCOME—Tendinitis and tenosynovitis are usually curable in about 6 weeks with heat treatments, corticosteroid injections and rest of the inflamed area. Recovery is usually quicker if the inflammation is caused by a direct blow rather than by a strain or sprain.

 HOW TO TREAT

NOTE—Follow your doctor's instructions. These instructions are supplemental.

FIRST AID—None. This problem develops slowly.

CONTINUING CARE
- Use a sling to rest the shoulder.
- Apply heat frequently. Use heat lamps, hot soaks, hot showers, heating pads or heat liniments and ointments.
- Take whirlpool treatments, if available.

MEDICATION—You may use nonprescription drugs such as acetaminophen for minor pain. Your doctor may prescribe:
- Stronger pain relievers. Don't take prescription pain medication longer than 4 to 7 days. Use only as much as you need.
- Injection of the tendon covering with a combination of a long-acting local anesthetic and a nonabsorbable corticosteroid such as triamcinolone.

ACTIVITY—Resume normal activities gradually.

DIET—During recovery, balance the amount of food you eat with any change in your level of physical activity. Eat a variety of foods to get the energy, protein, vitamins, minerals and fiber you need for good health and healing.

REHABILITATION
- Begin daily rehabilitation exercises when you can raise or work your hand overhead without pain and supportive wrapping is no longer needed.
- Use ice massage for 10 minutes before and after exercise. Fill a large styrofoam cup with water and freeze. Tear a small amount of foam from the top so ice protrudes. Massage firmly over the injured area in a circle about the size of a baseball.
- See Rehabilitation section for shoulder exercises.

 CALL YOUR DOCTOR IF

- You have symptoms of shoulder tendinitis or tenosynovitis.
- Any of the following occurs after surgery:
  Increased pain, swelling, redness, drainage or bleeding in the surgical area.
  Signs of infection (headache, muscle aches, dizziness or a general ill feeling and fever).
  New, unexplained symptoms. Drugs used in treatment may produce side effects.

SHOULDER, FROZEN
(Adhesive Capsulitis)

 GENERAL INFORMATION

DEFINITION—A general term used to describe pain and stiffness in the shoulder joint that progresses to inability to use the shoulder. Adhesive capsulitis is the medical term. Frozen shoulder occurs more often in people over age 40, in women more than in men, and can last a few months to a year or longer. Usually only one shoulder is involved, but with some patients, both shoulders are affected.

BODY PARTS INVOLVED—Shoulder capsule (tissues surrounding the ball and socket joint) and the ligaments that attach the shoulder bones to each other.

SIGNS & SYMPTOMS
• Stage 1 (painful)—Ache or pain in the shoulder, often slight, that progresses to severe pain that interferes with sleep and normal activities. Pain worsens with shoulder movement. This stage may last for 2-9 months.
• Stage 2 (adhesive)—Less pain occurs, but stiffness increases in the shoulder preventing normal range of motion movement. Reduced movement increases stiffness. This stage may last 4-12 months.
• Stage 2 (recovery)—The condition begins to resolve. For most patients, the range of motion begins to increase. This stage may last for 12 months or up to several years.

CAUSES—Exact cause is unknown. It may be due to an inflammatory process. In some cases, it may result from an injury that leads to lack of use due to pain. Adhesions (abnormal bands of tissue) grow between the joint surfaces, restricting motion. Also, there is less synovial fluid which normally lubricates the shoulder joint to help it move.

RISK INCREASES WITH
• Shoulder injury, fracture or trauma (could be very minor).
• Diabetes mellitus.
• Heart disease, stroke or lung conditions, thyroid problems, Parkinson's and depression.
• Immobilization (prolonged inactivity) due to trauma, overuse injuries, or surgery.

HOW TO PREVENT
• Obtain early medical treatment for any shoulder injury, pain or stiffness.
• See your doctor on a regular basis if you have any of the risk factors listed above.
• Do regular stretching exercises.

 WHAT TO EXPECT

APPROPRIATE HEALTH CARE
• Doctor's care.
• Physical therapy.
• Self-care during rehabilitation.
• Surgery in some cases.

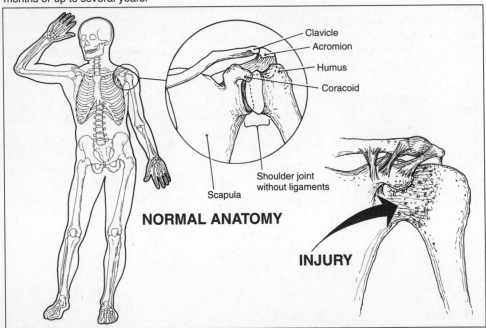

Clavicle
Acromion
Humus
Coracoid

Scapula

Shoulder joint without ligaments

NORMAL ANATOMY

INJURY

DIAGNOSTIC MEASURES
• Your own observation of symptoms.
• Medical history and physical exam by a doctor.
• Regular x-rays may be done or arthrography may be recommended. With arthrography, dye is injected into the shoulder and x-rays are taken. The results show the scarred and contracted tissue in the shoulder capsule. In some cases, an MRI scan is used to rule out other problems such as rotator cuff tear.

POSSIBLE COMPLICATIONS
• Some permanent shoulder disability and pain may occur despite treatment.
• If frozen shoulder is due to previous shoulder injury or surgery, treatment may be less successful.

PROBABLE OUTCOME—For the majority of patients, expect increased shoulder mobility and function with treatment and rehabilitation, but it may take many months to see the improvement.

 # HOW TO TREAT

NOTE—Follow your doctor's instructions. These instructions are supplemental.

FIRST AID—Not required. The problem develops slowly.

CONTINUING CARE
• The goal of treatment is to restore joint movement and reduce the pain. This is usually accomplished with medication and exercises.
• Application of heat (warm compresses or heating pad) to the affected area helps relieve pain. For some patients, ice may be more helpful.
• If conservative treatment is unsuccessful after several months, your doctor may recommend arthroscopic surgery to repair the shoulder.
• For some patients, manipulation may be recommended. In this procedure, while you are under a general anesthesia, the doctor stretches the shoulder joint capsule to break up the scar tissue.
• Other forms of treatment sometimes used along with exercise include acupuncture, ultrasound therapy and electrical stimulation.

MEDICATION
• Your doctor may prescribe:
Nonsteroidal anti-inflammatory drugs.
Muscle relaxers.
Injections of cortisone or local anesthesia into joints to reduce pain and inflammation.
• For minor pain, you may use nonprescription drugs such as ibuprofen or aspirin.

ACTIVITY
• Avoid activities which may increase the inflammation and pain. You may need help with accomplishing some daily activities.
• Some activity levels will depend on the underlying conditions (such as diabetes) that lead to the frozen shoulder.
• In most cases, you can resume your normal athletic or fitness activities as your symptoms ease and your shoulder feels comfortable. There may be some ongoing limitation in your range of motion.

DIET—During recovery, balance the amount of food you eat with any change in your level of physical activity. Eat a variety of foods to get the energy, protein, vitamins, minerals and fiber you need for good health and healing.

REHABILITATION
• Your doctor will prescribe supervised physical therapy.
• In addition to physical therapy, shoulder stretching exercises will be prescribed for you to do at home. These are done several times a day. Moist heat applied to the shoulder prior to the exercising and ice following helps some patients.
• Physical therapy and home exercises will be required following any surgical repair to help prevent a recurrence.

 # CALL YOUR DOCTOR IF

• You have any symptoms of a frozen shoulder. The longer a shoulder has been frozen, the more difficult it is to regain mobility and function.
• Several months of conservative treatment stops for your frozen shoulder are unsuccessful.
• New, unexplained symptoms develop. Drugs used in treatment may produce side effects.
• Following surgery, any signs of infection develop.

SKIN ABRASION

GENERAL INFORMATION

DEFINITION—Scraped skin or mucous membrane. An abrasion is usually a minor injury, but it can be serious if it covers a large area or if foreign materials become imbedded in it.

BODY PARTS INVOLVED—Skin or mucous membranes. The most common sites are usually over bone or other firm tissues.

SIGNS & SYMPTOMS
- Skin that looks scraped or irritated.
- Bleeding at the abrasion site.
- Immediate pain that lasts a short time.
- Crusting over the abraded area in 3 to 5 days.

CAUSES
- Falling on a hard, rough or jagged surface.
- Rough fabric, seams in clothing, ill-fitting shoes or other parts of athletic equipment such as helmets and shoulder pads that constantly irritate the skin.

RISK INCREASES WITH
- Athletic activity on rough terrain, such as bicycling or playing football or baseball (sliding).
- Skin that is not properly covered or protected, especially when playing on rough terrain.

HOW TO PREVENT
- Wear protective clothing, including long sleeves, high socks, knee and elbow pads and special clothing designed for your sport.
- Wear good-quality, well-fitting footgear to help avoid falls and to prevent foot abrasions.
- Choose athletic clothing wisely to avoid irritating fabric and poorly placed seams. A combination of cotton and synthetic may be the most comfortable. Seams of shorts on the inside of the thigh can be particularity irritating and should be checked for roughness before purchase.
- Avoid poor-quality playing fields.

WHAT TO EXPECT

APPROPRIATE HEALTH CARE
- Self-care for minor, noninfected wounds.
- Doctor's care for extensive contaminated abrasions.

DIAGNOSTIC MEASURES
- Your own observation of symptoms.
- Medical history and exam by a doctor.
- X-rays of underlying tissues (sometimes) to rule out other injuries.

PROBABLE COMPLICATIONS
- Infection.
- "Tattooing" if imbedded dark-colored foreign material is not carefully removed.

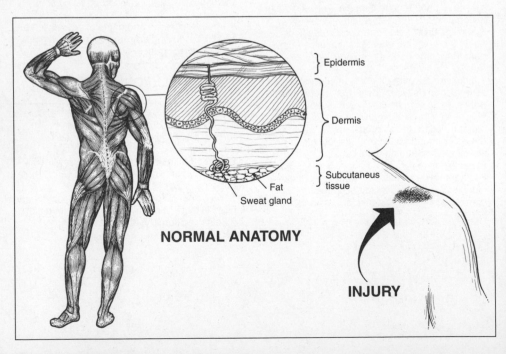

Epidermis

Dermis

Subcutaneus tissue

Fat

Sweat gland

NORMAL ANATOMY

INJURY

• Scarring if deeper layers of skin are affected (rare).

PROBABLE OUTCOME—The wound will heal in 3 to 10 days, depending on its location.

 ## HOW TO TREAT

NOTE—Follow your doctor's instructions. These instructions are supplemental.

FIRST AID
• For a scrape, wash the abraded area with plain soap and warm water as soon as possible. Scrub with a soft brush if possible. Soap acts as a solvent for imbedded dirt.
• For an irritation, protect the area against further abrasion. Use gauze or moleskin.

CONTINUING CARE
• If foreign material is imbedded too deeply or the wound is too painful to cleanse thoroughly, seek medical help.
• Cleanse lightly each day. If crusting or oozing occurs, soak in warm water with a little dishwashing or laundry detergent.
• Between soakings, apply nonprescription antibiotic ointment.
• Cover lightly with a bandage during the day, but leave the wound open to air at night.
• If infection occurs, use warm soaks more frequently. Keep the injured area elevated above the level of the heart, when possible.

MEDICATION
• Apply nonprescription antibiotic ointment to prevent infection.
• Spray with tincture of benzoin to reduce pain, if necessary.
• Don't use strong antiseptics such as iodine, Merthiolate, mercurochrome or alcohol. They will further irritate the skin.
• For minor discomfort, use aspirin, acetaminophen or ibuprofen.
• Your doctor may prescribe antibiotics if the abrasion becomes infected.

ACTIVITY—Resume normal activities as healing progresses, but don't overuse the abraded area until it heals. Protect it against repeated injury.

DIET—No special diet.

REHABILITATION—None.

 ## CALL YOUR DOCTOR IF

• You cannot clean all debris from an abrasion.
• Signs of infection begin (fever, headache or tenderness, increased oozing, redness, swelling and pain at the injury site).
• New, unexplained symptoms develop. Drugs used in treatment may produce side effects.

SKIN LACERATION

GENERAL INFORMATION

DEFINITION—A skin cut that has sharp or ragged edges. Athletic injuries are usually a combination of a contusion and a laceration, producing a bruised, jagged, irregular cut.

BODY PARTS INVOLVED—Any part of the body.

SIGNS & SYMPTOMS
- Cut of any type in the skin. Athletic injuries frequently produce lacerations at such a steep angle that they create flaps of skin.
- Pain at the lacerated site.
- Bleeding. This is especially heavy in lacerations of the scalp and forehead.
- Swelling, redness and tenderness around the laceration (sometimes).

CAUSES—Direct blow with a sharp or blunt object (boxer's glove, shoe, spike, cleat or sharp edge of another player's equipment).

RISK INCREASES WITH
- Contact sports.
- Auto, motorcycle or bicycle racing.
- Uneven terrain for a playing field.

HOW TO PREVENT
- Wear protective padding and equipment appropriate for your sport.
- Avoid playing on rough terrain when possible.
- Use seat belts in automobiles.

WHAT TO EXPECT

APPROPRIATE HEALTH CARE
- Doctor's treatment, which may include cleaning and evening of jagged edges as well as suturing (stitching) a laceration.
- Self-care after treatment.

DIAGNOSTIC MEASURES
- Your own observation of symptoms.
- Medical history and physical exam by a doctor.
- X-rays of bones adjacent to the laceration to rule out fractures.

POSSIBLE COMPLICATIONS
- Fluid collection under the sutures.
- Allergy to local anesthetics.
- Wound infection due to bacterial contamination of the laceration. If infection complicates healing, fever, pain and edema (collection of fluid) around the incision will occur. The edema may cause the sutures to become tighter and break.
- Scarring and disfigurement (sometimes).

PROBABLE OUTCOME—Lacerations usually heal in 2 weeks if they are sutured properly and do not become infected. Sutures are usually removed in about 10 days. Sutures for facial lacerations may be removed sooner. You will experience discomfort as the wound swells in the 6 to 20 hours after surgery.

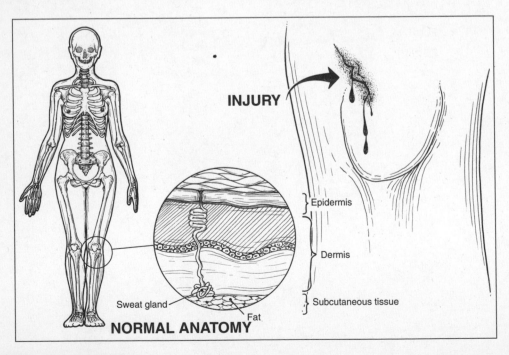

INJURY

Epidermis

Dermis

Subcutaneous tissue

Sweat gland

Fat

NORMAL ANATOMY

HOW TO TREAT

NOTE—Follow your doctor's instructions. These instructions are supplemental.

FIRST AID
For brisk bleeding:
- Cover the injured area with a cloth—or your bare hands if no cloth is available.
- Apply strong pressure directly to the laceration for 10 minutes while awaiting an ambulance or transportation to an emergency room.
- If direct pressure doesn't control brisk bleeding and bleeding is from an arm or leg, use a *light* tourniquet. Make a tourniquet from a length of cloth or similar material. Wrap and tie the tourniquet around the extremity above the wound. Place a stick or other rigid object between the cloth and the extremity. Twist the rigid object several times until the pressure is tight and bleeding stops. Note how long the tourniquet is in place so emergency medical personnel will know. Don't leave the tourniquet on longer than 20 minutes.

For wound care without brisk bleeding:
- Clean the wound carefully with soap and water.
- The wound will be cleaned again and sutured in the doctor's office or an emergency medical facility, usually under local anesthesia.

CONTINUING CARE
- Keep the wound covered with a bandage and moderate compression for 2 days to help prevent fluid collection under the sutures.
- If the bandage gels wet, replace it and apply nonprescription antibiotic ointment.
- If bleeding occurs after suturing, control it by applying firm pressure to the wound with a facial tissues or clean cloth. Hold the pressure for 10 minutes.
- Prevent tetanus by getting a booster dose of tetanus toxoid or human antitetanus serum.
- Protect a laceration with extra padding during contact sports until it heals.

MEDICATION
- For minor discomfort, you may use non-prescription drugs such as acetaminophen. Don't use aspirin, as it makes bleeding more likely.
- Your doctor may prescribe:
  Antibiotics to fight infection.
  Stronger pain medicine if needed.

ACTIVITY—Resume your normal activities gradually after treatment.

DIET—During recovery, balance the amount of food you eat with any change in your level of physical activity. Eat a variety of foods to get the energy, protein, vitamins, minerals and fiber you need for good health and healing.

REHABILITATION—None.

CALL YOUR DOCTOR IF

- You have a lacerated wound.
- You develop signs of a wound infection (fever, headache or increasing pain, redness and fluid with pus at the laceration site).
- A healed laceration leaves a scar and you would like to consider cosmetic surgery.

SKIN PUNCTURE WOUND

GENERAL INFORMATION

DEFINITION—Wound produced by any object that penetrates the skin to the soft tissues, bones or joint below.

BODY PARTS INVOLVED—Any part of the body.

SIGNS & SYMPTOMS—Hole in the skin with a puckered and discolored edge. The hole may appear smaller than the object that caused it due to partial reexpansion of the damaged tissues.

CAUSES—Any foreign body that penetrates the skin and underlying tissues (cleat, javelin, splinter, glass, etc.).

RISK INCREASES WITH
● Contact sports.
● Athletic activities on rough terrain.

HOW TO PREVENT—Avoid rough terrain for athletic activities.

WHAT TO EXPECT

APPROPRIATE HEALTH CARE—Doctor's treatment to clean the wound and sometimes to explore it surgically to determine the extent of damage.

DIAGNOSTIC MEASURES
● Your own observation of symptoms.
● Medical history and physical exam by a doctor.
● X-rays of the underlying area to rule out fractures and joint damage.

POSSIBLE COMPLICATIONS
● Fluid collection under a closed penetrating wound.
● Wound infection.

PROBABLE OUTCOME—With treatment, a puncture wound usually heals without complications.

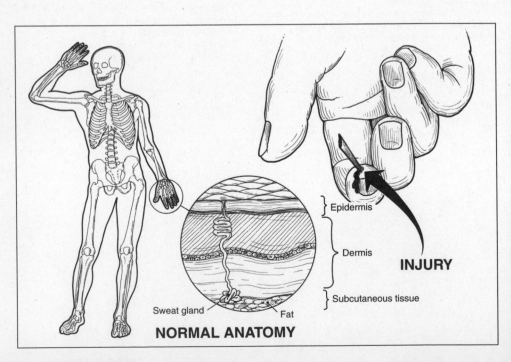

Epidermis

Dermis

Subcutaneous tissue

Sweat gland

Fat

INJURY

NORMAL ANATOMY

HOW TO TREAT

NOTE—Follow your doctor's instructions. These instructions are supplemental.

FIRST AID
• Remove any foreign material (splinter, glass, thorn or other) if you can.
• Clean the area with warm water and soap.

CONTINUING CARE
• Extensive or deep penetrating wounds may need to be enlarged and explored surgically under antiseptic conditions.
• If bleeding occurs, control it by applying firm pressure to the wound with a cloth.
• Use warm immersion soaks (see Glossary) to relieve pain and swelling.
• Rest the injured part until it heals.
• Wear a snug elastic bandage over the injured area if you can. This will decrease fluid collection under the wound and minimize further bleeding.

MEDICATION
• For minor discomfort, you may use non-prescription drugs such as acetaminophen
• Your doctor may prescribe antibiotics to fight infection.

ACTIVITY—Assume normal activity slowly after clearance by your doctor.

DIET—No special diet.

REHABILITATION—None

CALL YOUR DOCTOR IF

• You receive a puncture wound and have not had a tetanus booster in 10 years.
• You develop signs of a wound infection (fever, headache or increasing pain, redness and fluid with pus at the puncture site).

SPINE FRACTURE, LOWER THORACIC & LUMBAR REGION

GENERAL INFORMATION

DEFINITION—A complete or incomplete break in a bone in the lower thoracic or the lumbar spine. The lowest part of the thoracic spine and the first two bones of the lumbar spine are the most common sites for fractures in this region. This is due to the change in the spine's curvature and the lack of rib cage support.

BODY PARTS INVOLVED
- Bones of the lower thoracic and lumbar spine.
- Joints between segments of the spine.
- Soft tissues around the fracture site, including muscles, nerves, tendons, ligaments, periosteum (covering of bone), blood vessels and connective tissues.

SIGNS & SYMPTOMS
- Severe pain in the spine.
- Swelling and bruising around the fracture.
- Visible deformity if the fracture is complete and the bone fragments separate enough to distort normal back contours.
- Tenderness to the touch.
- Paralysis of legs and muscles in the pelvis if the spinal cord is injured.

CAUSES—Direct blow or indirect stress to the bone. Indirect stress can be excessive spinal flexing, extension, rotation or bending. Common situations that cause this fracture include:

- A hard fall in which the person lands on the heels.
- Falling into a sitting position, especially for an older person with osteoporosis.
- A heavy load falling on a bent back, such as someone jumping on a swimmer's back.

RISK INCREASES WITH
- Sledding or toboggan riding or ice skating.
- "Horseplay" around swimming pools and diving boards.
- Contact sports.
- History of bone or joint disease, especially osteoporosis.
- Obesity.
- Poor nutrition, especially calcium deficiency.
- If surgery or anesthesia is needed, risk increases with smoking and use of drugs, including mind-altering drugs, muscle relaxants, antihypertensives, tranquilizers, sleep inducers, insulin, sedatives, beta-adrenergic blockers or corticosteroids.

HOW TO PREVENT
- Participate in a strengthening, flexibility and conditioning program appropriate for your sport. Increased muscle mass helps protect bones and underlying tissues.
- Insure an adequate calcium intake (1000 mg to 1500 mg a day) with milk and milk products or calcium supplements.

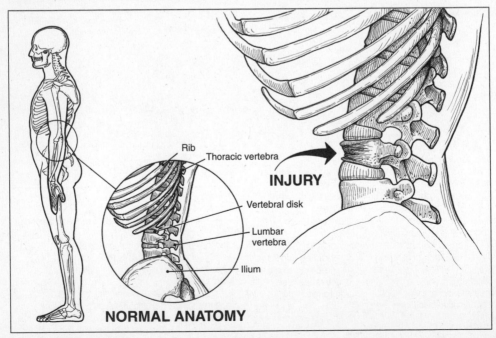

Rib
Thoracic vertebra
Vertebral disk
Lumbar vertebra
Ilium

INJURY

NORMAL ANATOMY

WHAT TO EXPECT

APPROPRIATE HEALTH CARE
• Traction.
• Surgery (sometimes) to set and immobilize the fracture.
• Long rehabilitation program and physical therapy if the spinal cord is damaged.

DIAGNOSTIC MEASURES
• Your own observation of symptoms.
• Medical history and exam by a doctor.
• X-rays of the spine.

POSSIBLE COMPLICATIONS
At the time of fracture:
• Shock.
• Pressure on or injury to the spinal cord, nearby nerves, ligaments, tendons, blood vessels or connective tissues.
After treatment or surgery:
• Excessive bleeding.
• Impaired blood supply to the healing bone.
• Arrested bone growth in a young person.
• Infection introduced during surgical treatment.
• Unstable or arthritic joint after repeated injury.
• Paralysis (sometimes).
• Deformity of the spine, with prominence (also referred to as a gibbus or hump).

PROBABLE OUTCOME—The average healing time for this fracture is 6 to 12 weeks. Healing is considered complete when there is no pain or motion at the fracture site and when x-rays show complete bone union.

HOW TO TREAT

NOTE—Follow your doctor's instructions. These instructions are supplemental.

FIRST AID
• Cut away clothing, if possible, but don't move the injured area to do so.
• Use a spine board to immobilize the back while transporting the injured person to an emergency facility.
• Elevate the injured part above the level of the heart to reduce swelling and prevent accumulation of excess fluid. To do so, elevate the foot of the spine board or the bed.
• Keep the patient warm with blankets to decrease the possibility of shock.
• Treatment consists of surgically or non-surgically realigning the spine and holding it in its correct position. Realignment should be done as soon as possible after injury. Many tissues lose their elasticity and become difficult to return to their normal positions.

CONTINUING CARE
• Immobilization will be necessary. This may mean immobilization of the patient in bed in a rehabilitation facility or immobilization of the fractured bones with internal wires or screws. A brace is common, while a cast is rarely used.
• After treatment, use ice massage if possible. Fill a large styrofoam cup with water and freeze. Tear a small amount of foam from the top so ice protrudes. Massage firmly over the injured area in a circle about the size of a softball. Do this for 15 minutes at a time 3 or 4 times a day.
• After 72 hours, you may apply heat instead of ice if it feels better. Use heat lamps, hot soaks, hot showers or heating pads.
• Take whirlpool treatments, if available.
• Massage gently and often to provide comfort and decrease swelling.

MEDICATION—Your doctor may prescribe:
• General anesthesia, local anesthesia or muscle relaxants to make bone manipulation possible.
• Special corticosteroids, such as dexamethasone, to reduce swelling and minimize spinal cord damage.
• Strong pain relievers for severe pain.
• Stool softeners to prevent constipation due to inactivity.
• Acetaminophen (available without prescription) for mild pain after initial treatment.
• Antibiotics to fight infection if needed.

ACTIVITY—Resume normal activities and begin rehabilitation after clearance from your doctor.

DIET
• Do not eat or drink before manipulation or surgery to treat fracture. Fluid or solid food in you stomach makes vomiting while under anesthesia more hazardous.
• During recovery, eat a well-balanced diet.

REHABILITATION—Begin daily rehabilitation exercise when movement is comfortable. Use ice massage for 10 minutes prior to exercise. See Rehabilitation section for low back exercises.

CALL YOUR DOCTOR IF

• You have signs or symptoms of a spine fracture.
• Any of the following occurs after treatment or surgery:
Numbness, complete loss of feeling or paralysis below the fracture site.
Increased pain, swelling or drainage in the surgical area.
Signs of infection (headache, muscle aches, dizziness or a general ill feeling and fever).
Nausea or vomiting; constipation.

SPINE FRACTURE, SACRUM

GENERAL INFORMATION

DEFINITION—A complete or incomplete break in the sacrum. This is a serious injury, because it frequently damages important nerves that supply the rectum, bladder and genitals. Signs of this nerve damage may not appear for several days after injury.

BODY PARTS INVOLVED
- Sacrum.
- Lumbosacral and sacroiliac joints.
- Soft tissues around the fracture site, including muscles, nerves, tendons, ligaments, periosteum (covering of bone), blood vessels and connective tissues.

SIGNS & SYMPTOMS
- Severe pain in the lower spine.
- Swelling and bruising of soft tissues around the fracture.
- Visible deformity if the fracture is complete and the bone fragments separate enough to distort normal body contours.
- Tenderness to the touch.
- Numbness beyond the fracture site (sometimes).

CAUSES
- Direct blow to the lower back.
- Indirect stress caused by twisting or other injury to the lower back.

RISK INCREASES WITH
- Skating.
- Contact sports.
- History of bone or joint disease, especially osteoporosis.
- Obesity.
- Poor nutrition, especially calcium deficiency.
- If surgery or anesthesia is needed, risk increases with smoking and use of drugs, including mind-altering drugs, muscle relaxants, antihypertensives, tranquilizers, sleep inducers, insulin, sedatives, beta-adrenergic blockers or cortisone.

HOW TO PREVENT
- Participate in a strengthening, flexibility and conditioning program appropriate for your sport. Increased muscle mass helps protect bones and underlying tissues.
- Use appropriate protective equipment, such as sacral or "tailbone" pads, when participating in contact sports.
- Ensure an adequate calcium intake (1000 mg to 1500 mg a day) with milk and milk products or calcium supplements.

WHAT TO EXPECT

APPROPRIATE HEALTH CARE
- Doctor's treatment to manipulate the broken bones or to prescribe bed rest and support with a sacral corset.

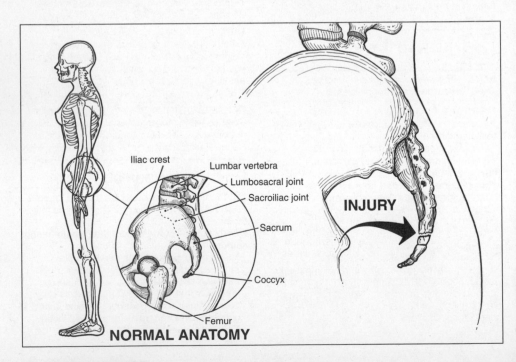

Iliac crest
Lumbar vertebra
Lumbosacral joint
Sacroiliac joint
Sacrum
Coccyx
Femur

INJURY

NORMAL ANATOMY

• Surgery (sometimes) to set the fracture if the fractured ends are displaced or to relieve pressure if there is evidence of nerve damage.

DIAGNOSTIC MEASURES
• Your own observation of symptoms.
• Medical history and exam by a doctor.
• X-rays of the lower back region, including the pelvis and hips.

POSSIBLE COMPLICATIONS
At the time of fracture:
• Shock.
• Pressure on or injury to nearby nerves, ligaments, tendons, blood vessels or connective tissues.
• Injury to the rectum.
After treatment or surgery:
• Excessive bleeding.
• Interference with bladder, rectal and sexual functions caused by postoperative swelling and pressure on nerves and blood vessels.
• Infection introduced during surgical treatment.
• Unstable or arthritic sacroiliac joint.

PROBABLE OUTCOME—The average healing time for this fracture is 6 to 12 weeks. Healing is considered complete when there is no pain at the fracture site and when x-rays show complete bone union.

HOW TO TREAT

NOTE—Follow your doctor's instructions. These instructions are supplemental.

FIRST AID
• Use a spine board to immobilize the back while transporting the injured person to an emergency facility.
• Keep the person warm with blankets to decrease the possibility of shock.
• The doctor may manipulate the broken bones in surgery to return them to their normal positions. Manipulation should be done as soon as possible after injury, particularly if there is evidence of injury to major nerves in the lower back region. Many tissues lose their elasticity and become difficult to return to their normal positions.

CONTINUING CARE
• Immobilization will be necessary. Non-displaced sacrum fractures usually require use of a corset. Displaced fractures may require more complicated immobilization techniques such as traction.
• After treatment, use ice massage if possible. Fill a large styrofoam cup with water and freeze. Tear a small amount of foam from the top so ice protrudes. Massage firmly over the injured area in a circle about the size of a softball. Do this for 15 minutes at a time 3 or 4 times a day.
• Apply heat instead of ice if it feels better. Use heat lamps, hot soaks, hot showers, heating pads or whirlpool treatments.
• Massage gently and often to provide comfort and decrease swelling.

MEDICATION—Your doctor may prescribe:
• General anesthesia, local anesthesia or muscle relaxants before joint manipulation.
• Narcotic or synthetic narcotic pain relievers for severe pain.
• Acetaminophen for mild pain.
• Stool softeners to prevent constipation due to inactivity.
• Antibiotics to fight infection if skin is broken or surgery is needed.

ACTIVITY
• Bed rest will be necessary for 2 to 6 weeks. You may need to wear a corset for support once you begin activity.
• During recovery, actively exercise all muscle groups not immobilized. Muscle contractions promote fracture alignment and hasten healing.
• Begin reconditioning and rehabilitation after clearance from your doctor.
• Resume normal daily activities gradually.

DIET
• Do not eat or drink before manipulation or surgery to treat the fracture. Fluid or solid food in your stomach makes vomiting while under anesthesia more hazardous.
• During recovery, balance the amount of food you eat with any change in your level of physical activity. Eat a variety of foods to get the energy, protein, vitamins, minerals and fiber you need for good health and healing.

REHABILITATION—Begin daily rehabilitation exercises when movement is comfortable. Use ice massage for 10 minutes prior to exercise. See Rehabilitation section for low back exercises.

CALL YOUR DOCTOR IF

• You have signs and symptoms of a sacrum fracture or observe these signs in someone else.
• Any of the following occurs after treatment or surgery:
Loss of feeling below the fracture site.
Increased pain, swelling or drainage in the surgical area.
Signs of infection (headache, muscle aches, dizziness or a general ill feeling and fever).
Impaired bladder, rectal or sexual function.

SPINE FRACTURE, TAILBONE (COCCYX)

GENERAL INFORMATION

DEFINITION—A complete or incomplete break in the coccyx (tailbone).

BODY PARTS INVOLVED
- Coccyx (lower tip of the spine).
- Joints connecting the coccyx to the sacrum.
- Soft tissues around the fracture site, including muscles, nerves, tendons, ligaments, periosteum (covering of bone), blood vessels and connective tissues.

SIGNS & SYMPTOMS
- Pain at the fracture site.
- Swelling and bruising of soft tissues around the fracture.
- Tenderness to the touch, especially when trying to sit down.

CAUSES
- Falling into a sitting position on the tailbone.
- Direct blow or kick to the tailbone.

RISK INCREASES WITH
- Skating, skiing and snowboarding.
- Contact sports.
- History of bone or joint disease, especially osteoporosis.
- Obesity.
- Poor nutrition, especially calcium deficiency.

- If surgery or anesthesia is needed, risk increases with smoking and use of drugs, including mind-altering drugs, muscle relaxants, antihypertensives, tranquilizers, sleep inducers, insulin, sedatives, beta-adrenergic blockers or corticosteroids.

HOW TO PREVENT
- Participate in a strengthening, flexibility and conditioning program appropriate for your sport.
- Use appropriate protective equipment, such as sacral or tailbone pads, during participation in contact sports.
- Ensure an adequate calcium intake (1000 mg to 1500 mg a day) with milk and milk products or calcium supplements.

WHAT TO EXPECT

APPROPRIATE HEALTH CARE
- Doctor's treatment to manipulate the broken coccyx.
- Hospitalization (sometimes) for anesthesia and surgery to remove the fractured coccyx.
- Physical therapy and rehabilitation exercises.
- Self-care during rehabilitation.

DIAGNOSTIC MEASURES
- Your own observation of symptoms.
- Medical history and exam by a doctor.
- X-rays of injured areas, including all of the lower back, pelvis and hips.

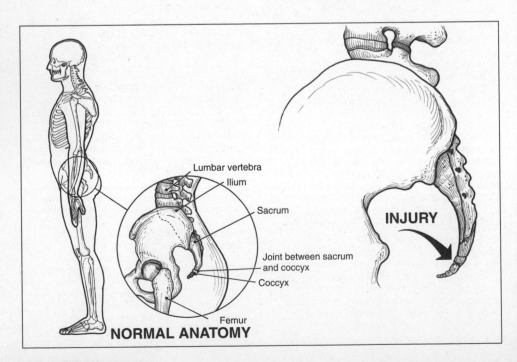

Lumbar vertebra
Ilium
Sacrum
Joint between sacrum and coccyx
Coccyx
Femur
NORMAL ANATOMY

INJURY

POSSIBLE COMPLICATIONS

At the time of fracture:
- Shock.
- Pressure on or injury to nearby nerves, ligaments, tendons, blood vessels or connective tissues.

After treatment or surgery:
- Excessive bleeding.
- Impaired blood supply to the healing bone.
- Infection introduced during surgical treatment.
- Unstable or arthritic tailbone joint following repeated injury.
- Continuing pain long after injury.

PROBABLE OUTCOME—The average healing time for this fracture is 8 to 12 weeks. Healing is considered complete when there is no motion at the fracture site and when x-rays show complete bone union.

 ## HOW TO TREAT

NOTE—Follow your doctor's instructions. These instructions are supplemental.

FIRST AID
- Cut away clothing, if possible, but don't move the injured area to do so.
- Apply ice packs to the injury site to decrease swelling and pain.
- Elevate the injured part above the level of the heart to reduce swelling and prevent accumulation of excess fluid. Use pillows to prop the lower part of the body, or elevate the foot of the bed.
- Keep the injured person warm. Cover with blankets to decrease the possibility of shock.
- The doctor will manipulate the broken coccyx into normal position in a "closed" procedure (without surgery) or will remove the coccyx surgically. Manipulation should be done as soon as possible after injury. Many tissues lose their elasticity and become difficult to return to their normal positions.

CONTINUING CARE—Treatment after manipulation or surgical removal:
- Use frequent ice massage. Fill a large styrofoam cup with water and freeze. Tear a small amount of foam from the top so ice protrudes. Massage firmly over the tailbone area in a circle about the size of a softball. Do this for 15 minutes at a time 3 or 4 times a day.

- Apply heat instead of ice if it feels better. Use heat lamps, hot soaks, hot towels, heating pads or heat liniments and ointments.
- Take whirlpool treatments, if available.
- Massage gently and often to provide comfort and decrease swelling.
- Use an air-filled or foam rubber donut-shaped pillow for sitting.

MEDICATION—Your doctor may prescribe:
- General, spinal or local anesthesia during surgery to remove the fractured coccyx.
- Narcotic or synthetic narcotic pain relievers for severe pain.
- Acetaminophen for mild pain.
- Stool softeners to prevent constipation due to inactivity.
- Antibiotics to fight infection it skin is broken or surgery is needed.

ACTIVITY—Begin reconditioning and rehabilitation after clearance from your doctor. Resume normal daily activities gradually after treatment.

DIET
- Do not eat or drink before manipulation or surgery to treat the fracture. Fluid or solid food in your stomach makes vomiting while under anesthesia more hazardous.
- During recovery, balance the amount of food you eat with any change in your level of physical activity. Eat a variety of foods to get the energy, protein, vitamins, minerals and fiber you need for good health and healing.

REHABILITATION—Begin daily rehabilitation exercises when movement is comfortable. Use ice massage for 10 minutes prior to exercise. See Rehabilitation section for low back exercises.

 ## CALL YOUR DOCTOR IF

- You have signs or symptoms of a fractured tailbone after a hard fall or injury.
- Any of the following occurs after surgery:
  Increased pain, swelling or drainage in the surgical area.
  Signs of infection (headache, muscle aches, dizziness or a general ill feeling and fever).
  Numbness or complete loss of feeling below the fracture site.
  Nausea or vomiting.
  Constipation.

SPINE STRESS FRACTURE, NECK OR BACK (Spondylolysis)

 GENERAL INFORMATION

DEFINITION—A hairline fracture of the spine in the neck or back (cervical, thoracic or lumbar spine) that develops after repeated stress. A stress fracture is sometimes called a fatigue fracture. x-ray changes may not appear clearly for several weeks after pain begins. The x-ray appearance may be similar to that of a bone tumor.

BODY PARTS INVOLVED
* Any segment of the spinal column in the neck or back, but most commonly the lower three lumbar vertebrae.
* Any joint connecting segments of the spinal column.
* Soft tissues surrounding the fracture site, including muscles, nerves, tendons, ligaments, periosteum (covering of bone), blood vessels and connective tissues.

SIGNS & SYMPTOMS
* Severe pain in the neck or back following injury, worsening with twisting and back extension.
* Swelling and bruising of soft tissues around the fracture.
* Tenderness to the touch.
* Warmth over the fracture site.

CAUSES—Direct or indirect stress to the bone. Indirect stress may be caused by twisting, marked hyperextension or violent muscle contraction.

RISK INCREASES WITH
* Weightlifting using poor technique.
* Contact sports such as football, wrestling, boxing or soccer.
* Gymnastics.
* History of bone or joint disease, especially osteoporosis.
* Congenital abnormality in shape of vertebrae.
* Oligomenorrhea or amenorrhea (decreased or absent menstrual periods) due to low percentage of body fat as seen in women with eating disorders and habitual exercisers.
* Obesity.
* Poor nutrition, especially insufficient calcium and protein.
* If surgery or anesthesia is needed, risk increases with smoking and use of drugs, including mind-altering drugs, muscle relaxants, antihypertensives, tranquilizers, sleep inducers, insulin, sedatives, beta-adrenergic blockers or corticosteroids.

HOW TO PREVENT
* Participate in a strengthening, flexibility and conditioning program appropriate for your sport. Increased muscle mass helps protect bones and underlying tissues.

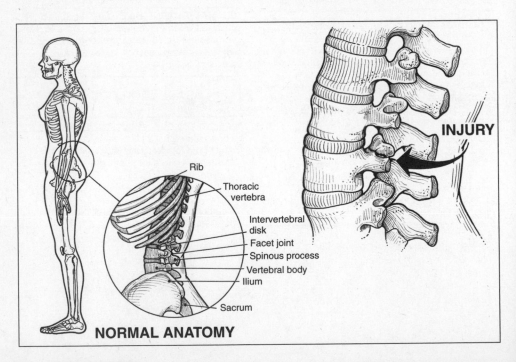

Rib
Thoracic vertebra
Intervertebral disk
Facet joint
Spinous process
Vertebral body
Ilium
Sacrum

INJURY

NORMAL ANATOMY

• Ensure an adequate calcium intake (1000 mg to 1500 mg a day) with milk and milk products or calcium supplements.

 ## WHAT TO EXPECT

APPROPRIATE HEALTH CARE
• Doctor's diagnosis and care.
• Physical therapy and rehabilitation.
• Self-care during rehabilitation.

DIAGNOSTIC MEASURES
• Your own observations of symptoms.
• Medical history and physical exam by a doctor.
• X-rays of the neck and back.
• Technetium bone scan (see Glossary) for continued symptoms when x-rays are normal.

POSSIBLE COMPLICATIONS
• Pressure on or injury to nearby nerves, ligaments, tendons, blood vessels or connective tissues from chronic stress fractures.
• Complete fracture and spinal cord damage from continued activity after symptoms begin.
• Problems arising from plaster casts, splints or other immobilizing materials. See Appendix 2 (Care of Casts).
• Arrest of bone growth in young people.
• Unstable or arthritic joint following repeated injury.
• Spondylolisthesis (slipping of one vertebra upon the next, which results in damage to the intervening disk and potential nerve injury).

PROBABLE OUTCOME
• It is impossible to predict exactly how long a fracture will take to heal. Variable factors include age, sex, previous health and general conditioning. The average healing time for this fracture is 3 months. Healing is considered complete when there is no pain at the fracture site and when x-rays show complete bone union.
• Commonly this injury does not heal permanently, but the symptoms may be lessened with flexibility and strengthening exercises.

 ## HOW TO TREAT

NOTE—Follow your doctor's instructions. These instructions are supplemental.

FIRST AID—None. This fracture develops gradually and does not require setting. The fractured bone is not displaced.

CONTINUING CARE—Treatment after manipulation or surgical removal:
• After cast removal, use frequent ice massage. Fill a large styrofoam cup with water and freeze. Tear a small amount of foam from the top so ice protrudes. Massage firmly over the injured area in a circle about the size of a softball. Do this for 15 minutes at a time 3 or 4 times a day.
• Apply heat instead of ice if it feels better. Use heat lamps, hot soaks, hot showers, heating pads or heat liniments and ointments.
• Take whirlpool treatments, if available.
• Massage gently and often to provide comfort and decrease swelling.

MEDICATION—Your doctor may prescribe:
• Pain relievers for severe pain.
• Stool softeners to prevent constipation due to inactivity.
• Acetaminophen (available without prescription) for mild pain after initial treatment.

ACTIVITY
• Actively exercise all muscles groups not immobilized. Muscle contractions promote fracture alignment and hasten healing.
• Resume normal daily activities gradually after treatment.
• Begin reconditioning and rehabilitation after clearance from your doctor.

DIET—During recovery, balance the amount of food you eat with any change in your level of physical activity. Eat a variety of foods to get the energy, protein, vitamins, minerals and fiber you need for good health and healing.

REHABILITATION—Begin daily rehabilitation exercises when movement is allowed. Use ice massage for 10 minutes prior to exercise. See Rehabilitation section for low back exercises and upper back exercises.

 ## CALL YOUR DOCTOR IF

You have symptoms of a spinal stress fracture, especially unexplained persistent numbness or pain in the neck or back.

SPLEEN RUPTURE

GENERAL INFORMATION

DEFINITION—Injury to the spleen, causing it to rupture. Bleeding of a ruptured spleen can be fatal. The spleen is vulnerable to injury, particularly if it is enlarged due to any underlying disorder (infectious mononucleosis is the most common). Spleen injuries are infrequent in athletes, but when they do occur, they can be disastrous.

BODY PARTS INVOLVED
- Spleen.
- Muscles of the abdominal wall.
- Peritoneum (membranous covering of the intestines).
- Ribs (sometimes) if fractured at the same time the spleen is injured.

SIGNS & SYMPTOMS
- Recent injury to the abdomen or flank.
- Rib fracture on the left side.
- Vomiting.
- Abdominal pain, rigidity and tenderness.
- Pain in the left shoulder or the left side of the neck.
- Rapid heart rate.
- Low blood pressure.
- Other signs of shock—pale, moist and sweaty skin; anxiety with feelings of impending doom; shortness of breath and rapid breathing; disorientation and confusion.

CAUSES—Direct injury to the left upper abdomen or the left side of the chest.

RISK INCREASES WITH
- Contact sports.
- Medical history of any bleeding disorder.
- Infectious mononucleosis or any other illness that causes spleen enlargement. If surgery is necessary, surgical risk increases with smoking, use of mind-altering drugs, muscle relaxants, tranquilizers, sleep induces, insulin, sedatives, beta-adrenergic blockers or corticosteroids.

HOW TO PREVENT—Avoid causes and risk factors when possible. Don't return to athletic activities until a spleen enlarged by disease has returned to normal.

WHAT TO EXPECT

APPROPRIATE HEALTH CARE
- Doctor's examination. When abdominal symptoms follow a blow to the abdomen, it is imperative that a diagnosis be established as soon as possible. Injury to any organ in the abdomen (spleen, liver, intestines, kidney, bladder, pancreas) causes an acute surgical emergency.
- Hospitalization for intravenous fluids or transfusions to treat shock.
- Surgery under general anesthesia to remove the ruptured spleen.

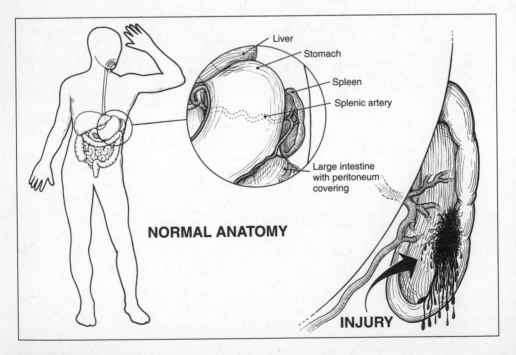

Liver
Stomach
Spleen
Splenic artery
Large intestine with peritoneum covering

NORMAL ANATOMY

INJURY

DIAGNOSTIC MEASURES

Before surgery:
- Blood and urine studies.
- X-rays of the abdomen and chest, CT scan (see Glossary).

After surgery:
- Examination of all tissues removed.
- Additional blood studies.

POSSIBLE COMPLICATIONS

At the time of injury:
- Rapid deterioration due to internal bleeding, possibly leading to death.

Following surgery:
- Excessive bleeding.
- Infection.
- Incisional hernia.
- Lung collapse.
- Inflammation of the pancreas.
- Deep vein blood clots.
- Pneumonia.

PROBABLE OUTCOME—Expect complete healing if no complications occur. Allow about 4 weeks for recovery from surgery.

 HOW TO TREAT

NOTE—Follow your doctor's instructions. These instructions are supplemental.

FIRST AID—Cover the victim with a blanket to combat shock, and take him or her to the nearest emergency facility. Do not give water, food or pain relievers.

CONTINUING CARE—No specific instructions except those under other headings. If surgery is required, your surgeon will supply postoperative instructions.

MEDICATION

- Do not give pain relievers at the time of injury. They may mask symptoms.

- After surgery, your doctor may prescribe:
  Pain relievers. Don't take prescription pain medication longer than 4 to 7 days. Use only as much as you need.
  Antibiotics to fight infection.
  Pneumonia vaccinations.
  Stool softeners to prevent constipation.
  Nonprescription drugs such as acetaminophen for minor pain.

ACTIVITY

- Avoid vigorous exercise for 6 weeks after surgery.
- Resume driving 4 weeks after returning home.

DIET

- Do not eat or drink before surgery. Fluid or solid food in your stomach makes vomiting while under anesthesia more hazardous.
- Drink a clear liquid diet until the gastrointestinal tract functions again. During recovery, balance the amount of food you eat with any change in your level of physical activity. Eat a variety of foods to get the energy, protein, vitamins, minerals and fiber you need for good health and healing.

REHABILITATION—Rehabilitation exercises must be individualized. Follow your doctor's or surgeon's directions.

 CALL YOUR DOCTOR IF

- You receive any abdominal injury and the symptoms last longer than a few minutes, worsen or recur within hours or days. This may be an emergency!
- Any of the following occurs after surgery:
  You develop signs of infection (headache, muscle aches, dizziness or a general ill feeling and fever).
  Pain, swelling, redness, drainage or bleeding increases in the surgical area.
  New, unexplained symptoms develop. Drugs used in treatment may produce side effects.

TESTICULAR TRAUMA

GENERAL INFORMATION

DEFINITION—Soft tissue damage and occasionally structural damage to the testicles. This type of injury is a relatively uncommon occurrence. In some cases, testicular injury is a complication of a larger trauma such as a pelvic fracture or hip dislocation. Young men (ages 15-40 years) are the most likely to experience testicular trauma. A more severe (but rare) injury, testicular rupture, occurs when the testicle receives a direct blow or is squeezed against the hard bones of the pelvis. This injury can cause blood to leak into the scrotum. Testicular torsion occurs when the spermatic cord gets twisted around a testicle, cutting off the blood supply to the testicle.

BODY PARTS INVOLVED—The testicles, also called testes, are located within the scrotum, which hangs outside of the body. Testes are suspended within the scrotum by the spermatic cord, allowing them to be freely mobile within the genital area. This allow testes to be protected from minor external trauma.

SIGNS & SYMPTOMS
- Mild to severe pain
- Bruising (discoloration) and/or swelling.
- Bleeding.
- Thickening of the skin.
- Symptoms of pressure.
- Frequently associated with nausea and vomiting, or feeling of faintness.

CAUSES—The testicles are struck, hit, kicked or crushed usually during participation in contact sports. The injury may result in a contusion, laceration, fracture, or dislocation. Injuries can be mild, from a slight cut or accidental hit, to more severe trauma.

RISK INCREASES WITH
- Contact sports such as football, soccer or hockey.
- Sports such as baseball and lacrosse.
- Horseback riding.
- Previous groin injury.

HOW TO PREVENT
- Use protective gear. Wear an athletic cup and supporter when practicing or playing sports or doing strenuous activity. Be sure the athletic supporter and cup you wear are the right size.
- Know what risks are associated with your sport.

WHAT TO EXPECT

APPROPRIATE HEALTH CARE
- Doctor's care, unless the injury is quite minor. Additional treatment depends on the severity and extent of the injuries.
- Surgery sometimes (for severe injury).
- With testicular torsion, if the testicle doesn't untwist on its own, your doctor will try to untwist it by hand, or, if that fails, surgery will be needed.

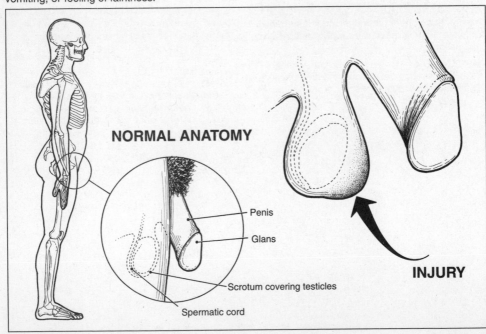

NORMAL ANATOMY

Penis

Glans

Scrotum covering testicles

Spermatic cord

INJURY

DIAGNOSTIC MEASURES
- Your own observation of symptoms.
- Medical history and exam by a doctor.
- Ultrasound, x-rays or other imaging studies of the testicles can help determine the nature and extent of injury.
- A urinalysis may be done to rule out urinary tract infection.

POSSIBLE COMPLICATIONS
- Problems with the testes can lead to serious illnesses, including hormonal imbalances, problems with sex, and infertility. Epididymus is where sperm maturation takes place, following which they are transported out during ejaculation. Obstruction of epididymus would inhibit sperm flow
- Without treatment, testicular infection, atrophy (shrinkage), and necrosis (tissue destruction) may occur.
- If the blood supply to the testicle is cut off for a long period of time, the testicle can become permanently damaged and may need to be removed.

PROBABLE OUTCOME
- Minor testicular injuries rarely have long-term effects.
- Most testicular trauma will heal completely. The usual treatment consists of scrotal support, ice packs, and bedrest for 24-48 hours. Sutures may be needed for any cuts. Surgery may be required to drain any accumulated blood and repair the testes.

 HOW TO TREAT

NOTE—Follow your doctor's instructions. These instructions are supplemental.

FIRST AID—Follow instructions for R.I.C.E., the first letters of *rest, ice, compression* and *elevation*. See Appendix 1 for details.

CONTINUING CARE
- Rest and apply ice packs to the area at least every 3-4 hours to decrease swelling.
- After the first 24 hours, apply heat instead of ice if it feels better. Use heat lamps, hot soaks, hot showers, heating pads.
- Wear a soft athletic support or jock strap to provide support and decrease the pain in the testicles.

MEDICATION
- For minor discomfort, you may use aspirin, acetaminophen or ibuprofen.
- Your doctor may prescribe:
  Stronger pain relievers.
  Antibiotics for infection if surgery is necessary.

ACTIVITY—Resume your normal activities gradually after clearance from your doctor. It can take weeks to months to recover from testicular surgery and resume normal sports activities.

DIET—During recovery, balance the amount of food you eat with any change in your level of physical activity. Eat a variety of foods to get the energy, protein, vitamins, minerals and fiber you need for good health and healing.

REHABILITATION—None required.

 CALL YOUR DOCTOR IF

- You have symptoms of a testicular injury (pain, bruising, swelling, or blood in your urine). Don't delay.
- Pain or swelling worsens despite treatment.
- Any of the following occurs after surgery:
  Increased pain, swelling, redness, drainage or bleeding in the surgical area.
  Signs of infection (headache, muscle aches, dizziness or a general ill feeling with fever).

THIGH BONE (FEMUR) FRACTURE

GENERAL INFORMATION

DEFINITION—A complete or incomplete break in the shaft of the femur (the large bone extending from the hip to the knee). This is a serious injury, but unusual in sports. The ankle, lower leg or knee will usually give way before the shaft of the femur does.

BODY PARTS INVOLVED
- Femur (usually in the middle of the bone).
- Soft tissues around the fracture site, including muscles, nerves, tendons, ligaments, periosteum (covering of bone), blood vessels and connective tissues.

SIGNS & SYMPTOMS
- Severe pain in the mid thigh at the time of injury.
- Swelling and bruising around the fracture.
- Visible deformity if the fracture is complete and the bone fragments separate enough to distort normal leg contours.
- Tenderness to the touch.
- Numbness and coldness in the leg and foot beyond the fracture site if the blood supply is impaired.

CAUSES
- Direct blow to the thigh.
- Indirect stress caused by twisting or violent muscle contraction.

RISK INCREASES WITH
- Physical therapy and rehabilitation.
- Contact sports (e.g., football).
- Field and track events.
- History of bone or joint disease, especially osteoporosis.
- Obesity.
- Poor nutrition, especially calcium deficiency.
- If surgery or anesthesia is needed, risk increases with smoking and use of drugs, including mind-altering drugs, muscle relaxants, antihypertensives, tranquilizers, sleep inducers, insulin, sedatives, beta-adrenergic blockers or corticosteroids.

HOW TO PREVENT
- Participate in a strengthening, flexibility and conditioning program appropriate for your sport. Increased muscle mass helps protect bones and underlying tissues.
- Ensure an adequate calcium intake (1000 mg to 1500 mg a day) with milk and milk products or calcium supplements.
- Use appropriate protective equipment, such as thigh pads, for participation in contact sports.

WHAT TO EXPECT

APPROPRIATE HEALTH CARE
- Doctor's care.
- Surgery to set the broken femur with use of a plate and screws or a rod and screws.

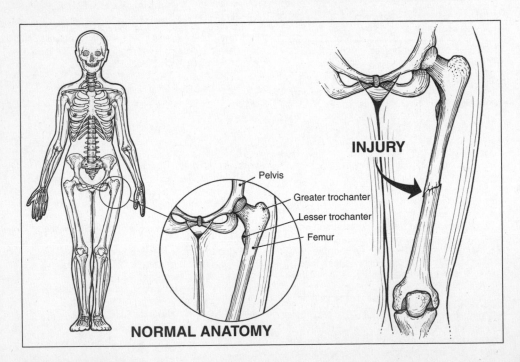

Pelvis
Greater trochanter
Lesser trochanter
Femur

INJURY

NORMAL ANATOMY

- Traction (sometimes) temporarily and then surgery to place an intramedullary rod in femur. No cast is necessary after surgery.
- Immobilization with a cast (sometimes) initially in small children.
- Physical therapy and rehabilitation.

DIAGNOSTIC MEASURES
- Your own observation of symptoms.
- Medical history and exam by a doctor.
- X-rays of the ankle, knee, femur and pelvis.

POSSIBLE COMPLICATIONS
At the time of fracture:
- Shock.
- Pressure on or injury to nearby nerves, ligaments, tendons, blood vessels or connective tissues.

After treatment or surgery:
- Excessive bleeding.
- Poor healing (nonunion) of the fracture.
- Impaired blood supply to the healing bone.
- Avascular necrosis (death of bone cells due to interruption of the blood supply).
- Shortening or deformity of fractured femur.
- Arrest of normal bone growth in children.
- Infection introduced during surgery.
- Problems caused by plaster casts. See Appendix 2 (Care of Casts).

PROBABLE OUTCOME—The average healing time for this fracture is 10 to 16 weeks. Healing is considered complete when there is no pain or motion at the fracture site and when x-rays show complete bone union.

 ## HOW TO TREAT

NOTE—Follow your doctor's instructions. These instructions are supplemental.

FIRST AID
- Keep the person warm with blankets to decrease the possibility of shock.
- Cut away clothing, if possible, but don't move the injured leg to do so.
- Follow instructions for R.I.C.E., the first letters of *rest, ice, compression* and *elevation.* See Appendix 1 for details.
- Use a padded splint or back board to immobilize the hip and leg before transporting the injured person to an emergency facility.
- The doctor will set (realign) the broken bones with surgery or, if possible, without. Realignment should be done as soon as possible after injury. Many tissues lose their elasticity and become difficult to return to their normal positions.

CONTINUING CARE
- Immobilization will be necessary, but is usually accomplished in surgery with metal screws, plates or a rod. Children are sometimes treated with immobilization preceding traction.

- After 48 hours, application of localized heat promotes healing by increasing blood circulation in the injured area. Use a heat lamp or heating pad so heat can penetrate the cast.
- When the cast is removed, take whirlpool treatments if available.

MEDICATION—Your doctor may prescribe:
- General anesthesia to make joint manipulation possible.
- Narcotic or synthetic narcotic pain relievers for severe pain.
- Stool softeners to prevent constipation due to inactivity.
- Acetaminophen for mild pain.
- Antibiotics to fight infection if necessary.

ACTIVITY
- Learn to walk with crutches. See Appendix 3 (Safe Use of Crutches) .
- Exercise the uninjured leg and the arms vigorously during recuperation. Muscle contractions promote fracture alignment and hasten healing.
- Resume normal daily activities gradually after treatment.

DIET
- Do not eat or drink before manipulation or surgery to treat the fracture. Fluid or solid food in your stomach makes vomiting while under anesthesia more hazardous.
- During recovery, eat a well-balanced diet.

REHABILITATION
- Begin daily prescribed rehabilitation exercises after clearance from your doctor when movement is comfortable.
- Use ice massage for 10 minutes before and after exercise. Fill a large styrofoam cup with water and freeze. Tear a small amount of foam from the top so ice protrudes. Massage firmly in a circle over the injured area.

 ## CALL YOUR DOCTOR IF

- You have signs or symptoms of a femur fracture. Call immediately if you have numbness or complete loss of feeling below the fracture site. This is an emergency!
- Any of the following occurs after surgery or other treatment:
  Increased pain, swelling or drainage in the surgical area.
  Signs of infection (headache, muscle aches, dizziness or a general ill feeling and fever).
  Swelling above or below the cast.
  Blue or gray skin color beyond the cast, especially under the toenails.
  Nausea or vomiting; constipation.

THIGH CONTUSION

GENERAL INFORMATION

DEFINITION—Bruising of skin and underlying tissues of the thigh (between knee and hip) due to a direct blow. Contusions cause bleeding from ruptured small capillaries that allow blood to infiltrate muscles, tendons and other soft tissues. The thigh is well suited to absorb direct blows, but contusions do occur here.

BODY PARTS INVOLVED—The thigh, including blood vessels, muscles, tendons, nerves, covering of bone (periosteum) and connective tissues.

SIGNS & SYMPTOMS
• Swelling of the thigh—either superficial or deep.
• Pain and tenderness in the thigh.
• Feeling of firmness when pressure is exerted at the injury site.
• Discoloration under the skin, beginning with redness and progressing to the characteristic "black-and-blue" bruise.
• Restricted activity of the injured leg proportional to the extent of injury.

CAUSES—Direct blow to the thigh, usually from a blunt object (frequently the edge of a thigh pad in football pants).

RISK INCREASES WITH
• Violent contact sports, especially football.
• Medical history of any bleeding disorder.
• Poor nutrition, including vitamin deficiency.
• Inadequate protection of exposed areas during contact spans.
• Use of anticoagulants or aspirin.

HOW TO PREVENT—Wear appropriate protective gear and equipment, such as thigh pads, during competition or other athletic activity if there is risk of a thigh contusion. Keep thigh pads strapped in position.

WHAT TO EXPECT

APPROPRIATE HEALTH CARE
• Doctor's care unless the contusion is quite small.
• Self-care for minor contusions and for serious contusions during the rehabilitation phase.
• Physical therapy following serious contusions.

DIAGNOSTIC MEASURES
• Your own observation of symptoms.
• Medical history and physical exam by a doctor for all except minor injuries.
• X-rays of the thigh, knee and hip to assess total injury to soft tissues and to rule out the possibility of underlying fractures. The total extent of injury may not be apparent for 48 to 72 hours.

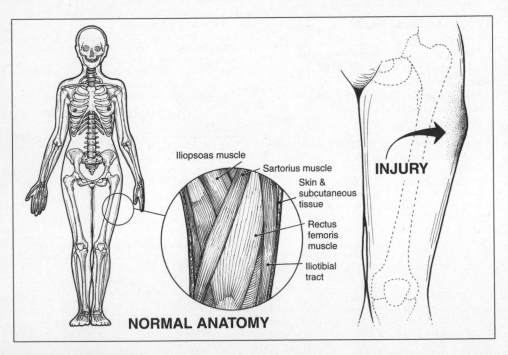

Iliopsoas muscle
Sartorius muscle
Skin & subcutaneous tissue
Rectus femoris muscle
Iliotibial tract
INJURY

NORMAL ANATOMY

POSSIBLE COMPLICATIONS
• Excessive bleeding, leading to disability. Infiltrative-type bleeding can often lead to calcification and impaired function of injured muscle (myositis ossificans).
• Prolonged healing time if usual activities are resumed too soon.
• Infection if skin over the contusion is broken.

PROBABLE OUTCOME—Healing time varies with the extent of injury, but average healing time for a thigh contusion is 1 to 2 weeks.

 HOW TO TREAT

NOTE—Follow your doctor's instructions. These instructions are supplemental.

FIRST AID—Use instructions for R.I.C.E., the first letters of *rest, ice, compression* and *elevation*. See Appendix 1 for details.

CONTINUING CARE
• Wrap an elasticized bandage over a felt pad placed on the injured area. Keep the area compressed for about 72 hours.
• Use ice massage. Fill a large styrofoam cup with water and freeze. Tear a small amount of foam from the top so ice protrudes. Massage gently over the injured area in a circle about the size of a softball. Do this for 15 minutes at a time 3 or 4 times a day, and also before workouts or competition.

• Massage gently and often to provide comfort and decrease swelling.

MEDICATION
• For minor discomfort, you may use: Acetaminophen or ibuprofen. Topical liniments and ointments.
• Your doctor may prescribe stronger medicine for pain.

ACTIVITY—Begin activities slowly, and stop exercise as soon as pain begins. Increase activity as healing progresses.

DIET—During recovery, balance the amount of food you eat with any change in your level of physical activity. Eat a variety of foods to get the energy, protein, vitamins, minerals and fiber you need for good health and healing.

REHABILITATION—Begin prescribed daily rehabilitation exercises when supportive wrapping is no longer needed.

 CALL YOUR DOCTOR IF

• You have a thigh contusion that doesn't improve in 1 or 2 days.
• Skin is broken and signs of infection (drainage, increasing pain, fever, headache, muscle aches, dizziness or a general ill feeling) occur.

THIGH HEMATOMA

GENERAL INFORMATION

DEFINITION—A collection of pooled blood in the thigh within a relatively constricted area. Thigh hematomas probably accompany all serious contusions of the thigh, but they are difficult to diagnose because of the large muscle mass in the thigh.

BODY PARTS INVOLVED—Thigh, including soft tissues (nerves, tendons, ligaments, muscles and blood vessels) surrounding the hematoma.

SIGNS & SYMPTOMS
- Swelling at the injury site.
- Fluctuance (feeling of mobile fluid beneath the skin).
- Tenderness.
- Redness that progresses through several color changes—purple, green-yellow, yellow—before it completely heals.

CAUSES—Direct injury, usually with a blunt object. Bleeding into tissues causes the surrounding tissues to be pushed away.

RISK INCREASES WITH
- Contact sports, especially if the thigh is not adequately protected.
- Medical history of any bleeding disorder.
- Poor nutrition, including vitamin deficiency.
- Use of anticoagulants or aspirin.

HOW TO PREVENT—Wear appropriate protective gear and equipment, such as thigh pads, during competition or other athletic activity if there is a risk of a thigh injury.

WHAT TO EXPECT

APPROPRIATE HEALTH CARE
- Doctor's care unless the hematoma is very small.
- Needle aspiration of blood from the hematoma if the hematoma is accessible. At the same time, hyaluronidase (an enzyme) can be injected into the hematoma space. Hyaluronidase may hasten absorption of blood.
- Self-care for minor hematomas or for serious hematomas during the rehabilitation phase.
- Physical therapy following serious hematomas.

DIAGNOSTIC MEASURES
- Your own observation of symptoms.
- Physical exam and medical history by a doctor for all except minor injuries.
- X-rays of the injured area to assess total injury and to rule out the possibility of an underlying bone fracture. Total extent of the injury may not be apparent for 48 to 72 hours following injury.

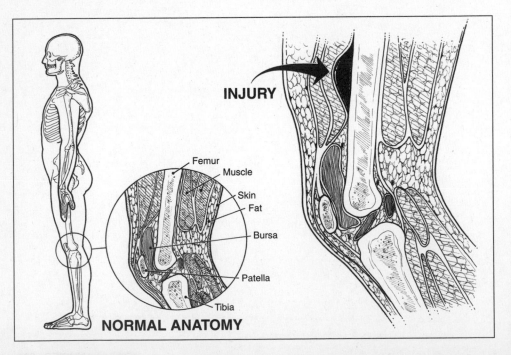

INJURY

Femur
Muscle
Skin
Fat
Bursa
Patella
Tibia

NORMAL ANATOMY

POSSIBLE COMPLICATIONS
- Infection introduced either through a break in the skin at the time of injury or during aspiration of the hematoma.
- Prolonged healing time if activity is resumed too soon.
- Calcification of the blood remaining in the hematoma if blood is not completely removed or absorbed. This may cause permanent stiffness of the knee joint and atrophy of the quadriceps muscle, since the calcification will occur within the injured muscle (myositis ossificans).

PROBABLE OUTCOME—Average healing time is 2 weeks to 2 months unless blood is removed with aspiration. Healing time may be lessened with this treatment.

 ## HOW TO TREAT

NOTE—Follow your doctor's instructions. These instructions are supplemental.

FIRST AID—Use instructions for R.I.C.E., the first letters of *rest, ice, compression* and *elevation*. See Appendix 1 for details.

CONTINUING CARE
- Directly after injury, keep the knee fully flexed rather than extended.
- Use frequent ice massage. Fill a large styrofoam cup with water and freeze. Tear a small amount of foam from the top so ice protrudes. Massage firmly over the injured area in a circle about the size of a softball. Do this for 15 minutes at a time 3 or 4 times a day.
- Don't massage the thigh. You may trigger bleeding again.

MEDICATION
- For minor discomfort you may use: Nonprescription medicines such as acetaminophen or ibuprofen. Topical liniments and ointments.
- Your doctor may prescribe stronger medicine for pain if needed.

ACTIVITY—Begin activities slowly, and stop exercise as soon as pain begins. Increase activity as healing progresses. To prevent a delay in healing, protect the hematoma area against excessive motion soon after injury. Motion breaks down the clot and causes irritation throughout the thigh, leading to possible scar formation, calcification and restricted movement after healing.

DIET—During recovery, balance the amount of food you eat with any change in your level of physical activity. Eat a variety of foods to get the energy, protein, vitamins, minerals and fiber you need for good health and healing.

REHABILITATION—Begin prescribed daily rehabilitation exercises when supportive wrapping is no longer needed. Use gentle massage for 10 minutes prior to exercise.

 ## CALL YOUR DOCTOR IF

- You have signs or symptoms of a thigh hematoma that doesn't begin to improve in 1 or 2 days.
- Skin is broken and signs of infection (drainage, increasing pain, fever, headache, muscle aches, dizziness or a general ill feeling) occur.

THIGH INJURY, HAMSTRING

GENERAL INFORMATION

DEFINITION—A strain injury to a hamstring muscle or tendon or their bony attachments. The hamstring muscles run from the pelvis and femur to the back and side of the knee. The hamstring tendons can be felt behind the knee on either side. They feel like tough rope. The hamstring tendons, muscles and their attached bones comprise contractile units that stabilize the knee and hip and allow their motion. The injury, usually a strain, occurs at the weakest part of a unit. Hamstring strains are of 3 types:
- Mild (Grade I)—Slightly pulled muscle without tearing of muscle or tendon fibers. There is no lose of strength.
- Moderate (Grade II)—Tearing of fibers of the muscle or tendon or at the attachment to bone. Strength is diminished.
- Severe (Grade III)—Rupture of the muscle-tendon-bone attachment, with separation of fibers. A severe strain may require surgical repair. Chronic strains are caused by overuse. Acute strains are caused by direct injury or overstress.

BODY PARTS INVOLVED
- Hamstring tendons and associated muscles.
- Bones in the pelvis and knee joints.
- Soft tissues surrounding the injury, including nerves, periosteum (covering of bone), blood vessels and lymph vessels.

SIGNS & SYMPTOMS
- Pain when moving or stretching the leg.
- Muscle spasm of the injured muscles.
- Swelling over the injury.
- Weakened leg (moderate or severe strain).
- Crepitation ("crackling" feeling and sound when the injured area is pressed with fingers).
- Calcification of the hamstring tendon or muscles (visible with x-rays).
- Inflammation of the sheath covering the hamstring tendon.

CAUSES
- Prolonged overuse of muscle-tendon units in the leg.
- Single violent injury or force applied to the muscle-tendons units in the leg.

RISK INCREASES WITH
- Contact sports.
- Running, jumping and quick-start sports.
- Medical history of any bleeding disorder.
- Obesity.
- Poor nutrition.
- Previous pelvic or knee injury.
- Poor muscle conditioning.

HOW TO PREVENT
- Participate in a strengthening, flexibility and conditioning program appropriate for your sport.
- Warm up adequately before practice or competition.
- Use proper protective equipment, such as knee pads and thigh pads, during participation in contact sports.

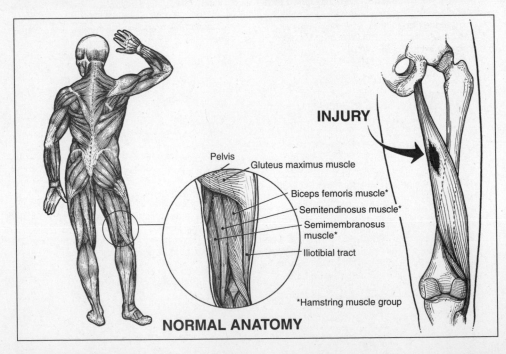

INJURY

Pelvis
Gluteus maximus muscle
Biceps femoris muscle*
Semitendinosus muscle*
Semimembranosus muscle*
Iliotibial tract

*Hamstring muscle group

NORMAL ANATOMY

WHAT TO EXPECT

APPROPRIATE HEALTH CARE
- Doctor's care.
- Application of tape or an elastic sleeve if a muscle ruptures or the muscle-tendon-bone attachment loosens.
- Self-care during rehabilitation.
- Physical therapy (moderate and severe injury).
- Surgery (severe injury).

DIAGNOSTIC MEASURES
- Your own observation of symptoms.
- Medical history and exam by a doctor.
- X-rays of the pelvis, femur and knee to rule out fractures.
- Diagnostic ultrasound or MRI (see Glossary for both) for a severe strain to establish the extent of the tear.

POSSIBLE COMPLICATIONS
- Prolonged healing time if activity is resumed too soon.
- Proneness to repeated injury.
- Loss of ability to quickly accelerate and decelerate.
- Inflammation at the attachment to bone (periostitis).
- Prolonged disability (sometimes).

PROBABLE OUTCOME—If this is a first-time injury, proper care and sufficient healing time before resuming activity should prevent permanent disability. Torn ligaments and tendons require as long to heal as fractured bones. Average healing times are:
- Mild strain—2 to 10 days.
- Moderate strain—10 days to 6 weeks.
- Severe strain—6 to 10 weeks.

If this is a repeat injury, complications listed above are more likely to occur.

HOW TO TREAT

NOTE—Follow your doctor's instructions. These instructions are supplemental.

FIRST AID—Use instructions for R.I.C.E., the first letters of *rest, ice, compression* and *elevation*. See Appendix 1 for details.

CONTINUING CARE
- Continue using an ice pack 3 or 4 times a day. Place ice chips or cubes in a plastic bag. Wrap the bag in a moist towel, and place it over the injured area. Use for 20 minutes at a time.
- After 72 hours, apply heat instead of ice if it feels better. Use heat lamps, hot soaks, hot showers, heating pads or heat liniments and ointments.
- Take whirlpool treatments, if available.
- Wrap the injured leg with an elasticized bandage between ice or heat treatments.
- Massage gently and often to provide comfort and decrease swelling.

MEDICATION
- For minor discomfort, you may use:
  Nonprescription medicines such as aspirin, acetaminophen or ibuprofen.
  Topical liniments and ointments.
- Your doctor may prescribe:
  Stronger medicine for pain, if needed.
  Injection of a long-acting local anesthetic to reduce pain.
  Injections of a corticosteroid, such as triamcinolone, to reduce inflammation.

ACTIVITY
- For a moderate or severe injury, use crutches for at least 72 hours.
- Resume your normal activities gradually.

DIET—During recovery, balance the amount of food you eat with any change in your level of physical activity. Eat a variety of foods to get the energy, protein, vitamins, minerals and fiber you need for good health and healing.

REHABILITATION
- Begin daily rehabilitation exercises when supportive wrapping is no longer needed. Participate in a stretching program.
- Use ice massage for 10 minutes before and after exercise. Fill a large styrofoam cup with water and freeze. Tear a small amount of foam from the top so ice protrudes. Massage firmly over the injured area in a circle about the size of a softball.
- See Rehabilitation section for hip and pelvis exercises.

CALL YOUR DOCTOR IF

- You have symptoms of a moderate or severe hamstring injury or a mild injury persists longer than 10 days.
- Pain or swelling worsens despite treatment.
- Either of the following occurs with splints, tight bracing or taping:
  Pain, numbness or coldness below the injury.
  Dusky, blue or gray toenails.

THIGH STRAIN

GENERAL INFORMATION

DEFINITION—Injury to the muscles or tendons of the thigh. Muscles, tendons and their attached bones comprise contractile units. These units stabilize the hip and knee and allow their motion. A strain occurs at the weakest part of a unit. Strains are of 3 types:
- Mild (Grade I)—Slightly pulled muscle without tearing of muscle or tendon fibers. There is no loss of strength.
- Moderate (Grade II)—Tearing of fibers in a muscle or tendon or at the attachment to bone. Strength is diminished.
- Severe (Grade III)—Rupture of the muscle-tendon-bone attachment, with separation of fibers. A severe strain may require surgical repair. Chronic strains are caused by overuse. Acute strains are caused by direct injury or overstress.

BODY PARTS INVOLVED
- Any tendons or muscles of the thigh.
- Bones of the thigh area, including the femur, pelvis, knee, tibia and fibula.
- Soft tissues surrounding the strain, including nerves, periosteum (covering of bone), blood vessels and lymph vessels.

SIGNS & SYMPTOMS
- Pain when moving or stretching the hip or knee.
- Muscle spasm of the injured muscle.
- Swelling over the injury.
- Weakened thigh muscles (moderate or severe strain).
- Crepitation ("crackling" feeling and sound when the injured area is pressed with fingers).
- Calcification of the muscle or tendon—visible with x-rays (myositis ossificans).
- Inflammation of sheath covering a tendon in the thigh.

CAUSES
- Prolonged overuse of muscle-tendon units in the thigh.
- Single episode of stressful overactivity in which muscles are under maximum stress and additional tension is applied when the knee is sharply flexed.
- Single violent blow or force applied to the thigh.

RISK INCREASES WITH
- Contact sports.
- Sports that require a quick start, such as running races, football and basketball.
- Medical history of any bleeding disorder.
- Obesity.
- Poor nutrition.
- Previous thigh injury.
- Poor muscle conditioning.

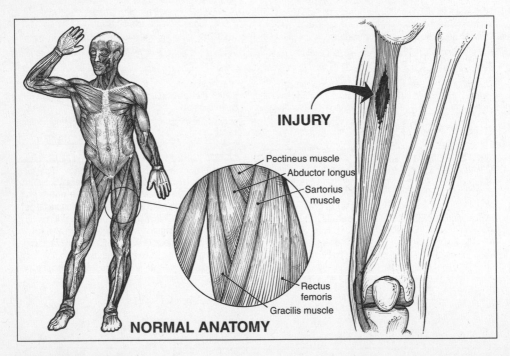

INJURY

Pectineus muscle
Abductor longus
Sartorius muscle
Rectus femoris
Gracilis muscle

NORMAL ANATOMY

HOW TO PREVENT
- Participate in a strengthening, flexibility and conditioning program appropriate for your sport.
- Warm up (include stretching exercises) before practice or competition.

WHAT TO EXPECT

APPROPRIATE HEALTH CARE
- Doctor's diagnosis.
- Application of tape or an elastic sleeve if the muscle ruptures or the muscle-tendon-bone attachment loosens.
- Self-care during rehabilitation.
- Physical therapy (moderate or severe strain).
- Surgery (severe strain).

DIAGNOSTIC MEASURES
- Your own observation of symptoms.
- Medical history and exam by a doctor.
- X-rays of the thigh area to rule out fractures.

POSSIBLE COMPLICATIONS
- Prolonged healing time if activity is resumed too soon.
- Proneness to repeated injury.
- Loss of ability to quickly accelerate and decelerate.
- Inflammation at the attachment to bone (periostitis).
- Prolonged disability (sometimes).

PROBABLE OUTCOME—If this is a first-time injury, proper care and sufficient healing time before resuming activity should prevent permanent disability. Torn ligaments and tendons require as long to heal as fractured bones do. Average healing times are:
- Mild strain—2 to 10 days.
- Moderate strain—10 days to 6 weeks.
- Severe strain—6 to 10 weeks.

If this is a repeat injury, complications listed above are more likely to occur.

HOW TO TREAT

NOTE—Follow your doctor's instructions. These instructions are supplemental.

FIRST AID—Use instructions for R.I.C.E., the first letters of *rest, ice, compression* and *elevation*. See Appendix 1 for details.

CONTINUING CARE
- Use ice massage 3 or 4 times a day for 15 minutes at a time. Fill a large styrofoam cup with water and freeze. Tear a small amount of foam from the top so ice protrudes. Massage firmly over the injured area in a circle about the size of a softball.
- After the first 72 hours, apply heat instead of ice if it feels better. Use heat lamps, hot soaks, hot showers, heating pads or heat liniments and ointments.
- Take whirlpool treatments, if available.
- Wrap the injured thigh area with an elastic bandage between treatments.
- Massage gently and often to provide comfort and decrease swelling.

MEDICATION
- For minor discomfort, you may use:
  Nonprescription medicines such as aspirin, acetaminophen or ibuprofen.
  Topical liniments and ointments.
- Your doctor may prescribe:
  Stronger medicine for pain, if needed.
  Injection of a long-acting local anesthetic to reduce pain.
  Injections of a corticosteroid, such as triamcinolone, to reduce inflammation.

ACTIVITY
- For a moderate or severe strain, walk with crutches for at least 72 hours—longer with a cast or splints. See Appendix 3 (Safe Use of Crutches).
- Resume normal daily activities gradually.

DIET—During recovery, balance the amount of food you eat with any change in your level of physical activity. Eat a variety of foods to get the energy, protein, vitamins, minerals and fiber you need for good health and healing.

REHABILITATION—Begin daily rehabilitation exercises when supportive wrapping is no longer needed. Use ice massage for 10 minutes prior to exercise. See Rehabilitation section for hip and pelvis exercises.

CALL YOUR DOCTOR IF

- You have symptoms of a moderate or severe thigh strain or a mild strain persists longer than 10 days.
- Pain or swelling worsens despite treatment.
- The following occur with splints, tight bracing or taping:
  Pain, numbness or coldness below the injury.
  Dusky, blue or gray toenails.

THIGH STRAIN, QUADRICEPS

GENERAL INFORMATION

DEFINITION—Injury to the quadriceps femoris muscle or its tendons. The quadriceps femoris is a large muscle at the front of the thigh. The muscle, tendon and their attached bones comprise a contractile unit. The unit stabilizes the hip and knee and allows their motion. A strain occurs at the weakest part of a unit. Strains are of 3 types:
- Mild (Grade I)—Slightly pulled muscle without tearing of muscle or tendon fibers. There is no loss of strength.
- Moderate (Grade II)—Tearing of fibers in a muscle or tendon or at the attachment to bone. Strength is diminished.
- Severe (Grade III)—Rupture of the muscle-tendon-bone attachment, with separation of fibers. A severe strain may require surgical repair. Chronic strains are caused by overuse. Acute strains are caused by direct injury or overstress.

BODY PARTS INVOLVED
- Quadriceps femoris muscle or its various tendons.
- Femur (thigh bone), patella (kneecap) or tibia (large lower leg bone).
- Soft tissues surrounding the strain, including nerves, periosteum (covering of bone), blood vessels and lymph vessels.

SIGNS & SYMPTOMS
- Pain when moving, stretching or flexing the thigh.
- Muscle spasm of the injured muscle.
- Swelling over the injury.
- Weakened leg (moderate or severe strain).
- Crepitation ("crackling" feeling and sound when the injured area is pressed with fingers).
- Calcification of the tendon or muscle (visible with x-rays).
- Inflammation of the sheath covering the tendon.

CAUSES
- Prolonged overuse of muscle-tendon units in the leg.
- Single violent injury or force applied to the knee or the quadriceps area of the thigh.

RISK INCREASES WITH
- Sports that require quick starts, such as running races and other track events.
- Contact sports.
- Medical history of any bleeding disorder.
- Obesity.
- Poor nutrition.
- Previous thigh, hip or knee injury.
- Poor muscle conditioning.

HOW TO PREVENT
- Participate in a strengthening, flexibility and conditioning program appropriate for your sport.
- Warm up before practice or competition.
- Use proper protective equipment, such as thigh pads, for contact sports.

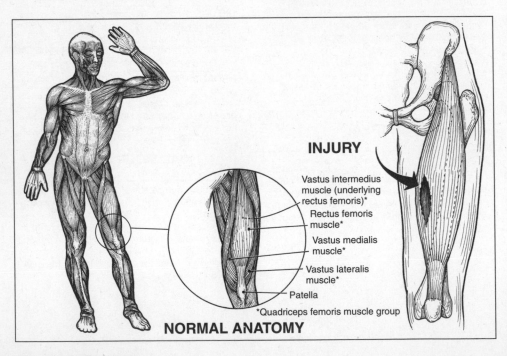

INJURY

Vastus intermedius muscle (underlying rectus femoris)*

Rectus femoris muscle*

Vastus medialis muscle*

Vastus lateralis muscle*

Patella

*Quadriceps femoris muscle group

NORMAL ANATOMY

WHAT TO EXPECT

APPROPRIATE HEALTH CARE
- Doctor's diagnosis.
- Self-care during rehabilitation.
- Physical therapy (moderate or severe strain).
- Surgery (severe strain).

DIAGNOSTIC MEASURES
- Your own observation of symptoms.
- Medical history and exam by a doctor.
- X-rays of the thigh area to rule out fractures.
- Diagnostic ultrasound or MRI (see Glossary for both) to demonstrate partial tears.

POSSIBLE COMPLICATIONS
- Prolonged healing time if activity is resumed too soon.
- Proneness to repeated injury.
- Loss of ability to quickly accelerate and decelerate.
- Inflammation at the attachment to bone (periostitis).
- Prolonged disability (weakness).

PROBABLE OUTCOME—If this is a first-time injury, proper care and sufficient healing time before resuming activity should prevent permanent disability. Torn ligaments and tendons require as long to heal as fractured bones do. Average healing times are:
- Mild strain—2 to 10 days.
- Moderate strain—10 days to 6 weeks.
- Severe strain—6 to 10 weeks.

If this is a repeat injury, complications listed above are more likely to occur.

 ## HOW TO TREAT

NOTE—Follow your doctor's instructions. These instructions are supplemental.

FIRST AID—Use instructions for R.I.C.E., the first letters of *rest, ice, compression* and *elevation*. See Appendix 1 for details.

CONTINUING CARE
- Use ice massage 3 or 4 times a day for 15 minutes at a time. Fill a large styrofoam cup with water and freeze. Tear a small amount of foam from the top so ice protrudes. Massage firmly over the injured area in a circle about the size of a softball.

- After the first 72 hours, apply heat instead of ice if it feels better. Use heat lamps, hot soaks, hot showers, heating pads or heat liniments and ointments.
- Take whirlpool treatments, if available.
- Wrap the injured quadriceps muscle loosely with an elastic bandage between treatments.
- Massage gently and often to provide comfort and decrease swelling.

MEDICATION
- For minor discomfort, you may use:
  Aspirin, acetaminophen or ibuprofen.
  Topical liniments and ointments.
- Your doctor may prescribe:
  Stronger pain relievers.
  Injection of a long-acting local anesthetic to reduce pain.
  Injections of a corticosteroid, such as triamcinolone, to reduce inflammation

ACTIVITY
- For a moderate or severe strain, walk with crutches for at least 72 hours—longer with a cast or splints. See Appendix 3 (Safe Use of Crutches).
- Resume normal daily activities gradually.

DIET—During recovery, balance the amount of food you eat with any change in your level of physical activity. Eat a variety of foods to get the energy, protein, vitamins, minerals and fiber you need for good health and healing.

REHABILITATION—Begin daily rehabilitation exercises when supportive wrapping is no longer needed. Use ice massage for 10 minutes prior to exercise. See Rehabilitation section for hip and pelvis exercises.

 ## CALL YOUR DOCTOR IF

- You have symptoms of a moderate or severe quadriceps strain or a mild strain persists longer than 10 days.
- Pain or swelling worsens despite treatment.

THUMB FRACTURE
(Thumb Metacarpal Fracture)

GENERAL INFORMATION

DEFINITION—A complete or incomplete break in the metacarpal bone of the thumb.

BODY PARTS INVOLVED
- Metacarpal bone of the thumb.
- Joint at the base of the thumb.
- Soft tissues around the fracture site, including nerves, tendons, ligaments and blood vessels.

SIGNS & SYMPTOMS
- Severe thumb pain at the fracture site.
- Swelling of soft tissues around the fracture.
- Visible deformity if the fracture is complete and the bone fragments separate enough to distort the thumb.
- Tenderness to the touch.
- Numbness or coldness in the thumb if the blood supply is impaired.

CAUSES
- Direct stress frequently caused by hitting with the fist or by catching the thumb on an object.
- Indirect stress that may be caused by twisting or violent muscle contraction.

RISK INCREASES WITH
- Contact sports such as hockey.
- Skiing (hand becomes caught in ski pole).
- History of bone or joint disease, especially osteoporosis.
- Poor nutrition, especially calcium deficiency.
- If surgery or anesthesia is needed, risk increases with smoking and use of drugs, including mind-altering drugs, muscle relaxants, antihypertensives, tranquilizers, sleep inducers, insulin, sedatives, beta-adrenergic blockers or corticosteroids.

HOW TO PREVENT
- Develop strength in your hands.
- Use appropriate taping, padding or protective equipment for the hand and thumb.

WHAT TO EXPECT

APPROPRIATE HEALTH CARE
- Doctor's treatment to manipulate the broken bones.
- Anesthesia and outpatient surgery to set the fracture and apply a cast.
- Self-care during rehabilitation.

DIAGNOSTIC MEASURES
- Your own observation of symptoms.
- Medical history and exam by a doctor.
- X-rays of the hand.

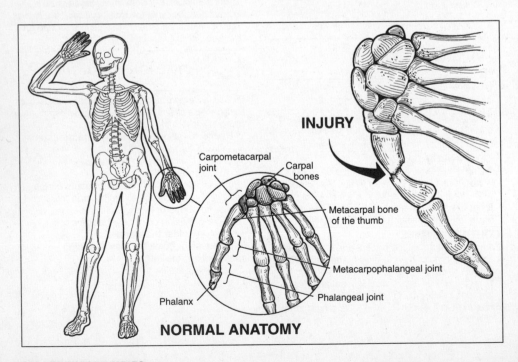

Carpometacarpal joint

Carpal bones

Metacarpal bone of the thumb

Metacarpophalangeal joint

Phalanx

Phalangeal joint

INJURY

NORMAL ANATOMY

POSSIBLE COMPLICATIONS

At the time of injury:
- Shock.
- Pressure on or injury to nearby nerves, ligaments, tendons, muscles, blood vessels or connective tissues.

After treatment or surgery:
- Delayed union or nonunion of the fracture.
- Impaired blood supply to the fracture site.
- Infection in open fractures (skin broken over fracture site) or at the incision if surgical setting was necessary.
- Shortening or angulation of the injured bones.
- Unstable or arthritic thumb following repeated injury.
- Prolonged healing time if activity is resumed too soon.
- Proneness to repeated thumb injury.
- Problems caused by plaster casts. See Appendix 2 (Care of Casts).

PROBABLE OUTCOME—The average healing time for this fracture is 6 to 8 weeks. Healing is considered complete when there is no pain or motion at the fracture site and when x-rays show complete bone union.

HOW TO TREAT

NOTE—Follow your doctor's instructions. These instructions are supplemental.

FIRST AID
- Use a padded splint or sling to immobilize the hand and wrist before taking the injured person to the doctor's office or emergency facility.
- Keep the person warm with blankets to decrease the possibility of shock.
- Follow instructions for R.I.C.E., the first letters of *rest, ice, compression* and *elevation*. See Appendix for details.
- The doctor will set the broken bones with surgery or, if possible, without. This manipulation should be done soon after injury. Many tissues lose their elasticity and become difficult to return to their normal positions.
- Shaft fractures of the metacarpal can sometimes be realigned without surgery, but the broken bones must be fixed in place with a wire or screws across the base of the metacarpal bone. This wire passes though the bone fragment into one of the bones of the hand.

CONTINUING CARE
- Immobilization will be necessary. A rigid cast is used to immobilize the thumb and wrist. This cast can usually be removed in 3 weeks.
- After 96 hours, application of localized heat promotes healing by increasing blood circulation in the injured area. Use a heat lamp or heating pad so heat can penetrate the cast.
- After the cast is removed, use frequent ice massage. Fill a large styrofoam cup with water and freeze. Tear a small amount of foam from the top so ice protrudes. Massage firmly over the injured area.

MEDICATION—Your doctor may prescribe:
- General anesthesia, local anesthesia, or muscle relaxants to make bone manipulation and fixation of bone fragments possible.
- Narcotic or synthetic narcotic pain relievers for severe pain.
- Acetaminophen (available without prescription) for mild pain after initial treatment.

ACTIVITY
- Actively exercise all muscle groups not immobilized. These muscle contractions promote fracture alignment and hasten healing.
- Begin reconditioning the thumb and hand after clearance from your doctor.
- Resume normal daily activities gradually after treatment.

DIET
- Do not eat or drink before manipulation or surgery to treat the fracture. Fluid or solid food in your stomach makes vomiting while under anesthesia more hazardous.
- During recovery, balance the amount of food you eat with any change in your level of physical activity. Eat a variety of foods to get the energy, protein, vitamins, minerals and fiber you need for good health and healing.

REHABILITATION—Begin daily rehabilitation exercises when movement is comfortable. Use ice massage for 10 minutes prior to exercise. See Rehabilitation section for wrist and hand exercises.

CALL YOUR DOCTOR IF

- You have signs or symptoms of a thumb fracture.
- Any of the following occurs after surgery or other treatment:
  Increased pain, swelling or drainage in the surgical area.
  Signs of infection (headache, muscle aches, dizziness or a general ill feeling and fever).
  Swelling above or below the cast.
  Blue or gray skin color beyond the cast, especially under the toenails.
  Numbness or complete loss of feeling anywhere in the hand.
  Nausea or vomiting.

THUMB SPRAIN
(Skier's Thumb; Gamekeeper's Thumb)

 GENERAL INFORMATION

DEFINITION—Violent overstretching of one or more ligaments in the joint of the thumb. Sprains involving two or more ligaments cause considerably more disability than single-ligament sprains. When the ligament is overstretched, it becomes tense and gives way at its weakest point, either where it attaches to bone or within the ligament itself. If the ligament pulls loose a fragment of bone, it is called an avulsion fracture. There are 3 types of sprains:
• Mild (Grade I)—Tearing of some ligament fibers. There is no loss of function.
• Moderate (Grade II)—Rupture of a portion of the ligament, resulting in some loss of function.
• Severe (Grade III)—Complete rupture of the ligament or complete separation of ligament from bone. There is total loss of function. A severe sprain may require surgical repair.

BODY PARTS INVOLVED
• Ligaments that hold the metacarpo-phalangeal joint of the thumb together.
• Tissues surrounding the sprain, including blood vessels, tendons, bone, periosteum (covering of bone) and muscles.

SIGNS & SYMPTOMS
• Severe pain at the time of injury.
• A feeling of popping or tearing inside the thumb.
• Tenderness at the injury site.
• Swelling and redness in the injured thumb.
• Bruising that appears soon after injury.

RISK INCREASES WITH
• Contact sports, especially catching sports such as baseball, football or basketball.
• Skiing (thumb becomes caught in ski pole)—gamekeeper's thumb (an older term for the injury).
• Previous thumb injury.
• Poor muscle conditioning.

HOW TO PREVENT—Tape vulnerable joints before practice or competition to prevent reinjury. Immobilization after healing can be provided by a slip-on protector devised by a bracemaker.

 WHAT TO EXPECT

APPROPRIATE HEALTH CARE
• Doctor's diagnosis.
• Self-care during rehabilitation.
• Application of a cast, tape or preformed brace for the thumb.
• Physical therapy (moderate or severe sprain).
• Surgery (severe sprain).

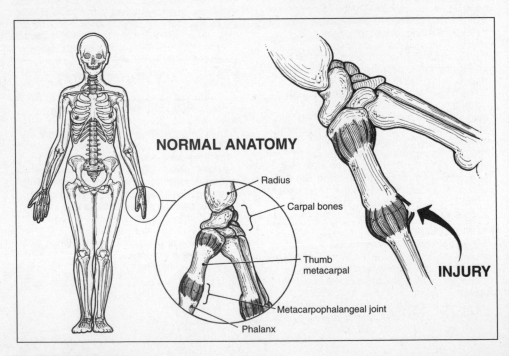

NORMAL ANATOMY

Radius

Carpal bones

Thumb metacarpal

Metacarpophalangeal joint

Phalanx

INJURY

DIAGNOSTIC MEASURES
- Your own observation of symptoms.
- Medical history and exam by a doctor.
- X-rays of the thumb, hand and wrist to rule out fracture.

POSSIBLE COMPLICATIONS
- Prolonged healing time if usual activities are resumed too soon.
- Proneness to repeated injury.
- Inflammation at the ligament attachment to bone (periostitis).
- Prolonged disability (sometimes), usually weakness of pinch strength.
- Unstable or arthritic thumb following repeated injury.

PROBABLE OUTCOME—If this is a first-time injury, proper care and sufficient healing time before resuming activity should prevent permanent disability. Ligaments have a poor blood supply, and torn ligaments require as much healing time as fractures. Average healing times are:
- Mild sprains—2 to 6 weeks.
- Moderate sprains—6 to 8 weeks.
- Severe sprains—8 to 10 weeks, but usually includes time for surgery.

HOW TO TREAT

NOTE—Follow your doctor's instructions. These instructions are supplemental.

FIRST AID—Use instructions for R.I.C.E., the first letters of *rest, ice, compression* and *elevation.* See Appendix 1 for details.

CONTINUING CARE—If the doctor does not apply a cast, tape or elastic bandage:
- Continue using an ice pack 3 or 4 times a day. Place ice chips or cubes in a plastic bag. Wrap the bag in a moist towel, and place it over the injured thumb. Use for 20 minutes at a time.
- After 72 hours, apply heat instead of ice if it feels better. Use heat lamps, hot soaks, hot showers, heating pads or heat liniments and ointments.
- Take whirlpool treatments, if available.
- Massage gently and often to provide comfort and decrease swelling.

MEDICATION
- For minor discomfort, you may use:
  Aspirin, acetaminophen or ibuprofen.
  Topical liniments and ointments.
- Your doctor may prescribe:
  Stronger pain relievers.
  Injection of a long-acting local anesthetic to reduce pain.
  Injections of a corticosteroid, such as triamcinolone, to reduce inflammation.

ACTIVITY—Resume your normal activities gradually after clearance from your doctor.

DIET—During recovery, balance the amount of food you eat with any change in your level of physical activity. Eat a variety of foods to get the energy, protein, vitamins, minerals and fiber you need for good health and healing.

REHABILITATION
- Begin daily rehabilitation exercises when the cast or supportive wrapping is no longer necessary.
- Use a gentle ice massage for 10 minutes before and after workouts. Fill a large styrofoam cup with water and freeze. Tear a small amount of foam from the top so ice protrudes. Massage firmly over the injured area in a circle about the size of a softball.
- See Rehabilitation section for wrist and hand exercises.

CALL YOUR DOCTOR IF

- You have symptoms of a moderate or severe thumb sprain or a mild sprain persists longer than 2 weeks.
- Pain, swelling or bruising worsens despite treatment.
- Any of the following occurs after casting or splinting:
  Pain, numbness or coldness in the tip of the thumb.
  Blue, gray or dusky thumbnail.
- Any of the following occurs after surgery:
  Increased pain, swelling, redness, drainage or bleeding in the surgical area.
  Signs of infection (headache, muscle aches, dizziness or a general ill feeling with fever).
- New unexplained symptoms develop. Drugs used in treatment may produce side effects.

TOE DISLOCATION

GENERAL INFORMATION

DEFINITION—Injury to any toe joint so that adjoining bones are displaced from their normal positions and no longer touch each other. Fractures and ligament sprains frequently accompany this dislocation. Toe dislocations are a common problem for athletes.

BODY PARTS INVOLVED
- Bones of the toes.
- Ligaments that hold toe bones in place.
- Soft tissues surrounding the dislocation site, including periosteum (covering of bone), nerves, tendons, blood vessels and connective tissues.

SIGNS & SYMPTOMS
- Excruciating pain in the toe at the time of injury.
- Walking difficulty.
- Severe pain when attempting to move the injured toe.
- Visible deformity if the dislocated toe has locked in the dislocated position. Bones may spontaneously reposition themselves and leave no deformity, but damage is the same.
- Tenderness over the dislocation.
- Swelling and bruising at the injury site.
- Numbness or paralysis beyond the dislocation from pinching, cutting or pressure on blood vessels or nerves.

- End result of a severe toe sprain.
- Congenital abnormality, such as a shallow or malformed joint surface.

RISK INCREASES WITH
- Contact or collision sports, especially those that require cleated shoes.
- Previous foot or toe dislocation or sprain.
- Repeated injury to any part of the foot.
- Poor muscle conditioning in the foot.

HOW TO PREVENT—Wear appropriate well-designed shoes during competition or other athletic activity. Tape the toes to prevent reinjury.

WHAT TO EXPECT

APPROPRIATE HEALTH CARE
- Doctor's treatment. This will include a local anesthetic block and manipulation of the joint to reposition the bones.
- Surgery (sometimes) to restore the joint to its normal position and repair torn ligaments and tendons. Acute or recurring dislocations may require surgical reconstruction of the joint.
- Self-care during rehabilitation.

DIAGNOSTIC MEASURES
- Your own observation of symptoms.
- Medical history and physical exam by a doctor.
- X-rays of the foot and ankle.

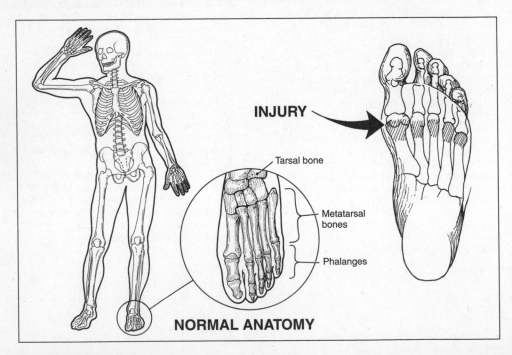

INJURY

Tarsal bone

Metatarsal bones

Phalanges

NORMAL ANATOMY

POSSIBLE COMPLICATIONS
- Pressure or damage to nearby nerves, ligaments, tendons, muscles, blood vessels or connective tissues.
- Excessive internal bleeding in the toe.
- Impaired blood supply to the dislocated area.
- Death of bone cells due to interruption of the blood supply (avascular necrosis).
- Infection introduced during surgical treatment.
- Continuing recurrent dislocations, often with progressively less severe provocation.
- Prolonged healing if activity is resumed too soon.
- Unstable or arthritic joint following repeated injury.

PROBABLE OUTCOME—After the dislocation has been corrected, the foot may require immobilization with a splint, tape or special shoe for 2 to 3 weeks. Injured ligaments require a minimum of 6 weeks to heal. The toe may lose some range of motion.

 HOW TO TREAT

NOTE—Follow your doctor's instructions. These instructions are supplemental.

FIRST AID
- Use instructions for R.I.C.E., the first letters of *rest, ice, compression* and *elevation*. See Appendix 1 for details.
- The doctor will manipulate the dislocated toes to return them to their normal positions. Manipulation should be accomplished within 6 hours, if possible. After that time, many tissues lose their elasticity and become difficult to return to their normal functional positions.

CONTINUING CARE
- Use an ice pack 3 or 4 times a day. Wrap ice chips or cubes in a plastic bag, and wrap the bag in a moist towel. Place it over the injured area for 20 minutes at a time.
- You may apply heat instead of ice if it feels better. Use heat lamps, hot soaks, hot showers, heating pads or heat liniments and ointments.
- Take whirlpool treatments, if available.
- Massage gently and often to provide comfort and decrease swelling. Stroke from the toes toward the heart.

MEDICATION—Your doctor may prescribe:
- Local anesthesia or muscle relaxants to make joint manipulation possible.
- Acetaminophen or aspirin to relieve moderate pain.
- Narcotic pain relievers for severe pain.
- Stool softeners to prevent constipation due to decreased activity.

ACTIVITY—Resume normal daily activities when comfortable.

DIET
- Do not eat or drink before manipulation or surgery to correct the dislocation. Fluid or solid food in your stomach makes vomiting while under general anesthesia more hazardous.
- During recovery, balance the amount of food you eat with any change in your level of physical activity. Eat a variety of foods to get the energy, protein, vitamins, minerals and fiber you need for good health and healing.

REHABILITATION
- Begin daily rehabilitation exercises when pain subsides.
- Use ice massage for 10 minutes prior to exercise. Fill a large styrofoam cup with water and freeze. Tear a small amount of foam from the top so ice protrudes. Massage firmly in a circle over the injured area.
- See Rehabilitation section for ankle and foot exercises.

 CALL YOUR DOCTOR IF

- You have symptoms of a dislocated toe, especially if the toe becomes numb, pale or cold. This is an emergency!
- Any of the following occurs after treatment or surgery:
  Swelling above or below the cast.
  Blue or gray skin color, particularly under the toenails.
  Numbness or complete loss of feeling below the dislocation.
  Increased pain, swelling or drainage in the surgical area.
  Signs of infection (headache, muscle aches, dizziness or general ill feeling and fever).
- New, unexplained symptoms develop. Drugs used in treatment may produce side effects.
- Toe dislocations that you can "pop" back into normal position occur repeatedly.

TOE EXOSTOSIS

 ## GENERAL INFORMATION

DEFINITION—A painful condition of the tip of the toe (usually the first or great toe) caused by an exostosis (overgrowth of bone) building up under the nailbed. An exostosis occurs at the site of repeated injury, usually from direct blows. This benign overgrowth of bone can be mistaken for a bone tumor.

BODY PARTS INVOLVED
* Toe (usually the big toe).
* Toenail.
* Soft tissues surrounding the exostosis, including muscles, nerves, lymph vessels, blood vessels and periosteum (covering of bone).

SIGNS & SYMPTOMS
* No symptoms for mild cases.
* Extreme pain at the tip of the toe and under the nail.
* Tenderness over the toe.
* Extreme sensitivity in the toe to pressure or minor injury.
* Change in the contour of the bone, ranging from a slight lump to the appearance of a large calcified spur (1 cm or more in length) in the toe.

CAUSES
* Repeated injury to the toe.
* Chronic irritation of an already damaged area.

RISK INCREASES WITH
* Contact sports, particularly those with quick stops and turns in which the toes are repeatedly jammed into the toes of the shoes.
* Ballet dancing in toe shoes.
* History of bone or joint disease, such as osteomyelitis, osteomalacia or osteoporosis.
* Vitamin or mineral deficiency.
* If surgery or anesthesia is needed, risk increases with smoking, use of mind-altering drugs, muscle relaxants, tranquilizers, sleep inducers, insulin, sedatives, beta-adrenergic blockers or corticosteroids.

HOW TO PREVENT
* Allow adequate recovery time for a toe injury before resuming sports participation.
* Wear adequate protective equipment, especially good shoes and toe padding if necessary, for participation in sports.
* Learn proper moves and techniques for your sport to minimize the risk of injury.

 ## WHAT TO EXPECT

APPROPRIATE HEALTH CARE
* Doctor's care.
* Surgery (sometimes) to remove the exostosis.
* Self-care during rehabilitation.
* Physical therapy.

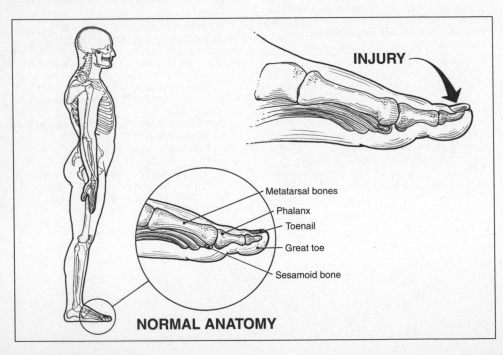

INJURY

Metatarsal bones
Phalanx
Toenail
Great toe
Sesamoid bone

NORMAL ANATOMY

DIAGNOSTIC MEASURES
- Your own observation of signs and symptoms.
- Medical history and physical exam by a doctor.
- X-rays of the toe.

POSSIBLE COMPLICATIONS
- Overlooking a mild exostosis that produces no symptoms, despite signs of diminished performance. Athletes and coaches frequently assume that decreased performance results from loss of competitive drive or emotional causes rather than from the physical disability that actually exists.
- Prolonged healing time if activity is resumed too soon.
- Proneness to repeated injury.
- Unstable or arthritic toe joints following repeated injury.
- Pressure on or injury to nearby nerves, ligaments, tendons, blood vessels or connective tissues.
- Impaired blood supply to the injured toe.

PROBABLE OUTCOME—Toe exostosis usually causes no disability if it is treated properly. Treatment usually involves resting the injured foot and toe for 2 to 4 weeks, heat treatments, corticosteroid injections and protection against additional injury. In a few cases, surgery is necessary to remove the toenail, nailbed, exostosis and tip of the toe.

 HOW TO TREAT

NOTE—Follow your doctor's instructions. These instructions are supplemental.

FIRST AID—None. This condition develops gradually.

CONTINUING CARE
- Rest the injured area. Use splints or crutches if needed.
- Apply heat frequently. Use heat lamps, hot soaks, hot showers, heating pads or heat liniments and ointments.
- Take whirlpool treatments, if available.
- Use proper shoes and extra toe padding, if possible, during competition and workouts to avoid recurrence of the injury.

MEDICATION
- Medicine usually is not necessary for this disorder. For minor pain, you may use non-prescription drugs such as aspirin.
- If surgery is necessary, your doctor may prescribe:
  Nonsteroidal anti-inflammatory drugs to help control swelling.
  Stronger pain relievers.
  Antibiotics to fight infection.

ACTIVITY—Decrease activity for 2 to 4 weeks. If surgery is necessary, resume normal activity gradually.

DIET—During recovery, balance the amount of food you eat with any change in your level of physical activity. Eat a variety of foods to get the energy, protein, vitamins, minerals and fiber you need for good health and healing. Your doctor may suggest vitamin and mineral supplements to promote healing.

REHABILITATION
- Begin daily rehabilitation exercises when movement is comfortable.
- Use ice massage for 10 minutes before and after exercise. Fill a large styrofoam cup with water and freeze. Tear a small amount of foam from the top so ice protrudes. Massage gently over the injured area. Do this for 15 minutes at a time 3 or 4 times a day, and also before workouts or competition.
- See Rehabilitation section for ankle and foot exercises.

 CALL YOUR DOCTOR IF

- You have symptoms of a toe exostosis.
- Any of the following occurs after surgery:
  Increased pain, swelling, redness, drainage or bleeding in the surgical area.
  Signs of infection (headache, muscle aches, dizziness or a general ill feeling and fever).
  New, unexplained symptoms. Drugs used in treatment may cause side effects.

TOE FRACTURE

GENERAL INFORMATION

DEFINITION—A complete or incomplete break in one or more bones of the toes.

BODY PARTS INVOLVED
- Any of the bones of the toes.
- Joints of the toes and joints between the foot and toe bones.
- Soft tissues around the fracture site, including nerves, tendons, ligaments and blood vessels.

SIGNS & SYMPTOMS
- Severe pain at the fracture site.
- Swelling of soft tissues around the fracture.
- Visible deformity if the fracture is complete and the bone fragments separate enough to distort normal toe and foot contours.
- Tenderness to the touch.
- Numbness or coldness in the toe if the blood supply is impaired.

CAUSES
- Direct blow to the toe, as from kicking or being stepped on.
- Indirect stress to the toe. Indirect stress may be caused by twisting.

RISK INCREASES WITH
- Sports that require shoes with cleats.
- History of bone or joint disease, especially osteoporosis.
- Obesity.
- Poor nutrition, especially calcium deficiency.

HOW TO PREVENT—Wear appropriate footgear for running and participation in contact sports.

WHAT TO EXPECT

APPROPRIATE HEALTH CARE
- Doctor's treatment to manipulate and set the broken bones. Surgery (occasionally) to place the bones in proper position and pin the bones.
- Self-care during rehabilitation.
- Whirlpool, ultrasound or massage (to displace excess fluid from the injured joint spaces).

DIAGNOSTIC MEASURES
- Your own observation of symptoms.
- Medical history and physical exam by a doctor.
- X-rays of the toe and the foot.

POSSIBLE COMPLICATIONS
- Pressure on or injury to nearby nerves, ligaments, tendons, muscles, blood vessels or connective tissues.
- Delayed union or nonunion of the fracture.
- Impaired blood supply to the fracture site.
- Infection in open fractures (skin broken over fracture site) or at the incision if surgical setting was necessary.
- Shortening of the injured bones.
- Unstable or arthritic toe joint following repeated injury.
- Prolonged healing time if activity is resumed too soon.
- Proneness to repeated toe injury.

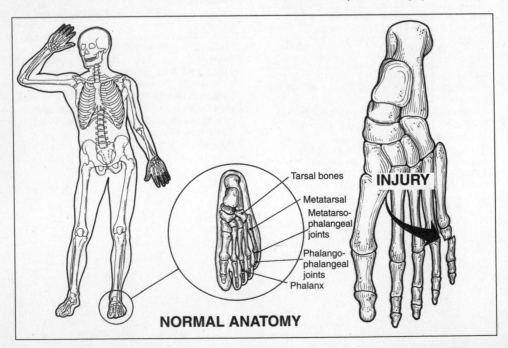

Tarsal bones
Metatarsal
Metatarso-
phalangeal
joints
Phalango-
phalangeal
joints
Phalanx

INJURY

NORMAL ANATOMY

PROBABLE OUTCOME—It is impossible to predict exactly how long it will take for any fracture to heal. Variable factors include age, sex and previous state of health and conditioning. The average healing time for this fracture is 4 to 6 weeks, but you may begin weight-bearing right away. Healing is considered complete when there is no motion at the fracture site and when x-rays show complete bone union.

 ## HOW TO TREAT

NOTE—Follow your doctor's instructions. These instructions are supplemental.

FIRST AID
• Cut away the shoe and sock, if possible, but don't move the injured toe to do so.
• Use instructions for R.I.C.E., the first letters of *rest, ice, compression* and *elevation*. See Appendix 1 for details.
• The doctor will realign the broken bones with surgery or, if possible without. This manipulation should be done as soon as possible after injury. Many tissues lose their elasticity and become difficult to return to their normal positions.

CONTINUING CARE
• Immobilization will be necessary. Place felt between the fractured toe and a good toe, then fix the two toes together with adhesive strips. Then bear weight on the foot as pain allows. Use a wooden-soled shoe or post-operative shoe with toes taped for weight-bearing.
• Use frequent ice massage. Fill a large styrofoam cup with water and freeze. Tear a small amount of foam from the top so ice protrudes. Massage firmly over the injured area in a circle about the size of a baseball. Do this for 15 minutes at a time 3 or 4 times a day, and also before workouts or competition.
• After 72 hours, application of localized heat promotes healing by increasing blood circulation in the injured area. Use hot baths, showers, compresses, heat lamps, heating pads, heat ointments and liniments or whirlpools.

MEDICATION—Your doctor may prescribe:
• General anesthesia to make joint manipulation possible.
• Narcotic or synthetic narcotic pain relievers for severe pain.
• Stool softeners to prevent constipation due to inactivity.
• Acetaminophen for mild pain.
• Antibiotics to fight infection if necessary.

ACTIVITY
• Elevate the foot whenever possible.
• Actively exercise all muscle groups in the foot that are not immobilized. Muscle contractions promote fracture alignment and hasten healing.
• Begin reconditioning the injured foot after clearance from your doctor.
• Resume normal activities gradually after treatment. Don't drive until healing is complete.

DIET—During recovery, balance the amount of food you eat with any change in your level of physical activity. Eat a variety of foods to get the energy, protein, vitamins, minerals and fiber you need for good health and healing.

REHABILITATION—Begin daily rehabilitation exercises when supportive wrapping is no longer needed. Use ice massage for 10 minutes prior to exercise. See Rehabilitation section for ankle and foot exercises.

 ## CALL YOUR DOCTOR IF

• You have signs of a toe fracture.
• Any of the following occurs after treatment or surgery:
  Blue or gray skin color, especially under the toenail.
  Numbness or complete loss of feeling in the toe.
  Increased pain, swelling or drainage in the surgical area.
  Signs of infection (headache, muscle aches, dizziness or a general ill feeling and fever).
  Swelling above the taped area.
  Nausea or vomiting.

TOOTH INJURY & LOSS
(Tooth Avulsion)

 GENERAL INFORMATION

DEFINITION—Damage to a tooth severe enough to separate it completely from the gum and bone without fracture. Children whose front teeth have short, slender roots are most likely to lose teeth through injury.

BODY PARTS INVOLVED
- Teeth.
- Bones that hold teeth.
- Gums and soft tissues surrounding the tooth, including nerves, blood vessels and covering of bone (periosteum).

SIGNS & SYMPTOMS
- Missing tooth.
- Pain and bleeding from the tooth site.
- Swelling of gum soon after injury.

CAUSES—Direct blow to the tooth and gum.

RISK INCREASES WITH
- Contact sports, especially football and boxing.
- Poor nutrition, especially calcium deficiency.
- Poor dental hygiene or gum disease.

HOW TO PREVENT—Wear a helmet, strong face guard and mouthpiece whenever possible during contact sports.

 WHAT TO EXPECT

APPROPRIATE HEALTH CARE
- Dentist's or oral surgeon's evaluation and replantation of an avulsed tooth.
- Blood studies (sometimes) after surgery to evaluate blood loss and infection.

DIAGNOSTIC MEASURES
- Your own observation of symptoms and signs.
- Medical history and physical exam by your dentist or oral surgeon.
- X-rays of the mouth and jaw to detect additional injuries.

POSSIBLE COMPLICATIONS
- Permanent tooth loss if the replantation fails.
- Excessive bleeding.
- Infection.

PROBABLE OUTCOME—Allow about 4 weeks for recovery from surgery if complications don't occur. After it heals, the tooth often appears normal. If it darkens, a plastic dental veneer can be applied to make it cosmetically acceptable.

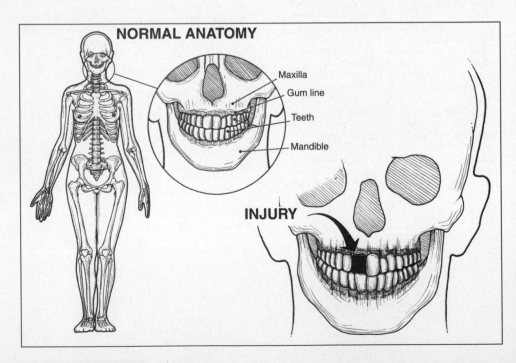

NORMAL ANATOMY

Maxilla

Gum line

Teeth

Mandible

INJURY

HOW TO TREAT

NOTE—Follow your doctor's or dentist's instructions. These instructions are supplemental.

FIRST AID
- Find and wash the missing tooth or teeth.
- Replace the tooth in its socket as soon as possible.
- If you cannot replace the tooth in its socket, wash it and keep it wet in a wet cloth until you reach a dentist or doctor. Put a moist cloth in the empty socket and have the patient bite on it.
- Go to the dentist or emergency room immediately. Hurry! The longer the tooth stays out of the mouth, the less chance there is of its being saved.

CONTINUING CARE
The dentist or oral surgeon will:
- Cleanse the socket.
- Remove the nerve from the tooth and fill the root canal with a plasticlike material before the tooth is replaced.
- Replace the tooth in its socket.
- Anchor the tooth to neighboring teeth with wire or plastic. The tooth must be held in place for 6 to 8 weeks.
Home care after replantation:
- Don't rinse your mouth, spit, smoke or suck on straws for 24 hours, after tooth replantation.
- After 24 hours brush your other teeth often with a soft toothbrush. A clean mouth heals faster. Don't brush the injured tooth until you have clearance from your dentist.

- Beginning 24 hours after surgery, rinse your mouth every 1 or 2 hours with a solution of 1/2 teaspoon salt in 8 oz. of lukewarm water.
- Don't bite down on the affected tooth until healing is complete.

MEDICATION
- You may use nonprescription drugs such as acetaminophen for minor pain.
- Your doctor may prescribe:
  Pain relievers. Don't take prescription pain medication longer than 4 to 7 days. Use only as much as you need.
  Antibiotics to fight infection.
  Mouthwashes.

ACTIVITY—Avoid vigorous physical exercise for 4 to 6 weeks following surgery. Wear a face mask after resuming sports activity.

DIET—Adequate food and fluid intake following surgery will promote more rapid healing. If you can't avoid putting pressure on the tooth while eating your normal diet, follow a liquid high-protein diet for 2 or 3 days. Avoid all alcoholic beverages during healing.

REHABILITATION—None.

CALL YOUR DENTIST IF

- You have a tooth knocked out.
- Any of the following occurs after surgery:
  Increased mouth pain, swelling, redness, drainage or bleeding.
  Signs of infection (headache, muscle aches, dizziness, or a general ill feeling and fever).
  New, unexplained symptoms. Drugs used in treatment may produce side effects.

TURF TOE

GENERAL INFORMATION

DEFINITION—Turf toe is a sprain injury at the base of the big toe, located at the ball of the foot. The name turf toe comes from the fact that this injury is common among athletes who play on artificial turf. Turf toe injuries are divided into three grades by severity:
- Grade I—Stretch of the joint capsule and ligaments.
- Grade II—Partial tear of the joint capsule and ligaments.
- Grade III—Complete tear of the joint capsule and ligaments.

BODY PARTS INVOLVED—The joint capsule and ligaments that connect the foot to the great (or big) toe. The joint is called the metatarsal phalangeal joint. and is composed of bones, ligaments and muscular attachments.

SIGNS & SYMPTOMS
- Pain, tenderness, bruising and swelling in the ball of the foot and the big toe.
- The joint pain may subside with rest and recur with increased activity. Symptoms may resolve in the off season and then recur with renewed exercise.
- Unable to put weight on ball of foot or push off on the big toe.
- Range of motion of the toe is reduced.

CAUSES—Direct injury to the joint. The sprain results from the toe being bent too far upward, (hyperextension) which is the most common or bent backward (hyperflexion). The condition is usually caused from either jamming the toe, or pushing off repeatedly when running or jumping.

RISK INCREASES WITH
- Playing sports on rigid surfaces such as artificial turf (it also occurs on grass surfaces).
- Turf toe is most commonly associated with football. Other sports that increase risk are soccer, rugby, basketball and running.
- Participating in martial arts.
- Ballet dancers.
- Wearing flexible lightweight athletic shoes.
- Poor coordination.
- Prior injury to the toe and joint area.

HOW TO PREVENT
- Often, turf toe cannot be prevented.
- To reduce risk, wear stiff-soled athletic shoes or a special shoe insert when playing sports.
- .Playing on natural grass.
- Taping of the big toe to prevent hyper-extension may prevent some cases of turf toe.

WHAT TO EXPECT

APPROPRIATE HEALTH CARE
- Doctor's treatment.
- Surgery (rarely) to restore the joint to its normal position and repair torn ligaments and tendons. Acute or recurring dislocations may require surgical reconstruction or replacement of the joint.

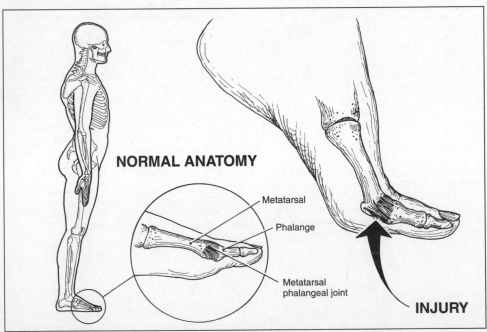

NORMAL ANATOMY

Metatarsal

Phalange

Metatarsal phalangeal joint

INJURY

DIAGNOSTIC MEASURES
• Your own observation of symptoms.
• Medical history and exam by a doctor.
• X-rays of the foot may be taken to rule out fractures. MRI or bone scan may be used to rule out other causes of foot pain.

POSSIBLE COMPLICATIONS
• Turf toe can return.
• Rehabilitation may be slow.
• Hallux limitus (a decreased range of motion due to arthritis developing in the joint).
• Surgery may be recommended if conservative treatment measures don't help.

PROBABLE OUTCOME
• Most sprains heal with time and conservative treatment allowing the individual to return to play pain free. For some players, there may be residual pain and some degree of limitation due to joint damage.
• If this is a first-time injury, proper care and sufficient healing time before resuming to the activity should prevent complications:
Mild strain 2 to 10 days.
Moderate strain 10 days to 6 weeks.
Severe strain 6 to 10 weeks.

 ## HOW TO TREAT

NOTE—Follow your doctor's instructions. These instructions are supplemental.

FIRST AID—Follow instructions for R.I.C.E., the first letters of *rest, ice, compression* and *elevation* (if possible). See Appendix 1 for details.

CONTINUING CARE
• For grade II and III injuries, rest and avoid using the injured toe. Patients with grade I injuries can often return to their activity if they wear stiff soled shoes and the great toe is taped.
• Use ice massage 3 or 4 times a day for 15 minutes at a time. Fill a large styrofoam cup with water and freeze. Tear a small amount of foam from the top so ice protrudes. Massage firmly over the injured area in a circle.
• After the first 24 hours, apply heat instead of ice if it feels better. Use heat lamps, hot soaks, heating pads or heat liniments and ointments.
• Wearing a brace to protect the toe or taping of the toe will help to prevent hyperextension. The doctor or physical therapist will provide instructions.

• Use a stiff insole insert in the shoe. Simple arch supports can help.
• In some cases, a cast may be necessary for a few days to promote healing.

MEDICATION—For minor pain and to reduce inflammation, you may use aspirin or ibuprofen. Steroid injections are usually not prescribed.

ACTIVITY
• Crutches may be needed for walking during recovery depending on the degree of injury. Usually any type of weight bearing can aggravate the injury.
• A return to activity level should progress from weight bearing to walking to jogging (depending on the amount of pain or discomfort).
• Resume sports participation after clearance from your doctor. Your toe should have full range of motion, be at full strength and be almost pain free when you run, jump, twist or do other movements necessary for your sports activity.
• Avoid vigorous exercise for 6 weeks after surgery. Then resume normal activities gradually.

DIET—During recovery, balance the amount of food you eat with any change in your level of physical activity. Eat a variety of foods to get the energy, protein, vitamins, minerals and fiber you need for good health and healing.

REHABILITATION
• The goal is to restore full painless range of motion of the big toe.
• Riding an exercise bike will help maintain aerobic conditioning while recovering.
• You can do non-weight bearing strength training on the affected limb.
• Once the pain subsides enough, begin gentle range of motion exercises for the foot and ankle as recommended by the doctor.
• Wear stiff-sole athletic shoes that fit properly or use an insert (orthotic) that replaces the flexible sole with a stiff steel or graphite plate in the forefoot.
• Ultrasound may be recommended to help decrease the inflammation in the acute stages.

 ## CALL YOUR DOCTOR IF

• You have symptoms of a turf toe injury.
• Any of the following occurs after treatment: Pain, swelling or bruising worsens.

WRIST CONTUSION

GENERAL INFORMATION

DEFINITION—Bruising of skin and underlying tissues of the wrist caused by a direct blow. Contusions cause bleeding from ruptured small capillaries that allow blood to infiltrate muscles, tendons or other soft tissues.

BODY PARTS INVOLVED—Wrist tissues, including blood vessels, muscles, tendons, nerves, covering of bone (periosteum) and connective tissues.

SIGNS & SYMPTOMS
- Wrist swelling—either superficial or deep.
- Wrist pain and tenderness.
- Feeling of firmness when pressure is exerted on the injury site.
- Discoloration under the skin, beginning with redness and progressing to the characteristic "black-and-blue" bruise.
- Restricted wrist motion proportional to the extent of injury.

CAUSES—Direct blow to the wrist, usually from a blunt object.

RISK INCREASES WITH
- Violent contact sports, especially with inadequate protection of the wrist.
- Medical history of any bleeding disorder.
- Poor nutrition, including vitamin deficiency.
- Use of anticoagulants or aspirin.

HOW TO PREVENT—Wear appropriate protective gear and equipment, such as wrapped elastic bandages, tape wraps or leather gauntlet gloves, during competition or other athletic activity if there is risk of a wrist contusion.

WHAT TO EXPECT

APPROPRIATE HEALTH CARE
- Doctor's care unless the contusion is quite small.
- Self-care for minor contusions and following serious contusions during the rehabilitation phase.
- Physical therapy following serious contusions.

DIAGNOSTIC MEASURES
- Your own observation of symptoms.
- Medical history and physical exam by a doctor for all except minor injuries.
- X-rays of the injured area to assess total injury to soft tissues and to rule out the possibility of underlying fracture. The total extent of injury may not be apparent and a MRI (see Glossary) may be necessary.

POSSIBLE COMPLICATIONS
- Excessive bleeding, leading to disability. Infiltrative-type bleeding can sometimes lead to calcification and impaired function of injured muscles and tendons.

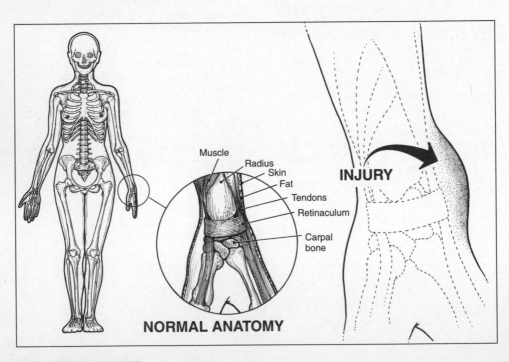

Muscle
Radius
Skin
Fat
Tendons
Retinaculum
Carpal bone

INJURY

NORMAL ANATOMY

- Prolonged healing time if usual activities are resumed too soon.
- Infection if skin over the contusion is broken.

PROBABLE OUTCOME—Healing time varies with the extent of injury, but the average healing time for a wrist contusion is 2 days to 2 weeks.

 ## HOW TO TREAT

NOTE—Follow your doctor's instructions. These instructions are supplemental.

FIRST AID—Use instructions for R.I.C.E., the first letters of *rest, ice, compression* and *elevation*. See Appendix 1 for details.

CONTINUING CARE
- Wrap an elastic bandage over a felt pad placed on the injured area. Keep the area compressed for about 72 hours.
- Continue ice massage. Fill a large styrofoam cup with water and freeze. Tear a small amount of foam from the top so ice protrudes. Massage firmly over the injured area in a circle about the size of a softball. Do this for 15 minutes at a time 3 or 4 times a day, and also before workouts or competition.
- After 72 hours, apply heat instead of ice if it feels better. Use heat lamps, hot soaks, hot showers, heating pads, heat liniments and ointments or whirlpool treatments.

- Massage gently and often to provide comfort and decrease swelling. Stroke from the fingers toward the heart.

MEDICATION
- For minor discomfort, you may use: Acetaminophen or ibuprofen. Topical liniments and ointments.
- Your doctor may prescribe stronger medicine for pain.

ACTIVITY—Begin activity slowly, and stop exercise as soon as pain begins. Increase activity as healing progresses.

DIET—During recovery, balance the amount of food you eat with any change in your level of physical activity. Eat a variety of foods to get the energy, protein, vitamins, minerals and fiber you need for good health and healing.

REHABILITATION—Begin daily rehabilitation exercises when supportive wrapping is no longer needed. See Rehabilitation section for wrist and hand exercises.

 ## CALL YOUR DOCTOR IF

- Injured wrist doesn't improve in 1 or 2 days.
- Skin is broken and signs of infection (drainage, increasing pain, fever, headache, muscle aches, dizziness or a general ill feeling) occur.

WRIST DISLOCATION, LUNATE

GENERAL INFORMATION

DEFINITION—Injury and displacement of the lunate bone of the wrist (usually) or of other bones in the hand and wrist (less commonly). The dislocated bone no longer touches the adjoining bones in the normal manner. The ligaments holding this bone in place have been torn.

BODY PARTS INVOLVED
- Joints in the hand adjoining primarily the lunate bone. Other hand bones are affected less frequently.
- Soft tissues surrounding the dislocation, including nerves, tendons, ligaments, muscles and blood vessels.

SIGNS AND SYMPTOMS
- Excruciating pain in the wrist at the time of dislocation.
- Loss of hand and wrist function, as well as severe pain when attempting to move them.
- Visible deformity if the dislocated bones have locked in the dislocation positions. Bones may spontaneously reposition themselves and leave no deformity, but damage is the same.
- Tenderness over the dislocation.
- Swelling and bruising at the injury site.
- Numbness or paralysis below the dislocation from pressure, pinching or traction on the median nerve.

CAUSES
- Direct blow to the wrist—usually from falling on an outstretched hand.
- End result of a severe wrist sprain.
- Congenital abnormality, such as shallow or malformed joint surfaces.

RISK INCREASES WITH
- Any sport in which falling on or stress to the arm or hand is a possibility.
- Previous wrist dislocation or sprain.
- Repeated wrist injury of any sort.
- Poor muscle conditioning.

HOW TO PREVENT
- Build strength and muscle tone with a long-term conditioning program appropriate for your sport.
- Wear protective devices, such as wrapped elastic bandages, tape wraps or leather gauntlet gloves, to protect vulnerable wrist joints.

WHAT TO EXPECT

APPROPRIATE HEALTH CARE
- Doctor's treatment. This may include manipulating the joint to reposition the bones.
- Surgery to restore the joint to its normal position. Usually requires placement of pins and repair of ligaments with cast immobilization. Acute or recurring dislocation may require surgical reconstruction or replacement of the joint.
- Self-care during rehabilitation.

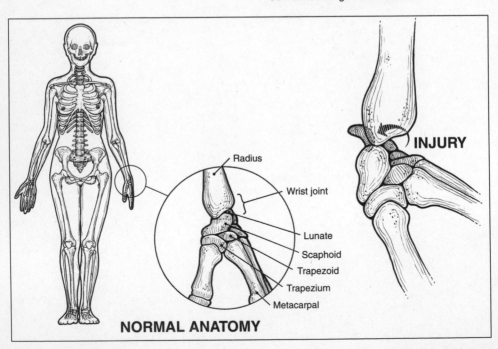

Radius
Wrist joint
Lunate
Scaphoid
Trapezoid
Trapezium
Metacarpal

INJURY

NORMAL ANATOMY

DIAGNOSTIC MEASURES
- Your own observation of symptoms.
- Medical history and physical exam by a doctor.
- X-rays of the joint and adjacent bones.

POSSIBLE COMPLICATIONS
- Injury to median nerve, causing numbness in the thumb, index finger and long fingers and weakness in thumb motion.
- Avascular necrosis (death of bone cells of the lunate bone) with possible collapse and development of arthritis.
- Excessive internal bleeding at the dislocation site.
- Chronic wrist ligament looseness, leading to abnormal carpal bone positions and ultimately to arthritis.
- Recurrent dislocations, particularly if the previous dislocation is not healed completely.

PROBABLE OUTCOME—After the dislocation has been corrected, the joint may require immobilization with a cast, splints or sling for 2 to 8 weeks. Complete healing of injured ligaments requires a minimum of 6 weeks.

 HOW TO TREAT

NOTE—Follow your doctor's instructions. These instructions are supplemental.

FIRST AID
- Keep the person warm with blankets to decrease the possibility of shock.
- Cut away clothing if possible, but don't move the injured area to remove clothing.
- Immobilize the wrist joint and the hand with padded splints.
- Follow instructions for R.I.C.E., the first letters of *rest, ice, compression* and *elevation*. See Appendix 1 for details.
- The doctor will manipulate the dislocated bones with surgery and maintain the correct positions with metal pins and a cast. Manipulation should be done as soon as possible after injury. Many tissues lose their elasticity and become difficult to return to their normal positions.

CONTINUING CARE
While in the cast:
- See Appendix 2 (Care of Casts).
- Actively exercise all muscle groups in the arm and hand that are not immobilized. The resulting muscle contractions promote proper alignment and hasten healing.
After the cast is removed:
- Use ice soaks 3 or 4 times a day. Fill a bucket with ice water, and soak the injured area for 20 minutes at a time.

- You may apply heat instead of ice if it feels better. Use heat lamps, hot soaks, hot showers, heating pads or heat liniments and ointments.
- Wrap the wrist with elasticized bandages between treatments.
- Massage gently and often from the fingers toward the heart to provide comfort and decrease swelling.

MEDICATION—Your doctor may prescribe:
- General anesthesia or muscle relaxants to make joint manipulation possible.
- Acetaminophen or aspirin for moderate pain.
- Narcotic pain relievers for severe pain.
- Antibiotics to fight infection.

ACTIVITY
- Begin reconditioning the wrist after clearance from your doctor.
- If surgery is necessary, resume your normal activities gradually.

DIET
- Do not eat or drink before manipulation or surgery to treat the fracture. Fluid or solid food in your stomach makes vomiting while under anesthesia more hazardous.
- During recovery, eat a well-balanced diet.

REHABILITATION
- Begin daily rehabilitation exercises after clearance from your doctor.
- Use ice massage for 10 minutes before and after exercise. Fill a large styrofoam cup with water and freeze. Tear a small amount of foam from the top so ice protrudes. Massage firmly in a circle over the injured area.
- See Rehabilitation section for wrist and hand exercises.

 CALL YOUR DOCTOR IF

- You have signs or symptoms of a dislocated wrist, especially if the hand becomes numb, pale or cold. This is an emergency!
- Any of the following occurs after treatment or surgery:
  Nausea or vomiting.
  Swelling above or below the cast.
  Blue or gray skin color beyond the cast, especially under the fingernails.
  Numbness or complete loss of feeling below the dislocation site.
  Increased pain, swelling or drainage in the surgical area.
  Signs of infection (headache, muscle aches, dizziness or a general ill feeling and fever).
- New, unexplained symptoms develop. Drugs used in treatment may produce side effects.
- Wrist dislocations that you can "pop" back into normal position occur repeatedly.

WRIST DISLOCATION, RADIUS OR ULNA

GENERAL INFORMATION

DEFINITION—An injury to the joint between the radius and the ulna in the wrist so that the adjoining bones no longer touch each other. Subluxation is a minor dislocation. The joint surfaces still touch, but not in normal relation to each other.

BODY PARTS INVOLVED
* Lower arm bones (radius and ulna).
* Bones in the hand.
* Ligaments that hold the bones in place.
* Soft tissues surrounding the dislocation site, including periosteum (covering of bone), nerves, tendons, blood vessels and connective tissues.

SIGNS & SYMPTOMS
* Excruciating pain in the wrist at the time of dislocation.
* Loss of hand and wrist function, as well as severe pain when attempting to move them.
* Visible deformity if the dislocated bones have locked in the dislocated positions. Bones may spontaneously reposition themselves and leave no deformity, but damage is the same.
* Tenderness over the dislocation.
* Swelling and bruising at the injury site.
* Numbness or paralysis below the dislocation from pressure, pinching or cutting of blood vessels or nerves.

CAUSES
* Direct blow to the wrist—usually from falling on an extended hand.
* End result of a severe wrist sprain.
* Congenital abnormality, such as shallow or malformed joint surfaces.
* This injury frequently occurs with a fracture of the radius.

RISK INCREASES WITH
* Contact sports such as football, basketball, soccer or hockey.
* Previous wrist dislocation or sprain.
* Repeated wrist injury of any sort.
* Poor muscle conditioning.

HOW TO PREVENT
* Participate in a strengthening, flexibility and conditioning program appropriate for your sport.
* Warm up adequately before physical activity.
* After healing, use protective devices such as wrapped elastic bandages or tape wraps to prevent reinjury during participation in sports.
* Consider avoiding contact sports if treatment does not restore a strong, stable wrist.

WHAT TO EXPECT

APPROPRIATE HEALTH CARE
* Doctor's treatment. This will include manipulation of the joint to reposition the bones and application of a cast to immobilize the wrist and forearm.
* Surgery (sometimes) to restore the joint to its normal position and repair torn ligaments and tendons. Acute or recurring dislocations may

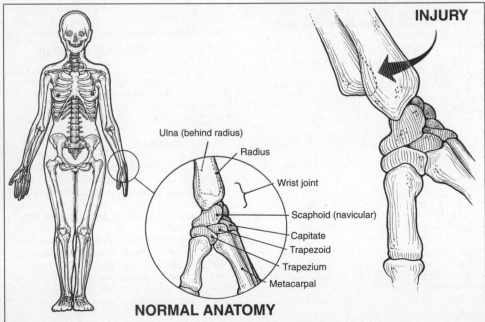

INJURY

Ulna (behind radius)

Radius

Wrist joint

Scaphoid (navicular)

Capitate

Trapezoid

Trapezium

Metacarpal

NORMAL ANATOMY

require surgical reconstruction or replacement of the joint.
- Self-care during rehabilitation.

DIAGNOSTIC MEASURES
- Your own observation of symptoms.
- Medical history and exam by a doctor.
- X-rays of the wrist, hand and elbow. An MRI scan may be done to rule out a fracture.

POSSIBLE COMPLICATIONS
At the time of fracture:
- Shock.
- Pressure on or injury to nearby nerves, ligaments, tendons, blood vessels or connective tissues.

After treatment or surgery:
- Excessive internal bleeding around the wrist.
- Impaired blood supply to the dislocation area.
- Infection introduced during surgical treatment.
- Prolonged healing if activity is resumed too soon.
- Inability to fully rotate the forearm from palm-up to palm-down position.
- Recurrent wrist dislocation.
- Unstable or arthritic wrist following repeated injury.

PROBABLE CAUSE—After the wrist dislocation has been corrected, the joint may require immobilization with a cast or splint for 4 to 8 weeks. Complete healing of injured ligaments requires a minimum of 6 weeks.

 HOW TO TREAT

NOTE—Follow your doctor's instructions. These instructions are supplemental.

FIRST AID
- Keep the person warm with blankets to decrease the possibility of shock.
- Cut away clothing if possible, but don't move the injured area to remove clothing.
- Immobilize the wrist joint and the hand with padded splints.
- Follow instructions for R.I.C.E., the first letters of *rest, ice, compression* and *elevation.* See Appendix 1 for details.

CONTINUING CARE
While in the cast:
- See Appendix 2 (Care of Casts).
- Actively exercise all muscle groups in the arm and hand that are not immobilized. The resulting muscle contractions promote proper alignment and hasten healing.
After the cast is removed:
- Use ice soaks 3 or 4 times a day. Fill a bucket with ice water, and soak the injured area for 20 minutes at a time.
- You may apply heat instead of ice if it feels better. Use heat lamps, hot soaks, hot showers, heating pads or heat liniments and ointments.

- Take whirlpool treatments, if available.
- Massage gently and often to provide comfort and decrease swelling. Stroke from the fingers toward the heart.
- Wrap the injured wrist with elasticized bandages between treatments.

MEDICATION—Your doctor may prescribe:
- General anesthesia or muscle relaxants to make joint manipulation possible.
- Acetaminophen to relieve moderate pain.
- Narcotic pain relievers for severe pain.
- Antibiotics to fight infection if surgery is necessary.

ACTIVITY
- Begin reconditioning the wrist after clearance from your doctor.
- If surgery is necessary, resume usual activities and reconditioning gradually after surgery.

DIET
- Do not drink or eat before manipulation or surgery to treat the fracture. Fluid or solid food in your stomach makes vomiting while under anesthesia more hazardous.
- During recovery, eat a well-balanced diet.

REHABILITATION
- Begin daily rehabilitation exercises after clearance from your doctor.
- Use ice massage for 10 minutes before and after exercise. Fill a large styrofoam cup with water and freeze. Tear a small amount of foam from the top so ice protrudes. Massage firmly in a circle over the injured area.
- See Rehabilitation section for wrist and hand exercises.

 CALL YOUR DOCTOR IF

- You have signs or symptoms of a dislocated wrist, especially if the hand becomes numb, pale or cold. This is an emergency!
- Any of the following occurs after treatment or surgery:
  Nausea or vomiting.
  Swelling above or below the cast.
  Blue or gray skin color beyond the cast, especially under the fingernails.
  Numbness or complete loss of feeling below the dislocation site.
  Increased pain, swelling or drainage in the surgical area.
  Signs of infection (headache, muscle aches, dizziness or a general ill feeling and fever).
  Constipation.
- New, unexplained symptoms develop. Drugs used in treatment may produce side effects.
- Wrist dislocations that you can "pop" back into normal position occur repeatedly.

WRIST FRACTURE, CARPAL BONES

GENERAL INFORMATION

DEFINITION—A break of the bone or bones that connect the forearm to the hand. The wrist is the most commonly injured region of the upper body. A simple fracture (closed) is when the bone has not broken through the skin. The compound (open) fracture is more serious since the bone breaks through the skin and there is also a risk of infection. Fractures can be displaced or not displaced. A displaced fracture means the bone has shifted its position.

BODY PARTS INVOLVED
- Wrist joint - where the bones of the forearm join the small bones of the hand. The wrist is what lets the hand move from side to side, up and down and rotate the hand so the palm can be either up or down.
- There are 8 carpal bones in each hand that extend from the wrist joint to the base of the fingers (the scaphoid [also called the navicular and the most frequently injured carpal bone], lunate, triquetrum, pisiform, trapezium, trapezoid, capitate, and hamate). These small bones work with the forearm bones and the finger bones. The carpal bones account for up to 10% of injuries to the structures of the hand.

SIGNS & SYMPTOMS
- Bruising, swelling and tenderness.
- Numbness and tingling.
- Limitation of movement.
- Pain (often severe that may get worse with time and movement).
- Deformity.
- Difficulty bearing weight.

CAUSES
- Direct blow to the wrist.
- Falling onto an outstretched hand (usually when trying to break a fall).
- Injury that causes the wrist to bend sharply backward.

RISK INCREASES WITH
- Contact sports (e.g., football, hockey. soccer).
- Rollerblading, skiing, iceskating, snowboarding, gymnastics.
- Bone loss due to aging and osteoporosis, certain medications, or chronic illness.

HOW TO PREVENT
- Build strength and flexibility before starting regular athletic practice or competition.
- Wear protective wrist guards.

WHAT TO EXPECT

APPROPRIATE HEALTH CARE
- Doctor's treatment to reposition the dislocated bone and manipulate the fractured bone.
- Hospitalization (sometimes) for surgical setting of the fracture.

DIAGNOSTIC MEASURES
- Your own observation of symptoms.
- Medical history and physical exam by a doctor.

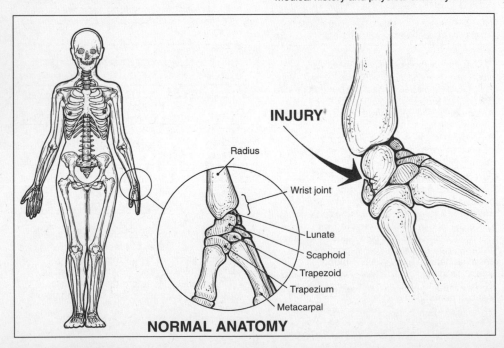

Radius

INJURY

Wrist joint

Lunate

Scaphoid

Trapezoid

Trapezium

Metacarpal

NORMAL ANATOMY

• X-rays of injured area to assess total injury. Rarely, a bone scan or MRI may be needed to detect hidden fractures.

POSSIBLE COMPLICATIONS
• Long-term problems may include arthritis, deformity, discomfort or stiffness, numbness or tingling in the hand or weakness.
• Infection in open fractures (skin broken over fracture site) or at the incision if surgical setting was necessary.
• Prolonged healing time if activity is resumed too soon.
• More complex fractures increase the risk of complications.

PROBABLE OUTCOME
• Over time (8-12 weeks), most wrist fractures heal without problems.
• Rehabilitation and physical therapy are important to help restore normal motion, function, and strength of the wrist.

 HOW TO TREAT

NOTE—Follow your doctor's instructions. These instructions are supplemental.

FIRST AID
• Keep the person warm with blankets to decrease the possibility of shock.
• Cut away clothing, if possible, but don't move the injured wrist to do so.
• Follow instructions for R.I.C.E., the first letters of *rest, ice, compression* and *elevation*. See Appendix 1 for details.
• There are many methods of treatment for fractures of the wrist. Your doctor will discuss the best options for your particular fracture.
• The doctor will set the broken bones with surgery or, if possible, without. The setting lines up the broken bones as close to their normal positions as possible. Manipulation should be done as soon as possible after injury. Six or more hours after the fracture, bleeding and displacement of body fluids may lead to shock. Also, many tissues lose their elasticity and become difficult to return to their normal positions.

CONTINUING CARE
• Immobilization will be necessary, usually with plaster, fiberglass or plastic cast or splint around the injured area to immobilize the wrist.
• External fixation may be required with metal pins or rods inserted into slits made in the skin.
• After 96 hours, application of localized heat promotes healing by increasing blood circulation in the injured area. Use a heat lamp or a heating pad for 30 minutes at a time so heat can penetrate the cast or splints.
• After the cast or splints are removed, use frequent ice massage. Fill a large styrofoam cup with water and freeze. Tear a small amount of foam from the top so ice protrudes. Massage firmly over the injured area in a circle about the size of a baseball. Do this for 15 minutes at a time 3 or 4 times a day.
• Apply heat instead of ice if it feels better. Use heat lamps, hot soaks, hot showers, heating pads or heat liniments and ointments.
• Use whirlpool treatments, if available.

MEDICATION—Your doctor may prescribe:
• General anesthesia, local anesthesia or muscle relaxants to make bone manipulation and fixation of bone fragments possible.
• Prescription pain relievers for severe pain.
• Acetaminophen for mild pain.

ACTIVITY
• Actively exercise all muscle groups not immobilized. Muscle contractions promote fracture alignment and hasten healing. Exercises to work the elbow, shoulder, and fingers may be prescribed while healing. Your age, the stability of the fracture, and how it was reset are all taken into consideration before giving you the exercises to do.
• Begin reconditioning the wrist area after clearance from your doctor.
• Resume normal activities gradually after treatment.

DIET
• Do not drink or eat before manipulation or surgery to treat the fracture. Fluid or solid food in your stomach makes vomiting while under anesthesia more hazardous.
• During recovery, balance the amount of food you eat with any change in your level of physical activity.

REHABILITATION
• Begin daily rehabilitation exercises when movement is comfortable. Use ice massage for 10 minutes prior to exercise.
• See Rehabilitation section for wrist and hand exercises.

 CALL YOUR DOCTOR IF

• You have signs of a wrist fracture.
• Any of the following occurs after surgery or other treatment:
  Increased pain, swelling or drainage in the surgical area.
  Signs of infection (headache, muscle aches, dizziness or a general ill feeling and fever).
  Swelling above or below the splints.
  Blue or gray skin color beyond the cast or splints, particularly under the fingernails.
  Numbness or complete loss of feeling below the fracture site.
  Nausea or vomiting.

WRIST FRACTURE, RADIUS OR ULNA

 GENERAL INFORMATION

DEFINITION—A break of the bone or bones that connect the forearm to the hand. The wrist is the most commonly injured region of the upper body. A simple fracture (closed) is when the bone has not broken through the skin. The compound (open) fracture is more serious since the bone breaks through the skin and there is also a risk of infection. Fractures can be displaced or not displaced. A displaced fracture means the bone has shifted its position.

BODY PARTS INVOLVED
• Wrist joint - where the two bones of the forearm join the small bones of the hand. The wrist is what lets the hand move from side to side, up and down and rotate the hand so the palm can be either up or down.
• The big bones associated with the wrist. The radius is the bone that runs on the thumb side of the arm, and the ulna is the one that runs along the small finger side. These bones account for approximately three quarters of bony injuries of the wrist.

SIGNS & SYMPTOMS
• Bruising, swelling and tenderness.
• Numbness and tingling.
• Limitation of movement.
• Pain (often severe that may get worse with time and movement).
• Deformity.
• Difficulty bearing weight.

CAUSES
• Direct blow to the wrist.
• Falling onto an outstretched hand (usually when trying to break a fall).
• Injury that causes the wrist to bend sharply backward.

RISK INCREASES WITH
• Contact sports (e.g., football, hockey. soccer).
• Rollerblading, skiing, iceskating, snowboarding, gymnastics.
• Bone loss due to aging and osteoporosis, certain medications, or chronic illness.

HOW TO PREVENT
• Build strength and flexibility before starting regular athletic practice or competition.
• Wear protective wrist guards.

 WHAT TO EXPECT

APPROPRIATE HEALTH CARE
• Doctor's treatment to reposition the dislocated bone and manipulate the fractured bone.
• Hospitalization (sometimes) for surgical setting of the fracture.

DIAGNOSTIC MEASURES
• Your own observation of symptoms.
• Medical history and physical exam by a doctor.
• X-rays of injured area to assess total injury. Rarely, a bone scan or MRI may be needed to detect hidden fractures.

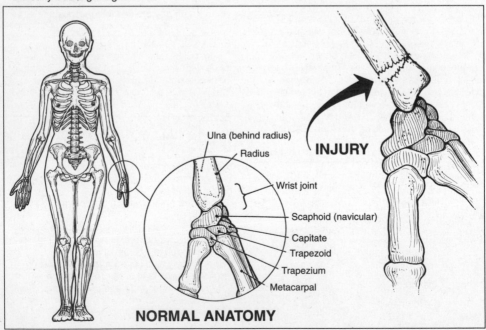

Ulna (behind radius)
Radius
INJURY
Wrist joint
Scaphoid (navicular)
Capitate
Trapezoid
Trapezium
Metacarpal

NORMAL ANATOMY

POSSIBLE COMPLICATIONS
- Long-term problems may include arthritis, deformity (shortening of one of the bones in the forearm), discomfort or stiffness, numbness or tingling in the hand or weakness.
- Infection in open fractures (skin broken over fracture site) or at the incision if surgical setting was necessary.
- Prolonged healing time if activity is resumed too soon.
- More complex fractures increase the risk of complications.

PROBABLE OUTCOME
- Over time (8-12 weeks), most wrist fractures heal without problems.
- Rehabilitation and physical therapy are important to help restore normal function, strength and motion of the wrist.

 HOW TO TREAT

NOTE—Follow your doctor's instructions. These instructions are supplemental.

FIRST AID
- Keep the person warm with blankets to decrease the possibility of shock.
- Cut away clothing, if possible, but don't move the injured wrist to do so.
- Follow instructions for R.I.C.E., the first letters of *rest, ice, compression* and *elevation*. See Appendix 1 for details.
- There are many methods of treatment for fractures of the wrist. Your doctor will discuss the best options for your particular fracture.
- The doctor will set the broken bones with surgery or, if possible, without. The setting lines up the broken bones as close to their normal positions as possible. Manipulation should be done as soon as possible after injury. Six or more hours after the fracture, bleeding and displacement of body fluids may lead to shock. Also, many tissues lose their elasticity and become difficult to return to their normal positions.

CONTINUING CARE
- Immobilization will be necessary, usually with plaster, fiberglass or plastic cast or splint around the injured area to immobilize the wrist.
- External fixation may be required with metal pins or rods inserted into slits made in the skin.
- After 96 hours, application of localized heat promotes healing by increasing blood circulation in the injured area. Use a heat lamp or a heating pad for 30 minutes at a time so heat can penetrate the cast or splints.
- After the cast or splints are removed, use frequent ice massage. Fill a large styrofoam cup with water and freeze. Tear a small amount of foam from the top so ice protrudes. Massage firmly over the injured area in a circle about the size of a baseball. Do this for 15 minutes at a time 3 or 4 times a day.
- Apply heat instead of ice if it feels better. Use heat lamps, hot soaks, hot showers, heating pads or heat liniments and ointments.
- Use whirlpool treatments, if available.

MEDICATION—Your doctor may prescribe:
- General anesthesia, local anesthesia or muscle relaxants to make bone manipulation and fixation of bone fragments possible.
- Prescription pain relievers for severe pain.
- Acetaminophen for mild pain.

ACTIVITY
- Actively exercise all muscle groups not immobilized. Muscle contractions promote fracture alignment and hasten healing. Exercises to work the elbow, shoulder, and fingers may be prescribed while healing. Your age, the stability of the fracture, and how it was reset are all taken into consideration before giving you the exercises to do.
- Begin reconditioning the wrist area after clearance from your doctor.
- Resume normal activities gradually after treatment.

DIET
- Do not drink or eat before manipulation or surgery to treat the fracture. Fluid or solid food in your stomach makes vomiting while under anesthesia more hazardous.
- During recovery, balance the amount of food you eat with any change in your level of physical activity. Eat a variety of foods to get the energy, protein, vitamins, minerals and fiber you need for good health and healing.

REHABILITATION
- Begin daily rehabilitation exercises when movement is comfortable. Use ice massage for 10 minutes prior to exercise.
- See Rehabilitation section for wrist and hand exercises.

 CALL YOUR DOCTOR IF

- You have signs or symptoms of a wrist fracture.
- Any of the following occurs after surgery or other treatment:
  Increased pain, swelling or drainage in the surgical area.
  Signs of infection (headache, muscle aches, dizziness or a general ill feeling and fever).
  Swelling above or below the splints.
  Blue or gray skin color beyond the cast or splints, particularly under the fingernails.
  Numbness or complete loss of feeling below the fracture site.
  Nausea or vomiting.

WRIST GANGLION
(Synovial Hernia; Ganglion Cyst)

 GENERAL INFORMATION

DEFINITION—A small, usually hard nodule lying directly over the tendon or joint capsule on the back or front of the wrist. Occasionally the nodule may become quite large. Wrist ganglions are fairly common.

BODY PARTS INVOLVED
• Back or front of the wrist.
• Tendon sheath (a thin membranous covering of any tendon).
• Any of the joint capsular ligaments in the wrist.

SIGNS & SYMPTOMS
• Hard lump over the tendon or joint capsule in the wrist. The nodule "yields" to heavy pressure because it is not solid.
• No pain usually, but overuse of the wrist may cause mild pain and aching.
• Tenderness if the lump is pressed hard.
• Discomfort with extremes of motion (flexing or extending) and with repetition of the exercises that produced the ganglion.

CAUSES
• Mild sprains and chronic sprains of the wrist, causing weakness of the joint capsule.
• A defect in the fibrous sheath of the joint or tendon that permits a segment of the underlying synovium (the thin membrane that lines the tendon sheath) to herniate through it.
• Irritation accompanying the herniated synovium, causing production of thickened fluid. The sac created by the herniated synovium gradually fills, enlarges and becomes hard, forming the ganglion.

RISK INCREASES WITH
• Repeated injury, especially mild sprains. Wrist ganglions frequently occur in bowlers, tennis players and those who play handball, racquetball and squash.
• Inadequate warmup prior to practice or competition.
• Poor muscle strength or conditioning.
• If surgery is necessary, surgical risk increases with smoking, poor nutrition, alcoholism and recent chronic illness.

HOW TO PREVENT
• Participate in a strengthening, flexibility and conditioning program appropriate for your sport.
• Warm up before practice or competition.

 WHAT TO EXPECT

APPROPRIATE HEALTH CARE
• Doctor's care for diagnosis and possible aspiration of cyst or injections of local anesthetic or corticosteriods.

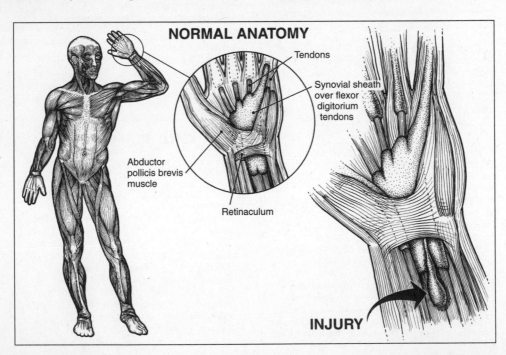

NORMAL ANATOMY

Tendons

Synovial sheath over flexor digitorium tendons

Abductor pollicis brevis muscle

Retinaculum

INJURY

- If needed, surgery will be conducted under local or general anesthesia in an outpatient surgical facility or hospital operating room.

DIAGNOSTIC MEASURES
- Your own observation of signs and symptoms.
- Medical history and physical examination by a doctor.
- X-rays of the area to rule out a bone tumor or unhealed bone fracture.
- Needle aspiration of cyst to inspect fluid content.

POSSIBLE COMPLICATIONS
- Calcification of the ganglion (rare).
- After surgery:
  Excessive bleeding.
  Surgical wound infection.
  Recurrence if surgical removal is incomplete.

PROBABLE OUTCOME—Ganglions sometimes disappear spontaneously, only to recur later. Surgery is frequently necessary if symptoms continue. Surgical removal has only an 80% cure rate, with 20% chance of recurrence. After surgery, allow about 3 weeks for recovery if no complications occur.

 HOW TO TREAT

NOTE—Follow your doctor's instructions. These instructions are supplemental.

FIRST AID—None. This condition develops gradually.

CONTINUING CARE
Immediately after surgery:
- The affected area is usually immobilized in a splint for 1 to 2 weeks following surgery.
After bandage or splints removed by doctor:
- A hard ridge should form along the incision. As it heals, the ridge will recede gradually.
- Bathe and shower as usual. You may wash the incision gently with mild unscented soap.
- You may apply nonprescription antibiotic ointment to the wound.
- Wrap the hand with an elasticized bandage until healing is complete.

- Use ice massage. Fill a large styrofoam cup with water and freeze. Tear a small amount of foam from the top so ice protrudes. Massage firmly over the injured area in a circle about the size of a baseball. Do this for 15 minutes at a time 3 or 4 times a day, and also before workouts or competition.
- You may apply heat instead of ice if it feels better. Use heat lamps, hot soaks, hot showers, heating pads or heat liniments and ointments.
- Take whirlpool treatments, if available.

MEDICATION
- Your doctor may prescribe pain relievers. Don't take prescription pain medication longer than 4 to 7 days. Use only as much as you need.
- You may use nonprescription drugs such as acetaminophen for minor pain.

ACTIVITY—Usually no restrictions.

DIET—During recovery, balance the amount of food you eat with any change in your level of physical activity. Eat a variety of foods to get the energy, protein, vitamins, minerals and fiber you need for good health and healing.

REHABILITATION
- Begin daily rehabilitation exercises when supportive wrapping is no longer needed. Use ice massage for 10 minutes before and after exercise.
- See Rehabilitation section for wrist and hand exercises.

 CALL YOUR DOCTOR IF

- You have signs or symptoms of a wrist ganglion.
- Any of the following occurs after surgery:
  Increased pain, swelling, redness, drainage or bleeding in the surgical area.
  Signs of infection (headache, muscle aches, dizziness or a general ill feeling and fever).
  New, unexplained symptoms. Drugs used in treatment may produce side effects.

WRIST SPRAIN

GENERAL INFORMATION

DEFINITION—Violent overstretching of one or more ligaments in the wrist joint. Sprains involving two or more ligaments cause considerably more disability than single-ligament sprains. When the ligament is overstretched, it becomes tense and gives way at its weakest point, either where it attaches to bone or within the ligament itself. If the ligament pulls loose a fragment of bone, it is called an avulsion fracture. There are 3 types of sprains:
● Mild (Grade I)—Tearing of some ligament fibers. There is no loss of function.
● Moderate (Grade II)—Rupture of a portion of the ligament, resulting in some loss of function.
● Severe (Grade III)—Complete rupture of the ligament or complete separation of ligament from bone. There is total loss of function. A severe sprain may require surgical repair.

BODY PARTS INVOLVED
● Ligaments of the wrist.
● Tissues surrounding the sprain, including blood vessels, tendons, bone, periosteum (covering of bone) and muscles.

SIGNS & SYMPTOMS
● Severe pain at the time of injury.
● A feeling of popping or tearing inside the wrist.
● Tenderness at the injury site.
● Swelling in the wrist.
● Bruising that appears soon after injury.

CAUSES—Stress on a ligament that temporarily forces or pries the wrist joint out of its normal location.

RISK INCREASES WITH
● Contact sports, such as boxing or wrestling.
● Bowling.
● Skiing.
● Pole vaulting.
● Previous wrist injury.
● Poor muscle conditioning.
● inadequate protection from equipment.

HOW TO PREVENT
● Build your strength with a conditioning program appropriate for your sport.
● Warm up before practice or competition.
● To prevent reinjury, tape vulnerable joints before practice or competition.

WHAT TO EXPECT

APPROPRIATE HEALTH CARE
● Doctor's diagnosis.
● Application of a cast, tape or elastic bandage.
● Self-care during rehabilitation.
● Physical therapy (moderate or severe sprain).
● Surgery (severe sprain).

DIAGNOSTIC MEASURES
● Your own observation of symptoms.
● Medical history and exam by a doctor.
● X-rays of the wrist and hand to rule out fractures.

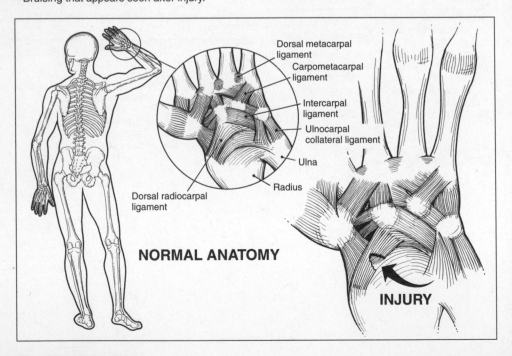

Dorsal metacarpal ligament
Carpometacarpal ligament
Intercarpal ligament
Ulnocarpal collateral ligament
Ulna
Radius
Dorsal radiocarpal ligament

NORMAL ANATOMY

INJURY

- Arthrogram or MRI (see Glossary for both) to evaluate the wrist ligaments for tears.

POSSIBLE COMPLICATIONS
- Prolonged healing time if usual activities are resumed too soon.
- Proneness to repeated injury.
- Inflammation at the ligament attachment to bone (periostitis).
- Prolonged disability (sometimes).
- Unstable or arthritic wrist following unrecognized repeated injury.

PROBABLE OUTCOME—If this is a first-time injury, proper care and sufficient healing time before resuming activity should prevent permanent disability. Ligaments have a poor blood supply, and torn ligaments require as much healing time as fractures. Average healing times are:
- Mild sprains—2 to 6 weeks.
- Moderate sprains—6 to 8 weeks.
- Severe sprains—8 to 10 weeks.

 ## HOW TO TREAT

NOTE—Follow your doctor's instructions. These instructions are supplemental.

FIRST AID—Use instructions for R.I.C.E., the first letters of *rest, ice, compression* and *elevation*. See Appendix 1 for details.

CONTINUING CARE—If the doctor does not apply a cast, tape or elastic bandage:
- Continue using an ice pack 3 or 4 times a day. Place ice chips or cubes in a plastic bag. Wrap the bag in a moist towel, and place it over the injured area. Use for 20 minutes at a time.
- Wrap the wrist with an elasticized bandage between ice treatments.
- After 72 hours, apply heat instead of ice if it feels better. Use heat lamps, hot soaks, hot showers, heating pads or heat liniments and ointments.
- Take whirlpool treatments, if available.
- Massage gently and often to provide comfort and decrease swelling.

MEDICATION
- For minor discomfort, you may use:
  Aspirin, acetaminophen or ibuprofen.
  Topical liniments and ointments.
- Your doctor may prescribe:
  Stronger pain relievers.
  Injection of a long-acting local anesthetic to reduce pain.
  Injections of a corticosteroid, such as triamcinolone, to reduce inflammation.

ACTIVITY—Resume your normal activities gradually after clearance from your doctor.

DIET—During recovery, balance the amount of food you eat with any change in your level of physical activity. Eat a variety of foods to get the energy, protein, vitamins, minerals and fiber you need for good health and healing.

REHABILITATION
- Begin daily rehabilitation exercises when the cast or supportive wrapping is no longer necessary.
- Use ice massage for 10 minutes before and after exercise. Fill a large styrofoam cup with water and freeze. Tear a small amount of foam from the top so ice protrudes. Massage firmly over the injured area in a circle.
- See Rehabilitation section for wrist and hand exercises.

 ## CALL YOUR DOCTOR IF

- You have symptoms of a moderate or severe wrist sprain or a mild sprain persists longer than 2 weeks.
- Pain, swelling or bruising worsens despite treatment.
- Any of the following occurs after casting or splinting:
  Pain, numbness or coldness beyond the wrist.
  Blue, gray or dusky fingernails.
- Any of the following occurs after surgery:
  Increased pain, swelling, redness, drainage or bleeding in the surgical area.
  Signs of infection (headache, muscle aches, dizziness or a general ill feeling with fever).
- New, unexplained symptoms develop. Drugs used in treatment may produce side effects.

WRIST STRAIN

GENERAL INFORMATION

DEFINITION—Injury to the muscles and tendons of the wrist. Muscles, tendons and their attached bones comprise contractile units. These units stabilize the hand and wrist and allow their motion. A strain occurs at the weakest part of the unit. Strains are of 3 types:
• Mild (Grade I)—Slightly pulled muscle without tearing of muscle or tendon fibers. There is no loss of strength.
• Moderate (Grade II)—Tearing of fibers of the muscle or tendon or at the attachment to bone. Strength is diminished.
• Severe (Grade III)—Rupture of the muscle-tendon-bone attachment, with separation of fibers. A severe strain may require surgical repair. Chronic strains are caused by overuse. Acute strains are caused by direct injury or overstress.

BODY PARTS INVOLVED
• Tendons and muscles of the forearm.
• Bones at the wrist, where the muscles and tendons attach.
• Soft tissues surrounding the injury, including nerves, periosteum (covering of bone), blood vessels and lymph vessels.

SIGNS & SYMPTOMS
• Pain when moving or stretching the wrist.
• Muscle spasm of the injured muscles.
• Redness and swelling over the injury.
• Loss of strength (moderate or severe strain).
• Crepitation ("crackling" feeling and sound when the injured area is pressed with fingers).
• Calcification of the tendon or muscles (visible with x-rays).
• Inflammation of the tendon sheath.

CAUSES
• Prolonged overuse of muscle-tendon units in the forearm.
• Single violent injury or force applied to the forearm.

RISK INCREASES WITH
• Contact sports such as boxing, wrestling or football.
• Gymnastics.
• Weightlifting.
• Recent forearm or wrist fracture.
• Medical history of any bleeding disorder.
• Obesity.
• Poor nutrition.
• Previous wrist injury.
• Poor muscle conditioning.

HOW TO PREVENT
• Participate in a strengthening, flexibility and conditioning program appropriate for your sport.
• Warm up before practice or competition.
• Tape the wrist area before practice or competition.
• Wear protective equipment.

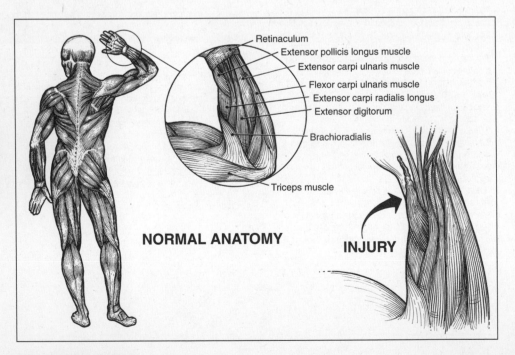

Retinaculum
Extensor pollicis longus muscle
Extensor carpi ulnaris muscle
Flexor carpi ulnaris muscle
Extensor carpi radialis longus
Extensor digitorum
Brachioradialis
Triceps muscle

NORMAL ANATOMY

INJURY

WHAT TO EXPECT

APPROPRIATE HEALTH CARE
- Doctor's diagnosis.
- Application of tape, plaster splints or cast (sometimes).
- Self-care during rehabilitation.
- Physical therapy (moderate or severe strain).
- Surgery (severe strain).

DIAGNOSTIC MEASURES
- Your own observation of symptoms.
- Medical history and exam by a doctor.
- X-rays of the wrist and forearm to rule out fractures.

POSSIBLE COMPLICATIONS
- Prolonged healing time if activity is resumed too soon.
- Proneness to repeated injury.
- Inflammation at the attachment to bone (periostitis).
- Prolonged disability (weakness).

PROBABLE OUTCOME—If this is a first-time injury, proper care and sufficient healing time before resuming activity should prevent permanent disability. Torn ligaments and tendons require as long to heal as fractured bones. Average healing times are:
- Mild strain—2 to 10 days.
- Moderate strain—10 days to 6 weeks.
- Severe strain—6 to 10 weeks.
If this is a repeat injury, complications listed above are more likely to occur.

 HOW TO TREAT

NOTE—Follow your doctor's instructions. These instructions are supplemental.

FIRST AID—Use instructions for R.I.C.E., the first letters of *rest, ice, compression* and *elevation*. See Appendix 1 for details.

CONTINUING CARE—If splints or a cast are used after injury or surgery, leave fingers free and exercise them regularly. If a cast or splints are not used:
- Use ice massage 3 or 4 times a day for 15 minutes at a time. Fill a large styrofoam cup with water and freeze. Tear a small amount of foam from the top so ice protrudes. Massage firmly over the injured area in a circle about the size of a softball.
- After the first 72 hours, apply heat instead of ice if it feels better. Use heat lamps, hot soaks, hot showers, heating pads or heat liniments and ointments.
- Take whirlpool treatments, if available.
- Wrap the injured wrist and forearm with an elasticized bandage between treatments.
- Massage gently and often to provide comfort and decrease swelling.

MEDICATION
- For minor discomfort, you may use:
  Aspirin, acetaminophen or ibuprofen.
  Topical liniments and ointments.
- Your doctor may prescribe:
  Stronger pain relievers.
  Injection of a long-acting local anesthetic to reduce pain.
  Injections of corticosteroids, such as triamcinolone, to reduce inflammation.

ACTIVITY
- For a moderate or severe strain, use a sling or wrist splint for at least 72 hours—longer with a cast. See Appendix 3 (Care of Casts).
- Resume your normal activities gradually.

DIET—During recovery, balance the amount of food you eat with any change in your level of physical activity. Eat a variety of foods to get the energy, protein, vitamins, minerals and fiber you need for good health and healing.

REHABILITATION
- Begin daily rehabilitation exercises when supportive wrapping (including a cast) is no longer needed. Use ice massage for 10 minutes prior to exercise.
- See Rehabilitation section for wrist and hand exercises.

 CALL YOUR DOCTOR IF

- You have symptoms of a moderate or severe wrist strain or a mild strain persists longer than 10 days.
- Pain or swelling worsens despite treatment.
- The following occur with a cast or splints:
  Pain, numbness or coldness below the injury.
  Dusky, blue or gray fingernails.

WRIST TENOSYNOVITIS

GENERAL INFORMATION

DEFINITION—Inflammation of the lining of a tendon sheath in the wrist. The lining secretes a fluid that lubricates the tendon. When the lining becomes inflamed, the tendon cannot glide smoothly in its covering.

BODY PARTS INVOLVED
* Any wrist-tendon lining and covering.
* Soft tissues in the surrounding area, including blood vessels, nerves, ligaments, periosteum (covering of bone) and connective tissues.

SIGNS & SYMPTOMS
* Constant pain or pain with motion of the wrist.
* Limited motion of the wrist and hand.
* Crepitation (a "crackling" sound when the tendon moves or is touched).
* Redness and tenderness over the inflamed tendon.

CAUSES
* Strain from overuse of the wrist.
* Direct blow or injury to muscles and tendons in the wrist and hand. Tenosynovitis becomes more likely with repeated injury to the wrist or hand.
* Infection introduced through broken skin at the time of injury or through a surgical incision after injury.
* Rheumatologic diseases, such as rheumatoid arthritis.

RISK INCREASES WITH
* Contact sports.
* Throwing sports.
* Use of constrictive taping or gloves that put pressure over the course of the tendon during repetitive use.
* If surgery is needed, surgical risk increases with smoking, poor nutrition, alcoholism, drug abuse and recent or chronic illness.

HOW TO PREVENT
* Engage in a vigorous program of physical conditioning before beginning regular sports participation.
* Warm up adequately before practice or competition.
* Wear protective gear appropriate for your sport.
* Learn proper moves and techniques for your sport.

WHAT TO EXPECT

APPROPRIATE HEALTH CARE
* Doctor's examination and diagnosis.
* Surgery (sometimes) to enlarge the tunnel of the tendon covering and restore a smooth, gliding motion. The surgical procedure is performed under anesthesia (local or general) in an outpatient surgical facility.

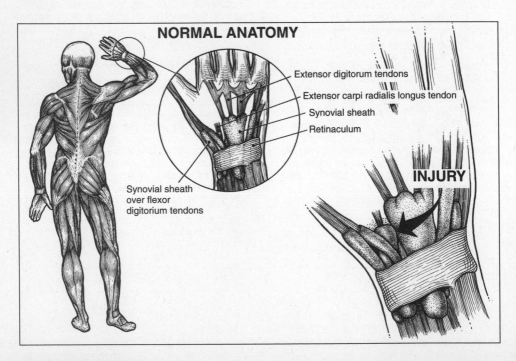

NORMAL ANATOMY

Extensor digitorum tendons
Extensor carpi radialis longus tendon
Synovial sheath
Retinaculum

Synovial sheath over flexor digitorium tendons

INJURY

DIAGNOSTIC MEASURES
- Your own observation of symptoms and signs.
- Medical history and physical examination by your doctor.
- X-rays of the wrist, arm and hand to rule out other abnormalities. An MRI may be done if diagnosis is uncertain.
- Laboratory studies:
  Blood and urine studies before surgery.
  Tissue examination after surgery.

POSSIBLE COMPLICATIONS
- Prolonged healing time if activity is resumed too soon.
- Proneness to repeated injury.
- Adhesive tenosynovitis—The tendon and its covering become bound together. Loss of motion may be complete or partial. Surgery is necessary to remove the covering or transfer the tendon to a new area.
- Constrictive tenosynovitis—The walls of the covering thicken and narrow, preventing the tendon from sliding through. Surgery may be necessary to cut away part of the covering.

PROBABLE OUTCOME—Tenosynovitis is usually curable in about 6 weeks with heat treatments, corticosteroid injections and rest of the inflamed area. Recovery is usually quicker if the inflammation is caused by a direct blow rather than by a strain or sprain.

 ## HOW TO TREAT

NOTE—Follow your doctor's instructions. These instructions are supplemental.

FIRST AID—None. This problem develops slowly.

CONTINUING CARE
- Wrap the hand and wrist with an elasticized bandage until healing is complete.
- Apply heat frequently. Use heat lamps, hot soaks, hot showers, heating pads or heat liniments and ointments.
- Take whirlpool treatments, if available.

MEDICATION—You may use nonprescription drugs such as acetaminophen or ibuprofen for minor pain.
Your doctor may prescribe:
- Stronger pain relievers. Don't take prescription pain medication longer than 4 to 7 days. Use only as much as you need.
- Injection of the tendon covering with a combination of a long-acting local anesthetic and a nonabsorbable corticosteroid such as triamcinolone.

ACTIVITY—Resume normal activities gradually.

DIET—During recovery, balance the amount of food you eat with any change in your level of physical activity. Eat a variety of foods to get the energy, protein, vitamins, minerals and fiber you need for good health and healing.

REHABILITATION
- Begin daily rehabilitation exercises when supportive wrapping is no longer needed.
- Use ice massage for 10 minutes before and after exercise. Fill a large styrofoam cup with water and freeze. Tear a small amount of foam from the top so ice protrudes. Massage firmly over the injured area in a circle about the size of a softball.
- See Rehabilitation section for wrist and hand exercises.

 ## CALL YOUR DOCTOR IF

- You have symptoms of wrist tenosynovitis.
- Any of the following occurs after surgery:
  Increased pain, swelling, redness, drainage or bleeding in the surgical area.
  Signs of infection (headache, muscle aches, dizziness or a general ill feeling and fever).
  New, unexplained symptoms. Drugs used in treatment may produce side effects.

Sports Medicine

ALTITUDE ILLNESS

GENERAL INFORMATION

DEFINITION—Altitude illness results from travel to higher than normal altitudes. It can affect anyone, no matter their age or how healthy they are. Types of altitude illness include:
• Acute mountain sickness (AMS); the most common.
• High-altitude pulmonary edema (HAPE) and high-altitude cerebral edema (HACE). These are less common.

SIGNS & SYMPTOMS
• Mild symptoms may begin when you climb or travel to around 7,000-8,000 feet.
  Headache, feeling lightheaded and weak.
  Nausea or vomiting.
  Sleeping problems.
• As you go higher, more severe symptoms may occur.
  Cough and trouble with breathing.
  Unsteady walk.
  Confusion; seeing things that aren't there.
  Coma (being unconscious).

CAUSES & RISK FACTOR
• There is less oxygen in the air at higher altitudes. Symptoms start to develop when the body tries to adjust to having less oxygen than it normally has. People who live at high altitudes have adapted to these lower oxygen levels and do not get sick.
Risk increases with:
• Some people are more susceptible. It is unclear why certain people get sick while others do not. At 14,000 feet, most people will have at least mild symptoms.
• People with severe heart or lung disease or people with sickle cell anemia.
• Going too high too fast.

HOW TO PREVENT
• Educate yourself before your trip. Find out how high the altitude will be. Know the symptoms of altitude illness. Check if medical help will be handy.
• Ask your health care provider for advice about high altitude travel for children, for pregnant women and for people with chronic health problems. It may be safe, but, find out for sure.
• While on the trip, slowly adjust to the change in altitude. Rest for a day or two at each 1,000-2,000 feet. Take it easy, don't overdo, drink fluids, but not alcohol.

WHAT TO EXPECT

DIAGNOSTIC MEASURES
• Your own observation of symptoms.
• Medical history and exam by a doctor.

SURGERY—Not necessary for these disorders.

NORMAL COURSE OF DISORDER—Most cases are mild and do not need medical treatment. Recovery takes only one to a few days.

POSSIBLE COMPLICATIONS—Serious outcomes, including death, are very rare. They are only likely to occur if unable to go down to a lower level, or not able to get medical help.

HOW TO TREAT

NOTE—Follow your doctor's instructions. These instructions are supplemental.

MEDICAL TREATMENT
• If symptoms do not improve or they get worse, seek medical help. Your health care provider will ask about your symptoms, may do a physical exam and have medical tests.
• Treatment steps will depend on your symptoms. You may be advised to go to a lower altitude. This is the most important and only sure treatment step.
• Symptoms should improve in a few days if you rest, drink plenty of fluids, don't drink alcohol, and avoid heavy exercise.
• For more severe symptoms, you will need to go to a lower altitude immediately. You may need pure oxygen breathed in through a mask for a period of time. A hospital stay might be necessary until you recover.

HOME TREATMENT—If mild symptoms occur, rest for a day or two at that altitude. You may want to go back down (to descend) to a lower altitude. Do not travel higher (to ascend) until the symptoms resolve or get much better.

MEDICATION
• Ask your health care provider's advice before you travel about drugs that can help prevent or treat symptoms. They do have side effects so be cautious.
• For mild symptoms, such as headache, you may use pain relievers such as ibuprofen or naproxen.
• In severe cases, drugs will be given to treat complications and help speed recovery.

ACTIVITY—Resume daily activities gradually upon returning to your normal altitude.

DIET—Increase fluid intake, avoid alcohol, eat small meals.

CALL YOUR DOCTOR IF

• You have symptoms of any altitude illness.
• New, unexplained symptoms develop. Drugs used in treatment may produce side effects.

AMENORRHEA

GENERAL INFORMATION

DEFINITION
Primary—Absence of menstruation in a young woman who is at least 16 years old or has reached age 14 with a lack of normal growth or absence of secondary sexual development.
Secondary—Cessation of menstruation in a woman who has previously menstruated.

SIGNS & SYMPTOMS
* Lack of menstrual periods after puberty. Most girls begin menstruating by age 14.
* Absence of menstrual periods for 3 months in a female who has menstruated at least once.

CAUSES & RISK FACTORS—Often unknown.
Possibly:
* Problems that a woman was born with, such as the absence or abnormal formation of female organs (vagina, uterus, ovaries).
* Strenuous athletic activities.
* Intact hymen (membrane covering the vaginal opening) that has no opening to allow passage of menstrual flow.
* Disorders (tumors, infections and others) of the endocrine system.
* Chromosome disorders.
* Emotional distress or eating disorders, including obesity, bulimia, anorexia nervosa, excessive dieting or starvation.
* Use of certain drugs, including mind-altering drugs, sedatives, hormones, oral contraceptives, anticancer drugs, barbiturates, narcotics, cortisone drugs and others.
Other causes of secondary amenorrhea:
* Pregnancy or breast-feeding.
* Discontinuing use of birth-control pills.
* Menopause (if woman is over 35 and not pregnant).
* Surgical removal of ovaries or uterus.
* Diabetes mellitus, tuberculosis, obesity.

HOW TO PREVENT
* Use drugs only if prescribed by your doctor.
* Reduce strenuous athletic activities.
* Medical treatment for underlying disorders.
* Maintain proper nutrition and body weight.

WHAT TO EXPECT

DIAGNOSTIC MEASURES
* Laboratory studies, such as chromosome studies, blood tests of hormone levels, thyroid and adrenal function tests.
* Pregnancy test and surgical diagnostic procedures, such as laparoscopy, hysteroscopy or dilatation and curettage.

SURGERY—Possibly minor surgery to create an opening in the hymen, if necessary, or to correct other problems of the reproductive system (sometimes).

NORMAL COURSE OF DISORDER
Primary—The absence of menstruation is not a health risk and is usually curable with hormone treatment or removal of the underlying cause. Treatment may be delayed to age 18 unless the cause can be identified and treated.
Secondary—If from pregnancy or breast-feeding, menstruation will resume when these conditions cease. If from discontinuing use of oral contraceptives, periods should begin in 2 months to 2 years. If from menopause, periods will become less frequent or may never resume. If from endocrine disorders, hormone replacement usually causes periods to resume. If from eating disorders, successful treatment of the disorder is necessary. If from diabetes or tuberculosis, menstruation may never resume. If from strenuous exercise, periods usually resume when exercise decreases.

POSSIBLE COMPLICATIONS—Feeling upset about sexual development. May experience estrogen deficiency symptoms, such as hot flashes, vaginal dryness. May affect fertility.

HOW TO TREAT

NOTE—Follow your doctor's instructions. These instructions are supplemental.

MEDICAL TREATMENT
* Will depend on the cause. If amenorrhea is temporary, treatment may not be necessary.
* Seek help in resolving any emotional stress.

HOME TREATMENT—Follow doctor's advice about exercise, diet or other lifestyle changes.

MEDICATION—Your doctor may prescribe progesterone (hormone) treatment to induce bleeding. If bleeding begins when progesterone is withdrawn, the reproductive system is functioning. If progesterone withdrawal does not induce bleeding, other hormone drugs may be used.

ACTIVITY
* Exercise regularly, but not to excess.
* Sleep at least 8 hours every night.

DIET—If overweight or underweight, a change in diet to correct the problem is recommended.

CALL YOUR DOCTOR IF

* You are 16 years old and have never had a period or periods have stopped for 3 months.
* Periods don't begin in 6 months, despite treatment, or new symptoms develop.

ANEMIA RELATED TO EXERCISE

GENERAL INFORMATION

DEFINITION—A decreased number of circulating red blood cells, or insufficient hemoglobin in the cells, caused by participation in exercise. Anemia is also a symptom of other disorders and may interfere with athletic performance. For proper treatment, the cause must be found.

SIGNS & SYMPTOMS
Signs of pronounced anemia:
* Decreased performance in maximum-effort activities.
* Tiredness and weakness.
* Paleness, especially in the hands and linings of the lower eyelids.
Less common signs:
* Tongue inflammation.
* Fainting.
* Feeling short of breath.
* Excessively rapid heartbeat with exercise.
* Appetite loss.

CAUSES & RISK FACTORS
* Taking part in exercise such as prolonged walking, running or cross-country skiing. The force exerted on the red blood cells in the capillaries of the feet may rupture the blood cells and lead to anemia.
* Other heavy physical exercise and exertion.
Contributing factors include:
* Heavy menstrual bleeding or pregnancy.
* Body does not absorb iron from food.
* Vegetarian diet or eating inadequate amounts of iron-rich foods.
* Profuse sweating.
* Age over 60.
* Recent illness with bleeding, such as an ulcer, diverticulitis, colitis, hemorrhoids or gastrointestinal tumor.

HOW TO PREVENT—Maintain adequate iron intake by eating a well-balanced diet or taking iron supplements.

WHAT TO EXPECT

DIAGNOSTIC MEASURES
* Your own observation of symptoms.
* Medical history and exam by a doctor.
* Laboratory blood studies every 2 months while involved in vigorous physical activity. Tests should include studies of hematocrit (see Glossary), hemoglobin and red blood cell counts.
* X-rays of the gastrointestinal tract.

SURGERY—Necessary only if the underlying cause, such as a tumor, requires surgery.

NORMAL COURSE OF DISORDER—Usually curable with iron supplements if the underlying cause can be identified and treated. Unless anemia is severe, you may continue training and vigorous physical activity while under treatment with iron supplements for anemia.

POSSIBLE COMPLICATIONS
* Failure to diagnose a bleeding malignancy.
* Without treatment, increasing weakness and eventual congestive heart failure.

HOW TO TREAT

NOTE—Follow your doctor's instructions. These instructions are supplemental.

MEDICAL TREATMENT—See your doctor to identify and treat the underlying cause.

HOME TREATMENT—Take iron supplements if prescribed and make diet changes if recommended.

MEDICATION—Your doctor may prescribe iron supplements:
* Take iron on an empty stomach (at least 1/2 hour before meals) for best results. If it upsets your stomach, you may take it with a small amount of food (except milk).
* If you take other medications, wait at least 2 hours after taking iron before taking them. Antacids and tetracycline especially interfere with iron being stored in the body.
* Continue iron supplements until 2 to 3 months after blood tests return to normal.
* Too much iron is dangerous. A bottle of iron tablets can poison a child. Keep iron supplements out of the reach of children.

ACTIVITY—No restrictions unless exercise-induced anemia is severe. In that case, you should reduce activity while undergoing treatment and iron levels are back to normal.

DIET
* Limit milk to 1 pint a day. It interferes with iron being stored in the body.
* Eat protein foods and iron-containing foods, including meat, beans and leafy green vegetables.
* Increase dietary fiber to prevent constipation (a common side effect of iron supplements).

CALL YOUR DOCTOR IF

* You have symptoms of anemia.
* Nausea, vomiting, severe diarrhea or constipation occurs during treatment.

ANIMAL BITES

GENERAL INFORMATION

DEFINITION—Bite wounds to humans from dogs, cats or other animals including humans. Animal bites most often occur on the hands, face or legs.

SIGNS & SYMPTOMS
• Bite wounds can be tears, punctures, scratches, ripping or crush injuries.
• Dog bites usually involve the hands, face or the lower extremities.
• Cat bites usually involve the hands, followed by lower extremities, face and trunk.

CAUSES & RISK FACTORS
• Bite wounds are often from a domestic pet known to the victim. Large dogs are the most common source.
• Human bites are often the result of one person striking another in the mouth with a clenched fist.
• Risk increases with exposure to domestic pets or wild animals.

HOW TO PREVENT
• Education on how to avoid animal bites for children as well as adults.
• Avoid stray animals and animals in the wild.

WHAT TO EXPECT

DIAGNOSTIC MEASURES
• Your own observations.
• Doctor's examination.
• Culture of wound fluids, x-rays (if wound is near a bone or joint), exploratory surgery sometimes to determine extent of injuries.

SURGERY
• Wound cleaning.
• Surgical closure if needed.
• Wound will usually be left open to heal to lessen risk of infection.

NORMAL COURSE OF DISORDER—Dog
bites rarely become infected. Cat bites and human bites frequently become infected. Wounds should steadily improve and close over by 7-10 days.

POSSIBLE COMPLICATIONS—Complications
from bites can included infection, extensive soft tissue injuries with scarring, hemorrhage, rabies, and sometimes death.

HOW TO TREAT

NOTE—Follow your doctor's instructions. These instructions are supplemental.

MEDICAL TREATMENT
• Wound will usually be left open to heal to lessen risk of infection.
• Splint hand if it is injured.
• Human bite wounds on the hands should not be primarily closed due to the high risk of infection.
• With human bites, tests for hepatitis or HIV infection may be recommended.

FIRST AID
• Elevate the injured extremity to prevent swelling.
• If wound is bleeding, apply pressure to area with clean towel or cloth until bleeding stops. Clean wound with soap and water, then dry area and cover with sterile gauze or clean cloth.
• Do not apply antiseptic or other medicine.
• Call doctor, or take patient to an emergency department if wound is severe, it won't stop bleeding, or bite was from a wild animal or one behaving strangely.
• Contact the local health department and consult about the prevalence of rabies in the species of animal involved.
• If possible the animal that caused the bite should checked for rabies. Call an animal control office for instructions.

HOME TREATMENT
• Will depend on the extent of the wound. Follow the doctor's recommendations for follow up wound care.
• Call the Health Department for your area to see if the animal bite should be reported.

MEDICATION—Your doctor may prescribe:
• Preventive antibiotic treatment.
• Antitetanus injection.
• Antirabies vaccine or serum (sometimes).

ACTIVITY—No restrictions, except those caused by the injury.

DIET—No special diet.

CALL YOUR DOCTOR IF

• You or your child suffers from an animal bite.
• The bite does not begin to heal within 2-3 days.
• New or unexplained symptoms develop. Drugs used in treatment may produce side effects.

ASTHMA, EXERCISE-INDUCED
(Exercise-Induced Bronchospasm)

 GENERAL INFORMATION

DEFINITION—Chronic asthma is a lung disease where a person has recurrent attacks of coughing, wheezing and shortness of breath. The symptoms are often brought on by exercising or sports activities. Many individuals experience these asthma symptoms only when they exercise and are they are not diagnosed as having chronic asthma.

SIGNS & SYMPTOMS
• Symptoms begin after 5 or more minutes of exercise, often worsen 5-10 minutes after stopping the exercise, and end in 20 -30 minutes.
• Coughing, wheezing and shortness of breath.
• Chest tightness or pain.

CAUSES & RISK FACTORS
• Symptoms are caused by the temporary shrinking and narrowing of the airways (bronchospasm) in your lungs during exercise. Breathing in air that is colder and drier than the air in your lungs causes the lungs to lose heat and water leading to the bronchospasm.
Contributing factors include:
• Allergens (such as pollen) and irritants (such as smoke) are the major triggers for asthma attacks. Allergens are more prevalent in the spring and fall.
• Exercise in smoggy or cold air. Bronchospasm can occur within minutes while exercising in cool air. Warm, humid air is less likely to trigger exercise-induced bronchospasm.
• Intense, prolonged activity.

HOW TO PREVENT
• Take your prescribed asthma medicines regularly—don't omit them when you feel well.
• Take any preventive asthma medication 15-30 minutes before exercising.
• Monitor your respiratory status while you exercise. Your doctor may have you use a peak flow meter to help you check how well your asthma is controlled.
• Warm up properly for 5-10 minutes before exercising and cool down following exercise.
• Wear a cold weather face mask or cover your mouth and nose with a scarf.
• Breathe through your nose as much as possible. This helps warms the air going into your lungs.
• Choose a less vigorous exercise (e.g., walking or swimming) if strenuous exercising causes symptoms.

 WHAT TO EXPECT

DIAGNOSTIC MEASURES
• Your own observation of symptoms.
• Medical history and exam by a doctor.
• Laboratory blood studies, pulmonary function tests and chest x-rays (sometimes).

NORMAL COURSE OF DISORDER— Symptoms can be controlled with treatment and adherence to preventive measures. Exercise or sports activity usually require no restrictions.

POSSIBLE COMPLICATIONS—None likely to occur if preventive measures are taken for exercised-induced asthma. People with chronic asthma may develop severe attacks due to exercise or other triggers.

 HOW TO TREAT

NOTE—Follow your doctor's instructions. These instructions are supplemental.

MEDICAL TREATMENT—Doctor's care to find medications that work best depending on your age, activity levels and physical condition.

HOME TREATMENT
• Eliminate allergens and irritants at home and at work, if possible. Avoid exposure to smoke, air pollutants and other irritants.
• Follow guidelines under How to Prevent.

MEDICATION—Your doctor may prescribe:
• Medications that will help prevent the symptoms, and' other medications that will treat the symptoms if they occur.
• Often a combination of medications that work differently are prescribed for chronic asthma.

ACTIVITY
• Stay active. If an attack follows heavy exercise, sit and rest.
• Continue sports activities if symptoms can be controlled. If not, decrease exercise levels temporarily until symptoms improve.

DIET—Avoid foods to which you are sensitive. Wait 2 hours after a meal before exercising.

 CALL YOUR DOCTOR IF

• You have symptoms of asthma during exercise.
• You have an asthma attack that doesn't respond to treatment. This is an emergency!
• New, unexplained symptoms develop. Drugs used in treatment may produce side effects.

ATHLETE'S FOOT
(Tinea Pedis; Ringworm of the Feet)

 GENERAL INFORMATION

DEFINITION—A common contagious fungus infection of the skin of the feet between the toes (usually 4th and 5th toes). It is especially common among athletes.

SIGNS & SYMPTOMS
• Moist, soft gray-white or red scales on feet, especially between toes.
• Dead skin between toes.
• Itching in inflamed areas.
• Damp, musty foot odor.
• Small blisters on the feet (sometimes).

CAUSES & RISK FACTORS—Infection by a *trichophyton* fungus or yeast. Contributing factors include:
• Infrequent washing of the feet.
• Infrequent changes of shoes or socks.
• Use of locker rooms and public showers.
• Hot, humid weather.
• Being at increased risk for infection due to illness or medications.
• Persistent moisture around the feet.

HOW TO PREVENT
• Bathe feet daily. Dry thoroughly, and apply drying or dusting powder.
• Go barefoot when possible.
• Change shoes and socks daily.
• Wear plastic or rubber sandals when using public showers.
• Wear socks made of cotton, wool or other natural, absorbent fibers. Avoid synthetics.

 WHAT TO EXPECT

DIAGNOSTIC MEASURES
• Your own observation of symptoms.
• Medical history and exam by a doctor.
• Laboratory culture and microscopic examination of scales.

SURGERY—Not necessary or useful for this condition.

NORMAL COURSE OF DISORDER—Usually curable in 3 weeks with treatment, but recurrence is common.

POSSIBLE COMPLICATIONS
• Secondary bacterial infection in the affected area.
• "Id" reaction (an allergic autoimmune response to the infection) on hands and face. This is rare.

 HOW TO TREAT

NOTE—Follow your doctor's instructions if provided. These instructions are supplemental.

MEDICAL TREATMENT—See your doctor if infection is severe or persistent.

HOME TREATMENT
• After soaking or bathing, carefully remove scales and material between the toes daily.
• Keep affected areas cool and dry. Go barefoot or wear sandals during treatment.

MEDICATION
• Use nonprescription antifungal powders, creams or ointments after each bath.
• For severe cases, your doctor may prescribe oral antifungal medications or more potent topical antifungal medications.

ACTIVITY—No restrictions. Temporarily avoid activities that cause feet to sweat.

DIET—No special diet.

 CALL YOUR DOCTOR IF

• You have severe symptoms of athlete's foot that persist, despite self-treatment.
• You develop fever or the infection seems to be spreading.

BACK PAIN

GENERAL INFORMATION

DEFINITION—Pain in the lower back usually caused by muscle strain. It often occurs along with sciatica (pain that radiates from the back to the buttock and down into the leg). Onset of pain may be immediate or occur some hours after exertion or an injury.

SIGNS & SYMPTOMS
- Pain. It may be continuous, or only occur when you are in a certain position. The pain may be made worse by coughing or sneezing, bending or twisting.
- Stiffness.

CAUSES & RISK FACTORS
- Exertion or lifting.
- Severe blow or fall.
- Back disorders, ruptured lumbar disk.
- Infections.
- Nerve dysfunction.
- Osteoporosis, tumors.
- Spondylosis (hardening and stiffening of the spinal column).
- Physical problems a person was born with.
- Childbirth.
- Often there is no obvious cause.
Contributing factors include:
- Using poor body mechanics (movements).
- Work that is either very physical or involves a lot of sitting.
- Gardening and other yard work.
- Sports and exercise activities.
- Obesity; aging.
- Poor muscle tone, poor posture.
- Wearing high heels (women).

HOW TO PREVENT
- Exercises to strengthen lower back muscles.
- Learn how to lift heavy objects.
- Sit properly.
- Back support in bed.
- Lose weight, if overweight.
- Choose proper footwear.
- Wear special back support devices.

WHAT TO EXPECT

DIAGNOSTIC MEASURES
- Your own observation of symptoms.
- Medical history and exam by a doctor.
- Laboratory blood studies to determine if there is an underlying disorder, x-rays of the spine, sometimes a CT or MRI scan.

SURGERY—May be recommended for damaged disk.

NORMAL COURSE OF DISORDER—Gradual recovery, but back troubles tend to recur.

POSSIBLE COMPLICATIONS—Chronic low back pain and restricted lifestyle.

HOW TO TREAT

NOTE—Follow your doctor's instructions. These instructions are supplemental.

MEDICAL TREATMENT
- Treatment will depend on severity of the pain and discomfort.
- Bed rest for first 24 hours. Additional bed rest will be determined by severity of the problem. Recent medical studies indicate that staying more active is better for back disorders than prolonged bed rest.
- Options are available such as electrical nerve stimulation, acupuncture, orthopedic care, physical therapy, treatment by a chiropractor, special exercise doctors and others.
- Massage therapy may help.

HOME TREATMENT—Some self-treatment guidelines include:
- Ice pack or cold massage or heat applied to affected area with heating pad or hot water bottle.
- Use a firm mattress (place a bed board under the mattress if needed). Sleep on your back with a pillow under your knees, or sleep on your side with a pillow between your knees.
- Wear a special back support device.
- Learn stress reduction techniques, if needed.
- Take breaks if you have to stand or sit for long periods.

MEDICATION
- Use mild pain medications such as aspirin or ibuprofen.
- Your doctor may prescribe stronger pain medicine or a muscle relaxant for severe pain.
- Note: Medications do not hasten healing. They only help to reduce symptoms.

ACTIVITY
- Try to continue with daily work or school schedules to the extent possible. Use care in resuming normal activities.
- Avoid strenuous activity for 6 weeks.
- After healing, an exercise program will help.

DIET—No special diet. A weight reduction diet is recommended if overweight is a problem.

CALL YOUR DOCTOR IF

- You have mild, low back pain that persists for 3 or 4 days after self-treatment.
- Back pain is severe or recurrent.
- New or unexplained symptoms appear.

BAROTITIS MEDIA
(Barotrauma)

 GENERAL INFORMATION

DEFINITION—Damage to the middle ear caused by pressure changes. This is very common in scuba divers.

SIGNS & SYMPTOMS
- Hearing loss (to varying degrees).
- A plugged feeling in the ear.
- Dizziness.
- Ringing noise in the ear.
- Mild to severe pain in the ear or over the cheekbone and forehead.

CAUSES & RISK FACTORS
- Damage caused by sudden increased pressure in the surrounding air such as occurs in the rapid descent of an airplane or while scuba diving. In these activities, air moves from passages in the nose into the middle ear to maintain equal pressure on both sides of the eardrum. If the tube leading from the nose to the ear (eustachian tube) doesn't function properly, pressure in the middle ear is less than outside pressure. The negative pressure in the middle ear sucks the eardrum inward. Blood and mucus may later appear in the middle ear. Additional factors that contribute include:
- Nose or throat infection or allergies.
- Airplane flight.
- Scuba diving; skydiving.
- High-altitude mountain climbing.
- High-impact sports.
- Smoking.
- In infants and young children, difficulty dilating the eustachian tube (by swallowing).

HOW TO PREVENT
- Don't fly or scuba dive when you have an upper respiratory infection. If you must fly anyway, use nonprescription decongestant tablets or sprays. Follow package instructions.
- During air travel, while ascending or descending suck on hard candy or chew gum to force frequent swallowing. Take a moderate-size breath, hold the nose and try to force air into the eustachian tube by gently puffing out the cheeks with the mouth closed (Valsalva maneuver). Give an infant a bottle of water or juice while ascending or descending.

 WHAT TO EXPECT

DIAGNOSTIC MEASURES
- Your own observation of symptoms.
- Medical history and exam by a doctor.

SURGERY—Sometimes necessary to open the ear drum and release fluid trapped in the middle ear. A plastic tube may be inserted through the surgically perforated ear drum to keep it open and equalize pressure. The tube falls out spontaneously in 9 to 12 months.

NORMAL COURSE OF DISORDER—With treatment, most cases of barotitis media are reversible without permanent damage or hearing loss.

POSSIBLE COMPLICATIONS
- Ruptured ear drum.
- Middle ear infection.
- Permanent hearing impairment.

 HOW TO TREAT

NOTE—Follow your doctor's instructions. These instructions are supplemental.

MEDICAL TREATMENT—See your doctor for prescription of medications and surgery (sometimes).

HOME TREATMENT—If fluid drains from the ear, place a small piece of cotton in the outer ear canal to absorb it.

MEDICATION
- For minor discomfort, you may use non-prescription decongestants and pain relievers, such as acetaminophen.
- Your doctor may prescribe:
  Stronger prescription decongestant nasal sprays or tablets. Use for at least 2 weeks after damage.
  Antibiotics if infection is present.

ACTIVITY—Resume normal activities as soon as symptoms improve. If surgery is necessary to insert tube in the ear, or if the eardrum is ruptured, keep water out of the ear. Consult your doctor about special ear plugs for use during swimming, bathing and shampooing.

DIET—No special diet.

 CALL YOUR DOCTOR IF

- You have symptoms of barotitis media.
- Severe ear pain, severe headache, fever or dizziness occurs during treatment.
- New, unexplained symptoms develop. Drugs used in treatment may produce side effects.

BLISTERS

GENERAL INFORMATION

DEFINITION—Collection of fluid in a "bubble" under the outer layer of skin.

SIGNS & SYMPTOMS
- Fluid collection under the superficial skin layer.
- Sensitivity to pressure over the blister.
- Redness and swelling around the blister.

CAUSES & RISK FACTORS—Repeated friction and pressure against the skin, especially during hot, humid weather. Examples of common sites for blisters include the hands of gymnasts, the feet of runners and dancers, the fingers of baseball pitchers and the buttocks of bicycle riders.

HOW TO PREVENT
- Apply 10% tannic acid to vulnerable areas of the skin once or twice daily for 2 to 3 weeks.
- Wear shoes that fit like a glove, but allow enough space for the forefoot and toes. Check for rough seams inside the shoe.
- Don't wear socks. Clean white cotton or cotton-wool socks are less likely to cause blisters than socks made of synthetic materials. Avoid tube socks.
- Try wearing no socks, but dusting shoes with talcum powder or rubbing feet and shoes with petroleum jelly.
- Put tape on vulnerable areas prior to exercise.
- Don't run in shoes still wet from previous use.
- Protect hands with gloves appropriate for your sport, if possible.

WHAT TO EXPECT

DIAGNOSTIC MEASURES—Your own observation of symptoms.

SURGERY—Not necessary or useful for this condition.

NORMAL COURSE OF DISORDER—Blisters usually heal in 3 to 7 days if they don't become infected.

POSSIBLE COMPLICATIONS—Infection. Fluid becomes pus, pain becomes worse and red streaks develop.

HOW TO TREAT

NOTE—Follow your doctor's instructions if provided. These instructions are supplemental.

MEDICAL TREATMENT—See your doctor if infection develops.

HOME TREATMENT—No treatment is necessary for small, painless blisters (less than 1 inch across). To treat painful blisters or blisters larger than 1 inch:
- Apply ice to the blister for 5 minutes.
- Wash the blistered area with warm, soapy water. Pat dry with a clean towel.
- Sterilize a pin or tip of a scissors by dipping in alcohol or by holding it in the flame of a lighted match until it becomes red.
- Puncture the blister in several places around the edge.
- Apply gentle pressure to the top of the blister to squeeze out fluid. Leave the skin in place.
- Repeat all steps above once a day if the blister persists.
- Place moleskin (see Glossary) over a blister pad on top of the blister. Pad blisters on the bottoms of the feet with adhesive felt foam with a hole cut slightly larger than the blister.

MEDICATION—You may use nonprescription antibiotic medicine such as Bacitracin or Neosporin on the skin of the blister.

ACTIVITY—No restrictions unless the blister becomes infected.

DIET—No special diet.

CALL YOUR DOCTOR IF

- Home treatment of blisters hasn't brought relief in 1 to 3 days.
- Signs of infection occur (increased heat, redness, swelling or pus in the blister).

BOIL
(Furuncle; Carbuncle)

 GENERAL INFORMATION

DEFINITION—A painful deep bacterial infection of a hair follicle. The infection—usually from *staphylococcus* bacteria—begins in the hair follicle and goes into the skin's deeper layers. Boils are common and contagious. Carbuncles are clusters of boils that occur when the infection spreads through small tunnels underneath the skin.

SIGNS & SYMPTOMS
- A domed nodule that is painful, tender and red and has pus at the surface. Boils appear suddenly and ripen in 24 hours. They are usually 1-1/2 cm to 3 cm in diameter; some are larger.
- Fever (rare).
- Swelling of the closest lymph glands.

CAUSES & RISK FACTORS—Boils are easily transmitted under crowded, unsanitary conditions. Members of athletic teams who work out with each other daily may have an outbreak of boils among members. Health clubs that do not keep showers clean or put adequate amounts of chemicals in pools or whirlpool hot tubs are particularly likely to harbor germs that cause boils. The following factors make a person more susceptible to boils:
- Poor nutrition.
- Illness that has lowered resistance.
- Diabetes mellitus.
- Use of drugs that affect the immune system.

HOW TO PREVENT
- Keep the skin clean.
- If someone in your household or on your team has a boil, don't share towels or washcloths or clothing with that person.
- If you have a chronic disease (such as diabetes mellitus), be sure to follow your medical regimen.

 WHAT TO EXPECT

DIAGNOSTIC MEASURES
- Your own observations of symptoms.
- Medical history and physical exam by a doctor.
- Laboratory culture of the pus to identify the germ.

SURGERY—Incision and drainage of the boil (sometimes).

NORMAL COURSE OF DISORDER—Without treatment, a boil will heal in 10 to 20 days. With treatment, the boil should heal in less time, symptoms will be less severe and new boils should not appear. The pus that drains when a boil opens spontaneously may infect nearby skin, causing new boils.

POSSIBLE COMPLICATIONS
- The infection may enter the bloodstream and spread to other body parts.
- Scarring.
- Boils may recur.
- Family or team members may need treatment.

 HOW TO TREAT

NOTE—Follow your doctor's instructions. These instructions are supplemental.

MEDICAL TREATMENT—Incision and drainage of the boil by a doctor may be necessary.

HOME TREATMENT
- Do not burst a boil, as this may spread bacteria.
- Taking showers instead of baths reduces chances of spreading infection.
- Relieve pain with gentle heat from warm-water soaks. Use 3 or 4 times daily for 20 minutes. Wash your hands carefully after touching the boil.
- Prevent the spread of boils by using clean towels only once or using paper towels and discarding them.

MEDICATION
- Your doctor may prescribe antibiotics.
- Don't use nonprescription antibiotic creams or ointments on the boil's surface. They are ineffective.

ACTIVITY—Decrease activity until the boil heals. Avoid sweating and avoid contact sports (such as wrestling) while lesions are present.

DIET—No special diet.

 CALL YOUR DOCTOR IF

- You have a boil.
- The following occur during treatment:
  Symptoms don't improve in 3 to 4 days, despite treatment.
  New boils appear.
  You have a fever.
  Other family/team members develop boils.
- New, unexplained symptoms develop. Drugs used in treatment may produce side effects.

BUNION

GENERAL INFORMATION

DEFINITION—A bony bulge on the outside edge of the joint at the base of the big (first or great) toe. A bunion often impairs athletic performance until it is corrected with medical treatment or surgery.

SIGNS & SYMPTOMS
- Thickened skin over the bony bulge at the base of the big toe.
- Fluid accumulation under the thickened skin (sometimes).
- Inflammation and swelling around the bunion.
- Foot pain and stiffness.
- An inward-turned big toe that may overlap the second—and sometimes the third—toe.

CAUSES & RISK FACTORS
- Family history of foot problems (inherited weakness in toe joints).
- Arthritis.
- Narrow-toed, high-heeled shoes that compress toes.

HOW TO PREVENT
- Exercise daily to keep the muscles of the feet and legs in good condition.
- Wear wide-toed shoes that fit well. Don't wear high heels or shoes without room for your toes in their normal positions.

WHAT TO EXPECT

DIAGNOSTIC MEASURES
- Your own observation of symptoms.
- Medical history and exam by a doctor or podiatrist.
- X-rays of the foot.

SURGERY—Often necessary to remove the overgrown tissue and correct the position of the bones.

NORMAL COURSE OF DISORDER—Usually improves with treatment and preventive measures to guard against recurrence.

POSSIBLE COMPLICATIONS
- Infection of the bunion, especially in persons with diabetes mellitus.
- Inflammation and arthritic changes in other joints caused by walking difficulty that places abnormal stress on the foot, hip and spine.
- Hallux valgus, a disorder that occurs if the big toe (hallux) has been forced by a bunion into a position where it overlaps one or more of the other toes.

HOW TO TREAT

NOTE—Follow your doctor's instructions if provided. These instructions are supplemental.

MEDICAL TREATMENT—None necessary for mild cases. Surgery may be required for persistent or severe cases.

HOME TREATMENT
- Before bedtime, separate the big toe from the others with a foam-rubber pad.
- When wearing shoes, place a thick, ring-shaped adhesive pad over the bunion.
- Use arch supports to relieve pressure on the bunion. These are available in shoe repair shops.

MEDICATION—Usually not necessary for this disorder unless infection develops.

ACTIVITY—No restrictions as long as the bunion is protected from irritation. If surgery is necessary, resume normal activities gradually afterward. Walk on your heel until the surgical site heals. Elevate the foot of the bed to reduce swelling over the incision. Avoid vigorous exercise for 6 weeks following surgery.

DIET—No special diet.

CALL YOUR DOCTOR IF

- You have a bunion that is interfering with normal activities.
- Signs of infection (fever, headache, heat, increased tenderness or pain) develop during treatment or after surgery.

CARPAL TUNNEL SYNDROME

GENERAL INFORMATION

DEFINITION—A nerve disorder that causes pain, loss of feeling and loss of strength in the hands. It may greatly decrease athletic performance in sports that require strong hand or wrist action, such as tennis, racquetball, squash, golf, skiing, weightlifting, baseball, football, horseshoes, bowling, archery, rowing, wrestling, boxing, gymnastics, hockey, judo or water skiing.

SIGNS & SYMPTOMS
- Tingling or numbness in part of the hand.
- Sharp pains that shoot from the wrist up the arm, especially at night.
- Burning sensations in the fingers.
- Thumb weakness.
- Frequent dropping of objects.
- Poor performance in any sports that requires a strong grip.
- Inability to make a fist.
- Shiny, dry skin on the hand.

CAUSES AND RISK FACTORS—Pressure on the median nerve of the wrist caused by swollen, inflamed or scarred tissue. The sources of pressure include:
- Inflammation of the wrist tendon sheaths, a likely result of any sport that requires gripping or squeezing.
- Fracture of the forearm.
- Sprain or dislocation of the wrist.
- Work that requires strong hand or wrist action (computer, factory and cashier work, some types of music).
Contributing factors include:
- Diabetes mellitus.
- Hypothyroidism (underactive thyroid gland).
- Raynaud's disease (a circulatory disorder).
- Menopause; obesity.
- Pregnancy.

HOW TO PREVENT
- Take a break at least once an hour when doing repetitive work involving hands.
- Wear a wrist brace or splint if your work involves doing repetitive work involving hands.

WHAT TO EXPECT

DIAGNOSTIC MEASURES
- Your own observation of symptoms. For a simple test, place the backs of your hands together with your fingers pointing straight down and your elbows pointing straight out to the side (wrists are at a 90° angle). If symptoms occur by you holding this position for one minute, you likely have carpal tunnel syndrome.
- Medical history and physical exam by a doctor.

- Electrophysiologic nerve tests (record electrical activity of muscles) and x-rays of the hand and wrist.

SURGERY—May be recommended to free the pinched nerve. It provides almost complete relief from all symptoms in 95% of patients. Procedure may be done on outpatient basis.

NORMAL COURSE OF DISORDER—Usually curable—sometimes spontaneously, sometimes with surgery. Surgery usually needed if muscle wasting or nerve changes have developed. If pregnancy is the cause, the problem usually clears up after delivery.

POSSIBLE COMPLICATIONS
- Permanent numbness and a weak thumb or fingers in the affected hand.
- Permanent paralysis of some of the hand and finger muscles.

HOW TO TREAT

NOTE—Follow your doctor's instructions. These instructions are supplemental.

MEDICAL TREATMENT—Surgery or medications listed below.

HOME TREATMENT
- Conservative treatment is usually tried first.
- Discomfort relieved by shaking hands or dangling arms. If you awaken at night with pain in your hand, hang it over the side of the bed; rub or shake it.
- Wearing a splint on the affected wrist may be recommended.
- For work at a computer terminal, be sure desk, keyboard and chair are at the proper heights. Take a break once an hour.

MEDICATION
- You may take aspirin or ibuprofen to reduce pain and inflammation.
- Your doctor may prescribe:
  Anti-Inflammatory drugs.
  Cortisone injections at the wrist to reduce inflammation.
  Vitamin B-6 injections or tablets.

ACTIVITY—Stay as active as your strength allows. If surgery has been necessary, allow 2 weeks for recovery. Exercises may be prescribed for the hand.

DIET—Eat a normal, well-balanced diet.

CALL YOUR DOCTOR IF

You have symptoms of carpal tunnel syndrome that don't disappear in 2 weeks.

COLD SORE
(Fever Blister; Herpes Simplex)

GENERAL INFORMATION

DEFINITION—A common, contagious viral infection of the lip and mouth areas and sometimes the area around the nose.

SIGNS & SYMPTOMS
- There may be a tingling or itchy feeling (prodrome) on the lip prior to an eruption of the cold sore.
- Eruption of very small, painful blisters that are grouped together and surrounded by a red ring. They fill with fluid, then dry up and disappear.

CAUSES & RISK FACTORS—Infection from the *herpes simplex* virus. The virus is transmitted through saliva, stools, urine or eye discharge from the infected eye of someone with active herpes. Most persons are exposed to the virus in childhood. The virus remains in the body indefinitely, becoming active occasionally and causing an outbreak of blisters. The following can trigger flare-ups:
- Injury to the skin from friction of clothing or protective gear.
- Previous eczema.
- Physical or emotional stress.
- Illness or excessive exercise that has lowered resistance.
- Excess sun exposure.
- Use of drugs that affect the immune system.
- Menstrual period.

HOW TO PREVENT
- Avoid physical contact with others who have active lesions.
- Avoid excess direct exposure to sun. Use zinc oxide or a sunscreen on your lips.
- To avoid spreading the virus to others: Wash your hands often during a flare-up. Avoid wrestling, judo, boxing and other sports involving physical contact until lesions heal. Don't use protective equipment such as a face mask until lesions heal.

WHAT TO EXPECT

DIAGNOSTIC MEASURES—Your own observation of symptoms.

NORMAL COURSE OF DISORDER—
Spontaneous recovery in a few days to a week, occasionally longer. Recurrence is common. The virus remains in the body for life, but it is usually dormant. Research continues in developing a vaccine.

POSSIBLE COMPLICATIONS—Usually none expected unless there is some underlying disorder.

HOW TO TREAT

NOTE—Follow your doctor's instructions if provided. These instructions are supplemental.

MEDICAL TREATMENT—Not usually necessary.

HOME TREATMENT
- Usually no treatment is needed. Just leave cold sore alone.
- Some people apply an ice cube to the lip for short periods when they first feel the tingling. This may help reduce inflammation.
- Avoid skin-to-skin contact with anyone while you have a cold sore, especially a newborn.

MEDICATION
- You may use the following nonprescription medications:
  Acetaminophen to relieve minor pain. Don't use aspirin, especially for children and adolescents. Use of aspirin for some viral illnesses has been linked to Reye's syndrome, a form of encephalitis.
  Cold sore medications that may help relieve symptoms, but may not hasten healing. Drying products, such as witch hazel or alcohol, applied to the cold sore may ease symptoms.
- Your doctor may prescribe antiviral medication at the earliest sign of a flare-up.

ACTIVITY—Avoid close contact—especially kissing or oral sex—until lesions heal.

DIET—No special diet.

CALL YOUR DOCTOR IF

The following occur with a cold sore:
- Signs of secondary bacterial infection, such as fever, pus instead of clear fluid in the lesions or headache and muscle aches.
- Eruption of lesions on the genitals similar to those around the mouth.
- Development of new, unexplained symptoms. Drugs used in treatment may produce side effects.

COLD, COMMON

 GENERAL INFORMATION

DEFINITION—A contagious viral infection of the upper-respiratory passages. Colds can affect the nose, throat, sinuses, trachea, larynx bronchial tubes, ears and eustachian tubes.

SIGNS & SYMPTOMS
- Runny or stuffy nose. Nasal discharge is watery at first, then becomes thick and greenish yellow.
- Sore throat.
- Hoarseness.
- Cough that produces little or no sputum.
- Low fever.
- Fatigue.
- Watering eyes.
- Appetite loss.

CAUSES & RISK FACTORS
- Colds are caused by any of at least 100 viruses. Virus particles spread through the air, from person-to-person contact, or by touching items that an infected person has left germs on.
Contributing factors include:
- Winter (colds are most frequent in cold weather).
- Contact with infected person at school, work, stores, health clubs or other crowded places.
- Household member who has cold.
- Touching one's nose or eyes with fingers that have germs on them.
- Stress, fatigue or allergic disorders may increase risk of infection.

HOW TO PREVENT
- To prevent spreading a cold to others, avoid unnecessary contact during the contagious phase (first 2 to 4 days).
- Wash hands frequently, especially after blowing your nose or before handling food.
- Avoid risks listed above if possible.
- Humidify your air.

 WHAT TO EXPECT

DIAGNOSTIC MEASURES
- Your own observation of symptoms.
- Medical history and physical exam by a doctor (sometimes).
- Laboratory throat culture to rule out bacterial infection with streptococcus or other germs (sometimes).

SURGERY—Not necessary for this disorder.

NORMAL COURSE OF DISORDER—Spontaneous recovery in 7 to 14 days.

POSSIBLE COMPLICATIONS—Lower respiratory infection, pneumonia, bronchitis, sinusitis, ear infection, worsening asthma, secondary bacterial infection.

 HOW TO TREAT

NOTE—Follow any doctor's instructions. These instructions are supplemental.

MEDICAL TREATMENT—Doctor's treatment if cold doesn't clear up in a week or so or if complications develop.

HOME TREATMENT
- Many remedies exist for treating colds.
- To relieve congestion, inhale steam from a pan of boiled water (after removing it from the heat); take hot showers; use salt-water drops (1/2 teaspoon salt to 1 cup of warm water).
- Use a cool-mist, ultrasonic humidifier to increase air moisture. Clean humidifier daily.
- Don't smoke if you have a cough.
- For a sore throat, drink warm liquids, use medicated throat lozenges or suck on hard candies.

MEDICATION
- No medicine, including antibiotics, can cure the common cold.
- To relieve symptoms, you may use nonprescription drugs, such as acetaminophen, decongestants, nose drops or sprays, cough remedies and throat lozenges. Don't give a child under age 18 aspirin for cold symptoms.

ACTIVITY—Bed rest is not necessary, but avoid vigorous activity. Rest often.

DIET—Drink extra fluids, including water, fruit juice, tea and carbonated drinks.

 CALL YOUR DOCTOR IF

The following occurs during the illness:
- Increased throat pain, or white or yellow spots on the tonsils or other parts of the throat.
- Coughing episodes that last longer than intervals between coughing; cough that produces thick, yellow-green or gray sputum; cough that lasts longer than 10 days; or difficult or labored breathing between coughing bouts.
- You cannot distinguish a cold from the flu.
- Fever that lasts several days; shaking chills.
- Chest pain or shortness of breath.
- Earache, headache or skin rash.
- Pain in the teeth or over the sinuses.
- Unusual lethargy or irritability.
- Delirium.
- Enlarged, tender glands in the neck.
- Dusky blue or gray lips, skin or nail beds.
- Inability to bottle-feed or breast-feed (infant).

CONJUNCTIVITIS
(Pink Eye)

GENERAL INFORMATION

DEFINITION—An inflammation of the eyelid's underside and the white part of the eye. It is contagious and easily transmitted, particularly to athletes on the same team who have close daily contact or in crowded or unsanitary athletic facilities. Conjunctivitis is the most common eye disease.

SIGNS & SYMPTOMS—The following symptoms may affect one or both eyes:
● Clear, green or yellow discharge from the eye.
● After sleeping, crusts on lashes that cause eyelids to stick together.
● Eye pain.
● Swollen eyelids.
● Sensitivity to bright light.
● Redness and gritty feeling in the eye.
● Intense itching (allergic conjunctivitis only).

CAUSES & RISK FACTORS
● Viral infection. Conjunctivitis may occur with colds or diseases such as measles.
● Bacterial infection.
● Chemical irritation, wind, dust, smoke and other types of air pollution.
● Allergies caused by cosmetics, pollen or other allergens.
● A partially closed tear duct.
● Intense light, such as from sunlamps, snow or water reflection or electric arcs in welding.
● Crowded or unsanitary living conditions.
● Exposure to others in public places, such as day care centers and public schools.

HOW TO PREVENT
● Wash hands frequently with soap and warm water to avoid spreading germs to the eye area.
● Don't use anyone else's towel.
● Avoid exposure to eye irritants.
● Never share or borrow eye makeup.

WHAT TO EXPECT

DIAGNOSTIC MEASURES
● Your own observation of symptoms.
● Medical history and physical exam by a doctor.
● Laboratory culture of the eye discharge (sometimes).

SURGERY—Not necessary or appropriate for this disorder.

NORMAL COURSE OF DISORDER
● Bacterial or viral conjunctivitis is curable in 1 to 2 weeks with treatment.
● Allergic conjunctivitis can be cured if the allergen is removed. It is likely to recur.

POSSIBLE COMPLICATIONS—Usually none expected.

HOW TO TREAT

NOTE—Follow your doctor's instructions. if provided. These instructions are supplemental.

MEDICAL TREATMENT—Doctor's examination and medication.

HOME TREATMENT
● Wash hands often with antiseptic soap, and use paper towels to dry. Don't touch eyes. Gently wipe the discharge from the eye using disposable tissues. Infections are frequently spread by germs on fingers, towels, handkerchiefs or washcloths that have touched the infected eye.
● Use cool or warm-water soaks (see Soaks in Appendix) to reduce discomfort.
● Don't use eye makeup.
● You are no longer contagious once symptoms are gone.

MEDICATION—Your doctor may prescribe:
● Antibiotic or antiviral eye drops, sulfa eye drops or ointment to fight infection. Most eye care specialists believe steroid eyedrops should not be used until a diagnosis is definite. If the infection is caused by *herpes simplex* virus, steroids may spread it from the conjunctiva to the cornea, damaging the eye.
● Oral antibiotics.

ACTIVITY—Resume vigorous physical activities when symptoms improve.

DIET—No special diet.

CALL YOUR DOCTOR IF

● You have symptoms of conjunctivitis.
● The infection does not improve in 48 hours despite treatment.
● Fever occurs.
● Eye pain increases.
● Vision is affected.

CONSTIPATION

GENERAL INFORMATION

DEFINITION—Difficult, uncomfortable or infrequent bowel movements that are hard and dry. In most people, constipation is harmless, but it can indicate an underlying disorder.

SIGNS & SYMPTOMS—People vary widely in bowel activity. Any of the following may be a sign of constipation:
- Infrequent bowel movements,.
- Hard stool.
- Straining during bowel movements.
- Pain or bleeding with bowel movements.
- Sensation of continuing fullness after a bowel movement.
- Bloated feeling.

CAUSES & RISK FACTORS
- Not enough fluid intake.
- Insufficient fiber in the diet. Fiber adds bulk, holds water and creates easily passed, soft stool.
- Hypothyroidism; hypercalcemia.
- Anal fissure.
- Chronic kidney failure.
- Back pain.
- Colon or rectal cancer; irritable bowel syndrome.
- Depression or stress.
- Illness requiring complete bed rest.
- Use of certain drugs, including: belladonna; calcium-channel blockers; beta-adrenergic blockers; tricyclic antidepressants; narcotics; atropine; aspirin and others.
- Travel.
- Not being active or fit.

HOW TO PREVENT
- Eat a well-balanced, high-fiber diet.
- Exercise regularly.
- Drink at least 8 glasses of water a day.

WHAT TO EXPECT

DIAGNOSTIC MEASURES
- Your own observation of symptoms. Tell your doctor of any major change in your bowel pattern that lasts longer than 1 week (though unlikely, it could be a sign of cancer).
- Medical history and physical exam by a doctor.
- Laboratory tests of blood and stool to detect internal bleeding.
- Colon exam (rarely needed).

NORMAL COURSE OF DISORDER—Usually curable with exercise, diet and adequate fluids.

POSSIBLE COMPLICATIONS—Hemorrhoids, laxative dependency, hernia from excessive straining, uterine or rectal prolapse, spastic colitis, bowel obstruction, chronic constipation.

HOW TO TREAT

NOTE—Follow your doctor's instructions if provided. These instructions are supplemental.

MEDICAL TREATMENT—Doctor's treatment may be necessary for prolonged constipation, or if medications are causing the problem or if other complications develop.

HOME TREATMENT
- Set aside a regular time each day for bowel movements. The best time is often within 1 hour after breakfast. Don't try to hurry. Sit at least 10 minutes, whether or not a bowel movement occurs.
- Enemas may help some people.
- Drinking hot water, tea or coffee may help stimulate bowel.

MEDICATION—For occasional constipation, you may use mild nonprescription laxatives such as bulk-formers, lubricants, stool softeners and enemas. Don't use laxatives or enemas regularly as this can cause dependency. Avoid harsh laxatives and cathartics, such as Epsom salts. The best laxatives are bulk-formers, such as bran, psyllium, polycarbophil and methylcellulose.

ACTIVITY—Exercise and good physical fitness helps maintain healthy bowel patterns.

DIET—Drink at least 8 glasses of water each day. Include bulk foods, such as bran and raw fruits and vegetables, in your diet.

CALL YOUR DOCTOR IF

- You have constipation that persists, despite self-care—especially if the constipation represents a change in your normal bowel patterns.
- Constipation along with fever or severe abdominal pain.

CORN OR CALLUS

GENERAL INFORMATION

DEFINITION
- A corn is a painful thickening (bump) of the outer skin layer, usually over bony areas such as toe joints.
- A callus is a painless (usually) thickening of skin caused by repeated pressure or irritation. Corns and calluses form to protect a skin area from injury caused by repeated irritation (rubbing or squeezing). Pressure causes cells in the irritated area to grow at a faster rate, leading to overgrowth. They are frequent problems for all athletes.

SIGNS & SYMPTOMS
- Corn—Small, tender, painful raised bump on the side of or over the joint of a toe. A corn is usually 3 mm to 10 mm in diameter and has a hard center.
- Callus—A rough, thickened area of skin that appears after repeated pressure or irritation.

CAUSES & RISK FACTORS—Repeated injury to the skin, particularly on the feet. These occur frequently in athletes due to excessive perspiration, increased heat, friction of clothing and protective gear or poorly fitting shoes. Athletic activities that cause pressure on the hands or knees include throwing sports, gripping sports and wrestling.

HOW TO PREVENT
- Don't wear shoes that fit poorly.
- Avoid activities that create constant pressure on specific skin areas.
- When possible, wear protective gear such as gloves or knee pads.
- Use corn and callus pads on the feet to reduce pressure on irritated areas.

WHAT TO EXPECT

DIAGNOSTIC MEASURES
- Your own observation of symptoms.
- Medical history and physical exam by a medical doctor or a podiatrist.

SURGERY—Avoid surgery. It does not remove the cause. Postsurgical scarring is painful and may complicate healing.

NORMAL COURSE OF DISORDER—Usually curable if the underlying cause can be removed. Allow 3 weeks for recovery. Recurrence is likely—even with treatment—if the cause is not removed.

POSSIBLE COMPLICATIONS—Back, hip, knee or ankle pain caused by a change in one's gait due to severe discomfort.

HOW TO TREAT

NOTE—Follow your doctor's instructions if provided. These instructions are supplemental.

MEDICAL TREATMENT—Not usually necessary. For resistant cases, your doctor may inject cortisone medication into the corn or callus to reduce inflammation.

HOME TREATMENT
- If you have diabetes or poor circulation, consider consulting a podiatrist for treatment.
- Remove the source of pressure, if possible. Discard ill-fitting shoes.
- Use corn and callus pads to reduce pressure on irritated areas.
- Peel the thickened area or rub it with a pumice stone to remove it. Don't cut it with a razor. Soak the area in warm water to soften it before peeling.
- Ask the shoe repairman to sew a metatarsal bar onto your shoe to use while a corn is healing.

MEDICATION
- After peeling the upper layers of a corn once or twice a day, apply ointment. Use a non-prescription 5% or 10% salicylic ointment. Cover with adhesive tape.
- Your doctor may inject a corn or callus with cortisone medicine to suppress inflammation or pain.

ACTIVITY—Resume your normal activities as soon as symptoms improve.

DIET—No special diet.

CALL YOUR DOCTOR IF

- You have a corn or callus that persists despite self-treatment.
- Any signs of infection, such as redness, swelling, pain, heat or tenderness, develop around a corn or callus.

CORNEAL ULCER

GENERAL INFORMATION

DEFINITION—An open sore in the thin clear layers that cover the eye. It is particularly likely to occur in sports activities in areas with lots of wind, sand or gravel.

SIGNS & SYMPTOMS
- Eye pain.
- Sensitivity to bright light.
- Eyelid spasm.
- Tearing.
- Blurred vision.
- Redness in the white of the eye.

CAUSES & RISK FACTORS
- Injury to the cornea or the imbedding in the cornea of a foreign body, such as a small piece of steel, sand or glass. A bacterial infection—usually pneumococcal, streptococcal or staphylococcal—may follow the injury.
- Ill-fitting or prolonged use of contact lenses (especially soft lenses).
- Complications of the virus, *herpes simplex*, that produces cold sores on the mouth and can affect the eye.
- Infections of the eyelids and conjunctiva.
- Defective closure of the lid.
- Smoking or other environmental eye irritants.

HOW TO PREVENT
- Wash hands frequently.
- Avoid injury. Use appropriate equipment such as protective goggles, helmets and face masks to prevent injury to the head, face and eyes.
- Don't touch your eyes if you have cold sores.
- Handle contact lenses properly.

WHAT TO EXPECT

DIAGNOSTIC MEASURES
- Your own observation of symptoms.
- Medical history and physical exam by a doctor (ophthalmologist).
- Sometimes a visual acuity test and a laboratory culture study of a corneal scraping.

SURGERY—Not necessary or useful for this disorder unless a corneal transplant becomes necessary (rare).

NORMAL COURSE OF DISORDER—A corneal ulcer is a serious eye problem. It is usually curable in 2 to 3 weeks if treated by an ophthalmologist. If scars from previous corneal ulcers impair vision significantly, a corneal transplant (grafting a new cornea onto the eye) may make vision nearly normal.

POSSIBLE COMPLICATIONS—Neglected corneal ulcers may go into the cornea, allowing infection to enter the eyeball. This can cause permanent vision impairment.

HOW TO TREAT

NOTE—Follow your doctor's instructions. These instructions are supplemental.

MEDICAL TREATMENT—None is usually necessary after diagnosis and treatment with prescription medications.

HOME TREATMENT—Apply cool-water compresses to the eye as often as they feel good.

MEDICATION
- Your doctor may prescribe antibiotic eye drops, ointments or oral antibiotics for bacterial infections. Your doctor will administer medication for virus and fungus infections.
- For minor pain, you may use nonprescription drugs such as acetaminophen.

ACTIVITY—After treatment, resume normal activity as soon as possible.

DIET—No special diet.

CALL YOUR DOCTOR IF

- You have symptoms of a corneal ulcer.
- The following occur during treatment:
  Fever over 101 F° (38.3°C).
  Pain that is not relieved by acetaminophen.
  Changed vision.
- New, unexplained symptoms develop. Drugs used in treatment may produce side effects.

COSTOCHONDRITIS
(Tietze's Syndrome)

 GENERAL INFORMATION

DEFINITION—An inflammation of the cartilage of one or more ribs, most commonly the second or third ribs. The pain that results is often increased by movements that change the position of the ribs, such as lying down, bending over, coughing or sneezing. Pain may mimic that of heart disease or digestive disorders. It is more common in young adults, but can occur in any age group.

SIGNS & SYMPTOMS
• Pain in the chest wall, usually sharp in nature.
• Pain worsens with movement.
• Pain may occur in more than one location and may radiate into the arm.
• Tightness in the chest.
• Affected area is sensitive to the touch.

CAUSES & RISK FACTORS
• Inflammation of the cartilage that attaches ribs to the sternum. Cause of the inflammation is often unknown.
Contributing factors include:
• Trauma, such as a severe blow to the chest or repetitive minor trauma.
• Any physical activity that causes strain to the ribcage.
• Upper respiratory infection.

HOW TO PREVENT—Avoidance of activities that may strain or cause trauma to the rib cage.

 WHAT TO EXPECT

DIAGNOSTIC MEASURES
• Your own observation of symptoms.
• Medical history and physical exam by a doctor. There is no specific test or study for diagnosing costochondritis. X-rays or a bone scan may be recommended to rule out other disorders.

SURGERY—Not necessary for this disorder.

NORMAL COURSE OF DISORDER—Complete healing. The disorder is benign and the course is usually of a short duration.

POSSIBLE COMPLICATIONS—It may recur or become persistent.

 HOW TO TREAT

NOTE—Follow your doctor's instructions if provided. These instructions are supplemental.

MEDICAL TREATMENT—None usually required. Once the diagnosis is confirmed, your doctor will provide reassurance about the benign aspects of the condition.

HOME TREATMENT
• Heating pad or ice massage applied to the affected area (whichever feels best).
• Avoidance of sudden movements that will intensify the pain.
• Gentle stretching of the chest muscles several times a day may be helpful.

MEDICATION
• You may use mild pain medications, such as aspirin or ibuprofen to help relieve discomfort.
• Your doctor may prescribe stronger pain medicines or steroid injections (rare).

ACTIVITY—As tolerated. Rest is important.

DIET—No special diet.

 CALL YOUR DOCTOR IF

• You have symptoms of costochondritis.
• Pain continues or worsens despite treatment.

DECOMPRESSION SICKNESS (Bends)

 GENERAL INFORMATION

DEFINITION—A painful, sometimes life-threatening condition of the blood gases that is caused by a sudden drop in environmental pressure.

SIGNS & SYMPTOMS—The following may occur immediately or up to 24 hours after the pressure change:
- Mild to severe joint pain, especially in the shoulders, elbows, hips and knees.
- Chest pain; shortness of breath; a burning sensation behind the breastbone.
- Chokes (severe breathing difficulty experienced by scuba divers and others who go from high to normal air pressure too rapidly. Bubbles of nitrogen develop in the bloodstream and obstruct blood supply to vital organs, sometimes resulting in severe injury or death).
- Coughing.
- Weakness, loss of normal sensation, paralysis, being unconscious and coma (rare).
- Inability to speak, see or hear.
- Abdominal pain.
- Difficult urination.

CAUSES & RISK FACTORS—Formation of nitrogen bubbles in the blood. Nitrogen is a normal blood component. If the pressure around the body drops rapidly—as in surfacing too quickly while scuba diving or climbing too rapidly in a nonpressurized aircraft—the nitrogen collects in bubbles in the blood vessels, blocking them and depriving the body of essential blood nutrients.
- Commercial diving or recreational scuba diving. Repeated dives in one day increase the risk.
- Flying in some kinds of high-performance aircraft.
- Working in compression chambers; tunnel work (caisson disease).

HOW TO PREVENT
- Obtain professional instruction before scuba diving.
- Don't dive if you are not in good general health. You are at risk if you are obese or have a medical history of:
  - Lung conditions, such as asthma.
  - Spontaneous pneumothorax.
  - Heart disease.
  - Chronic sinusitis.
  - Emotional instability.
  - Alcoholism.
- Allow for a slow, gradual change to normal air pressure in situations listed above. (The U.S. Navy has tested and established guidelines.)
- Avoid air travel for 24 hours after diving.

 WHAT TO EXPECT

DIAGNOSTIC MEASURES
- Your own observation of symptoms.
- Medical history and physical exam by a doctor.
- Laboratory blood studies, oxygen levels, EEG (see Glossary), chest x-ray, CT scan (see Glossary).

SURGERY—Not necessary or appropriate for this condition.

NORMAL COURSE OF DISORDER—Excellent prognosis for patients who receive early treatment; in others, it depends on duration and severity of symptoms prior to treatment.

POSSIBLE COMPLICATIONS
- Permanent brain damage.
- Permanent bone destruction caused by reduced blood supply.

 HOW TO TREAT

NOTE—Follow your doctor's instructions. These instructions are supplemental.

MEDICAL TREATMENT
- Hospitalization in a decompression chamber to force nitrogen bubbles to dissolve into the blood.
- Treatment is best when it is accomplished early; however, some patients may benefit even 6 to 9 days after the incident. Referral is critical even if symptoms resolve, since 25% of patients will experience relapse.

HOME TREATMENT—Self-care is impossible for this condition. If you observe someone with symptoms of decompression sickness, obtain emergency medical care immediately.

MEDICATION—Medicine usually is not necessary for this disorder. Don't take pain relievers. These may further decrease normal breathing efficiency.

ACTIVITY—Resume your normal activities as soon as symptoms improve after treatment.

DIET—No special diet.

 CALL YOUR DOCTOR IF

You develop any symptoms of decompression sickness within 24 hours after scuba diving or rapid ascent without pressurization.

DEHYDRATION

GENERAL INFORMATION

DEFINITION—Loss of water and essential body salts (electrolytes) needed for normal body function. Necessary salts contain sodium, potassium, calcium, bicarbonate and phosphate. Water accounts for about 60% of a man's weight and 50% of a woman's weight and needs to be kept within fairly narrow limits to maintain cells and body tissue.

SIGNS & SYMPTOMS
- Dry mouth and swollen tongue.
- Decreased or absent urination; urine color may be deep yellow.
- Sunken eyes and wrinkled skin.
- Inability to sweat.
- Fatigue.
- Dizziness; confusion; coma.
- Low blood pressure.
- Severe thirst.
- Increase in heart rate and breathing.

CAUSES & RISK FACTORS
- Heavy sweating; too much exercise.
- Persistent vomiting or diarrhea from any cause.
- Persistent high fever.
- Use of drugs that deplete fluids and electrolytes, such as diuretics ("water pills").
- Overexposure to sun or heat.
- Not taking in a sufficient amount of water.
- Diabetes mellitus, chronic lung disease, chronic kidney disease or adrenal disease.
- Injuries to the skin, such as burns, can cause fluid loss through the damaged skin.

HOW TO PREVENT
- Obtain medical treatment for underlying causes of dehydration.
- If you are vomiting or have diarrhea, drink enough water to keep urine consistently pale (you may not feel thirsty, but fluid intake is essential).
- If you use diuretics, weigh daily.
- Carry water with you to outdoor activities; drink plenty of water while exercising and avoid exercising outdoors in very hot weather.
- Avoid drinking alcohol in hot weather.

WHAT TO EXPECT

DIAGNOSTIC MEASURES
- Your own observation of symptoms.
- Medical history and physical exam by a doctor if needed.
- Laboratory blood studies, including blood counts and electrolyte measurement (see Glossary).

SURGERY—Not necessary or useful for this disorder.

NORMAL COURSE OF DISORDER—Curable with control of the underlying cause and replacement of necessary fluids.

POSSIBLE COMPLICATIONS
- Depends on seriousness of underlying cause. Usually with mild to moderate symptoms, no complications are expected.
- Severe dehydration or electrolyte imbalance may lead to heartbeat irregularities, cardiac arrest and death.

HOW TO TREAT

NOTE—Follow your doctor's instructions if provided. These instructions are supplemental.

MEDICAL TREATMENT—Hospitalization to be sure you get enough fluids (with a severe or prolonged illness only).

HOME TREATMENT
- For minor dehydration, take frequent small amounts of clear liquids. Sip through a straw or suck on ice chips. Large amounts may trigger vomiting.
- Take off excess clothing and loosen any other clothes. Place a wet towel around the person. Don't use ice packs on the skin; they can actually raise a person's temperature.
- Get the person to an air conditioned area, or near a fan. If outside, get the person to a shady area.

MEDICATION—Your doctor may prescribe fluids given through a vein (IV) to replace lost water, anti-emetic drug if vomiting is severe, drugs for diarrhea if it is persistent or to lower fever.

ACTIVITY—Rest in bed until you recover.

DIET—Drink carbohydrate/electrolyte solutions. For adults, diluting commercial solutions such as Gatorade or Recharge with an equal amount of water may be adequate. Suck on popsicles made from juices or sports drinks. For children, use special commercial products (Pedialyte or Ricelyte). Instructions are on the labels.

CALL YOUR DOCTOR IF

- If symptoms are severe, seek emergency care.
- You have mild to moderate symptoms of dehydration that are not relieved by self-treatment.
- Fever is over 101°F (38.3°C).
- Diarrhea or vomiting continues for over 2 days.

DERMATITIS, CONTACT

GENERAL INFORMATION

DEFINITION—A common skin inflammation caused by contact with an irritating or an allergenic substance. When an irritant causes the dermatitis, the discomfort usually begins immediately after exposure. With an allergen-caused dermatitis, the reaction may take several hours or more to develop. Contact dermatitis is not contagious.

SIGNS & SYMPTOMS
- Itching (sometimes).
- Slight redness in milder cases.
- Bright red weeping areas in some cases.
- Cracks and fissures in the skin.

CAUSES & RISK FACTORS
- There are many causes of contact dermatitis. It may take time and effort to determine the exact cause for each individual. Sometimes the causes may be from a mix of allergens and irritants, especially dermatitis on the hands.
- Irritants include ingredients in soaps, detergents, bleaches, cleaners; bromine or chlorine used in swimming pools; certain oils, tars; a variety of plants including poinsettia; and numerous other items.
- Allergic reaction may come from nickel found in earrings, rings and watches; glues; household cleansers; leather; paints, rubber; ingredients in hair dyes, perfumes, deodorants and cosmetics; plants such as poison ivy, oak or sumac; and there are numerous other possibilities.
- Reaction to topical drugs such as antibiotics or anesthetics.

HOW TO PREVENT
- Avoid contact with any irritant or allergen that has caused dermatitis in the past.
- Wear protective clothing if you might be at risk for exposure to plants (such as poison ivy) or other allergens or irritants. A product such as Ivyblock may offer some protection. If you are exposed, bathe as soon as possible, and wash all clothing thoroughly including shoes.
- Protect skin from sunburn and other burns.

WHAT TO EXPECT

DIAGNOSTIC MEASURES
- Your own observation of symptoms.
- Medical history and physical exam by a doctor (sometimes).

SURGERY—Not necessary or useful for this disorder.

NORMAL COURSE OF DISORDER—Symptoms can often be controlled with treatment and avoidance of the irritant or allergen.

POSSIBLE COMPLICATIONS
- Recurrence is common, so some treatment may be necessary for years.
- Secondary bacterial infection or more generalized skin eruption.
- Rarely, an allergic response may lead to anaphylactic shock and death if untreated.

HOW TO TREAT

NOTE—Follow your doctor's instructions if provided. These instructions are supplemental.

MEDICAL TREATMENT—Usually not necessary unless infection develops. Testing for specific skin allergies may be recommended in some cases.

HOME TREATMENT
- Avoid the chemical or material causing the skin eruption.
- Reduce water temperature to lukewarm for bathing or other uses. Use Aveeno (a commercial product for soaking). Use wet compresses with an astringent such as Burrow solution. Pat skin dry rather than rubbing it.

MEDICATION
- Use nonprescription cream, lotion or ointment products to help relieve symptoms. These can add moisture to the skin, have an anti-itching ingredient and may include a mild topical anesthetic. Follow instructions on the label.
- Oral antihistamines may help relieve itching.
- Your doctor may prescribe:
  Other topical skin care products. These may include superpotent steroid preparations to reduce inflammation or lubricants to preserve moisture.
  Oral steroids for severe cases.
  Antibiotics (topical or oral) for secondary infections.

ACTIVITY—Resume your normal activities gradually as irritation subsides.

DIET—No special diet.

CALL YOUR DOCTOR IF

- Severe pain develops.
- You develop a fever.
- Signs of infection (swelling, tenderness, redness, warmth) develop at the site of irritation.
- Treatment does not relieve symptoms in 1 week.

DIARRHEA, ACUTE

GENERAL INFORMATION

DEFINITION—The passage of many loose, watery or unformed bowel movements. The diarrhea may be mild to severe. It is a symptom, not a disease.

SIGNS & SYMPTOMS
- Cramping abdominal pain.
- Loose, watery or unformed bowel movements.
- Lack of bowel control (sometimes).
- Fever (sometimes).

CAUSES & RISK FACTORS
- There are many causes including infections (viral, parasitic or bacterial).

Contributing factors include:
- Emotional upsets or acute stress.
- Food poisoning or food allergy.
- Recent illness.
- Regional enteritis; diverticulitis; irritable bowel syndrome, inflammatory bowel disease.
- Pancreas or liver disorders.
- Foods, such as prunes or beans.
- Use of drugs, such as laxatives, antacids, antibiotics, quinine or anticancer drugs.
- Children in day care.
- Radiation treatments for cancer.
- Excess alcohol drinking.
- Immunosuppression due to illness or drugs.
- Travel to foreign country.
- Ingestion of water from streams, springs or untested wells.
- Inability to tolerate lactose or sorbitol.

HOW TO PREVENT
- If diarrhea is recurrent and a cause can be identified, treatment or avoidance of the cause should prevent recurrence.
- Everyone is likely to have bouts of diarrhea occasionally from minor causes that disappear and leave no lasting effects. Most cases of acute diarrhea last a short time and a search for the cause may not be necessary.
- Avoid undercooked or raw seafood, buffet or picnic foods left out several hours and food served by street vendors.
- Wash hands frequently, especially after using the toilet.

WHAT TO EXPECT

DIAGNOSTIC MEASURES
- Your own observation of symptoms.
- Medical history and exam by a doctor (sometimes).
- Laboratory stool studies (for prolonged diarrhea).

SURGERY—Not necessary for this disorder.

NORMAL COURSE OF DISORDER—Spontaneous recovery in 24 to 48 hours.

POSSIBLE COMPLICATIONS
- Dehydration if diarrhea is prolonged, especially in infants.
- Rarely, diarrhea may become chronic, or other serious complications may occur.

HOW TO TREAT

NOTE—Follow your doctor's instructions if provided. These instructions are supplemental.

MEDICAL TREATMENT—Doctor's treatment (if symptoms persist longer than 2 to 3 days).

HOME TREATMENT
- Self-care. Diarrhea is a symptom. If possible, the underlying disorder should be treated.
- If you think a prescription drug is causing the diarrhea, consult with the doctor before discontinuing it.
- If cramps are present, place hot compresses, a hot-water bottle or an electric heating pad on the abdomen.
- Maintain fluid intake. Severe diarrhea may require urgent fluid and electrolyte replacement to correct dehydration.

MEDICATION
- For minor discomfort, you may use nonprescription drugs such as bismuth subsalicylate (Pepto-Bismol).
- Your doctor may prescribe antibiotic or antiparasitic medications or other drugs depending on any laboratory findings.

ACTIVITY—Decrease activity until diarrhea stops.

DIET
- Replace lost fluids and electrolytes with a commercial rehydration product (e.g., Gatorade). There are special products for infants. Follow product instructions.
- A special diet (such as bananas, rice, applesauce, toast) is usually not needed. Resume a normal diet after the diarrhea stops. Avoid alcohol and highly seasoned foods for several more days.

CALL YOUR DOCTOR IF

- Diarrhea lasts more than 48 hours, especially in a child.
- Mucus, blood or worms appear in the stool.
- Fever rises to 101°F (38.3°C) or higher.
- Severe pain develops in the stomach or rectum, or dehydration occurs.(dry mouth; wrinkled skin; excess thirst; little or no urine).

DROWNING, NEAR

GENERAL INFORMATION

DEFINITION—The immediate aftereffects of prolonged period of time under water. These may occur with or without aspiration (breathing water into the lungs). Approximately 10% to 15% of all drownings or near drownings occur without aspiration. There have been a few reports of survival after up to 40 minutes under water when the water was very cold. Warm or hot water can result in more rapid death.

SIGNS & SYMPTOMS
- Confusion.
- Unconscious (not awake and aware).
- Little or no breathing or heartbeat.
- Bluish-white paleness.

CAUSES & RISK FACTORS—Prolonged time under water, resulting in either of the following:
- Spasm of the larynx (the tube from the throat to the lungs). After rescue, this spasm prevents oxygen from reaching the lungs unless air is forced through the spasm by a respirator or CPR procedures.
- Water in the lungs, causing life-threatening changes in the circulation of blood.

Risk is increased by:
- Excess alcohol drinking.
- Accidents—especially head injury—while swimming.
- Poor supervision of children or lack of fencing of swimming pools.

HOW TO PREVENT
- Learn cardiopulmonary resuscitation (CPR).
- Encourage all family members—including infants—to learn to swim. Never leave a child, even one who can swim, alone near the water.
- Never swim alone.
- Install a fence around a home swimming pool.
- Don't drink alcohol and swim.

WHAT TO EXPECT

DIAGNOSTIC MEASURES
- Your own observation of symptoms.
- Medical history and physical exam by a doctor.
- Laboratory blood tests.

SURGERY—Not necessary or useful for this disorder.

NORMAL COURSE OF DISORDER—Depends on the length of time under water. With early rescue and treatment, full recovery is possible. Special actions by the body may permit full recovery from near drowning in icy water.

POSSIBLE COMPLICATIONS
- Pulmonary edema (body fluid in the lungs) followed by acute respiratory failure.
- Permanent brain damage.
- Lung infection.
- Heart irregularities, including cardiac arrest and death.

HOW TO TREAT

NOTE—Follow your doctor's instructions. These instructions are supplemental.

FIRST AID
- If the victim is unconscious and not breathing, yell for help. Don't leave the victim.
- Call 911 (emergency) for an ambulance or medical help (if the victim is a child, give 1 minute of CPR and then call 911).
- Begin mouth-to-mouth breathing immediately.
- If there is no heartbeat, give external cardiac massage.
- Don't stop CPR until help arrives.
- The near drowning victim should be taken to the nearest hospital for intensive care even if the victim is awake and aware (conscious). Complications or death may occur 24 to 48 hours after the accident due to heart rhythm disturbances.
- Remain with a recovering patient to provide support and reassurance. Near drowning is a traumatic experience.

MEDICAL TREATMENT
- Immediate cardiopulmonary resuscitation (CPR). Rewarming for patient with hypothermia.
- Hospitalization (sometimes) to lower body temperature, to induce coma with medicines and to monitor spinal fluid pressure.
- Hospitalization for observation for serious delayed reactions.

HOME TREATMENT—None appropriate.

MEDICATION—Your doctor may prescribe:
- Oxygen.
- Bronchodilators to enable oxygen to enter the lungs.
- Antibiotics if pneumonia develops.

ACTIVITY—Complete bed rest is necessary until activity is permitted by the doctor.

DIET—Liquid nutrient (food) given through a vein (IV) if the victim is unconscious upon hospitalization. After recovery, no special diet is necessary.

CALL YOUR DOCTOR IF

- Someone appears to have drowned. Call for emergency help immediately.
- Signs of infection (fever, cough, muscle aches and fatigue) appear after apparent recovery.

EAR INFECTION, OUTER
(Swimmer's Ear; Otitis Externa)

 GENERAL INFORMATION

DEFINITION—Inflammation or infection of the ear canal that extends from the ear drum to the exterior of the ear. This is a particularly common problem in athletes when the ear canal remains moist due to perspiration running into the ear. It is also very likely to be a problem in swimmers, divers and water polo players.

SIGNS & SYMPTOMS
• Ear pain that worsens when the earlobe is pulled.
• Itching and plugging of the ear.
• Slight fever (sometimes).
• Discharge of pus from the ear.
• Temporary hearing loss on affected side.

CAUSES & RISK FACTORS
• Bacterial or fungal infection or eczema of the delicate skin lining of the ear canal.
• Excess moisture from any cause.
• Swimming in dirty, polluted water.
• Frequent swimming in hot or warm chlorinated pools. Chlorinated water dries out the ear canal, allowing bacteria or fungi to enter the skin.
• Irritation from swabs, metal objects such as bobby pins, or ear plugs, especially if they are left in a long time.
• Previous ear infections.
• Skin allergies.
• Use of hearing aid.
• Diabetes mellitus or other disorders that predispose one to infections.
• Use of hair spray or hair dye that may enter the ear canal.

HOW TO PREVENT
• Don't clean your ears with any object or chemical. A small amount of ear wax helps protect against infection.
• Avoid prolonged exposure to moisture.
• After you have had otitis externa, keep the ear drops prescribed on hand. If the ear canals get wet for any reason, such as swimming or shampooing, put drops in both ears at bedtime.

 WHAT TO EXPECT

DIAGNOSTIC MEASURES
• Your own observation of symptoms.
• Medical history and physical exam by a doctor.

SURGERY—Not necessary or useful for this disorder.

NORMAL COURSE OF DISORDER—Usually curable with treatment in 7 to 10 days.

POSSIBLE COMPLICATIONS
• Severe pain.
• Chronic inflammation that is difficult to cure.
• A boil in the ear canal.
• Cellulitis (deep tissue infection).

 HOW TO TREAT

NOTE—Follow your doctor's instructions. These instructions are supplemental.

MEDICAL TREATMENT
• Your doctor will probably cleanse the ear canal and may insert a cotton wick. The wick allows medication to reach all infected parts.
• Severe cases may require treatment by an ear, nose and throat specialist.

HOME TREATMENT
• If your doctor has inserted a wick, moisten the wick with medication every hour for the first 24 hours. Continue to use drops according to your doctor's instructions after the wick is removed. Clean the tip of the dropper with alcohol after each use. Don't let other persons use the medicine.
• After you have had otitis externa, keep the prescription ear drops on hand. If the ear canals get wet for any reason, such as swimming, showering or shampooing, put drops in both ears at bedtime.

MEDICATION
• You may use nonprescription drugs, such as acetaminophen or aspirin, for minor pain.
• Your doctor may prescribe:
  Other pain medication.
  Ear drops that contain acetic acid solution to control inflammation and fight infection.
  Topical creams or ointments for fungal or bacterial infections.
  Oral antibiotics for severe infection.

ACTIVITY—Resume your normal activities as soon as symptoms improve. Avoid getting water in the ears for 3 weeks after all symptoms disappear. Any moisture—even from showering or washing hair—can trigger a recurrence.

DIET—No special diet.

 CALL YOUR DOCTOR IF

• You have symptoms of otitis externa.
• Pain persists despite treatment.
• You feel your ears need cleaning.

EYE, FOREIGN BODY IN

GENERAL INFORMATION

DEFINITION—Imbedding of a small speck of dirt, stone, sand, paint, an eyelash or other foreign material in the eye. This is particularly likely to occur in athletes who cycle, box, wrestle, or play football, soccer or any other field sport.

SIGNS & SYMPTOMS
- Severe pain, irritation and redness in the eye.
- Scratchy feeling with blinking.
- Blurred vision or loss of vision.
- Bleeding into the white of the eye.
- Foreign body visible with the naked eye (usually). Sometimes the foreign body is small or trapped under the eyelid and invisible except with medical examination.

CAUSES & RISK FACTORS
- Windy weather.
- Sports activity in which the eye may come into contact with foreign material.

HOW TO PREVENT—Wear protective eye coverings if possible.

WHAT TO EXPECT

DIAGNOSTIC MEASURES
- Your own observation of symptoms.
- Medical history and physical exam by a doctor if needed. This may include staining the eye with a harmless fluorescent dye to outline the object and examination of the eye through a magnifying lens.

SURGERY—Necessary only for deeply imbedded particles or other eye serious injury.

NORMAL COURSE OF DISORDER—Most foreign objects can be removed simply with home care or in a doctor's office or emergency room. Most heal within 48 hours.

POSSIBLE COMPLICATIONS
- Infection, especially if the foreign body is not removed completely.
- Severe, permanent vision damage caused by damage of deeper eye layers.

HOW TO TREAT

NOTE—Follow your doctor's instructions if provided. These instructions are supplemental.

MEDICAL TREATMENT
- For larger foreign bodies or metal pieces or if the object went deeper into the eye, a doctor's or emergency room care is needed to remove the particle.

- Ask someone else to drive you to the doctor's office. Don't try to drive.
- Keep the eye closed if possible. Cover the eye, but do not apply compression.

HOME TREATMENT
For minor foreign bodies:
- Don't rub the eye.
- Flush the eye using one of these options:
  Use a saline solution (a small amount of salt and water) or plain water. Pour the warm (not hot) solution from a pitcher over the eye. Keep eye open.
  Use a water fountain to flush out the eye. Stand at a sink with water running and cup your hands and put face in running water. Get in a shower and tip head back.
  If outside, use a garden hose. Use great amounts of water, but don't use high pressure.
- Check the eye periodically to see if object is removed.
- If flushing is not effective, you may consider trying to remove the object with the tip of a tissue or cotton-tipped applicator. Lift upper or lower eyelid (someone else may need to help you). Don't scrape tissue or applicator across the cornea (middle portion of eye).
- If you removed the object, but it was large, or the patient is a child, a health care provider should be seen for follow up evaluation.
- Use moist compresses to relieve discomfort after removal of particle. Prepare by folding a clean cloth in several layers. Dip in warm water, wring out slightly and apply to the eye. Dip the compress often to keep it moist. Apply the compress for 1 hour, rest 1 hour, then repeat.

MEDICATION—Your doctor may prescribe:
- Antibiotic eye drops or ointment to prevent infection or to dilate the pupil.
- Pain relievers.
- Local anesthetic eye drops may be applied by the doctor.

ACTIVITY—Resume your normal activities gradually after removal of the foreign body.

DIET—No special diet.

CALL YOUR DOCTOR IF

- You have a foreign body in your eye that you are unable to remove.
- You are bleeding from the eye.
- The following occur after removal:
  Pain increases or does not disappear in 2 days.
  You develop a fever.
  Your vision changes.

EYE, SUBCONJUNCTIVAL HEMORRHAGE OF

GENERAL INFORMATION

DEFINITION—Sudden appearance of blood in the white area of the eye (conjunctiva). Although the bleeding may be frightening, it is not painful or serious. It is often discovered in the morning when you first look in a mirror.

SIGNS & SYMPTOMS—A small, painless collection of bright red blood in the white of the eye. It may first appear as a patch, but may then spread to cover the entire white area of the eye. The condition doesn't interfere with vision.

CAUSES & RISK FACTORS—Sometimes caused by injury to the eye, but usually is spontaneous bleeding with no known cause. It may follow coughing, sneezing or vomiting or rubbing of the eyes. Certain disorders such as high blood pressure or diabetes can be a risk factor.

HOW TO PREVENT—There is no known prevention. Always use appropriate equipment to protect the head and face from injury.

WHAT TO EXPECT

DIAGNOSTIC MEASURES
- Your own observation of symptoms.
- Medical history and physical exam by a doctor if needed.

SURGERY—Not necessary or useful for this disorder.

NORMAL COURSE OF DISORDER—The blood will go away by itself (should be absorbed in 1-3 weeks). The blood may change color gradually from red to yellow before disappearing.

POSSIBLE COMPLICATIONS—None expected.

HOW TO TREAT

NOTE—Follow your doctor's instructions if provided. These instructions are supplemental.

MEDICAL TREATMENT—Consult a doctor if there has been injury to the eye or a change in vision.

HOME TREATMENT—No treatment is necessary except time. Cool compresses may be applied at first. After 24 hours, you may use warm compresses applied to the eye to help hasten the removal of the blood.

MEDICATION—Medicine is usually not necessary for this disorder. Your doctor may prescribe artificial tears if irritation is present.

ACTIVITY—No rest is necessary and you may continue with your regular activities.

DIET—No special diet.

CALL YOUR DOCTOR IF

- You have symptoms of subconjunctival hemorrhage with eye pain or your vision changes or both eyes are affected.
- Your subconjunctival hemorrhage does not get better within 3 weeks or it recurs often.

FAINTING
(Syncope)

 GENERAL INFORMATION

DEFINITION—Sudden temporary loss of consciousness (not aware or awake) due to insufficient oxygen reaching the brain. This is most likely to occur in an athlete involved in prolonged physical exertion in warm weather. It sometimes occurs after exercising.

SIGNS & SYMPTOMS
- Sudden lightheadedness.
- General weakness, then falling.
- Blurred vision (sometimes).
- Nausea (sometimes).
- Paleness and sweating.
- Rapid heartbeat and rapid breathing. If heartbeat or breathing is not present, this may be cardiac arrest rather than fainting.

CAUSES & RISK FACTORS—A sudden decrease in blood pressure, which temporarily deprives the brain of blood. The drop in blood pressure may result from:
- Pooled blood in the extremities caused by a long run.
- Prolonged straining, such as from lifting heavy weights, coughing forcefully or attempting a bowel movement when constipated.
- Sudden emotional stress.
- Standing after squatting (orthostatic hypotension). This can occur in weightlifting when also holding breath ("weightlifter's blackout").
- Hot, humid weather.
- Low blood sugar.
- Some drugs, such as alcohol.
- Heart disease, diabetes mellitus.
- Heart attack (rare).
- Use of certain drugs, such as heart medications that slow the heartbeat. These include digitalis, beta-adrenergic blockers and other antihypertensive drugs.

HOW TO PREVENT
- Avoid any of the causes or risk factors listed above if possible.
- Avoid sudden changes in physical activity.
- If fainting episodes are caused by medication, consult your doctor about changing drugs.

 WHAT TO EXPECT

DIAGNOSTIC MEASURES
- Observation of symptoms by those nearby.
- Medical history and physical exam by a doctor if needed.
- Diagnostic tests for an underlying cause may include a CT scan or MRI of the head and an EEG (see Glossary for all).

SURGERY—Not necessary for this disorder.

NORMAL COURSE OF DISORDER—Simple fainting disappears in 1 to 3 minutes. It may seem longer to bystanders.

POSSIBLE COMPLICATIONS
- Injury while fainting.
- Mistaking cardiac arrest for fainting.

 HOW TO TREAT

NOTE—Follow your doctor's instructions if provided. These instructions are supplemental.

FIRST AID
- If someone faints, check for breathing and a neck pulse. If neither is present:
  Dial 911 (emergency) for an ambulance or medical help. (If the victim is a child, perform 1 minute of CPR first, then call 911).
  Begin cardiac massage and mouth-to-mouth breathing (CPR). Don't stop until help arrives.
- If someone faints, is breathing and has a pulse, leave the person on the ground and elevate both legs. This helps return blood to the heart. Person should remain lying down for 10 to 15 minutes.

MEDICAL TREATMENT—Doctor's treatment if fainting is caused by an underlying disorder.

HOME TREATMENT
- If you feel faint, sit down immediately and bend over, or lie down.
- If you are subject to frequent fainting spells, avoid activities in which fainting may endanger your life, such as climbing to high places, driving vehicles or operating dangerous machinery.

MEDICATION—Medication usually is not necessary for fainting. Medication may be necessary for underlying disorders.

ACTIVITY—You may resume full activities unless your doctor recommends changes.

DIET—No special diet unless fainting episodes are caused by low blood sugar. If so, eat 5 or 6 small meals a day. The meals should be high in protein, high in complex carbohydrates and low in simple carbohydrates (sugar). Drink adequate fluids, and avoid alcohol.

 CALL YOUR DOCTOR IF

You have had a fainting event.

FEMALE ATHLETE TRIAD

GENERAL INFORMATION

DEFINITION—Female athlete triad is a result of three related conditions. The conditions can occur in females of any age, or athletic skill level. An athlete may have one, two or all three of these conditions that make up the triad:
- Disordered eating (harmful eating behavior) combined with excessive exercise.
- Menstrual period stops (amenorrhea).
- Loss of bone density (osteoporosis).

SIGNS & SYMPTOMS
- Weight loss and fatigue.
- Not having monthly periods or periods that are not regular.
- Young females may not start their first period.
- Stress fractures (bones break for no apparent reason).
- Injuries to muscles.
- Eating only small amounts of food. May overeat (binge) and then throw up or use laxatives (purge).

CAUSES & RISK FACTORS
- Not eating enough food for the energy being spent. Muscles and bones soon start wearing down. Estrogen hormone levels decrease causing problems with menstrual periods and loss of bone density.
Risk increases with:
- Compulsive exercising. Workouts become the most important part of life.
- Over concern with reaching goals.
- Pushed by coach or parents to lose weight for improved performance.
- Stress (emotional as well as physical stress).
- Activities where low body weights and thin body shape seem to be important. These include track and field, swimming, rowing, cycling, basketball, body-building, ballet, and gymnastics.

HOW TO PREVENT
- Eat a healthy, well-balanced diet. Don't skip meals.
- Maintain a healthy body weight for your height.
- Keep track of your menstrual periods.
- Do not over exercise or over train.
- Educate athletes on good eating and exercise habits.

WHAT TO EXPECT

DIAGNOSTIC MEASURES
- Symptoms noticed by you or others.
- Medical history and physical exam by a doctor. if needed. Blood tests and a bone density test may be done.

SURGERY—None expected.

NORMAL COURSE OF DISORDER—Outcome will vary for each athlete. With prompt diagnosis and early treatment, menstrual periods can return to normal, and further bone loss can be halted.

POSSIBLE COMPLICATIONS
- A decrease in athletic performance.
- Permanent bone loss and risk of bone fractures.
- Serious medical problems, including death.

HOW TO TREAT

NOTE—Follow your doctor's instructions if provided. These instructions are supplemental.

MEDICAL TREATMENT
- Treatment involves an increase in the amount of food you eat, weight gain, and sometimes reducing physical activity. Small changes may be all that is needed.
- Parents, along with trainers and coaches should be included in treatment plans. This is important with adolescent (early teens) patients.
- Some may benefit from seeing a mental health provider for any stress or emotional problems.

HOME TREATMENT—The treatment steps are not easy and will take time, but female athletes need to make the changes to improve their overall health now and for the future.

MEDICATION
- Hormones may be prescribed to stop bone loss.
- Take calcium pills to help prevent more bone loss.

ACTIVITY—Try for a balance in activity levels that will still allow you to train, compete, and achieve your goals, while not harming your health. Ask your health care provider and coach to help you make specific plans.

DIET—It is important to get adequate calories, protein and calcium and eat foods you enjoy. Proper nutrition can enhance athletic performance. Consult an expert in nutrition to help you in making the right choices.

CALL YOUR DOCTOR IF

- You or a family member has symptoms of any of the conditions that make up the female athlete triad.
- Symptoms don't improve after a few months of treatment

FIBROMYALGIA
(Fibrositis)

 GENERAL INFORMATION

DEFINITION—Fibromyalgia is a painful condition that involves muscles, tendons and joints. It may affect the muscle areas of the low back, neck, shoulder, chest, arms, hips and thighs. It is a chronic problem that can come and go for years. Symptoms may be brought on by a change in the weather, being in cold or damp places, stress, hormone changes, or in response to activity. It most often affects women ages 20-50.

SIGNS & SYMPTOMS
- Pain and aches in the muscles, often described as "hurting all over all the time."
- Fatigue and sleep problems.
- Areas of the body are tender to the touch (tender points). Common tender points are the front of the knees, the elbows, the hip joints and around the neck.
- Feeling stiffness in mornings; having swollen joints. Hands and feet may be numb and tingly.
- Headache, anxiety and depression.
- Other symptoms may also occur, such as digestion, bowel and urinary problems; vision changes; emotional or mental changes; allergies; dry eyes and mouth; and painful menstrual periods.

CAUSES & RISK FACTORS—The cause is unknown and there are many theories. Research is ongoing into finding possible causes and cures.
Risk increases with:
- Females ages 20-50.
- Having a relative with the condition. It appears to run in families.

HOW TO PREVENT—There are no steps that will prevent fibromyalgia.

 WHAT TO EXPECT

DIAGNOSTIC MEASURES
- Your own observation of symptoms.
- Medical history and physical exam by a doctor.
- Laboratory blood studies to measure inflammation and tests to rule out rheumatoid arthritis or polymyalgia. There is no specific test for fibromyalgia.

SURGERY—None useful or necessary for this disorder.

NORMAL COURSE OF DISORDER—The symptoms vary and may improve on their own or can be helped with treatment. The condition does not lead to more serious illness, nor is it life-threatening.

POSSIBLE COMPLICATIONS—Stress or other problems may cause the pain symptoms to worsen or flare up, usually only for a short time.

 HOW TO TREAT

NOTE—Follow your doctor's instructions. These instructions are supplemental.

MEDICAL TREATMENT—May include prescribed medications and exercise; mental health or behavioral therapy to reduce stress and anxiety, and promote well-being.

HOME TREATMENT
- There is no cure for fibromyalgia. Taking steps to reduce the symptoms is the main goal.
- Treatment steps vary. They may include prescribed medications and injections, exercise, physical therapy, acupuncture, chiropractic care or massage therapy.
- Counseling can help reduce stress and anxiety and promote well-being.
- Make changes in your life that may be needed to help you cope day to day. Maintain your social life and contact with friends.
- Join a local support group so you can talk with others about self help ideas that work.
- Keep your activity levels about the same each day. Get the right amount of sleep each night.
- Don't smoke.

MEDICATION
- For minor pain, use over-the-counter drugs such as acetaminophen or ibuprofen.
- Drugs may be prescribed for symptoms of pain, depression, anxiety and sleep problems. They will take a few weeks to work and side effects are common.

ACTIVITY—A daily exercise program is important. It will improve your fitness level, help reduce muscle pain, and let you sleep better. Talk to your health care provider about an exercise routine that will suit your needs.

DIET—Eat a healthy diet. Avoid caffeine and alcohol.

 CALL YOUR DOCTOR IF

- You have symptoms of fibromyalgia that last more than 2 or 3 days.
- Symptoms continue or worsen despite treatment.

FROSTBITE
(Cold Injury)

 GENERAL INFORMATION

DEFINITION—Temporary or permanent tissue damage from exposure to subfreezing temperature. Ice crystals form in the skin and blood vessels, leading to tissue injury or tissue death, depending on the temperature and length of exposure.

SIGNS & SYMPTOMS
During exposure:
• Gradual numbness, hardness and paleness in the affected area.
• Whiteness or yellowness of the skin.
After rewarming:
• Pain and tingling or burning (sometimes severe) in the affected area, with color change from white to red, then purple.
• Blisters (severe cases).
• Shivering.
• Slurred speech, memory loss.

CAUSES & RISK FACTORS—The following factors make frostbite more likely:
• Windy weather, which increases the chill factor; cold water, snow and rain.
• Poor health; poor physical condition; poor nutrition.
• Persons with a previous cold injury.
• Health problems such as diabetes mellitus blood vessel disease such as Raynaud's phenomenon (a circulatory system disorder), peripheral neuropathy and others.
• Smoking; excess alcohol drinking.
• Dehydration.
• Advanced age.

HOW TO PREVENT
• Anticipate sudden temperature changes. Carry a jacket, gloves, socks, hat, knit face mask and scarf. Get treatment for cold injury.
• Don't drink alcohol or smoke prior to anticipated exposure.

 WHAT TO EXPECT

DIAGNOSTIC MEASURES
• Your own observation of symptoms.
• Medical history and physical exam by a doctor.
• X-rays of damaged areas.

SURGERY—Sometimes necessary to remove permanently damaged (gangrenous) tissue.

NORMAL COURSE OF DISORDER—For mild cases, full recovery is possible with treatment. You may be sensitive to cold and experience burning and tingling. Healing process may take 6 to 12 months.

POSSIBLE COMPLICATIONS
• Gangrene; amputation of dead or infected tissue, especially fingers, toes, nose or ears, following severe exposure.
• Cardiac arrest if frostbite occurs with total body hypothermia.

 HOW TO TREAT

NOTE—Follow your doctor's instructions. These instructions are supplemental.

MEDICAL TREATMENT
• Doctor's care for all but the mildest cases.
• Hospitalization (sometimes).

FIRST AID—The following instructions apply to emergency care until medical care is available:
• Don't thaw tissue if there is chance of refreezing. Upon reaching shelter, remove clothing from the frostbitten parts.
• Never massage damaged tissue and don't warm injury over a fire or by a heater.
• Immerse the affected parts in warm water (about 104-108°F [or 40-42.8°C]). Use a thermometer, if available. Higher temperatures may cause further injury. Pat the skin dry.
• Drink warm fluids (no alcohol). Don't smoke.
• After rewarming, cover the affected areas with soft cloth bandages.
• Don't use affected limbs until you have medical care (if feet are involved, don't walk).

HOME TREATMENT—Appropriate for mildest cases only.

MEDICATION
• Your doctor may prescribe:
Fluids given through a vein (IV) and oxygen.
Analgesics, including narcotics, to relieve severe pain.
Antibiotics to fight infection.
Antitetanus toxoid.
• You may use nonprescription drugs, such as acetaminophen, for minor pain.

ACTIVITY—Physical therapy may be recommended. Resume normal activities slowly after treatment.

DIET—No special diet.

 CALL YOUR DOCTOR IF

• You have symptoms of frostbite or observe them in someone else.
• The following occur during treatment: increased pain, swelling, redness or drainage at the site of injury, fever, muscle aches, dizziness or a general ill feeling.

GASTROENTERITIS ("Stomach Flu"; "Intestinal Flu")

GENERAL INFORMATION

DEFINITION—Irritation and infection of the digestive tract that can often cause sudden and sometimes violent upsets. Gastroenteritis is a generic term and often is used when there is a nonspecific, uncertain or unknown cause. Infectious causes can be spread by contact with an infected person or eating or drinking infected food or water. It affects all ages, but most severe in young children (1 to 5 years) and adults over 60.

SIGNS & SYMPTOMS
• Nausea; vomiting.
• Diarrhea that ranges from 2 or 3 loose stools to many watery stools.
• Abdominal cramps, pain or tenderness.
• Appetite loss; fever; weakness.
• Headache; loss of appetite.

CAUSES & RISK FACTORS
• A viral infection is the most common cause. Types includes Norwalk virus (second only to the common cold in prevalence of viral infections), rotavirus (causes about 50% of diarrheal illnesses among infants and children), adenovirus and enterovirus.
• Bacterial or parasitic infection.
• Food poisoning or food allergy.
• Excess alcohol drinking.
• Use of drugs, such as aspirin, nonsteroidal anti-inflammatories, antibiotics, harsh laxatives, cortisone or caffeine.
• Travel to foreign countries.

HOW TO PREVENT
• There are no specific preventive measures. If you or someone around you has symptoms of gastroenteritis, be extra careful about personal hygiene. Wash hands frequently.
• Medical researchers are experimenting with various vaccines that may be effective against some viruses.

WHAT TO EXPECT

DIAGNOSTIC MEASURES
• Medical history and exam by a doctor.
• Laboratory studies, such as blood counts and stool studies (sometimes.).

SURGERY—None useful or necessary for this disorder.

NORMAL COURSE OF DISORDER—The prognosis is excellent. Vomiting and diarrhea usually disappear in 2 to 5 days, but adults may feel somewhat weak and fatigued and possibly, depressed for about 1 week.

POSSIBLE COMPLICATIONS—Serious dehydration that requires special treatment. Other complications are rare.

HOW TO TREAT

NOTE—Follow your doctor's instructions if provided. These instructions are supplemental.

MEDICAL TREATMENT
• Treatment in a hospital if severe dehydration.
• Consult your doctor if you are a breast-feeding mother and your infant has gastroenteritis.

HOME TREATMENT
• It is not necessary to isolate persons with gastroenteritis.
• Supportive care is the most important aspect of treatment (rest, fluids, close proximity to bathroom or bedpan).

MEDICATION
• Nonprescription medications such as Pepto Bismol may help some patients.
• If gastroenteritis is severe or prolonged, your doctor may prescribe antinausea and antidiarrhea medication. Antibiotics help if the cause is found to be bacterial.

ACTIVITY—Rest in bed until nausea, vomiting, diarrhea and fever are gone.

DIET
• Suck ice chips or drink small amounts of clear fluids frequently.
• Replace lost fluids and electrolytes with commercial products such as Pedialyte or Ricelyte for infants and children; diluted rehydration fluids (Gatorade) for adults.
• After diarrhea and vomiting stop, a diet of complex carbohydrates is recommended (e.g., rice, wheat, potatoes, bread and cereal) plus lean meats, yogurt, fruit and vegetables. Milk and dairy products do not need to be restricted.
• Avoid foods with a lot of sugar or fatty foods for several days.

CALL YOUR DOCTOR IF

• Symptoms of gastroenteritis persist longer than 2 to 3 days.
• The following occurs during treatment:
  Mucus or blood in the stool.
  Fever of 101°F (38.3°C) or higher.
  Abdominal swelling.
  Severe pain in the abdomen or rectum, especially pain that begins in the center and moves to the lower right side.
• Signs of dehydration develop.

HEADACHE, MIGRAINE, RELATED TO EXERTION (Effort Migraine)

 GENERAL INFORMATION

DEFINITION—An intense headache, along with other symptoms, that occurs after physical effort in various sports, such as running, football, basketball, boxing, wrestling or soccer. Migraines related to exertion are most common in persons with a family history of migraines.

SIGNS & SYMPTOMS—The nature of attacks varies between persons and from time to time in the same person. Symptoms of a classic migraine attack appear in the following sequence:
• Inability to see clearly, followed by seeing bright spots and zigzag patterns. Visual disturbances may last several minutes or several hours, but they disappear once the headache begins.
• Dull, boring pain in the temple that spreads to the entire side of the head. Pain becomes intense and throbbing. Sometimes the pain may affect both temples simultaneously.
• Nausea and vomiting.
In other types of migraine attacks, the above symptoms (vision disturbances, headache or vomiting) may be absent, or other symptoms may be present. Some persons become pale, with bloodshot eyes and a runny nose or eyes.

CAUSES & RISK FACTORS—The blood vessels that go to the scalp and brain become narrow and then widen. Vision disturbances occur when blood vessels narrow. Headache begins when they widen again. Effort migraine attacks may be triggered by:
• Physical activity that is prolonged and moderately intense.
• Excessive fatigue.
• Not warming up properly before exercising.
• Dehydration
• Exercise at high altitude.
• Hot humid weather or cold weather.
• There are a number of triggers for migraine headaches including certain foods, alcohol, changes in sleep schedules, excessive caffeine, stress, hunger and others.

HOW TO PREVENT
• Be sure to balance your activities with the proper amount of rest. Avoid fatigue. Eat a nutritional diet. Avoid alcohol and smoking.
• Warm up before you work out.
• Talk to your doctor about various medications that are available and are helpful for some people. Be sure to discuss how the drug might impact your ability to exercise.
• Avoid those factors that seem to trigger attacks.

 WHAT TO EXPECT

DIAGNOSTIC MEASURES
• Your own observation of symptoms.
• Medical history and exam by a doctor.
• Laboratory blood studies.
• CAT scan (see Glossary) of the head.

SURGERY—Not necessary or useful for this disorder.

NORMAL COURSE OF DISORDER—Symptoms can usually be controlled with treatment.

POSSIBLE COMPLICATIONS—None expected.

 HOW TO TREAT

NOTE—Follow your doctor's instructions if provided. These instructions are supplemental.

MEDICAL TREATMENT
• Doctor's examination and medication for persistent migraines.
• Relaxation exercises may help some patients.

HOME TREATMENT—At the first sign of a migraine attack:
• Apply a cold cloth or ice pack to your head, or splash your face with cold water.
• Lie down in a quiet, dark room for several hours. Wedge pillows to support head. Relax and sleep, if possible. Listen to music or meditate, but don't read. Minimize noise and odors (especially cooking odors and tobacco smoke).

MEDICATION—Your doctor may prescribe:
• Medications for the migraine pain.
• Medications that are to be taken at the first symptom of a migraine.
• Medications that are for prophylactic (preventive) purposes.

ACTIVITY—Rest during attacks. Otherwise exercise regularly to achieve maximum fitness.

DIET—Because some attacks are triggered by foods such as cheese or chocolate, keep a record of what you ate before each attack. Avoid foods that seem to trigger migraine attacks. Otherwise, no special diet is necessary.

 CALL YOUR DOCTOR IF

• You have a migraine attack that persists longer than 24 hours, despite treatment.
• Recurrent migraine attacks interfere with normal life.

HEADACHE, TENSION OR VASCULAR

GENERAL INFORMATION

DEFINITION—Tension headaches are the most common type of headache. These headaches can occur infrequently, such as one brought on by a stressful event, or they can occur on a chronic basis (15 or more times a month for 6 months). Symptoms may be mild to severe.

SIGNS & SYMPTOMS—Any of the following:
• Dull, aching feeling on both sides of the head.
• Tight muscles in the neck or scalp.
• Not preceded by warnings (aura or prodrome; see Glossary).
• Feelings of fatigue, weakness.
• Nausea, light and sound sensitivity (if severe).

CAUSES & RISK FACTORS
• Severe overexertion.
• Tension, producing strain on muscles of the neck, scalp, face and jaw.
• Sleep disturbance.
• Excessive eating, drinking or smoking.
• Anxiety or depression.
• Sun glare.
• Use of drugs or alcohol.
• Low blood sugar.
• Hormone changes during menstrual cycle.
• Allergic reactions.
• Stress, either mental or physical.
• Environments that are noisy, stuffy, hot or poorly lit or have irritating odors.
• Exposure to, or the eating of, nitrites, sulfites, monosodium glutamate or other food additives.

HOW TO PREVENT
• Get enough sleep—an average of 8 hours for men and 7 hours for women.
• Don't skip meals, especially breakfast.
• Don't overeat.
• Exercise regularly to reduce tension and improve circulation. But don't exercise to the point of headache.
• Don't smoke cigarettes, and avoid smoky environments.
• Don't use mood-altering, mind-altering, stimulant or sedative drugs.
• Avoid foods that contain nitrites or other additives to which you are sensitive.

WHAT TO EXPECT

DIAGNOSTIC MEASURES
• Your own observation of symptoms.
• Medical history and exam by a doctor.
• Diagnostic tests are usually not needed, but may be indicated if a serious underlying cause is suspected.

NORMAL COURSE OF DISORDER—Most tension or vascular headaches can be relieved with simple treatment.

POSSIBLE COMPLICATIONS—None expected for a simple headache.

HOW TO TREAT

NOTE—Follow your doctor's instructions if provided. These instructions are supplemental.

MEDICAL TREATMENT
• Doctor's treatment if headache persists or worsens despite self-care.
• Biofeedback training, relaxation therapy and hypnotherapy are sometimes useful.

HOME TREATMENT
• If possible, take a break.
• Massage shoulders, neck, jaw and scalp.
• Take a hot bath or long shower.
• Lie down. Place a warm or cold cloth (or ice packs), whichever feels better, over the aching area.
• For jobs requiring long hours of sitting, be sure to get up and move around at least hourly.
• Identify your headache triggers: Keep a record of the time and duration of each headache, what foods or drinks you consumed in the previous 12 hours and any physical, emotional or personal upsets that occurred prior to onset of headache.

MEDICATION
• You may take acetaminophen or aspirin to relieve pain.
• Your doctor may prescribe:
  Nonsteroidal anti-inflammatory medications.
  Antianxiety drugs if anxiety is a problem.
  Antidepressants if headaches are chronic.
  Stronger pain medicines; muscle relaxants.

ACTIVITY—Rest in a quiet room until headache subsides.

DIET
• Most people feel better if they don't eat, unless the headache is from low blood sugar.
• Don't drink alcohol.

CALL YOUR DOCTOR IF

You have a headache and any of the following:
• Fever of 101°F (38.3°C) or higher.
• Recent head injury.
• Drowsiness, nausea and vomiting.
• Pain in one eye; blurred vision.
• High blood pressure.
• Pain and tenderness around the eyes and cheekbones that worsens when you lean forward. This may indicate a sinus infection.
• Vision disturbances and vomiting prior to the headache.
• Persistent headache pain for longer than 24 hours without other symptoms.

HEAT ILLNESS
(Heatstroke; Heat Exhaustion; Heat Cramps)

 ## GENERAL INFORMATION

DEFINITION—Illness caused by prolonged exposure to hot temperatures, high humidity, slow air movement and increased physical activity. Long runs are responsible for most heat illness in athletes. Heat exhaustion is caused by a loss of body fluids. Heatstroke represents failure of the body's heat-regulating mechanism, leading to a heat buildup in the body.

SIGNS & SYMPTOMS
Heat exhaustion:
- Dizziness, fatigue, faintness, headache.
- Skin that is pale and clammy.
- Rapid and weak pulse.
- Fast and shallow breathing.
- Muscle cramps.
- Intense thirst.

Heatstroke:
- Often preceded by heat exhaustion and its symptoms.
- Skin that is hot, dry and flushed.
- No sweating.
- High body temperature.
- Rapid heartbeat.
- Confusion.
- Becomes unconscious (not awake or aware).

CAUSES & RISK FACTORS
- Excessive sweating.
- Failure to drink enough fluid.
- Recent illness involving fluid loss from vomiting or diarrhea.
- Hot, humid weather.
- Working or exercising in a hot environment.
- Alcohol or other drug abuse.
- Chronic illness, such as diabetes or blood vessel disease.

HOW TO PREVENT
- Wear light, loose-fitting clothing in hot weather.
- Drink water often; don't wait until thirsty.
- Drink extra water if you sweat heavily. If urine output decreases, increase your water intake.
- Splash water on the body during a race or heavy exercise.
- Don't take salt tablets.
- Pay attention to early symptoms of heat illness. Reduce exercise if necessary.

 ## WHAT TO EXPECT

DIAGNOSTIC MEASURES
- Your own observation of symptoms.
- Medical history and physical exam by a doctor if needed.

- Laboratory studies of blood and urine to measure electrolyte levels.

SURGERY—Not necessary or useful for this disorder.

NORMAL COURSE OF DISORDER—Prompt treatment usually brings full recovery in 1 to 2 days.

POSSIBLE COMPLICATIONS
- Can involve any major organ system (heart, lungs, kidneys, brain).
- Related to duration and intensity of heat and to speed and effectiveness of treatment.

 ## HOW TO TREAT

NOTE—Follow your doctor's instructions if provided. These instructions are supplemental.

MEDICAL TREATMENT
- For heatstroke—Hospitalization to lower body temperature and provide replacement fluids.
- For heat exhaustion—Call your doctor for advice.

FIRST AID
- If someone with symptoms is very hot and not sweating:
  Cool the person rapidly. Use a cold-water bath, or wrap in wet sheets.
  Arrange for transportation to the nearest hospital. This is an emergency!
- If someone is faint, but sweating:
  Give the person liquids (water, soft drinks or fruit juice). Don't give salt pills.
  Arrange for transportation to the hospital, except in mild cases. Call your doctor for advice.

HOME TREATMENT—Not appropriate, except for mildest cases of heat exhaustion.

MEDICATION—Medicine usually is not necessary for this disorder.

ACTIVITY—Activity may be resumed slowly when symptoms improve.

DIET—No special diet.

 ## CALL YOUR DOCTOR IF

You have symptoms of heatstroke or heat exhaustion or observe them in someone else. Call immediately! These conditions may be serious or fatal.

HEEL PAIN
(Heel Contusion; Heel Spur; Plantar Fasciitis; Heel Bursitis)

 GENERAL INFORMATION

DEFINITION—Heel pain or discomfort of the following types:
- Contusion or bruise of the heel bone—Inflammation of the tissue (periosteum) that covers the heel bone (calcaneus).
- Heel spur—A hard, bony shelf as wide as the heel bone caused by repeated pulling away of the periosteum from the calcaneus. The repeated stress or injury causes inflammation and other problems in tendons and ligaments in the foot.
- Plantar fasciitis—Inflammation of the fibrous band that encloses muscles on the sole of the foot. This hurts worse when running faster or when weight is on the ball of the foot.
- Heel bursitis—Formation in the heel area of an irritated or inflamed protective sac of fluid due to irritation caused by a heel spur.

SIGNS & SYMPTOMS—Pain and tenderness in the heel and sole of the foot under the heel bone. Pain often occurs after resting or after rising in the morning. There may be no pain when sitting. One or both feet can be affected.

CAUSES & RISK FACTORS
- Running, jogging or fast walking.
- Previous, or recent, foot or leg injury.
- Poorly cushioned shoes; lack of arch support.
- Prolonged standing; sciatica (leg nerve pain).
- Overweight.

HOW TO PREVENT
- Avoid activities that put constant strain on the foot. Switch to swimming or cycling.
- Wear a shoe with inserts.
- Wear athletic shoes with good shock support in the heels, good flexibility and good support to control side-to-side motion.
- Don't wear everyday shoes with more than 1-1/2-inch heels.

 WHAT TO EXPECT

DIAGNOSTIC MEASURES
- Your own observation of symptoms.
- Medical history and exam by a doctor or podiatrist.
- X-rays, bone scan or MRI of the heel.

SURGERY—Occasionally recommended.

NORMAL COURSE OF DISORDER—Usually curable with conservative treatment. Different types of treatment work for different people.

POSSIBLE COMPLICATIONS—Inflammation and arthritic changes in the heel that place abnormal stress on previously pain-free joints, such as those in the knee, hip and spine.

 HOW TO TREAT

NOTE—Follow your doctor's instructions if provided. These instructions are supplemental.

MEDICAL TREATMENT—Most people try home treatment first. Medical care may include physical therapy, casts, taping, night splints, injections, orthotics, and surgery.

HOME TREATMENT
- Use ice massage. Fill a large styrofoam cup with water and freeze. Tear a small amount of foam from the top so ice protrudes. Massage firmly over the heel in a circle. Do this for 15 minutes at a time 3 or 4 times a day.
- Lightly massage the heel and calf before getting out of bed. Apply heat with heating pad.
- Taping helps some people. Apply athletic tape as directed on the product's instructions.
- Try heel cushions or lifts, arch supports or medial wedge support (available at sporting-goods stores and drug stores). Use products in both shoes so other problems don't develop. Custom orthotics (inserts designed for an individual) may be helpful.
- Purchase well-fitting shoes. Sandals help some people. Break in new shoes slowly by wearing a few minutes a day to start.
- Stretching exercises will help. Repeat each one 10-15 times several times a day. 1)While sitting, grab a towel with your toes. 2)Stand on ball of foot on edge of step and raise and lower leg. 3)Calf stretches.

MEDICATION
- To relieve minor pain and inflammation, you may use nonprescription drugs, such as ibuprofen or aspirin.
- Your doctor may inject steroids into the inflamed area to reduce inflammation.

ACTIVITY
- Rest often. Elevate the heel above the heart. Stay off your feet as much as possible.
- Use ice massage before warmup and after exercise.

DIET—No special diet, unless you are overweight. If so, lose weight to reduce stress on the foot.

 CALL YOUR DOCTOR IF

- You have symptoms of a heel problem.
- Pain or disability persists, despite treatment.

HEPATITIS, ACUTE VIRAL

 GENERAL INFORMATION

DEFINITION—Inflammation of the liver caused by a virus. Hepatitis can be a devastating illness for an athlete and may prevent sports participation for a long period of time. It can be transmitted among teammates who share locker facilities.

SIGNS & SYMPTOMS
Early stages:
• Flulike symptoms, such as fever, fatigue, nausea, vomiting, diarrhea and loss of appetite.
Several days later:
• Jaundice (yellow eyes and skin) caused by a buildup of excess bile in the blood.
• Dark urine from bile in the urine.
• Light, "clay-colored" or whitish stools.

CAUSES & RISK FACTORS
• Types A and E—The virus usually enters the body through water or food, especially raw shellfish, that has been infected by sewage (fecal-oral contact). This type can occur in epidemics.
• Type B—Usually transmitted sexually. Contracted through contact with body fluids of an infected person, through a blood transfusion infected with the virus or through injection with a nonsterile needle or syringe. An infected mother can pass it to her newborn. Some cases appear sporadically.
• Type C—Usually transmitted through intravenous (IV) drug use, blood transfusions and other exposure to infected blood or its products. In 40% of the cases, the mode of transmission is unknown.
• Type D—Always associated with an infection of hepatitis type B.
Additional risk factors include:
• Travel to areas with poor sanitation.
• Oral-anal sexual practices.
• Use of intravenous (IV) mind-altering drugs.
• Alcoholism.
• Blood transfusions.
• Work in hospitals, day care centers or residential programs; kidney dialysis treatment.
• Poor nutrition; illness that has lowered resistance.

HOW TO PREVENT
• If you are exposed to someone with hepatitis, consult your doctor about receiving gamma globulin injections to prevent or decrease risk.
• If you are in a high-risk group, such as hospital workers, dentists, dental workers, male homosexuals, sexually promiscuous men and women or intravenous (IV) drug abusers, consider vaccination for Type-A and B hepatitis. Vaccines are in development for other forms.
• Routine hepatitis B vaccinations for newborns.

 WHAT TO EXPECT

DIAGNOSTIC MEASURES
• Medical history and exam by a doctor.
• Laboratory blood tests to identify infection Other tests may include urine and stool examination, CT, MRI and liver biopsy.

NORMAL COURSE OF DISORDER—Jaundice and other symptoms peak and then gradually disappear over 3-6 weeks. Most people in good general health recover fully in 1-4 months. A small percentage (1-2%) with hepatitis B or C may proceed to chronic hepatitis. Recovery from other viral hepatitis types usually provides immunity.

POSSIBLE COMPLICATIONS—Chronic hepatitis (lasts 6 months or longer), liver failure, cirrhosis of the liver, liver cancer, even death.

 HOW TO TREAT

NOTE—Follow your doctor's instructions. These instructions are supplemental.

MEDICAL TREATMENT—Hospitalization (severe cases).

HOME TREATMENT
• Most persons with hepatitis can be cared for at home without undue risk. Bed rest, time and good nutrition are essential for recovery. Strict isolation is not necessary, but the ill person should have separate eating and drinking utensils or use disposable ones.
• People with hepatitis A or E shouldn't prepare food or handle food for others.
• If you are caring for someone with hepatitis or have hepatitis, wash your hands often—especially after bowel movements. Wear disposable gloves when handling body fluids.

MEDICATION—Your doctor may prescribe interferon and ribavirin for some types of hepatitis. Other drugs are being researched.

ACTIVITY
• Bed rest is necessary until jaundice and fever disappear and appetite returns.
• Resume normal activities slowly. Fatigue may limit some physical activities or exercises.

DIET—Despite poor appetite, small well-balanced meals help promote recovery. Drink at least 8 glasses of water daily. Avoid alcohol.

 CALL YOUR DOCTOR IF

• You have symptoms of hepatitis or have been exposed to someone who has it.
• During treatment, any new or unusual symptoms develop.

HERNIA

GENERAL INFORMATION

DEFINITION—A part of the intestine bulges through a weak area in the muscles of the abdomen. The most common types that affect athletes include inguinal hernia (more common in males), incisional hernia, femoral hernia (more common in females), umbilical hernia (more common in children). Athletic performance will be impaired until the hernia is repaired.

SIGNS & SYMPTOMS—One of the following:
• A lump in the groin or umbilical area that usually returns to its normal position with gentle pressure or when lying down.
• A bulge at the site of a previous surgery.
• Scrotal swelling, with or without pain.
• Fullness or swelling in lips of the vagina.
All types of hernias can cause mild discomfort or pain at the site of the lump, particularly with exercise or participation in competitive sports.

CAUSES & RISK FACTORS—Weakness in connective tissue or a muscle wall. This may be present at birth or acquired later in life. In athletes, hernias are usually associated with straining. Weightlifters are especially susceptible. In the general population, premature infants, obese persons and pregnant women are most vulnerable to hernias.

HOW TO PREVENT—A weak area may not herniate until it ruptures with heavy lifting or straining. Don't strain when having bowel movements. Don't use weightlifting equipment until the hernia has been repaired surgically. If you must lift something, lift properly. Bend your knees, lift the object and rise using your leg muscles. Keep the object close to your body. Don't bend from the waist and lift. Prevent complications by having surgery to repair the hernia.

WHAT TO EXPECT

DIAGNOSTIC MEASURES
• Your own observation of symptoms.
• Medical history and physical exam by a doctor.
• Laboratory blood studies.
• X-rays of the abdomen.

SURGERY—Necessary to repair the opening caused by weakened muscle or connective tissue. Most hernias are now repaired by endoscopic (laparoscopic) surgery that involves 3-4 small incisions in the abdomen. No abdominal muscles need to be cut.

NORMAL COURSE OF DISORDER—Umbilical hernias (more common in children) usually heal spontaneously by age 4 and rarely require surgery. Other hernias can be repaired with surgery that is followed by a short recovery period.

POSSIBLE COMPLICATIONS—If the hernia becomes strangulated (loses its blood supply), it may cause severe illness (intestinal obstruction, fever, severe pain and shock).

HOW TO TREAT

NOTE—Follow your doctor's instructions. These instructions are supplemental.

MEDICAL TREATMENT—Necessary for diagnosis and surgery.

HOME TREATMENT
• Whenever you lie down prior to surgery, push your hernia gently into place if it protrudes visibly.
• If hernia is causing only mild discomfort and can readily be pushed back, a supportive garment or truss may be an option. This is usually a temporary measure.
• Don't strain to have bowel movements.

MEDICATION—For minor discomfort, you may use nonprescription drugs such as acetaminophen.

ACTIVITY
• Avoid heavy lifting either before or after surgery.
• Speed of recovery will depend on general health and type of hernia repaired. Light activities can usually be resumed in a few days.
• Don't return to exercise program until you have medical approval.

DIET—Eat a high-fiber diet and increase fluid intake to prevent constipation and straining with bowel movements.

CALL YOUR DOCTOR IF

You have symptoms of a hernia. If you have fever or severe pain, call immediately!

HIDRADENITIS SUPPURATIVA

GENERAL INFORMATION

DEFINITION—A skin disorder where a person has nodules in the armpit. Athletes are more likely to develop the disorder because of excessive sweating and moisture.

SIGNS & SYMPTOMS—Nodules have the following description:
• Nodules are firm, tender and domed.
• Nodules are 1 cm to 3 cm in diameter.
• Larger nodules soften in the center and become painful. When pressed, they feel like an overfilled innertube.
• Nodules open and drain pus spontaneously.
• Individual nodules (with or without drainage) heal slowly over 10 to 30 days.
• Nodules leave scars.
• Severity of the disorder varies from a few lesions per year to a constant succession of lesions that form as old ones heal. Lesions frequently recur at the same site.

CAUSES & RISK FACTORS
• Hormonal influences that activate the apocrine glands under the arms. Substances in these glands enlarge the glands. The outlets become blocked, probably by heat, sweat or incomplete gland development. The substances that are blocked in the glands force sweat and bacteria into surrounding tissue, which becomes infected.
• Repeated injury to the skin of athletes due to excessive heat, perspiration and friction of clothing and protective gear.
• Obesity.
• Smoking may be a triggering factor.
• Exposure to environmental heat and moisture.
• Disorders such as Crohn's disease, irritable bowel syndrome, certain forms of arthritis, some thyroid disorders, Down syndrome, herpes simplex, Sjoren syndrome, diabetes.
• Genetic factors. This disorder is most common in black females.

NOW TO PREVENT—No specific preventive measures. Consider weight loss if overweight; minimize heat exposure and sweating if possible.

WHAT TO EXPECT

DIAGNOSTIC MEASURES
• Your own observation of symptoms.
• Medical history and physical exam by a doctor.
• Laboratory culture of the discharge from a draining abscess.
• Thyroid function studies in some cases.

SURGERY—May be necessary to open and drain abscesses. Surgery is necessary to remove involved skin in rare cases only.

NORMAL COURSE OF DISORDER—This disorder may last many years–from puberty through the following 10 to 20 years. Symptoms can be controlled with treatment.

POSSIBLE COMPLICATIONS—Scarring.

HOW TO TREAT

NOTE—Follow your doctor's instructions. These instructions are supplemental.

MEDICAL TREATMENT—None is usually necessary after diagnosis and prescription of medications. Surgery is helpful in some cases.

HOME TREATMENT
• Don't use commercial underarm deodorants or antiperspirants.
• Wear cotton shirts or shirts without sleeves to prevent accumulation of sweat in the armpits during exercise.
• Avoid clothing that is extremely tight.
• Lose weight if you're overweight.
• Apply warm-water compresses to soothe pain or inflammation. Cool-water soaks feel better for itching.

MEDICATION
• Your doctor may prescribe:
  Injection of cortisone drugs directly into the lesions.
  Antibiotics to fight infection.
  Hormones to help subdue inflammation.
  Isotretinoin (has been effective in some patients). This is a potent drug and must be given under doctor's supervision.
• For minor discomfort, you may use non-prescription drugs such as acetaminophen.

ACTIVITY—Restrict your actively in extremely hot weather. Swimming is an excellent substitute exercise.

DIET—No special diet unless you need to lose weight. Obesity is a main risk factor for this disorder.

CALL YOUR DOCTOR IF

• You have symptoms of hidradenitis suppurativa.
• Lesions don't improve after 5 days of treatment.
• Your temperature rises to 101°F (38.3°C).
• Lesions appear that become soft and seem to have pus, but don't drain spontaneously.
• New, unexplained symptoms develop. Drugs used in treatment may produce side effects.

HIV INFECTION & AIDS
(Human Immunodeficiency Virus; Acquired Immunodeficiency Syndrome)

 GENERAL INFORMATION

DEFINITION—A major failure of the body's immune system (immunodeficiency). This decreases the body's ability to fight infection and stop the increase of abnormal cells, such as cancer. It affects the immune system, including special blood cells (lymphocytes) and cells of the organs (bone marrow, spleen, liver and lymph glands). These cells manufacture antibodies to protect against disease and cancer. AIDS is a secondary immunodeficiency syndrome resulting from HIV infection. Both sexes can be affected and all ages; most common in young males ages 25-44.

SIGNS & SYMPTOMS
- Initial HIV infection may produce no symptoms.
- Fatigue; unexplained weight loss; mouth sores.
- Night sweats; fever; diarrhea.
- Recurrent respiratory and skin infections.
- Swollen lymph glands throughout the body.
- Genital changes; enlarged spleen.

CAUSES & RISK FACTORS
- HIV is a virus that invades and destroys cells of the immune system, resulting in lowered resistance to infections and some cancers.
- The virus is transmitted by:
  Sexual contact among infected persons.
  Using infected needles for IV drug use.
  Transfusions of blood or blood products from a person with acquired immune deficiency syndrome (rare).
  Children born to an HIV infected mother.
  Note: Usual nonsexual contact does not transmit the disease.
  Contributing factors include:
- Multiple male-to-male sexual partners or male-to-female sexual partners (less likely).
- Exposure of hospital workers and laboratory technicians to blood, feces and urine of HIV positive patients. Greatest risk is with an accidental needle injury.
- Infants born to mothers with HIV infection.
- Intravenous (IV) drug abuse.

HOW TO PREVENT
- Avoid sexual contact with affected persons or known intravenous (IV) drug users.
- Sexual activity should be restricted to partners whose sexual histories are known.
- Use condoms for vaginal and anal intercourse.
- The risk of oral sex is not fully known. Ejaculation into the mouth should be avoided.
- Avoid intravenous (IV) self-administered drugs. Do not share unsterilized needles.
- Avoid unscreened blood products.

- Infected people or those in risk groups are not to donate blood, sperm, organs or tissue.

 HOW TO TREAT

DIAGNOSTIC MEASURES—Laboratory studies of blood cells and HIV antibody test (may not become positive for 6 months after contact).

SURGERY—Not usually needed.

NORMAL COURSE OF DISORDER—This condition is currently considered incurable. However, symptoms can be relieved or controlled and scientific research into causes and treatment continues. AIDS may not develop for years following a positive HIV test. Once ill, survival averages vary.

POSSIBLE COMPLICATIONS—Serious infection; cancer; death.

 HOW TO TREAT

NOTE—Follow your doctor's instructions. These instructions are supplemental.

MEDICAL TREATMENT—Early diagnosis is helpful. If you are at risk, get a medical evaluation even if you feel well. Follow your doctor's recommended treatment plan.

HOME TREATMENT
- Contact AIDS support groups.
- Avoid exposure to infections.

MEDICATION
- A variety of drugs are used to treat HIV infection and AIDS. Your doctor will recommend the best regimen for you.
- In an HIV infected pregnant woman, drugs reduce the risk of HIV infection in the newborn.
- Studies continue for new drugs and vaccines.

ACTIVITY
- No restrictions on normal activity.
- Get adequate rest, and exercise.

DIET
- Try to maintain good nutrition. Poor diet, changed metabolism and weight loss are common; take vitamin supplements.
- Avoid raw eggs, unpasteurized milk or other potentially problem-causing foods.

 CALL YOUR DOCTOR IF

- Infection occurs after diagnosis. Symptoms include fever, cough, diarrhea.
- New symptoms develop.

HIVES
(Urticaria; Giant Urticaria)

 GENERAL INFORMATION

DEFINITION—An allergic disorder that involves skin changes with raised areas, redness and itching. It may occur anywhere on the body including the scalp, lips, palms and soles.

SIGNS & SYMPTOMS—Itchy skin papules (small, raised bumps) with the following signs:
- They swell and produce pink or red lesions called wheals. Wheals have clearly defined edges and flat tops. They measure 1cm to 5cm in diameter.
- Wheals join together quickly and form large, flat plaques (larger areas of raised, skin-colored lesions).
- Wheals and plaques change shape, resolve and reappear in minutes or hours. This rapid change is unique to hives.

CAUSES & RISK FACTORS—Release of histamines, sometimes for unknown reason. Following are the most common causes:
- Medications. Nearly every drug causes hives in some persons.
- Insect bites; viral infections; some chronic medical disorders.
- Exposure to cold, heat, water or sunlight.
- Cancer, especially leukemia.
- Exposure to animals, especially cats.
- Eating eggs, fruits, nuts and shellfish. Other foods sometimes cause hives in infants, but not in adults.
- Food dyes and preservatives (possibly).
- Infection (bacterial, viral, fungal).
Contributing factors include:
- Stress.
- Other allergies or a family history of allergies.

HOW TO PREVENT
- If you have had hives and identified the cause, avoid the source.
- Keep an anaphylaxis kit if you experience severe reactions.

 WHAT TO EXPECT

DIAGNOSTIC MEASURES
- Your own observation of symptoms.
- Medical history and exam by a doctor.
- Diagnostic tests may include laboratory blood studies, urinalysis, chest x-ray and others to rule out inflammatory infection.

SURGERY—None necessary for this disorder.

NORMAL COURSE OF DISORDER—
Unpredictable, depending on the cause. If a medication or acute viral infection is responsible, hives usually disappear within hours or days. Some cases become chronic and last for months or years. Most eventually go into spontaneous remission—even if the cause is not identified.

POSSIBLE COMPLICATIONS
- Swelling of the larynx and inability to breathe.
- Hives may be the first sign of life-threatening anaphylaxis. If so, it will be followed by itching, runny nose, wheezing, paleness, cold sweats and low blood pressure. Without prompt treatment, coma and cardiac arrest can occur.

 HOW TO TREAT

NOTE—Follow your doctor's instructions. These instructions are supplemental.

MEDICAL TREATMENT
- Emergency-room care for life-threatening reactions.
- Allergy skin tests and injections.

HOME TREATMENT
- Don't take drugs (including aspirin, laxatives, sedatives, vitamins, antacids, pain killers or cough syrups) not prescribed for you.
- Don't wear tight underwear or foundation garments. Any skin irritation may trigger new outbreaks.
- Don't take hot baths or showers.
- Apply cold-water compresses or soaks.

MEDICATION—Your doctor may prescribe:
- Antihistamines, ephedrine, or cortisone drugs to relieve itching and rash.
- Sedatives or tranquilizers for anxiety.
- Epinephrine by injection for severe symptoms.

ACTIVITY—Decrease activities until several days after hives disappear. Avoid getting hot, sweaty or excited.

DIET
- If foods are suspected as a cause, keep a food diary to help identify the offending food.
- Avoid alcohol and coffee or other caffeine-containing beverages.

 CALL YOUR DOCTOR IF

- The following occurs during an episode of hives:
  Swollen lips.
  Shortness of breath or wheezing.
  A tight or constricted feeling in the throat.
  This is an emergency!
- New, unexplained symptoms develop. Drugs used in treatment may produce side effects.

HYPERTENSION
(High Blood Pressure)

 GENERAL INFORMATION

DEFINITION—Blood is forced through the arteries under systolic pressure; when the heart rests between beats, a diastolic pressure remains. Blood pressure is a measure of these two pressures. Normal pressure is considered 120/80. Blood pressure normally goes up as a result of stress or physical activity, but a person with hypertension has high blood pressure at rest. The diagnosis of hypertension is made when the readings are consistently high. Hypertension is sometimes called "the silent killer" because it often has no early symptoms.

SIGNS & SYMPTOMS—Usually no symptoms unless disease is severe. Following are symptoms of a hypertensive crisis:
- Headache; drowsiness; confusion.
- Numbness and tingling in the hands and feet.
- Coughing blood; nosebleeds.
- Severe shortness of breath.

CAUSES & RISK FACTORS—Usually unknown. A small number of cases result from:
- Chronic kidney disease.
- Severe narrowing of the aorta (major artery of the heart).
- Disorders of some endocrine glands.
- Hardening of the arteries.
Contributing factors include:
- Adults over 60; sedentary lifestyle.
- Obesity; smoking; stress; alcoholism.
- Diet that is high in salt or saturated fat.
- Genetic factors. Hypertension is most common among blacks.
- Family history of hypertension, stroke, heart attack or kidney failure.
- Use of contraceptive pills, steroids and some appetite suppressants or decongestants.

HOW TO PREVENT—Essential hypertension (from unknown causes) cannot be prevented at present. If you have a family history of hypertension, obtain frequent blood-pressure checks. If hypertension is detected early, treatment that includes diet, exercise, stress management and medication can usually prevent complications.

 WHAT TO EXPECT

DIAGNOSTIC MEASURES
- Medical history and exam by a doctor.
- Laboratory studies such as blood studies of kidney function, urinalysis and ECG (a test that records the electrical activity of the heart).
- X-rays of the chest and kidneys.

SURGERY—None useful or necessary for this disorder.

NORMAL COURSE OF DISORDER
- With treatment, complications are preventable (except for possible side effects of drugs). Life expectancy is near normal.
- Without treatment, life expectancy is reduced because of likelihood of heart attack or stroke.

POSSIBLE COMPLICATIONS
- Stroke; heart attack; kidney failure.
- Congestive heart failure and pulmonary edema.

 HOW TO TREAT

NOTE—Follow your doctor's instructions. These instructions are supplemental.

MEDICAL TREATMENT—Overall treatment goals will be decided and may involve weight loss; smoking cessation; exercise program; reduction in alcohol drinking; and lifestyle changes to reduce stress.

HOME TREATMENT
- Consider lifestyle changes and practice relaxation techniques to reduce stress.
- Learn to take your own blood pressure. Your doctor or nurse can teach you.
- Smokers should stop smoking and heavy alcohol users should stop or reduce drinking.

MEDICATION
- Blood pressure lowering drugs can reduce blood pressure if more conservative measures don't work.
- Don't take nonprescription cold and sinus remedies. These contain drugs, such as ephedrine and pseudoephedrine, that raise blood pressure.

ACTIVITY—Normal activity with exercise program at least 3 times a week. This helps reduce stress and maintain normal body weight; and it may lower blood pressure. Seek medical advice (your doctor or an exercise doctor) about an exercise prescription.

DIET—Your doctor may recommend a low-salt diet and/or reducing diet if overweight.

 CALL YOUR DOCTOR IF

- High-blood pressure continues (according to your home monitoring system) despite treatment steps.
- Chest pain or sudden severe headache occurs. This may be an emergency. Seek help immediately!
- New, unexplained symptoms develop.

IMPETIGO
(Pyoderma)

GENERAL INFORMATION

DEFINITION—A common infectious, contagious bacterial skin infection that affects the superficial layers of the skin. This is more common in athletes and those who participate in vigorous physical activity that causes excessive sweating.

SIGNS & SYMPTOMS
• A red rash with many small blisters. Some blisters contain pus, and yellow crusts form when they break. The blisters don't hurt, but they may itch.
• Slight fever (sometimes).

CAUSES & RISK FACTORS—Usually *Staphylococci* bacteria or *streptococci* bacteria growing in the upper skin layers. The following conditions make a person more susceptible to impetigo infections:
• Increased perspiration from physical exertion.
• Crowded or unsanitary conditions, such as locker rooms, or sharing of towels.
• Constant friction of clothing and athletic equipment.
• Fair complexion.
• Skin that is sensitive to sun and irritants such as soap and makeup.
• Warm, moist weather.
• Poor hygiene.
• Recent illness that has lowered resistance.

HOW TO PREVENT
• Bathe daily with soap and water.
• Keep fingernails shot. Don't scratch impetigo blisters.
• If there is an outbreak in your team or family, urge all members to use antibacterial soap.
• Use separate towels for each person, or substitute paper towels temporarily.

WHAT TO EXPECT

DIAGNOSTIC MEASURES
• Your own observation of symptoms.
• Medical history and physical exam by a doctor.
• Laboratory skin culture to identify the germ causing the infection.

SURGERY—Not necessary or useful for this illness.

NORMAL COURSE OF DISORDER—Rarely becomes serious and is curable in 10 days with treatment, usually leaving no scars.

POSSIBLE COMPLICATIONS
• Spread of the infection to deeper skin layers (ecthyma or cellulitis). This may cause scarring. Treatment is the same as for impetigo.
• Acute glomerulonephritis (kidney disease) if impetigo has been caused by a streptococcal infection that has not been adequately treated.

HOW TO TREAT

NOTE—Follow your doctor's instructions. These instructions are supplemental.

MEDICAL TREATMENT—None usually necessary after diagnosis and prescription of medication.

HOME TREATMENT
• Follow the suggestions listed under How to Prevent.
• Scrub lesions with gauze and antiseptic soap. Break any pustules. Remove all crusts, and expose and cleanse all lesions. If crusts are difficult to remove, soak them in warm soapy water and scrub gently.
• Cover impetigo soars with gauze and tape to keep hands away from them.
• Treat new lesions the same way, even if you are not sure they are impetigo.
• Separate and boil bed linen, towels, clothes and other items that have touched sores.
• Men should shave around sores on the face, not over them. Use an aerosol shaving cream and change razor blades each day. Don't use a shaving brush—it may harbor germs.

MEDICATION—Your doctor may prescribe:
• Oral antibiotics, such as dicloxacillin or erythromycin. To avoid complications, take antibiotics for 10 days even if symptoms disappear.
• Antibiotic ointments for small areas of infection. Rub antibiotic ointment into the lesions for 60 seconds at least 4 times a day. If your doctor has not prescribed an ointment, you may use a nonprescription ointment containing neomycin and bacitracin.

ACTIVITY—No restrictions.

DIET—No special diet.

CALL YOUR DOCTOR IF

• You have symptoms of impetigo.
• Fever of 101°F (38.3°C) or higher develops.
• The sores continue to spread or don't begin to heal in 3 days despite treatment.

INSECT BITES AND STINGS

GENERAL INFORMATION

DEFINITION—Skin eruptions and other symptoms caused by insect bites or stings from mosquitoes, fleas, chiggers, bedbugs, ants, spiders, bees and other insects. The victim often doesn't remember being bitten or stung.

SIGNS & SYMPTOMS—Red lumps in the skin. The lumps usually appear within minutes after the bite or sting, but some don't appear for 6 to 12 hours. Skin reactions fall into 2 kinds:
• A toxic reaction with pain and sometimes fever, such as from bee stings.
• A toxic reaction with itching due to the body's release of histamine at the bite site, such as from mosquitoes.

CAUSES & RISK FACTORS—Bites or stings are most likely in areas with heavy insect infestations and during outdoor activity in the warm weather of spring and summer.

HOW TO PREVENT
• Apply an insect repellent on exposed skin. Use one with diethyltoluamide (DEET). Permethrin is an insecticide that stuns or kills insects that come in contact with it. Apply it to your clothing (it is not intended for the skin).
• Wear protective clothing.
• Treat animals for fleas, and spray the house or kennel.

WHAT TO EXPECT

DIAGNOSTIC MEASURES
• Your own observation of symptoms.
• Medical history and physical exam by a doctor if needed.

SURGERY—Not necessary or useful for this problem.

NORMAL COURSE OF DISORDER—Most troublesome symptoms disappear in 2 to 3 days, but scratching may prolong symptoms for several weeks or introduce a bacterial infection. Treatment helps, but it doesn't cure quickly.

POSSIBLE COMPLICATIONS
• Secondary bacterial infection at the site of the bite. This may cause swollen lymph glands in the neck, armpit, groin or elbow.
• Anaphylaxis (severe allergic response in hypersensitive persons).
• Rarely, one of the numerous diseases (bacterial, parasitic and viral) that are caused by insects (including malaria, West Nile virus, leishmaniasis, relapsing fever, and Lyme disease) may result.

HOW TO TREAT

NOTE—Follow your doctor's instructions if provided. These instructions are supplemental.

MEDICAL TREATMENT—If you have had anaphylaxis (severe allergic reaction) following an insect bite, ask your doctor for an anaphylaxis kit to treat any future recurrence.

HOME TREATMENT
• If anaphylaxis occurs, give CPR if the victim is not breathing and has no heartbeat. Ask someone to get emergency medical help.
• For less severe cases, apply compresses to the bite or sting to relieve itching and hasten healing. Warm-water compresses are usually more soothing for pain or inflammation. Cool-water compresses feel better for itching.

MEDICATION
• For minor discomfort, you may use:
  Nonprescription oral antihistamines to decrease itching.
  Nonprescription topical steroid drugs. Preparations to reduce inflammation and decrease itching. Use according to label directions. For face and groin, use only low-potency steroid products without fluorine.
• For serious symptoms, your doctor may prescribe:
  Stronger topical or oral steroid drugs if the reaction is severe.
  Epinephrine or steroid drugs (orally or by injection) to prevent or diminish anaphylaxis symptoms.

ACTIVITY—Usually no restrictions.

DIET—No special diet.

CALL YOUR DOCTOR IF

• You have symptoms of anaphylaxis. This is an emergency!
• Self-care doesn't relieve symptoms or symptoms don't improve after 2 to 3 days of medical treatment.
• A bitten area becomes red, swollen, warm and tender, indicating infection.
• Temperature rises to 101°F (38.3°C)

INSOMNIA (Sleep Disorder)

GENERAL INFORMATION

DEFINITION—Sleep problems that include difficulty in falling asleep, remaining asleep, being awake off and on, early morning awakening or a combination of these. Insomnia affects all age groups but is more common in the elderly. Insomnia may be for a short period due to a life crisis or lifestyle change; or chronic, due to medical or mental health problems or other situations.

SIGNS & SYMPTOMS
• Restlessness when trying to fall asleep.
• Brief sleep followed by wakefulness.
• Normal sleep until very early in the morning (3 a.m. or 4 a.m.), then wakefulness (often with frightening thoughts).
• Periods of sleeplessness, alternating with periods of excessive sleep or sleepiness at inconvenient times.

CAUSES & RISK FACTORS
• Depression. This is usually characterized by early-morning wakefulness.
• Overactivity of the thyroid gland.
• Anxiety caused by stress.
• Sexual problems, such as impotence or lack of a sex partner.
• Daytime napping.
• Noisy environment (including a snoring partner).
• Allergies and early-morning wheezing.
• Heart or lung conditions that cause shortness of breath when lying down.
• Painful disorders, such a fibromyositis or arthritis.
• Urinary or stomach problems that require urination or bowel movements during the night.
• Use of stimulants, such as caffeine.
• Use of some medications, including dextroamphetamines, cortisone drugs or decongestants.
• Odd hours for work schedule.
• New environment or location; jet lag after travel; lack of physical exercise.
• Alcoholism; drug abuse, including overuse of sleep-inducing drugs; withdrawal from addictive substances.
• Stress, obesity, smoking.

HOW TO PREVENT—Establish a lifestyle that fosters healthy sleep patterns.

WHAT TO EXPECT

DIAGNOSTIC MEASURES
• Medical history and exam by a doctor.
• Laboratory thyroid studies, EEG (see Glossary).

• Tests in a sleep-study laboratory (sometimes).

SURGERY—Not necessary for this disorder.

NORMAL COURSE OF DISORDER—Most persons can establish good sleep patterns if the underlying cause of insomnia is treated or eliminated.

POSSIBLE COMPLICATIONS
• Off and on insomnia becomes chronic.
• Increased daytime sleepiness that can affect all aspects of your life.

HOW TO TREAT

NOTE—Follow your doctor's instructions if provided. These instructions are supplemental.

MEDICAL TREATMENT—Usually not necessary.

HOME TREATMENT
• Seek ways to minimize stress. Learn and practice relaxation techniques.
• Don't use stimulants close to bedtime.
• Treat any underlying or medical cause.
• Relax in a warm bath before bedtime.
• Don't turn your bedroom into an office or a den. Create a comfortable sleep setting.
• Turn off your mind. Focus on peaceful and relaxing thoughts. Play soft music or relaxation tapes. Set a rigid sleep schedule.
• Use mechanical aids such as ear plugs, eye shades or electric blanket.

MEDICATION—Your doctor may prescribe sleep-inducing drugs for a short time if:
• Temporary insomnia is interfering with your daily activities.
• You have a medical disorder that regularly disturbs sleep.
• You need to establish regular sleep patterns. Long-term use of sleep inducers may be counter-productive or addictive.

ACTIVITY—Exercise regularly to create healthy fatigue, but not within 2 hours of going to bed.

DIET
• No special diet, but don't eat within 3 hours of bedtime if indigestion has previously disturbed your sleep.
• Drinking warm milk before bedtime helps some. Limit coffee and caffeine use.

CALL YOUR DOCTOR IF

• You have insomnia and self-help methods are ineffective.
• New, unexplained symptoms develop.

ISCHEMIA DURING EXERCISE

 ## GENERAL INFORMATION

DEFINITION—Decreased blood flow to the brain, spinal cord and other parts of the body during exercise. In younger people, this is a warning sign that risk factors may exist for stroke. Symptoms may cease, but underlying problems will not. In older persons, ischemia is often a sign of impending stroke.

SIGNS & SYMPTOMS
* Dizziness or falling.
* Leg pain brought on by exercise and relieved by rest.
* Impaired gait or legs "giving out."
* Nystagmus (irregular, involuntary movement of the eyes).
* Vomiting.
* Speech impairment.
* Partial, temporary or permanent paralysis of arm, leg and neck muscles on one or both sides.
* Diminished vision.
* Breathing difficulty.

CAUSES & RISK FACTORS
* Excessive exercise, such as prolonged walking or running, that tires the heart and decreases the amount of blood it can pump.
* Excessive turning or bending of the neck backward or forward that can affect the blood vessels in the neck. This may occur occasionally in people who participate in gymnastics, exercising, wrestling, football and yoga.
Underlying conditions that make ischemia during exercise more likely:
* Hardening of the arteries.
* Cervical spondylosis (degenerative changes in bones of the neck, causing pressure on nerves, blood vessels and muscles).
* Having been born with problems in the blood vessels to the brain (aneurysms, for example).
* High blood pressure; diabetes mellitus.
* Obesity.
* Family history of strokes.

HOW TO PREVENT
* Try to avoid specific exercises or activities that bring on ischemia.
* Follow measures to prevent hardening of the arteries:
  Don't smoke.
  Reduce stress to a manageable level.
  Follow a low-fat, low-salt, high-fiber diet.
  Maintain your ideal weight.
* If you have diabetes or high blood pressure, keep it under control.
* If you are over 40, ask your doctor about taking 1 aspirin tablet daily to decrease the likelihood of platelet clumping (see Glossary).

 ## WHAT TO EXPECT

DIAGNOSTIC MEASURES
* Medical history and physical exam by a doctor.
* X-rays of the head and spine, CAT scan (see Glossary) of the brain and spinal cord.

SURGERY—May be necessary to clear out or bypass blocked or narrowed arteries.

NORMAL COURSE OF DISORDER—In some cases, symptoms of ischemia disappear within 1 or 2 days without residual effects. In most cases, an underlying disorder is causing the ischemia, and it must be treated. Ischemia symptoms may improve, but they may not disappear entirely.

POSSIBLE COMPLICATIONS—Severe stroke and death.

 ## HOW TO TREAT

NOTE—Follow your doctor's instructions. These instructions are supplemental.

MEDICAL TREATMENT
* Consult your doctor after the first incident of ischemia, *even if symptoms disappear.* Diagnosis of the underlying cause is essential.
* Hospitalization and surgery may be needed to correct serious underlying disorders.
* If ischemia leaves residual disability, physical therapy will be helpful until recovery is complete.

HOME TREATMENT—No self-treatment. Seek professional care for any signs of ischemia.

MEDICATION—Your doctor may prescribe blood thinning drugs such as warfarin, aspirin or others.

ACTIVITY
* Rest in bed until symptoms improve.
* Resume your normal activities gradually, but consult your doctor before resuming the activity that brought on the ischemia.
* If you have lost a great deal of muscle control, physical therapy will help you to use affected limbs to regain basic skills, such as eating dressing and using the toilet.

DIET—Follow a low-fat, low-salt, high-fiber, low-cholesterol diet. This will help minimize the chance of stroke.

 ## CALL YOUR DOCTOR IF

You have symptoms of ischemia during or following exercise.

JET LAG

GENERAL INFORMATION

DEFINITION—Jet lag results from travel between different time zones. The degree of severity depends on the number of time zones crossed and the direction traveled. Most people find traveling eastward and adapting to a shorter work day is more difficult than traveling westward and adapting to a longer work day. North-South travel does not normally cause jet lag.

SIGNS & SYMPTOMS
- Extreme fatigue.
- Sleep disturbances.
- Loss of concentration.
- Feeling tired.
- Disorientation (loss of sense of time, place and personal identity).
- Stomach upset.
- Loss of appetite.
- Swollen feet.

CAUSES
- Changes in the body's normal actions that control not only sleep and wakefulness, but also alertness, hunger, digestion, urine production, temperature and hormone secretion.
- Risk increases with frequent travel in short periods of time.

HOW TO PREVENT—Numerous specific preventive measures have been studied and written about including special diets. Some measures may work for some people. See the suggestions in Home Treatment, Medications, Activity and Diet.

WHAT TO EXPECT

DIAGNOSTIC MEASURES—Your own observation of symptoms.

SURGERY—None useful or necessary for this disorder.

NORMAL COURSE OF DISORDER—Symptoms usually resolve themselves after a short period of time in the same geographic location.

POSSIBLE COMPLICATIONS—Depending on the individual, symptoms may last up to a week. For some, sleep patterns may be affected for several weeks after a trip.

HOW TO TREAT

NOTE—Follow your doctor's instructions if provided. These instructions are supplemental.

MEDICAL TREATMENT—No medical care is necessary for typical mild cases of jet lag. For severe cases doctor's treatment may be necessary.

HOME TREATMENT
- Plan destination activities so you will adjust to the time differences. Don't plan meetings or athletic events that first day abroad.
- Try to get plenty of rest before you leave.
- Take a daytime flight if possible.
- Adjust your bed and mealtimes to the new timetable as soon as possible
- Set your watch to local time as soon as possible after takeoff.
- Avoid smoking; it can worsen jet lag symptoms.
- At your destination, spend some time every day in natural sunlight.

MEDICATION
- Your doctor may prescribe short-acting benzodiazepines for sleep in transit.
- The hormone melatonin has been used for this condition, but long-term data are lacking.

ACTIVITY
- Exercise as much as possible.
- Don't operate motor vehicles or swim alone if you feel tired.

DIET
- Eat a normal well-balanced diet, even if you have no appetite. Avoid overeating.
- Avoid caffeine. Do drink plenty of water.
- Avoid or limit any alcoholic drinks.

CALL YOUR DOCTOR IF

You or a family member has symptoms of jet lag and they don't subside after one week.

JOCK ITCH
(Tinea Cruris)

 ## GENERAL INFORMATION

DEFINITION—Infection of the skin in the groin with one of several fungus germs. These fungi thrive in the groin, where darkness, warmth and moisture stimulate their growth. Jock itch is more likely to occur in men than in women. It is contagious from person to person.

SIGNS & SYMPTOMS—Scaling patches on the skin of the groin, thighs and buttocks. Patches have well-defined edges. Occasionally small, pus-filled blisters appear.
* Itching of involved areas.
* Pain (if the skin becomes secondarily infected with bacteria).

CAUSES & RISK FACTORS
* Fungus infection.(often referred to as dermatophyte infections).
Risk is increased by:
* Contact with infected surfaces, such as towels or benches.
* Hot, humid weather.
* Excessive sweating.
* Obesity, which fosters sweating.
* Friction of skin against skin from constant movement.

HOW TO PREVENT
* Dry thoroughly after bathing.
* Don't sit around in a wet bathing suit.
* Wear absorbent, loose cotton underwear.
* Wear clean, dry athletic supporters and underwear for each workout.
* Use nonprescription tolnaftate (Tinactin) after bathing if you have had jock itch. This powder discourages recurrence.

 ## WHAT TO EXPECT

DIAGNOSTIC MEASURES
* Your own observation of symptoms.
* Medical history and physical exam by a doctor if needed.
* May perform laboratory studies, including microscopic examination of scraped-off scales suspended in potassium hydroxide liquid.

SURGERY—Not necessary or useful for this disorder.

NORMAL COURSE OF DISORDER—Symptoms can be controlled in 2 to 3 weeks with treatment. Recurrences are common.

POSSIBLE COMPLICATIONS
* A contact or allergic dermatitis that occurs with the jock itch requires additional treatment, usually with topical steroid treatment.
* Slow healing.
* Secondary bacterial infection in the affected area.
* Rash from an "id reaction" (allergic immune system response to the disorder) on the hands and face (rare).

 ## HOW TO TREAT

NOTE—Follow your doctor's instructions if provided. These instructions are supplemental.

MEDICAL TREATMENT—None is usually necessary unless there are complications.

HOME TREATMENT
* Bathe with clear water only. Don't use soaps until the skin clears completely. Soap irritates infected skin.
* Wear loose cotton underwear.
* Change to dry clothes immediately after swimming.
* If you have an athlete's foot infection also, treat both areas with equal care.

MEDICATION
* Topical treatment with antifungal medicines such as clotrimazole, ketoconazole or miconazole or others.
* Your doctor may prescribe oral antifungal medication such as griseofulvin for severe cases.

ACTIVITY—No restriction.

DIET—No special diet.

 ## CALL YOUR DOCTOR IF

* You have symptoms of jock itch that don't clear spontaneously in 5 days.
* New, unexplained symptoms develop. Drugs used in treatment may produce side effects.

KERATOSIS, ACTINIC

GENERAL INFORMATION

DEFINITION—A sharply outlined, red or skin-colored, flat or elevated growth that may develop into squamous cell skin cancer. Actinic keratoses can be a problem for athletes who spend a lot of time in the sun. It is the most common sun-related growth.

SIGNS & SYMPTOMS—Brownish or reddish scaly patches on exposed areas of skin. The patches are painless.

CAUSES & RISK FACTORS—Keratoses (lesions) occur after prolonged exposure to the sun's radiation (may develop years after the person's most intense sun exposure). The following factors contribute to their formation:
- Outdoor athletic activities and sports.
- Outdoor occupations such as farming.
- Light complexion and blue eyes.
- Being at increased risk for infection due to illness or medications.

HOW TO PREVENT—Protect yourself against direct sun exposure. When outdoors, wear a hat and protective clothing. Use sunscreen lotions and creams (with SPF ratings of 15 or more), and reapply them often during prolonged exposure.

WHAT TO EXPECT

DIAGNOSTIC MEASURES
- Your own observation of symptoms.
- Medical history and physical exam by a doctor.
- Biopsy of the lesions in some cases, such as those that recur frequently and those that do not respond to treatment.

SURGERY
Several different surgical options are available and one may be recommended by your doctor.
- Cryosurgery is the application of liquid nitrogen to the skin.
- Curettage is the scraping away of the lesions with a sharp instrument.
- Excisional surgery removes the lesions.
- Laser surgery may be used to destroy the cells.
- Dermabrasion is a treatment where the top layers of the skin are ground away.
- Chemical peels may be used for facial lesions.

NORMAL COURSE OF DISORDER—There are several types of effective treatment and outcome is usually excellent. New lesions do sometimes occur following treatment. Be sure to follow guidelines in preventive measures.

POSSIBLE COMPLICATIONS
- Skin damage.
- Skin cancer (squamous cell carcinoma), which is curable when treated early.

HOW TO TREAT

NOTE—Follow your doctor's instructions. These instructions are supplemental.

MEDICAL TREATMENT
- Treatment with medications.
- Photodynamic therapy (medicine is applied to the lesions and then exposed to a special light).
- Surgery.

HOME TREATMENT
- Minimize direct sun exposure.
- See your doctor for checkups every 6 months to ensure early detection and treatment of skin cancers.

MEDICATION—Your doctor may use:
- Liquid nitrogen to freeze the affected tissue.
- Applications of 5-fluorouracil to the affected area. This causes uncomfortable inflammation, but it is very effective.
- Other topical or oral drugs.

ACTIVITY—No restrictions.

DIET—No special diet.

CALL YOUR DOCTOR IF

You have signs of an actinic keratosis. Even though this causes no symptoms, it can be a risk for cancer.

LABYRINTHITIS
(Inner Ear Disorder)

 GENERAL INFORMATION

DEFINITION—Inflammation of the inner ear. Because dizziness is the main symptom of labyrinthitis, this problem can impair performance in any sport until it clears.

SIGNS & SYMPTOMS
• Vertigo (sensation that you or your surroundings are spinning around).
• Extreme dizziness, especially with head movement, that begins gradually and peaks in 48 hours.
• Involuntary eye movement.
• Nausea and vomiting (sometimes).
• Loss of balance, especially falling toward the affected side.
• Temporary hearing loss (sometimes).
• Ringing in the ear (tinnitus).

CAUSES & RISK FACTORS
• Virus infection (usually) in the inner ear.
• Other recent viral illness, especially respiratory infection.
• Bacterial infection in the inner ear.
• Spread of a chronic middle ear infection.
• Head injury.
• Heavy exercise in hot weather, causing dehydration or electrolyte imbalance from excessive sweating.
• Stress, fatigue or overwork.
• Use of medication or toxic drugs, including aspirin.
• Allergy or family history of allergies.
• Cholesteatoma (an accumulation of debris covered by skin in the outer ear canal).
• Smoking.
• Excess alcohol drinking.
• Heart or blood circulation disease.

HOW TO PREVENT
• Obtain prompt medical treatment for ear infections.
• Don't take medication that has produced dizziness without consulting your doctor.

 WHAT TO EXPECT

DIAGNOSTIC MEASURES
• Your own observation of symptoms.
• Medical history and physical exam by a doctor.
• Diagnostic tests may include hearing studies, culture of any purulent drainage and other studies as needed to determine any underlying disorder.

SURGERY—Surgical removal of cholesteatoma (an infected collection of debris in the middle ear) and drainage of infected areas may be necessary if conservative measures fail.

NORMAL COURSE OF DISORDER—Recovery—either spontaneously or with treatment—in 1 to 3 weeks.

POSSIBLE COMPLICATIONS—Permanent hearing impairment on the affected side.

 HOW TO TREAT

NOTE—Follow your doctor's instructions. These instructions are supplemental.

MEDICAL TREATMENT
• See your doctor for diagnosis and treatment. Hearing tests may be required.
• Your doctor may recommend medications or special exercises or maneuvers to help speed your recovery.

HOME TREATMENT
• Follow any doctor instructions. This disorder can be frightening and debilitating, but complete recovery is usual.
• Perform the special exercises or maneuvers as directed by your doctor.
• Try to keep low-noise levels in your home.
• Stop smoking.

MEDICATION—Your doctor may prescribe:
• Antinausea medications (oral or suppositories).
• Sedatives to reduce dizziness.
• Diuretics to decrease fluid accumulation in the inner ear.
• Antibiotics if bacterial infection is present.
• Antihistamines to help relieve symptoms.

ACTIVITY—Keep your head as still as possible. Rest in bed until dizziness subsides. Then resume your normal activities gradually. Avoid heavy exercise, competition or hazardous activities, such as driving, climbing or working around dangerous machinery, until 1 week after symptoms disappear.

DIET—Decreasing salt and fluid intake may help. Also avoiding chocolate, coffee and alcohol may help in some cases.

 CALL YOUR DOCTOR IF

• You get dizzy for more than 1 or 2 minutes.
• The following occur during treatment:
Decreased hearing in either ear.
Persistent vomiting.
Convulsions.
Fainting.
Fever of 101°F (38.3°C) or higher.
New, unexplained symptoms. Drugs used in treatment may produce side effects.

LEGG-CALVÉ PERTHES DISEASE
(Legg Perthes Disease; Coxa Plana)

 GENERAL INFORMATION

DEFINITION—Gradual weakening of the head of the thighbone (femur) where it meets the pelvis due to interrupted blood flow. The disorder occurs in several stages and usually affects one leg, but sometimes, both are affected. It occurs in children ages 3 to 12 years, of both sexes, but is more common in boys. Caucasians are more frequently affected than other races.

SIGNS & SYMPTOMS
- Pain and stiffness in the hip and thigh. Sometimes both sides are involved.
- Pain in the leg—often the knee—even though the disorder is in the hip.
- Limping or other difficulty in walking.
- Difference in leg length.
- Symptoms usually have a gradual onset.

CAUSES & RISK FACTORS
- The cause is unknown. Prior injury is usually not a factor.
- Obesity and a family history of the disorder are possible risk factors.
- Increased incidence in children with low birth weight, abnormal presentation at birth, and delayed development.

HOW TO PREVENT—No specific preventive measures.

 WHAT TO EXPECT

DIAGNOSTIC MEASURES
- Your own observation of symptoms, especially a limp or knee pain in your child.
- Medical history and physical exam by a doctor.
- X-ray of the hip, MRI or bone scan.

SURGERY—Surgery may be done to reinforce the bone's attachment to the joint and prevent further deformity, or to replace hip bone in the hip socket.

NORMAL COURSE OF DISORDER—Most patients can expect a favorable outcome within 1-3 years. New bone formation takes place during this healing time. The younger the patient is at the time of diagnosis, the better the outcome.

POSSIBLE COMPLICATIONS
- Delayed treatment may cause permanent bone injury.
- Osteoarthritis may develop later in life.

 HOW TO TREAT

NOTE—Follow your doctor's instructions. These instructions are supplemental.

MEDICAL TREATMENT
- Doctor's treatment, including consultation with an orthopedist.
- Treatment may involve only observation at first for children younger than 6 with no limitations of hip motion, or older children who maintain good range of motion.
- Other treatment steps are aimed at maintaining the range of motion and keeping the hip bone in the hip socket. These may include casting, bracing or physical therapy.
- Hospital treatment (sometimes) for traction (a steady pull on the leg), or for surgery.

HOME TREATMENT
- Youngsters often have difficulty accepting the need for bed rest, casts, braces or other treatment. Enlist the help of your doctor, a counselor, school nurse or other significant persons, if necessary, to discuss the situation with your child.
- Help your child find activities and interests that don't involve athletics.
- Use heat to relieve pain. Warm compresses, heating pads, whirlpool baths, heat lamps, diathermy and ultrasound are effective.

MEDICATION—For minor discomfort, you may use nonprescription drugs, such as ibuprofen.

ACTIVITY—Bed rest may be necessary for 6 months to 1 year until the condition improves or until after surgery. When the bones can bear weight, crutches, braces, casts or splints are usually necessary. After that, activities may be resumed gradually.

DIET—No special diet, unless the child is overweight.

 CALL YOUR DOCTOR IF

- Your child has hip pain, knee pain, stiffness or a limp.
- The following occurs during treatment:
  Symptoms don't improve in 4 weeks, despite treatment.
  Pain increases.
  Temperature rises to 101°F (38.3°C).

LICE
(Pediculosis; Head Lice; Body Lice; "Crabs")

 ## GENERAL INFORMATION

DEFINITION—Skin inflammation caused by tiny parasites (lice) that live on the hairy areas of the body, especially the genital area, scalp, eyelashes, eyebrows and skin in close contact with clothing. The tiny (1 to 2 mm) parasites bite through skin to obtain blood that they feed on. The bites cause itching and inflammation. Some lice live in clothing near skin. Eggs (nits) adhere to hairs.

SIGNS & SYMPTOMS
- Itching and scratching, sometimes intense and usually in hair-covered areas.
- Eggs (nits) on hair shafts.
- Scalp inflammation and matted hair.
- Enlarged lymph glands at the back of the scalp or in the groin (sometimes).
- Red bite marks and hives.
- Eye inflammation if eyelashes are infected.

CAUSES & RISK FACTORS
- Crowded or unsanitary living conditions or locker rooms.
- Sexual intercourse (genital or oral) with an infected person.
- Contact with infected objects such as combs, hats or clothing or with infected person.

HOW TO PREVENT
- Bathe and shampoo often.
- Avoid wearing the same clothing more than a day or two.
- Don't share combs, brushes, towels, helmets or hats with others.

 ## WHAT TO EXPECT

DIAGNOSTIC MEASURES
- Your own observation of symptoms. You may see nits (like tiny footballs) on hair shafts.
- Medical history and physical exam by a doctor.

SURGERY—Not necessary or useful for this disorder.

NORMAL COURSE OF DISORDER—Usually curable with medicated creams, lotions and shampoos. Allow 5 days after treatment for symptoms to disappear. Lice often recur.

POSSIBLE COMPLICATIONS—Infection at the site of deep scratching.

 ## HOW TO TREAT

NOTE—Follow your doctor's instructions if provided. These instructions are supplemental.

MEDICAL TREATMENT—Home care is usually sufficient. Lice on eyebrows and eyelashes must be removed by a doctor.

HOME TREATMENT—The following measures apply to all members of the household and to any sexual partners of household members:
- Use medicated shampoo, cream or lotion prescribed by your doctor.
- Machine wash all clothing and linen in hot water. Dry in the dryer's hot air cycle. Iron the clothing and linen, if possible. Washing removes the lice, and ironing destroys the nits.
- If you don't have a washing machine, iron the clothes and linen, or seal for 10 days in a plastic bag to kill lice and nits.
- Dry clean nonwashable items or seal in a plastic bag for 10 days.
- Boil articles such as combs, curlers, hairbrushes and barrettes.
- Spray (with Lysol or similar product) all furniture that comes in contact with infected body areas.

MEDICATION—Your doctor may prescribe anti-lice (pediculicide) cream, lotion or shampoo. Apply creams or lotions to infected body parts according to instructions. To use the shampoo:
- Wet the hair. Apply 1 tablespoon of shampoo. Lather for 4 minutes, working the lather into the scalp well.
- If shampoo gets in eyes, wash out immediately with water.
- Rinse hair thoroughly, and towel dry. Don't use this towel again without laundering and boiling.
- Comb the hair with a fine comb dipped in hot vinegar to remove the lice. The comb must run through the hair repeatedly from the scalp outward until the hair is completely free of nits.
- A single application of shampoo is effective in more than 90% of cases. Don't use more frequently than recommended, because the shampoo may cause skin irritation or be absorbed into the body.
- If the lice infect eyelashes or eyebrows, they must be removed carefully by your doctor. The prescribed medications should not go into the eyes or onto the eyelashes. You may apply petroleum jelly to the eyelashes for 7 or 8 days after removal.

ACTIVITY—No restrictions.

DIET—No special diet.

 ## CALL YOUR DOCTOR IF

- You, your sexual partner or anyone in your household has symptoms of lice.
- Symptoms recur after treatment.

LYME DISEASE
(Lyme Arthritis)

 GENERAL INFORMATION

DEFINITION—An inflammatory disorder that starts with a skin rash, followed in weeks to months by symptoms in the central nervous system, joints and the heart. Most people who get Lyme disease do not become seriously ill. It can be a self-limited illness that goes away without treatment.

Named for Lyme, Connecticut, where it was first described, it's often confused with juvenile rheumatoid arthritis of children.

SIGNS & SYMPTOMS
First stage:
● A red papule (small, raised bump) on the skin of the thighs, buttocks or armpits that grows as large as 50cm, usually with clearing of the center area. They may be multiple.
Later stages—any or some of the following:
● Muscle aches and pains.
● Fatigue and lethargy.
● Chills and fever.
● Stiff neck with headache.
● Backache.
● Nausea and vomiting.
● Sore throat.
● Enlargement of the spleen and lymph glands.
● Migrating joint pain, followed by skin redness and warmth.
● Enlarged heart and heart rhythm disturbances.

CAUSES & RISK FACTORS
● Infection with a spirochete (term for organism or germ), Borrelia burgdorferi, transmitted by a deer tick bite. Many patients report a tick bite at the site of the lesion 3 days to 4 weeks prior to the rash.
● Risk increases in areas where ticks are numerous, such as long grass or brush.

HOW TO PREVENT
● Wear protective clothing with tight collars and cuffs.
● Use effective insect repellents, such as DEET, in areas with ticks.
● Have dogs and cats wear tick-repellant collars.
● Careful skin inspection; removal of any ticks.
● A vaccine is no longer available.

 WHAT TO EXPECT

DIAGNOSTIC MEASURES
● Your own observation of symptoms.
● Medical history and physical exam by a doctor.

● Laboratory blood studies and sometimes a skin biopsy.

NORMAL COURSE OF DISORDER—The skin rash is curable in some patients in 10 days with treatment, and this may prevent development of other symptoms. If not, symptoms in the joints, central nervous system and the heart usually subside slowly over 2 to 3 years. Symptoms often recur after several years—without another tick bite.

POSSIBLE COMPLICATIONS
● Congestive heart failure.
● Permanent joint deformity.
● Permanent brain damage (rare).
● Nerve disorder (peripheral neuropathy).

 HOW TO TREAT

NOTE—Follow your doctor's instructions. These instructions are supplemental.

MEDICAL TREATMENT—Your doctor will prescribe medications and provide follow up care for the duration of your illness.

HOME TREATMENT
● Early treatment is important to prevent progression.
● Use crutches to keep weight off affected joints, if necessary.
● Heat relieves joint pain. Take hot baths or use heating pads, heat lamps or whirlpool treatments.

MEDICATION—Your doctor may prescribe:
● An oral antibiotic for 14-21 days for early stage of the disease.
● Antibiotics given through a vein (IV) for later stages.
● Nonsteroidal anti-inflammatory drugs.
● Steroid drugs to reduce the inflammatory response in the heart or central nervous system.

ACTIVITY—Rest in bed until symptoms of active inflammation subside. Then resume normal activities gradually.

DIET—No special diet.

 CALL YOUR DOCTOR IF

● You have symptoms of Lyme disease.
● New, unexplained symptoms develop. Drugs used in treatment may produce side effects.

MONONUCLEOSIS, INFECTIOUS
(Mono)

 GENERAL INFORMATION

DEFINITION—An infectious viral disease that affects the respiratory system, liver and lymphatic system. Mononucleosis causes spleen enlargement, making athletic activity dangerous.

SIGNS & SYMPTOMS
• Fever.
• Sore throat (sometimes severe).
• Appetite loss.
• Fatigue.
• Swollen lymph glands, usually in the neck, underarms or groin.
• Enlarged spleen.
• Enlarged liver.
• Jaundice, with yellow skin and eyes (sometimes).
• Headache.
• General aching.

CAUSES & RISK FACTORS—A contagious virus (Epstein-Barr virus) that is transmitted from person to person by close contact, such as kissing, sharing food or coughing. The following factors increase the risk of getting mononucleosis:
• Stress.
• Illness that has lowered resistance.
• Fatigue or overwork. The high incidence among college students, athletes and military recruits may result from inadequate rest and crowded living conditions.
• High school or college attendance.

HOW TO PREVENT
• Avoid contact with persons who have infectious mononucleosis.
• If you have mononucleosis, avoid contact with persons with immune deficiencies to prevent them from getting mononucleosis.

 WHAT TO EXPECT

DIAGNOSTIC MEASURES
• Your own observation of symptoms.
• Medical history and exam by a doctor.
• Laboratory blood tests.

SURGERY—Not necessary or useful for this illness, unless a ruptured spleen must be removed (rare).

NORMAL COURSE OF DISORDER—
Spontaneous recovery in 10 days to 6 months. Most previously healthy athletes usually have about 3 weeks of disability. Fatigue frequently persists for 3 to 6 weeks after other symptoms disappear.

POSSIBLE COMPLICATIONS
• Ruptured spleen, resulting in emergency surgery (rare).
• In rare cases, the heart, lungs or central nervous system may become involved, and the disease may prove to be serious.
• A few patients experience a chronic form in which symptoms persist for months or years.

 HOW TO TREAT

NOTE—Follow your doctor's instructions. These instructions are supplemental.

MEDICAL TREATMENT—Not usually necessary after diagnosis.

HOME TREATMENT
• No specific cure is available. Extra rest and a healthy diet are important. No need for quarantine.
• To relieve the sore throat, gargle frequently with double-strength tea or warm salt water (1 teaspoon of salt to 8 oz. of water).
• Don't strain hard for bowel movements. This may injure an enlarged spleen.
• If you are a student, check on ways to continue school work while you are recovering.

MEDICATION
• For minor discomfort, you may use non-prescription drugs such as acetaminophen. Don't give aspirin to children under age 18.
• If symptoms are severe, your doctor may prescribe a short course of cortisone drugs.

ACTIVITY
• Rest in bed while you have fever. Complete bed rest is normally not necessary or beneficial. Resume activity gradually.
• Don't participate in contact sports until at least 1 month after complete recovery or when your doctor gives approval.
• Avoid heavy lifting.

DIET—No special diet. You may not feel like eating while you are ill. Maintain an adequate fluid intake. Drink at least 8 glasses of water or juice a day—more during periods of high fever.

 CALL YOUR DOCTOR IF

• You have symptoms of infectious mononucleosis.
• Any of the following occurs during treatment: fever over 102°F (35.9°C); constipation, which may cause straining; severe pain in the upper left abdomen that lasts for 5 minutes or more; swallowing or breathing difficulty from severe throat inflammation.

MOTION SICKNESS
(Car, Sea or Air Sickness)

 GENERAL INFORMATION

DEFINITION—An unpleasant, temporary disorder that occurs while traveling, that causes dizziness and stomach upset. The semicircular canals in the inner ear are affected. These fluid-filled canals maintain a person's balance.

SIGNS & SYMPTOMS
- Loss of appetite.
- Nausea and vomiting.
- Spinning sensation.
- Weakness and being unsteady.
- Confusion; anxiety; sweating.
- Paleness.
- Yawning.

CAUSES & RISK FACTORS
—Motion, especially airplane, boat or car; amusement park ride or swinging. Irregular motion causes fluid changes in the semicircular canals of the inner ear, which transmit signals to the brain's vomiting center.

HOW TO PREVENT
- Don't eat large meals or drink alcohol before and during travel.
- Sit in areas of the airplane (usually over the wings) or boat with the least motion.
- Recline in your seat, if possible.
- Breathe slowly and deeply.
- Avoid areas where others are smoking, if possible.
- On an airplane or bus, turn on the overhead air vent to improve air circulation.
- Don't read.
- Take medication to prevent motion sickness before you travel.
- Some airlines have developed behavior-modification techniques for those who are afraid to fly or have motion sickness. Contact the airline or your travel agent for information.
- Mental and emotional factors contribute to motion sickness. Try to resolve concerns about travel before leaving home. Maintain a positive attitude.
- Consider preventive therapy. One technique involves special training for using your eyes that may help avoid the symptoms of motion sickness.

 WHAT TO EXPECT

DIAGNOSTIC MEASURES
- Your own observation of symptoms.
- Medical history and physical exam by a doctor, if motion sickness is recurrent and interferes with your life.

SURGERY—None needed for this disorder.

NORMAL COURSE OF DISORDER—Spontaneous recovery when the trip is over or soon thereafter.

POSSIBLE COMPLICATIONS
- Dehydration from vomiting, fainting, low blood pressure.
- Falls and injuries from being unsteady.

 HOW TO TREAT

NOTE—Follow your doctor's instructions if provided. These instructions are supplemental.

MEDICAL TREATMENT
- Doctor's treatment, if you have a chronic illness that may be worsened by vomiting.
- Mental health therapy or counseling, if your occupation or lifestyle requires travel and you usually develop motion sickness.

HOME TREATMENT
- Once you have the symptoms, try to rest in a dark room with a cool cloth over the eyes and forehead.
- Allowing yourself to vomit can help the nausea. Don't make yourself vomit.

MEDICATION
- For minor discomfort, you may use nonprescription drugs, such as dimenhydrinate (Dramamine), or meclizine (Bonine) before and during travel.
- Your doctor may prescribe scopolamine patches to control symptoms. Remove promptly after travel is completed; long-term use is not recommended.

ACTIVITY—To minimize symptoms during travel, rest in a reclining position and fix your gaze on a distant object.

DIET—Eat lightly or not at all before and during brief trips. For longer trips, sip frequently on beverages—don't take large drinks—to maintain your fluid intake. Avoid alcohol, carbonated drinks and extra-cold beverages.

 CALL YOUR DOCTOR IF

You plan to travel and have had disabling motion sickness in the past.

MUSCLE CRAMPS

GENERAL INFORMATION

DEFINITION—Painful involuntary contractions of muscles in swimmers and others caused by abnormal conditions of the nervous system or exercise-related changes in muscle cell chemistry.

SIGNS & SYMPTOMS—Painful involuntary contraction (spasm) of muscles, usually in the legs. Swimming more than other sports causes leg cramps in athletes during exercise.

CAUSES & RISK FACTORS
• Vigorous physical activity.
• Inadequate warm-up before engaging in strenuous physical activity.
• Calcium deficiency.
• Nerve disorders, such as pressure on nerve roots near the spinal cord, or problems of the nerve fibers after they leave the spinal cord.
• Enzyme deficiency (temporary).
• Diabetes, alcoholism, chronic kidney disease, a variety of medications, hardening of the arteries and Burger's disease (see Glossary), all of which can cause damage to peripheral nerves and thereby cause muscle cramps.
• In swimmers the cause of leg cramps is frequently unknown, and their presence does not suggest an underlying disorder.

HOW TO PREVENT
• Undertake a slow, thorough conditioning program, and warm up properly prior to beginning vigorous physical activity, including swimming.
• Consult your doctor if you take any medicine and develop cramps. Discontinuing or modifying the dosage may prevent recurrent cramps.
• Don't smoke. Avoid polluted air while exercising. Both may decrease oxygen flow to muscles. Oxygen is needed in the muscles to avoid cramps.

WHAT TO EXPECT

DIAGNOSTIC MEASURES
• Your own observation of symptoms and signs.
• Medical history and exam by a doctor if needed.

SURGERY—None useful or necessary for this disorder.

NORMAL COURSE OF DISORDER—Muscle cramps usually resolve spontaneously. In some cases, they can be controlled by treating any underlying medical disorder, increasing fluid intake and starting a better fitness program.

COMPLICATIONS—Muscle cramps may become more frequent and interfere with sports activities.

HOW TO TREAT

NOTE—Follow your doctor's instructions if provided. These instructions are supplemental.

MEDICAL TREATMENT—Physical therapy including warm soaks, applications of ice or heat, whirlpool use, or gentle massage may help relieve residual pain and soreness in cramped muscles.

HOME TREATMENT
• Stretch and rub the cramping muscles.
• Voluntarily contract the muscles that directly oppose those that are cramping. For example, if cramp affects the calf of the leg, force the front of the foot upward toward the knee and hold it until the cramp is diminished.

MEDICATION—Your doctor may prescribe the following medications:
• Aspirin or acetaminophen for pain following a muscle cramp.
• Special drugs for muscle cramps due to nerve damage.

ACTIVITY—Decrease or discontinue vigorous physical activity until muscle cramp relaxes.

DIET
• Drink plenty of fluids, especially water, during exercise periods. Electrolyte solutions help some people.
• If you have frequent muscle cramps from any cause, ask your doctor about eating foods high in potassium, such as dried apricots, whole-grain cereal (hot or cold), dried lentils, dried peaches, bananas, peanuts, citrus fruits or fresh vegetables.
• Follow a diet that is high in complex carbohydrates to maintain or reach a good level of health and fitness.
• Make sure you have sufficient calcium in your diet with dairy foods or calcium supplements.

CALL YOUR DOCTOR IF

• You have persistent or recurrent muscle cramps despite self-treatment.
• You develop new symptoms after starting any prescribed medicine. All effective medicines have possible undesired side effects. These can frequently be controlled by changing the dosage.

MUSCLE WEAKNESS

GENERAL INFORMATION

DEFINITION—Profound muscle weakness or paralysis following hard or unaccustomed exercise.

SIGNS & SYMPTOMS
• Symptoms that appear following a period of rest after the exercise, an hour or 2 later or the next day. Frequently a high-carbohydrate meal is eaten after competition or vigorous physical exercise, followed by a night's sleep. The muscle weakness appears the next day.
• Weakness that begins in the legs and progresses to the arms or other muscles in the body. Disabling fatigue occurs with the muscle weakness.

CAUSES & RISK FACTORS—Decreased potassium levels in the circulating blood and muscle cells. The decreased potassium levels can be brought about by any of the following:
• An underlying inherited disorder called *periodic paralysis* (see Glossary) that interferes with muscle cell metabolism.
• Excessive exercise in hot weather with loss of water, sodium and potassium, leading to dehydration.
• Diuretic medications that cause sodium loss and excessive potassium loss through the kidneys. The sodium loss is desirable; the potassium loss is a major adverse side effect that may lead to severe symptoms. The usual doses of diuretics may require reduction during hot weather.

HOW TO PREVENT
• Prevent potassium loss, increase fluid intake and adjust exercise programs and medication dosages during hot weather.
• Avoid the combination of diuretic medications, alcohol and heavy exercise during exceptionally hot weather. This combination can be lethal, causing strokes and life-threatening episodes of irregular heart rhythms.
• Increase potassium-rich foods in your diet.
• Take potassium supplements (with a doctor's prescription) prior to vigorous exercise if you have had an exercise-induced muscle weakness in the past.
• Modify your activity level to one below that which triggers attacks.

WHAT TO EXPECT

DIAGNOSTIC MEASURES
• Your own observation of symptoms and signs.
• Medical history and exam by a doctor.
• Blood studies (sometimes) to measure potassium levels.
• Electromyography (see Glossary).

SURGERY—None useful or necessary for this disorder.

NORMAL COURSE OF DISORDER—Curable and preventable without long-lasting complications by modifying one's exercise program, taking potassium supplements if recommended and avoiding dehydration.

COMPLICATIONS—None expected with proper diagnosis and treatment.

HOW TO TREAT

NOTE—Follow your doctor's instructions. These instructions are supplemental.

MEDICAL TREATMENT—Must be individualized according to the underlying disorder.

HOME TREATMENT
• Replace lost potassium with supplements or increase high-potassium foods in the diet.
• Replace fluids lost with water instead of soft drinks.
• After vigorous exercise, avoid a high-carbohydrate meal.

MEDICATION—Your doctor may prescribe potassium supplements or potassium-sparing medications that keep potassium levels in your heart elevated.

ACTIVITY—If exercise-induced muscle weakness is a recurrent problem, it may be necessary to cut back on your activity level permanently.

DIET
• If you have a potassium deficiency, eat foods high in potassium, such as dried apricots, whole-grain cereal (hot or cold), dried lentils, dried peaches, bananas, peanuts, citrus fruits or fresh vegetables.
• Follow a diet that is high in complex carbohydrates to maintain or reach a good level of health and fitness. However, do not eat such a meal within 3 to 5 hours before competition, and eat only lightly directly afterward.

CALL YOUR DOCTOR IF

• You have persistent or recurrent muscle weakness following exercise.
• You develop new symptoms after starting any prescribed medicine. All effective medicines have possible unwanted side effects. These can frequently be controlled by changing the dosage.

NOSEBLEED
(Epistaxis)

 GENERAL INFORMATION

DEFINITION—Bleeding from the nose. This is common in athletes who participate in contact or collision sports, especially football, boxing, wrestling or hockey.

SIGNS & SYMPTOMS
- Blood oozing from the nostril. If the nosebleed is close to the nostril, the blood is bright red. If the nosebleed is deeper in the nose, the blood may be bright or dark.
- Lightheadedness from heavy blood loss.
- Rapid heartbeat, shortness of breath and pallor (with significant blood loss only).
- Black stool from swallowed blood.

CAUSES & RISK FACTORS
- Injury to the nose.
- Nasal or sinus infection.
- Nasal polyps or a foreign body in the nose.
- Use of certain drugs, such as anticoagulants or aspirin, or prolonged use of nose drops.
- Exposure to irritating chemicals.
- High altitude or dry climate.
- Dry nasal membranes from any cause.
- Dry air in airplanes or air conditioned buildings.
- Atherosclerosis (hardening of the arteries).
- High blood pressure. Bleeding tendencies associated with aplastic anemia, leukemia, hemophilia, thrombocytopenia or liver disease.
- Hodgkin's disease, scarlet fever or rheumatic fever.

HOW TO PREVENT
- Avoid injury if possible. Use appropriate equipment to protect your face and head.
- Obtain medical treatment for any known underlying cause.
- Humidify the air if you live in a dry climate or at high altitude.

 WHAT TO EXPECT

DIAGNOSTIC MEASURES
- Your own observation of symptoms.
- Medical history and physical exam by a doctor if needed.

SURGERY—May be necessary in cases of severe bleeding to tie off the artery feeding the area bleeding.

NORMAL COURSE OF DISORDER—
Symptoms can be controlled with treatment or time. Severe bleeding requires emergency care.

POSSIBLE COMPLICATIONS—Rarely, bleeding severe enough to require transfusion.

 HOW TO TREAT

NOTE—Follow your doctor's instructions if provided. These instructions are supplemental.

MEDICAL TREATMENT
- Doctor's or emergency room treatment if there is a nose fracture or other injury or if home treatment is unsuccessful. Gauze packing may be inserted to absorb blood, stop dripping and exert pressure on the ruptured blood vessels. Continued bleeding may require cauterization (see Glossary) and packing.
- Surgery (for severe bleeding only).

HOME TREATMENT—If there has been no serious injury to the nose:
- Sit up with your head bent forward.
- Clamp your nose closed with your fingers for 5 uninterrupted minutes. During this time, breathe through your mouth. If blood is coming from one nostril, press firmly on that nostril.
- If bleeding stops and recurs, repeat, but pinch your nose firmly on both sides for 8 to 10 minutes. Holding your nose tightly closed allows the blood to clot and seal the damaged blood vessels.
- You may apply cold compresses at the same time.
- Don't blow your nose for 12 hours after bleeding stops to avoid dislodging blood clot.
- Don't swallow blood. It may upset your stomach or make you gag, causing you to inhale blood.
- Don't talk (also to avoid gagging).

MEDICATION—Your doctor may prescribe drugs to treat any underlying serious disorder.

ACTIVITY—Resume your normal activities as soon as symptoms improve.

DIET—No special diet.

 CALL YOUR DOCTOR IF

- You have a nosebleed that won't stop with home treatment described above.
- After the nosebleed, you become nauseated or vomit.
- After the nose has been packed, your temperature rises to 101°F (35.3°C) or higher.
- Renewed bleeding or signs of infection (fever and a general ill feeling) begin after surgery.

OSGOOD-SCHLATTER DISEASE
(Osteochondrosis)

 GENERAL INFORMATION

DEFINITION—A temporary condition of the leg at the knee that involves swelling, tenderness and pain. The powerful quadriceps muscles of the thigh attach to the lower leg bone (tibia) at a growth zone (tibial tubercle), a relatively vulnerable area of bone. Pain, tenderness and swelling occur at this point with repeated stress. Sometimes both knees are affected.

SIGNS & SYMPTOMS
* Pain following an extended period of vigorous exercise in an adolescent. In more severe cases, pain occurs during less vigorous activity, especially straightening the leg against force, as in stair climbing, jumping, doing deep knee bends or weightlifting.
* A slightly swollen, warm and tender bump below the knee.

CAUSES & RISK FACTORS—Probably results from stress or injury of the tibial tubercle (which is still developing during adolescence). Repeated stress or injury interferes with development, causing inflammation. Other risk factors include:
* Repeated overzealous conditioning routines, such as running, jumping or jogging.
* Overweight.
* Being a male between 11 and 18.
* Rapid skeletal growth.

HOW TO PREVENT
* Help an overweight child or adolescent to lose weight.
* Encourage your child to exercise moderately, avoiding extremes.

 WHAT TO EXPECT

DIAGNOSTIC MEASURES
* Your own observation of symptoms.
* Medical history and physical exam by a doctor.
* X-ray or bone scan of the knee.

SURGERY—Necessary only in severe cases in which a bone fragment forms and remains painful after growth has ceased.

NORMAL COURSE OF DISORDER
* Usually resolves within 2 years after reaching full skeletal growth.
* Moderate to severe cases may require significantly reduced activity and immobilization for several months.
* No permanent defects are expected.

POSSIBLE COMPLICATIONS
* Bone infection.
* Recurrence of the condition in adulthood (rare).

 HOW TO TREAT

NOTE—Follow your doctor's instructions. These instructions are supplemental.

MEDICAL TREATMENT—Not necessary for mild cases. For moderate or severe cases, the knee may be immobilized with a cast for approximately 2 months.

HOME TREATMENT
* Use heat to relieve pain. Warm compresses, heating pads, warm whirlpool baths and heat lamps are effective.
* Wear a knee pad below the knee during exercise.
* Apply ice to the affected area immediately before and after exercise (if your doctor has cleared you for increased activity).
* Avoid kneeling.

MEDICATION
* For minor discomfort, you may use non-prescription drugs such as ibuprofen.
* Your doctor may prescribe steroid drug injections if other treatment fails. Injections may weaken tendons. Avoid them if possible to allow the condition more time to heal with rest and simpler treatment.

ACTIVITY
* If pain is severe, resting the affected leg is the most important treatment. This is done with:
  Crutches.
  A leg cast or splint.
  An elastic knee brace that prevents the knee from bending fully.
* During treatment, don't participate in sports that cause pain. Consider switching to a sport that does not cause the same stresses on the knee. The problem is usually temporary, and normal activity can be resumed when inflammation subsides. Mild to moderate activity up to the point of pain may be done during treatment phase. Check with your doctor.

DIET—No special diet. Lose weight to normal if you are overweight.

 CALL YOUR DOCTOR IF

* You have symptoms of Osgood-Schlatter disease.
* Symptoms worsen or don't improve in 4 weeks, despite treatment.

OSTEOARTHRITIS
(Degenerative Joint Disease)

 GENERAL INFORMATION

DEFINITION—Degeneration of cartilage at a joint and growth of bone "spurs" that inflame surrounding tissue. It can affect all joints, but is most common in the fingers, feet, knees, hips and spine in adults over 45.

SIGNS & SYMPTOMS
- Joint stiffness and pain, including backache. Weather changes, especially cold, damp weather, may increase aching.
- Limited movement and loss of dexterity in affected joints.
- No redness, heat or fever in joints (usually).
- Swelling of affected joints (sometimes), especially finger joints.
- Cracking or grating sounds with joint movement (sometimes).

CAUSES & RISK FACTORS—Exact cause is
unknown. Appears to be a combination or interaction of mechanical, biologic, inflammatory and immune system factors. Other factors include:
- Obesity.
- Occupations that put stress on joints.
- Stress on joints caused by activity and aging. Most people over age 50 have some osteoarthritis.
- Injury to the joint lining.

HOW TO PREVENT
- Maintain a normal weight for your height and body structure.
- Be physically active, but avoid activities that lead to joint injury, especially after age 40. Try regular stretching or yoga exercises.

 WHAT TO EXPECT

DIAGNOSTIC MEASURES
- Medical history and exam by a doctor.
- Laboratory blood studies to rule out inflammatory forms of arthritis.
- X-rays of painful joints.

SURGERY—Surgery for osteoarthritis includes arthroplasty (joint replacement) and arthrodesis (immobilization of a joint).

NORMAL COURSE OF DISORDER—
Symptoms can usually be relieved, but joint changes are permanent. Pain may begin as a minor irritant, but it can become severe enough to interfere with daily activities and sleep.

POSSIBLE COMPLICATIONS
- Crippling (sometimes).

- Muscles around affected joints may become smaller and weaker because of decreased use.
- Tends to be progressive.

 HOW TO TREAT

NOTE—Follow your doctor's instructions. These instructions are supplemental.

MEDICAL TREATMENT—An overall treatment plan will involve understanding the disorder, seeking rehabilitation, adapting activities of daily living and using medications if needed.

HOME TREATMENT
- To relieve pain, apply heat to painful and stiff joints for 20 minutes 2 or 3 times a day. Use hot towels, hot tubs, infrared heat lamps, electric heating pads or deep heating ointments or lotions. Swim often in a heated pool or spa.
- If osteoarthritis of the neck causes pain in the arms, wear a soft, immobilizing collar (Thomas collar).
- Massage the muscles around painful joints. Massaging the joint itself is not helpful.
- If osteoarthritis affects the spine, sleep on your back on a very firm mattress or place 3/4-inch plywood slab between your box spring and mattress. Waterbeds help some people.
- Avoid chilling. Wear thermal underwear or avoid outdoor activity in cold weather.
- Keep a positive outlook on life. Remain active to prevent wasting of muscles.

MEDICATION—Your doctor may prescribe:
- Aspirin or other nonsteroidal anti-inflammatory drugs or acetaminophen for pain.
- Cortisone injections into painful, stiff joints. These may provide temporary relief.
- Other medications as needed.

ACTIVITY
- Rest is important only during acute phases when joints are very painful. Resume normal activity as soon as symptoms improve.
- A general fitness program is important.
- Seek physical therapy for muscle and joint rehabilitation (severe cases only).
- May need to protect joints from overuse by using crutches or a cane, walker or elastic knee support.

DIET—If you are overweight, lose weight.

 CALL YOUR DOCTOR IF

- You have joint pain or stiffness.
- New, unexplained symptoms develop. Drugs used in treatment may produce side effects.

OSTEOPOROSIS

GENERAL INFORMATION

DEFINITION—Loss of normal bone density, bone mass and strength, leading to increased thinning and increased risk of bone fractures. It is most likely to develop in women after menopause, particularly women who lead inactive lives and have insufficient calcium intake. Conversely, osteoporosis at an early age is also likely in women who exercise so strenuously (such as marathon runners) that menstrual periods cease and estrogen production declines. Osteoporosis does occur in men, but is less common.

SIGNS & SYMPTOMS
Early stages:
- Backache.
- No symptoms (often).
Later stages:
- Sudden back pain with a cracking sound indicating fracture.
- Deformed spinal column with humps.
- Loss of height.
- Fractures, especially of the hip or arm, occurring with minor injury.

CAUSES & RISK FACTORS—Loss of bony structure and strength. Factors include:
- Prolonged lack of adequate calcium and protein in the diet.
- Low estrogen levels after menopause.
- Decreased activity with increased age.
- Use of steroid (cortisone) drugs.
- Prolonged disease, including alcoholism.
- Vitamin deficiency (especially of vitamin C).
- Hyperthyroidism.
- Cancer.
- Family history of osteoporosis.
- Surgery to remove the ovaries.
- Radiation treatment for ovarian cancer.
- Body type. Thin women with a small frame are more susceptible.
- Smoking.
- Use of thyroid medications.

HOW TO PREVENT
- Ensure an adequate calcium intake—up to 1500 mg a day—with milk and milk products or calcium supplements.
- Engage in regular weight-bearing exercise, such as brisk walking, which may be better at preventing osteoporosis than swimming.
- Seek medical advice about taking estrogen, calcium and bone-building medications after menopause begins or the ovaries have been removed.
- Avoid risk factors where possible.

WHAT TO EXPECT

DIAGNOSTIC MEASURES
- Your own observation of symptoms.
- Medical history and exam by a doctor.
- Bone density tests.

NORMAL COURSE OF DISORDER—Diet, calcium, vitamin D, estrogen, bone-building drugs and exercise can halt progress of the disease. Fractures heal slowly with treatment.

POSSIBLE COMPLICATIONS—Bone fracture after a fall. The hip and spine are most vulnerable. Fractured hips require surgery. Sometimes a bone will break or collapse without injury or a fall.

HOW TO TREAT

NOTE—Follow your doctor's instructions. These instructions are supplemental.

MEDICAL TREATMENT—If estrogen is prescribed, visit your doctor for regular pelvic exams, breast exams and pap smears, and have follow-up bone density tests.

HOME TREATMENT
- If you already have osteoporosis, avoid all circumstances that may lead to injury. Stay off icy streets and wet or waxed floors.
- Use heat or ice in any form to ease pain.
- Sleep on a firm mattress.
- Use a back brace if prescribed by your doctor.
- Use correct posture when lifting.

ACTIVITY—Stay active, but avoid the risk of falls. Exercise—especially weight-bearing exercise, such as weightlifting, walking or running—helps maintain bone strength.

MEDICATION
- You may use nonprescription drugs such as acetaminophen to relieve minor pain.
- Your doctor may prescribe:
  Calcium and vitamin D.
  Bone-building medications.
  Estrogen replacement therapy.

DIET—Eat a normal, well-balanced diet high in protein, calcium and vitamin D.

CALL YOUR DOCTOR IF

- You have symptoms of osteoporosis.
- Pain develops, especially after injury.
- New, unexplained symptoms develop, such as vaginal bleeding. Drugs used in treatment may produce side effects.

PHOTOSENSITIVITY

GENERAL INFORMATION

DEFINITION—Abnormal sensitivity to sunlight (a reaction may occur after only a few minutes exposure). This is likely to be a problem for those engaging in any hot-season sport such as swimming, surfing, sailing, tennis or water skiing. Some people react to winter daylight as well.

SIGNS & SYMPTOMS
- Red skin rash, sometimes with small blisters, in areas exposed to sunlight.
- Fever.
- Fatigue or dizziness.

CAUSES & RISK FACTORS—Exposure to sun during hot seasons when ultraviolet light is strongest. It is triggered by exposure to the sun, usually in conjunction with sunburn. Risks increase with any of the following:
- Use of medications or herbs that cause photosensitivity (increased sensitivity to ultraviolet light). The most common drugs include tetracycline antibiotics, thiazide diuretics, sulfa drugs and oral contraceptives. The herb St. John's Wort can cause the problem. Some sunscreens and some cosmetics, including lipstick, perfume and soaps, can also cause a photosensitive reaction.
- Underlying infection.
- Previous episodes of sun poisoning.
- Metabolic disorders, such as diabetes mellitus or thyroid disease.
- Use of drugs that affect the immune system.

HOW TO PREVENT
- Stay out of the sun when possible if you have a history of photosensitivity. Change the time vigorous workouts to a part of the day when you will be less exposed to sunlight (before 10 a.m. or after 2 p.m.).
- Avoid the medications or products known to cause photosensitivity. It is important to remember that not all individuals who use these medications will have a photosensitive reaction. Also, a reaction will be different in different people, and a person may have a one time reaction and not experience it again.

WHAT TO EXPECT

DIAGNOSTIC MEASURES
- Your own observation of symptoms.
- Medical history and physical exam by a doctor.

SURGERY—Not necessary or useful for this disorder.

NORMAL COURSE OF DISORDER—Symptoms can be controlled with treatment if you stay out of the sun. For most people, it will take up to 1 week for recovery, but in some cases, complete recovery may take weeks to months.

POSSIBLE COMPLICATIONS—Recurrence of the rash and other symptoms when exposed to the sun—even for short periods—especially in spring and summer.

HOW TO TREAT

NOTE—Follow your doctor's instructions. These instructions are supplemental.

MEDICAL TREATMENT—If a medication is the cause, your doctor will discuss alternative therapies or other options for treatment for the disorder being treated.

HOME TREATMENT
- Stay out of the sun during the hours of strongest ultraviolet light (10 a.m. to 2 p.m.).
- Apply cool moist compresses to the affected area.
- If you must go out in the sun for your athletic workouts, wear protective clothing and the most protective sunscreen preparation available. Beware of heat exhaustion and dehydration.

MEDICATION
- You may take aspirin or acetaminophen to relieve mild pain or itching.
- Beta carotene taken orally helps some people.
- Your doctor may prescribe steroid drugs for severe cases or other drugs which can reduce the photosensitivity.

ACTIVITY—No restrictions, except to avoid prolonged sun exposure.

DIET—No special diet. Drink extra fluids to prevent dehydration.

CALL YOUR DOCTOR IF

- You have symptoms of photosensitivity.
- New, unexplained symptoms develop. Drugs used in treatment may produce side effects.

PLANTAR NEUROMA (Morton's Toe)

 GENERAL INFORMATION

DEFINITION—A small benign tumor in the nerve that serves the 2nd, 3rd and 4th toes. It may affect one or both feet and is more common in women.

SIGNS & SYMPTOMS
Early stages:
- Excruciating pain, numbness or tingling in the front part of the foot, particularly when running or bearing weight while jumping, turning or dancing.

Later stages:
- Localized pain in the sides of the 3rd and 4th toes (usually). Pain occurs suddenly when least expected. Removing the shoe and massaging the painful area brings dramatic relief almost immediately. Pain is less when barefooted.
- Tenderness at the base of the 3rd and 4th toes.
- Feelings of electric shock or numbness running out into one or both toes.

CAUSES & RISK FACTORS
- Relaxation of the ligaments of the foot, causing thickening of the plantar nerve.
- Ill-fitting shoes (possibly), particularly shoes used for athletic activity.
- Repeated foot injuries.
- Obesity and poor nutrition.
- Recent or chronic illness.

HOW TO PREVENT—Unknown.

 WHAT TO EXPECT

DIAGNOSTIC MEASURES
- Your own observation of symptoms.
- Medical history and physical exam by a doctor.
- Your doctor may inject an anesthetic into the area. If the pain stops, it helps confirm the diagnosis and location of the problem.
- X-rays of the foot; for some cases, ultrasound or MRI may be recommended.

SURGERY—May be necessary to remove the neuroma if conservative treatment fails. Several different surgical options are available. Your doctor will discuss these with you.

NORMAL COURSE OF DISORDER
- Treatment with a metatarsal bar in the shoe usually relieves pain, although the tumor will remain until removed surgically. If surgery is necessary, allow about 3 weeks for recovery.
- For some patients, there may be footwear restrictions and activity limitations.

POSSIBLE COMPLICATIONS—Continuous pain and partial disability if the tumor is untreated. Even with surgical treatment, some patients have sensitivity, tenderness or numbness in the area. In most cases, these were not disabling or causing major problems.

 HOW TO TREAT

NOTE—Follow your doctor's instructions. These instructions are supplemental.

MEDICAL TREATMENT—Your doctor may prescribe a trial treatment with a metatarsal bar in the shoe and other restrictions. If this type of therapy fails, surgery will be recommend.

HOME TREATMENT
- Footwear changes and restrictions will help 20-30% of the patients.
- Following any surgery, the foot will be snugly wrapped in a bandage. Keep the bandage dry and the foot elevated as much as possible during recovery. After removal of bandages, apply heat with soaks, tub baths or heat lamps. You will be able to bear weight in a postoperative shoe. When foot has healed, massage with ice for 10 minutes before and after vigorous physical activity.

MEDICATION—After surgery, your doctor may prescribe:
- Pain relievers.
- Antibiotics to fight infection.
- Nonprescription drugs, such as acetaminophen, for minor pain.

ACTIVITY—No restrictions except those imposed by foot pain. After surgery, avoid vigorous exercise for 6 weeks. Gradually return to light activity after clearance from your doctor once the bandage is removed.

DIET—No special diet.

 CALL YOUR DOCTOR IF

- You have signs and symptoms of plantar neuroma.
- Any of the following occur after surgery:
  Pain, swelling, redness, drainage or bleeding increases in the surgical area.
  You develop signs of infection (headache, muscle aches, dizziness or a general Ill feeling and fever).
  New, unexplained symptoms develop. Drugs used in treatment may produce side effects.

PNEUMOTHORAX

GENERAL INFORMATION

DEFINITION—Collapse of part or all of a lung caused by pressure from free air in the chest between the two layers of the pleura (thin membranes that cover the lung). Peak incidence is in males from ages 20 to 40.

SIGNS & SYMPTOMS—The following symptoms vary according to the degree of lung collapse and extent of underlying lung disease. Symptoms may be less acute if the pneumothorax develops slowly:
* Sharp chest pain. Pain may extend to a shoulder or across the chest or abdomen.
* Shortness of breath and rapid breathing.
* Dry, hacking cough (occasionally).
* Bluish nails.
* Coughing bloody sputum (sometimes).
* Rapid pulse.
* In worst cases (tension pneumothorax), fainting and shock.

CAUSES & RISK FACTORS
Spontaneous pneumothorax:
* Physical exertion in a healthy individual, with no obvious preceding injury, infection or disease. Activities most likely to produce pneumothorax include:
  Ascent while scuba diving.
  Diving or high-altitude flying.
  Activities that require stretching the chest and rib cage, such as track and field events, throwing sports and bowling.
* Rupture of small air sacs in the lung. Asthma, emphysema, chronic bronchitis, lung abscess, empyema or other lung disease may cause the rupture of air sacs.
Pneumothorax due to trauma:
* A wound to the chest area, which permits outside air to rush into the pleural space and causes the lung to collapse.
* Complication of removing fluid from the lung (thoracentesis).

HOW TO PREVENT
* Learn and use proper techniques for activities listed above (especially ascending in scuba diving).
* Obtain medical treatment for lung disorders such as asthma or emphysema.
* Don't smoke.

WHAT TO EXPECT

DIAGNOSTIC MEASURES
* Your own observation of symptoms.
* Medical history and physical exam by a doctor.
* X-rays of the chest to confirm the diagnosis.

SURGERY—Sometimes necessary to close a persistent air leak.

NORMAL COURSE OF DISORDER—A small pneumothorax is not a major problem and heals itself. However, if the collapse is extensive and it occurs in middle-aged or older adults whose lungs are damaged by asthma, chronic bronchitis or emphysema, it can lead to respiratory failure and critical illness. Treatment depends on the size of the pneumothorax and the condition of the lungs.

POSSIBLE COMPLICATIONS
* Respiratory failure.
* Lung infection.
* Recurrence of pneumothorax. If it is going to recur, in 20% to 40% of cases it does so within 2 years of initial pneumothorax.

HOW TO TREAT

NOTE—Follow your doctor's instructions. These instructions are supplemental.

MEDICAL TREATMENT—Hospitalization usually required. An extensive lung collapse may require treatment with special equipment to suck out the air.

TREATMENT
* Don't exercise during healing, but resume normal activities—including the one that triggered the pneumothorax—after clearance from your doctor.
* Don't smoke.
* Try not to cough.
* Avoid loud talking, laughing or singing.
* You may be more comfortable if you rest in a sitting or semireclining position.

MEDICATION—Medication usually is not necessary. However, you may use non-prescription drugs such as acetaminophen for minor pain. For severe pain, your doctor may prescribe stronger pain relievers.

ACTIVITY—Bed rest. Your doctor will advise you when to resume your normal activities. Allow about 2 to 3 weeks for lung to re-expand. Allow 6 weeks before returning to maximum exercise.

DIET—No special diet.

CALL YOUR DOCTOR IF

* You have symptoms of pneumothorax.
* The following occur during treatment: temperature rises to 101°F (38.3°C); chest pain or shortness of breath increases; painful, debilitating coughing or sputum production begins.

POISON IVY, OAK, SUMAC

 GENERAL INFORMATION

DEFINITION—A type of contact dermatitis. The skin reaction (sometimes severe) results from contact with an oily substance (resin) produced by these three plants. This particular allergic reaction is the most common in the U.S. and about 50% of the population has developed an allergy to these plants.

SIGNS & SYMPTOMS—Skin rash with the following signs:
• Bright red papules and plaques that develop 24 to 48 hours (sometimes may take several days) after contact.
• Weeping, crusting and swelling.
• Intense itching and burning.
• The rash forms a linear pattern.
• Blistering (the fluid in blisters is not contagious).
• Enough of the oily resin remains on hands or clothing so that the rash is carried to other body parts, such as the face or genitalia.

CAUSES & RISK FACTORS
• Allergic reaction from contact with any part of poison ivy, poison oak or poison sumac plants. They grow as vines or bushes and have three leaflets (poison ivy and poison oak) or a row of paired leaflets (poison sumac). They produce a potent resin (or oil) that is responsible for the problem. A reaction may also occur from touching the poison substance on clothing, equipment (hunting, golf or athletic), or animals such as pets; and from any smoke these plants give off when burned (may affect the face, eyelids, throat and lungs).
• Risk increases in spring and summer (though plants are dangerous year round) and when not wearing protective clothing.

HOW TO PREVENT
• Learn to identify and avoid contact with these plants.
• When walking in areas where these plants grow, wear shoes, socks, long pants, long sleeved shirts and sometimes, gloves. Wash this clothing as soon thereafter as possible.
• If you are exposed, washing the skin immediately with soap and water and sponging with rubbing alcohol may prevent the rash.

 WHAT TO EXPECT

DIAGNOSTIC MEASURES
• Your own observation of symptoms.
• Medical history and physical exam by a doctor (sometimes).

SURGERY—None useful for this disorder.

NORMAL COURSE OF DISORDER—Itching, redness and swelling are often improved by the second day, and complete healing occurs within 7-14 days.

POSSIBLE COMPLICATIONS—Development of a secondary bacteria infection.

 HOW TO TREAT

NOTE—Follow your doctor's instructions. These instructions are supplemental.

MEDICAL TREATMENT—Doctor's treatment for severe cases.

HOME TREATMENT
• Sweating and heat make the itching worse, so stay cool if possible.
• Apply cool compresses to the affected area.
• A soothing bath helps. Use Aveeno (a commercial product) or baking soda (about a half cup) per bath.
• Wash all clothing and shoes and any equipment that came in contact with the plant oils with soap and water.
• Give pets a warm, soapy bath to remove any oil from the fur.

MEDICATION
• You may use calamine lotion to relieve the itching; oral antihistamines may be helpful also.
• Your doctor may prescribe topical or oral steroid drugs for severe symptoms.

ACTIVITY—No restrictions. Avoid activities that can cause sweating. This can worsen itching.

DIET—No special diet.

 CALL YOUR DOCTOR IF

• If the rash seems severe.
• If swelling or pain develops around the eyes, nose or genitals.
• Rash worsens or doesn't improve with self-care methods.

POTASSIUM IMBALANCE

GENERAL INFORMATION

DEFINITION—Above-normal levels (hyperkalemia) or below-normal levels (hypokalemia) of potassium in the blood, body fluids and body cells.

SIGNS & SYMPTOMS
Hyperkalemia:
- Weakness and paralysis.
- Dangerously rapid, irregular heartbeat or slow heartbeat (sometimes).
- Nausea and diarrhea.

Hypokalemia:
- Muscle cramps, particularly following or during exercise.
- Weakness and paralysis.
- Low blood pressure.
- Life-threatening rapid, irregular heartbeat. This is more severe than with hyperkalemia.

CAUSES & RISK FACTORS
Hypokalemia:
- The use of diuretic drugs for any purpose. Taking diuretics is a frequent—but unwise and unethical—practice among athletes who must meet a certain weight limit before competing (jockeys, boxers, wrestlers).
- Prolonged loss of body fluids from vomiting or diarrhea.
- Chronic kidney disease with kidney failure. At certain stages, this may cause the body to lose potassium.
- Uncontrolled diabetes mellitus.
- Adrenal disease.
- Use of drugs, including diuretics, potassium supplements and digitalis. Low potassium levels—especially in persons who take digitalis—often lead to serious heartbeat disturbances.

Hypokalemia:
- Chromic kidney disease with kidney failure. Failing kidneys eliminate potassium too slowly, causing an excess in the body.
- Use of oral potassium supplements without monitoring of potassium levels.
- Burns or crushing injuries. These may cause potassium to be released from body tissues into body fluids.

HOW TO PREVENT
- If you have a disorder or take drugs that affect potassium levels (see Causes & Risk Factors), learn as much as you can about your condition, your drugs and how you can prevent a potassium imbalance.
- If you take digitalis and diuretics, have frequent blood studies to monitor potassium levels.
- For prolonged vomiting or diarrhea, reduce athletic activities and seek medical care.

OTHER—A medium to high blood level of potassium (in the normal range) may help protect against coronary artery disease.

WHAT TO EXPECT

DIAGNOSTIC MEASURES
- Your own observation of symptoms, especially muscle weakness and heart rhythm changes.
- Medical history and exam by a doctor.
- Laboratory blood and urine studies of potassium, sodium and other electrolytes.
- EKG (see Glossary).

NORMAL COURSE OF DISORDER—Usually can be corrected with replacing lost fluids in the body and treatment of the underlying disorder.

POSSIBLE COMPLICATIONS—Cardiac arrest and possibly death.

HOW TO TREAT

NOTE—Follow your doctor's instructions. These instructions are supplemental.

MEDICAL TREATMENT
- Monitoring of blood potassium levels, treatment of underlying disorders and prescription of medications by a doctor.
- Hospitalization (severe cases).

HOME TREATMENT—If you take diuretics and digitalis, your friends and family members should learn cardiopulmonary resuscitation (CPR). Learn to count your own pulse at the wrist or neck, and report major changes to your doctor.

MEDICATION—Your doctor may prescribe:
- Oral potassium supplements to raise low levels.
- Diuretics to increase urination and decrease high potassium levels.
- Fluids given through a vein (IV) to correct a serious loss.
- Medications appropriate for the underlying disease.

ACTIVITY—Resume your normal activities after clearance from your doctor when symptoms improve.

DIET—Depends on the condition. Mild hypokalemia can be corrected by increasing potassium-containing foods in your diet, such as apricots, cantaloupes, bananas and citrus. There is no special diet for hyperkalemia.

CALL YOUR DOCTOR IF

You have symptoms of a potassium imbalance or are having problems with a disorder that affects potassium levels.

PRICKLY HEAT
(Miliaria Rubra)

 ## GENERAL INFORMATION

DEFINITION—A skin disorder that starts with a itchy rash caused by obstructed sweat-gland ducts. It tends to affect areas of the body where sweat collects (armpits, waist, upper trunk, insides of the elbows).

SIGNS & SYMPTOMS
- Clusters of vesicles (small, fluid-filled skin blisters that may come and go within a matter of hours) or red rash without vesicles in areas of heavy perspiration.
- Lack of sleep due to the irritation of the rash.

CAUSES & RISK FACTORS
- Obstruction of sweat-gland ducts for reasons not clearly known.
Risk increases with:
- Obesity.
- Stress.
- Fever.
- Hot, humid weather.
- Plastic undersheets.

HOW TO PREVENT
- Avoid wearing heavy tight clothing or garments that cause friction on the skin.
- Avoid situations that cause excessive sweating if possible.
- Avoid contact with skin irritants or excessive use of soap.
- In hot weather, use air conditioning, fans and take cool showers or baths.

 ## WHAT TO EXPECT

DIAGNOSTIC MEASURES
- Your own observation of symptoms.
- Medical history and physical exam by a doctor (severe cases only).

SURGERY—None useful or necessary for this disorder.

NORMAL COURSE OF DISORDER—Usually will clear up on its own if affected area is kept cool and dry. Recurrence is common.

POSSIBLE COMPLICATIONS—Secondary skin infection.

 ## HOW TO TREAT

NOTE—Follow your doctor's instructions if provided. These instructions are supplemental.

MEDICAL TREATMENT—Doctor's treatment, if home care fails.

HOME TREATMENT
- Take frequent cool showers or tub baths.
- Avoid the use topical products on the skin that may trap more sweat (e.g., powder, lotion, antiperspirant).
- Use cool-water soaks to relieve itching and hasten healing. Pat skin dry, and dust with cornstarch after and between soaks.
- Wear cotton socks and leather-soled footwear rather than shoes made of man-made materials.
- Expose the affected skin to air as much as possible.
- Don't use binding materials, such as adhesive tape, or wear tight clothing.
- Change diapers on infants as soon as they are wet.
- Avoid sunburn once you have had prickly heat. The body's inflammatory reaction to sunburn may trigger a new outbreak of prickly heat.
- Provide cool, dry environment.

MEDICATION
- To relieve itching, you may try calamine lotion or nonprescription 1% steroid cream (apply 2 or 3 times a day).
- Oral antibiotics may be prescribed if there is a secondary bacterial infection.

ACTIVITY—Decrease activity during hot, humid weather or until skin heals.

DIET—No special diet.

 ## CALL YOUR DOCTOR IF

- Prickly heat doesn't improve in a few days, despite home care.
- You develop a skin infection in the area where you have prickly heat.

RINGWORM
(Tinea Infection)

GENERAL INFORMATION

DEFINITION—Fungus (tinea) infection of the skin or scalp. The infection results from contact with infected person or animal, or by contact with infected surfaces, such as combs, brushes, towels, shoes, shower stalls or children's toys. *Tinea corporis* affects the nonhairy skin of the body. *Tinea capitis* affects the scalp.

SIGNS & SYMPTOMS—Red, itchy, circular, flat, scaling lesions with well-defined borders. They cause patchy hair loss on the scalp.

CAUSES & RISK FACTORS—Fungus infection. It is more likely to occur when combined with the following:
- Diabetes mellitus.
- Exposure to darkness, moisture and warmth.
- Crowded or unsanitary locker room or living conditions.
- Existing cuts or scratches on the skin.
- Repeated abrasion of the skin or scalp from friction with clothing and protective gear. An athlete is especially vulnerable during hot weather when exercising while wearing an athletic uniform or head covering such as a swimming cap, football helmet or baseball cap.

HOW TO PREVENT—The fungi are so prevalent that total prevention is impossible. To minimize risk:
- Avoid continuous exposure to overheated humid environments.
- Avoid close contact with infected person and don't share personal items such as brushes or clothing or hats.
- Don't touch pets that have skin problems.

WHAT TO EXPECT

DIAGNOSTIC MEASURES
- Your own observation of symptoms.
- Medical history and physical exam by a doctor if needed.
- Microscopic exam of skin scrapings suspended in potassium hydroxide solution.
- Laboratory culture of skin scrapings.

SURGERY—Not necessary or useful for this disorder

NORMAL COURSE OF DISORDER—Usually curable in several weeks with treatment, but recurrence is common.

POSSIBLE COMPLICATIONS
- Secondary bacterial infection of ringworm lesions.
- Ringworm becomes chronic in some cases.

HOW TO TREAT

NOTE—Follow your doctor's instructions if provided. These instructions are supplemental.

MEDICAL TREATMENT—None necessary after diagnosis.

HOME TREATMENT
- Practice good locker room hygiene (wear thong sandals for showering, don't share towels or other personal items).
- Boil or chemically sterilize all clothing, towels or bed linens that have touched the lesions.
- Keep the skin dry. Moist, dark areas favor fungus growth.
- Wear cotton underwear. Change more than once a day if necessary. Avoid tight clothes.
- If the area is red, swollen and weeping, use saltwater compresses (1 teaspoon salt to 1 pint water). Apply 4 times a day for 2 to 3 days before starting the local antifungal medication.
- For scalp infections: Shampoo the hair every day. Have the hair cut short, but don't shave the scalp. Place large sheets of paper under and around the hair and chair to catch all the clippings. Place a cloth drape around the shoulders, chest and back. Don't wear street clothes for a haircut. Wear something that can be sterilized, such as pajamas, a housecoat or smock. Repeat this procedure every 2 weeks for 6 months.

MEDICATION—Your doctor may prescribe topical antifungal drugs in creams, lotions or ointments to be used for 2-4 weeks. For severe cases, an oral antifungal medication may be prescribed.

ACTIVITY—No restrictions

DIET—No special diet.

CALL YOUR DOCTOR IF

- You have symptoms of ringworm.
- Ringworm lesions become redder and painful and ooze pus.
- Symptoms don't improve in 3 or 4 weeks, despite treatment.
- New, unexplained symptoms develop. Drugs used in treatment may produce side effects.

RUNNER'S KNEE
(Patellofemoral Pain Syndrome)

 GENERAL INFORMATION

DEFINITION—Aching pain behind the kneecap (patella). Pain begins and progresses slowly. It appears in healthy, physically active young people between 12 and 36 years of age, and is twice as common in women as in men.

SIGNS & SYMPTOMS
- Soreness and aching pain around or under the kneecap, especially on the inner side. Symptoms worsen after walking or running up ramps or hills, squatting or jumping up and running.
- A rubbing or clicking sound may be heard.
- "Giving way" at the knee (sometimes).

CAUSES & RISK FACTORS
- Usually caused by the kneecap's not "tracking" properly.
- Having physical problem such as leg length difference, thigh bone that turns inward, "knock knee" or flat foot.
- Lack of strength or flexibility in surrounding muscles.
- Imbalance in the leg muscles that causes the kneecap to be pulled sideways.
- Overstress of the knee, as can occur in any running sport, such as jogging, sprinting, football, basketball or soccer.

HOW TO PREVENT
- Strengthen and condition upper leg and hip muscles for maximum strength, flexibility and endurance before you start competition or vigorous physical activity.
- Avoid deep squats or activities that compress the kneecap.
- Don't use knee wraps for weightlifting. Wraps increase knee compression.

 WHAT TO EXPECT

DIAGNOSTIC MEASURES
- Your own observation of symptoms.
- Medical history and exam by a doctor.
- Sometimes, x-rays, CT or MRI of the knee.
- Rarely, arthroscopy helps confirm the diagnosis and may provide treatment as well.

SURGERY—Rarely necessary. In surgery, cartilage is shaved using an arthroscope (see Glossary). Open-knee surgery may be necessary to realign the kneecap.

NORMAL COURSE OF DISORDER—Full function of the knee with successful treatment. Adherence to the prescribed exercise program is necessary for recovery. Allow 4-6 weeks for healing.

POSSIBLE COMPLICATIONS—Nonhealing with conservative measures.

 HOW TO TREAT

NOTE—Follow your doctor's instructions. These instructions are supplemental.

MEDICAL TREATMENT
- Often none is necessary after diagnosis and recommendations for strength and flexibility training.
- Therapists may recommend changes alternatives or restrictions to your physical activities, until the knee is healed.
- Taping of the knee may be recommended.
- For some, orthotics (shoe inserts) or a knee brace help correct the physical problems.

HOME TREATMENT
For acute pain or discomfort:
- Trying to "work through" or "run through" pain worsens the condition.
- Apply ice bags for 10 minutes for 4 times a day for 2 to 4 days.
- After ice treatments end, apply heat frequently. Use heat lamps, hot soaks, hot showers, heating pads or heat liniments and ointments.
- Your doctor may prescribe orthotic shoe devices, knee straps or braces. Proper footwear is important.

MEDICATION—You may use ibuprofen or other nonsteroidal anti-inflammatory medicine for pain.

ACTIVITY
- When pain has subsided, start on quadriceps exercises for rehabilitation.
- Stay active even though you may not be able to participate in your sport of choice for a period of time. Swimming is a good alternative.
- Resume athletic training when the injured leg reaches 75% of the strength of the other leg.

DIET—Eat a well-balanced diet. Increase fiber and fluid intake to prevent constipation that may result from decreased activity.

 CALL YOUR DOCTOR IF

You have symptoms of runner's knee that don't improve after resting for 2 or 3 days.

SCABIES

GENERAL INFORMATION

DEFINITION—A disease of the skin caused by a parasitic mite (the "itch" mite) involving the skin of the finger webs and folds under the arms, breasts, elbows, genitals and buttocks. Scabies is contagious from person to person (by shared clothing or bed linen) and from one site to another in the same person. Outbreaks are likely among teammates using crowded locker room facilities.

SIGNS & SYMPTOMS
- Small, itchy blisters on several parts of the body. The blisters break easily when scratched.
- Broken blisters leave scratch marks and thickened skin, crisscrossed by grooves and scaling.

CAUSES & RISK FACTORS—Infestation by a mite (*Sarcoptes scabiei*) that burrows into deep skin layers, where the female mite deposits eggs. Eggs mature into adult mites in 3 weeks. Mites are 0.1 mm in diameter and can be seen only under a microscope. Scratching collects mites and eggs under the fingernails, so they spread to other parts of the body. Spreading increases with crowded or unsanitary living conditions.

HOW TO PREVENT
- Avoid contact with persons or linen and clothing that you suspect may be infected with scabies.
- Maintain personal cleanliness: Bathe daily, or at least 2 or 3 times a week.
- Wash hands before eating.
- Launder clothes often.
- Observe good locker room hygiene.

WHAT TO EXPECT

DIAGNOSTIC MEASURES
- Your own observation of symptoms.
- Medical history and physical exam by a doctor. The diagnosis is confirmed by discovering the mite, lifting it with a needle or sharp scalpel point from its burrow, and identifying it under a microscope. Other simple diagnostic tests are available and may be used for children or those with few burrows.

SURGERY—Not necessary or useful with this disease.

NORMAL COURSE OF DISORDER—Itching usually disappears quickly, and evidence of the disease is gone in 1 to 2 weeks with treatment. If skin irritation persists longer than this, oral antihistamines or topical steroids may be necessary to break the itch-scratch cycle. When untreated, scabies can last for years.

POSSIBLE COMPLICATIONS—Secondary bacterial infection of mite-infested areas of inflammation.

HOW TO TREAT

NOTE—Follow your doctor's instructions. These instructions are supplemental.

MEDICAL TREATMENT—For diagnosis and follow up to be sure treatment is effective.

HOME TREATMENT
- All family members and those in close contact with the infected person should receive treatment.
- Bathe thoroughly before applying the prescribed medicine.
- Apply medicine from the neck down, and cover the entire body.
- Wait 15 minutes before dressing.
- Carefully wash all clothes used prior to or during treatment. You don't need to clean furniture or floors with special care.
- Leave medicine on the skin for 8-14 hours (or as directed) before bathing. Usually a one time treatment is sufficient, but some medications may be applied for 2-3 successive nights.
- You may need to repeat the treatment in 1 week. Ask your doctor.
- If many members of a team are infested, it will be most effective to treat the entire team, including those without symptoms, at one time. Lockers should also be disinfected.

MEDICATION
- Topical medications such as permethrin or lindane to clear up the infection. Infants, young infants and pregnant women may need a treatment that is considered less toxic. Oral medication may be prescribed for some cases where topical therapy is difficult or not practical.
- Antipruritic medications, such as antihistamines, if needed to help relieve the itching.
- Steroid or antibiotic treatment in rare cases.

ACTIVITY—No restrictions. Avoid skin-to-skin contact with others until healing is complete.

DIET—No special diet.

CALL YOUR DOCTOR IF

- You have symptoms of scabies.
- After treatment, the lesions show signs of infection (redness, pus, swelling or pain).
- New, unexplained symptoms develop. Drugs used in treatment may produce side effects.

SKIN CANCER, BASAL CELL

GENERAL INFORMATION

DEFINITION—Skin cancer affecting the skin's basal layer (the 5th layer). Basal cell skin cancer invades areas under the skin and it rarely spreads (metastasize) to distant areas. Skin of the face, ears, backs of hands, shoulders and arms is most frequently affected.

SIGNS & SYMPTOMS
- A small skin lesion that does not heal in 3 weeks.
- The lesion appears flat and "pearly." Its edges are translucent and rounded or rolled. The edges may have small, curvy, new blood vessels. The ulcer in the center is dimpled. Lesion size varies from 4 mm to 6 mm, but it may grow larger if untreated.
- The lesion occurs on skin that is exposed to the sun and shows evidence of sun damage.
- The lesion grows slowly. It does not hurt or itch.

CAUSES & RISK FACTORS—Skin damage from sun that occurs many years prior to the cancer's appearance. Persons most at risk include:
- Athletes who exercise, train and play outdoors.
- Persons over age 60.
- Previous radiation treatment.
- Chronic inflammation of the skin.
- Those with family history of skin cancer.
- Use of tobacco products (lip and oral cancers).
- Persons with a fair complexion.

HOW TO PREVENT
- Limit exposure to sun. Protect skin from sun exposure with a head covering, clothing and sunscreen. Protection is important in children.
- Doctor visits for skin examination and your own self-examination. Can help detect and often treat skin conditions that could be a cancer risk.
- Seek treatment for any chronic skin inflammation or skin trauma.

WHAT TO EXPECT

DIAGNOSTIC MEASURES
- Your own observation of symptoms.
- Medical history and physical exam by a doctor.
- Skin biopsy. Pathological exam of tissue after removal to confirm diagnosis.

SURGERY—Usually necessary and can be fairly minor. See Medical Treatment below.

NORMAL COURSE OF DISORDER—Curable with treatment. Surgery is the usual treatment. Other nonsurgery options are sometimes recommended and newer treatment methods are being researched and tested. Long term follow up after treatment is important.

POSSIBLE COMPLICATIONS
- Without treatment, cancers may enlarge and change in the way they look.
- 2-6% skin cancers spread to other sites. Recurrence is a possibility (most happen within 5 years). New skin cancers may develop.
- Rarely, infection or excessive bleeding may occur after surgical treatment.

HOW TO TREAT

NOTE—Follow your doctor's instructions. These instructions are supplemental.

MEDICAL TREATMENT—Removal of cancer by one of several methods. The treatment method is chosen in a doctor-patient conference:
- Surgery in the doctor's office or an outpatient surgical unit of the hospital. Surgical options include simple excision, electrosurgery, cryosurgery, Moh's surgery, laser surgery and others. Skin grafting may be necessary.
- Radiation treatment.
- Follow up evaluation every 2-12 months for skin check up. Frequency will depend on individual risk of recurrence, new skin cancers and chances of cancer spreading.

HOME TREATMENT—After surgery, follow the instructions provided by your doctor for wound care.

MEDICATION—After surgery:
- For minor pain, you may use nonprescription drugs, such as acetaminophen.
- Your doctor may prescribe an antibiotic ointment to prevent wound infection.

ACTIVITY—Depending on the type of surgery and the work you do, your activity may be restricted one or more days. Your doctor will provide specific instructions. After the wound heals, there are usually no restrictions.

DIET—No special diet.

CALL YOUR DOCTOR IF

- You have symptoms of basal cell skin cancer.
- The wound bleeds after surgery and the bleeding cannot be stopped by applying pressure for a few minutes.
- The wound shows signs of infection, such as pain, redness, swelling or increased tenderness.

SKIN CANCER, SQUAMOUS CELL

GENERAL INFORMATION

DEFINITION—A malignant growth of the epithelial layer (external surface) of the skin, especially in areas exposed to the sun, such as the face, ears, hands or arms.

SIGNS & SYMPTOMS—A small, firm, scaling raised bump on the skin with a crusting ulcer in the center. The bump doesn't hurt or itch.

CAUSES & RISK FACTORS—Skin damage from sun that occurs many years prior to the cancer's appearance. Persons most at risk include:
* Athletes who exercise, train and play outdoors.
* Persons over age 60.
* Previous radiation treatment.
* Chronic inflammation of the skin.
* Those with family history of skin cancer.
* Use of tobacco products (lip and oral cancers).
* Persons with a fair complexion.

HOW TO PREVENT
* Limit exposure to sun. Protect skin from sun exposure with a head covering, clothing and sunscreen. Protection is important in children.
* Doctor visits for skin examination and your own self-examination. Can help detect and often treat skin conditions that could be a cancer risk.
* Seek treatment for any chronic skin inflammation or skin trauma.

WHAT TO EXPECT

DIAGNOSTIC MEASURES
* Your own observation of symptoms.
* Medical history and physical exam by a doctor.
* Skin biopsy. Pathological exam of tissue after removal to confirm diagnosis.

SURGERY—Usually necessary and can be fairly minor. See Medical Treatment below.

NORMAL COURSE OF DISORDER—Curable with treatment. Surgery is the usual treatment. Other nonsurgery options are sometimes recommended and newer treatment methods are being researched and tested. Long term follow up after treatment is important.

POSSIBLE COMPLICATIONS
* Without treatment, cancers may enlarge and change in the way they look.
* 2-6% skin cancers spread to other sites. Recurrence is a possibility (most happen within 5 years). New skin cancers may develop.
* Rarely, infection or excessive bleeding may occur after surgical treatment.

HOW TO TREAT

NOTE—Follow your doctor's instructions. These instructions are supplemental.

MEDICAL TREATMENT—Removal of skin cancer by one of several methods. The treatment method is chosen in a doctor-patient conference:
* Surgery in the doctor's office or an outpatient surgical unit of the hospital. Surgical options include simple excision, electrosurgery, cryosurgery, Moh's surgery, laser surgery and others. Skin grafting may be necessary.
* Radiation treatment.
* Follow up evaluation every 2-12 months for skin check up. Frequency will depend on individual risk of recurrence, new skin cancers and chances of cancer spreading.

HOME TREATMENT—After surgery, follow the instructions provided by your doctor for wound care.

MEDICATION—After surgery:
* For minor pain, you may use nonprescription drugs, such as acetaminophen.
* Your doctor may prescribe an antibiotic ointment to prevent wound infection.

ACTIVITY—Depending on the type of surgery and the work you do, your activity may be restricted one or more days. Your doctor will provide specific instructions. After the wound heals, there are usually no restrictions.

DIET—No special diet.

CALL YOUR DOCTOR IF

* You have symptoms of basal cell skin cancer.
* The wound bleeds after surgery and the bleeding cannot be stopped by applying pressure for a few minutes.
* The wound shows signs of infection, such as pain, redness, swelling or increased tenderness.

SODIUM IMBALANCE

GENERAL INFORMATION

DEFINITION—Above-normal level (hypernatremia) or below-normal level (hyponatremia) of sodium in the blood.

SIGNS & SYMPTOMS—Any of the following:
- Muscle cramps (usually in the legs), particularly following or during exercise.
- Confusion.
- Restlessness and anxiety.
- Weakness.
- Changes in pulse rate and blood pressure.
- Tissue swelling (edema).
- Stupor or coma. Sodium imbalance may be part of a disease with other symptoms that predominate, such as fever, vomiting, diarrhea or excessive sweating.

CAUSES & RISK FACTORS
Hypernatremia:
- Inability to drink water, as with stroke or gastrointestinal diseases.
- Use of cortisone drugs or anabolic steroids.
- Excessive intake of salty food or liquid, as in near drowning in salt water.
- Diabetes mellitus.
- Congestive heart failure.
- Kidney diseases. Healthy kidneys can usually control sodium levels.
Hyponatremia:
- Use of diuretics. Diuretics are used for serious medical problems such as hypertension and disorders of the kidney, liver and heart. They are sometimes used unwisely and not appropriately by athletes who need to meet a certain weight limit (boxers, wrestlers, jockeys). Coupled with excessive sweating, heat and exercise, diuretics can cause severe sodium imbalance.
- Poor kidney function.
- Excessive fluid intake.
- Prolonged loss of body fluids from vomiting or diarrhea.
- Infections with high fever.

HOW TO PREVENT—If you take diuretics for any reason and exercise strenuously, make sure you drink extra water, but not too excess. Eat a generous diet. Do not drink salt mixtures such as Gatorade or take salt tablets. They may compound any developing problem.

WHAT TO EXPECT

DIAGNOSTIC MEASURES
- Your own observation of symptoms.
- Medical history and physical exam by a doctor.
- Laboratory blood and urine studies of sodium and other electrolytes.

SURGERY—Not necessary or useful for this disorder.

NORMAL COURSE OF DISORDER—Usually can be corrected by replacing lost fluids and treatment of the underlying disorder.

POSSIBLE COMPLICATIONS—Shock and death from severe fluid and sodium imbalance following vigorous exercise in hot weather.

HOW TO TREAT

NOTE—Follow your doctor's instructions. These instructions are supplemental.

MEDICAL TREATMENT—Hospitalization (sometimes).

HOME TREATMENT—If you have a disorder or take drugs that cause sodium balance, learn as much as possible about your drugs, your condition and how to prevent a sodium imbalance.

MEDICATION—Your doctor may prescribe:
- Sodium given through a vein (IV) if sodium levels are low.
- Medications to correct underlying disorders.

ACTIVITY—Resume your normal activities after recovery.

DIET
- No special diet usually for low sodium levels. Your doctor may recommend fluid restriction.
- If high sodium is a problem, your doctor may prescribed a low-salt diet.
- If you take diuretics, don't drink alcohol. Diuretics combined with alcohol use and excessive sweating can cause life-threatening shock.

CALL YOUR DOCTOR IF

- You have symptoms of a sodium imbalance.
- You are having problems with a disorder that affects sodium levels.

STRESS INCONTINENCE

GENERAL INFORMATION

DEFINITION—A leaking of urine that occurs with any action that increases pressure in the abdomen. This is most common when jumping, running or straining (as with lifting weights).

SIGNS & SYMPTOMS—Loss of urine (in drops or spurts or larger amount) with exercise, lifting, sneezing, singing, coughing, laughing, crying or straining to have a bowel movement.

CAUSES & RISK FACTORS
• Loss of the normal muscle support for the bladder and floor of the pelvis. For women, this happens during pregnancy and after childbirth. In men, prostate surgery or radiation may cause the problem. The pelvic muscles also weaken as a natural part of aging. The problem is made worse by obesity or chronic constipation.
• Problems of the urethra (tube that carries urine from the bladder to the outside). It does not close properly or it moves too easily in the body.

HOW TO PREVENT
• Empty your bladder before exercise.
• Eat a normal, well-balanced diet and exercise regularly to build and maintain muscle strength.
• Learn and practice Kegel exercises (see Home Treatment).

WHAT TO EXPECT

DIAGNOSTIC MEASURES
• Your own observation of symptoms.
• Medical history and physical exam by a doctor.
• Urinalysis to check for infection.

SURGERY—Sometimes needed for men or women to correct the problem. Different options are used. For women, this surgery may be done along with other female surgery.

NORMAL COURSE OF DISORDER—Treatment will help improve the symptoms for many patients and cure the problem for some. If it is severe, it can be treated with surgery.

POSSIBLE COMPLICATIONS
• Feelings of embarrassment and shame about the problem can affect all areas of your life.
• Bladder infection.
• Vaginal irritation in women.

HOW TO TREAT

NOTE—Follow your doctor's instructions. These instructions are supplemental.

MEDICAL TREATMENT
Your doctor may recommend one or more of a variety of treatments. Details about each one will be discussed with you. You need to be involved with the treatment plan and follow it. Progress may be slow, but stick with the plan.
• A pessary (support device) made of plastic, rubber or other material to fit inside the vagina to support the uterus and the lower muscle layer of the bladder.
• Kegel exercises for pelvic muscles.
• Weighted cones to be placed in the vagina for help in making pelvic muscles stronger.
• Bladder training exercises.
• Electrical stimulation for the pelvic muscles.
• Implanted electrodes to stimulate nerves.
• Inserts placed in the urethra to block urine.
• Medications.

HOME TREATMENT—Learn to recognize, control and develop the muscles of the pelvic floor. These are the ones you use to interrupt the urine in midstream. The following exercises (Kegel exercises) strengthen these muscles so you can control or relax them completely:
• To identify which muscles are involved, first start and then stop urination when using the toilet. Another method is to place a finger just inside the opening of your vagina and squeeze the finger with your vaginal muscles.
• Practice tightening and releasing these muscles while sitting, standing, walking, driving, watching TV or listening to music.
• Tighten the muscles a small amount at a time "like an elevator going up to the 10th floor." Then release very slowly, "one floor at a time."
• Tighten the muscles from front to back, including the anus, as in the previous exercise.
• Practice exercises every morning, afternoon and evening. Gradually work up to doing the exercises a total of 150 to 200 times a day.
• Wear pads or underwear made to absorb urine. Use other products for beds, chairs, etc.

MEDICATION—Your doctor may prescribe:
• Antibiotics if you have a urinary tract infection.
• Drugs to relax the bladder, increase its volume, stop bladder spasms, or improve muscle strength.
• Estrogen therapy for women.
• Collagen injection (helps urethra close tightly).

ACTIVITY—No restrictions.

DIET—Follow a weight-loss diet if you are overweight.

CALL YOUR DOCTOR IF

• You have symptoms of stress incontinence.
• Signs of infection develop (e.g., fever, painful or frequent urination, or a general ill feeling.
• Symptoms don't improve with one type of treatment and you want to discuss a different treatment step.

SUNBURN

GENERAL INFORMATION

DEFINITION—Skin inflammation and damage that follows overexposure to the sun, sun lamps or occupational light sources.
- First-degree burn consists of mild redness.
- Second-degree burn has redness and blisters.
- Third-degree burn includes redness, blisters and skin ulceration. Sunburn is common in athletes because of frequent exposure to sunlight for long periods. Sunburn can result also from exposure to winter sun, especially at high altitudes.

SIGNS & SYMPTOMS
- Red, swollen, painful, stinging, blistered and sometimes ulcerated skin.
- Chills and fever.
- Nausea and vomiting (severe burns).
- Severe, extensive burns may cause fever, headache, nausea, vomiting and dehydration.
- Tanning or peeling of the skin after recovery, depending on severity of the burn.

CAUSES & RISK FACTORS—Excess
exposure to ultraviolet (UV) light. The following factors make a person more susceptible to sunburn:
- Genetic factors, especially fair skin, blue eyes and red or blonde hair.
- Use of drugs, including sulfa, tetracyclines, amoxicillin or oral contraceptives.

HOW TO PREVENT
- Avoid sun exposure from 11 a.m. to 3 p.m.
- Use a sun-block preparation for outdoor activity. Use products with a sun protective factor of 15 or more. Reapply after swimming or after prolonged exposure. Baby oil, mineral oil or cocoa butter offer no protection from the sun.
- For maximum protection, use a physical barrier agent such as zinc oxide ointment. Reapply after swimming and at frequent intervals during exposure. Barrier agents are especially helpful on skin areas that are most susceptible to burns, such as the nose, ears, backs of the legs and back of the neck.
- Wear clothes that have colors, such as tan, to protect skin from sun. Avoid brilliant colors and whites, which reflect the sun into your face.
- Wear a wide-brimmed hat and sunglasses.
- If you insist on tanning, limit your sun exposure on the first day to 5 or 10 minutes on each side. Add 5 minutes per side each day.

WHAT TO EXPECT

DIAGNOSTIC MEASURES
- Your own observation of symptoms.
- Medical history and exam by a doctor if needed.

NORMAL COURSE OF DISORDER—
Recovery in 3 days to 3 weeks, depending on the severity of the sunburn.

POSSIBLE COMPLICATIONS
- Usually no complications from mild sunburn; if sunburn is severe, the symptoms may need a doctor's treatment.
- Long term sun exposure can cause a variety of sun-damage-related disorders, such as erythema multiforme, vitiligo, heatstroke, porphyria, lupus erythematosus or photosensitivity and skin changes leading to skin cancer, including life-threatening malignant melanoma.

HOW TO TREAT

NOTE—Follow your doctor's instructions if provided. These instructions are supplemental.

MEDICAL TREATMENT—A doctor's care will be necessary for severe burns and for complications of sun exposure.

HOME TREATMENT
- To reduce heat and pain, dip gauze or towels in cool water and lay these on the burn.
- Take cool (not cold) showers or baths. Using vinegar in bathwater helps take the sting out. Aveeno (a commercial oatmeal product).

MEDICATION
- Use nonprescription drugs, such as aspirin (do not give to children) or acetaminophen, to relieve pain and reduce any fever.
- Use a moisturizing product for the skin if there are no blisters. An aloe vera lotion may help.
- Avoid remedies that contain benzocaine or lidocaine as they produce allergic reactions in some. Avoid petroleum jelly as it does not allow sweat and heat to escape from the skin.
- Your doctor may prescribe pain relievers or cortisone drugs to use briefly.

ACTIVITY—No restrictions except as needed to protect the sunburned areas from any further irritation. Stay out of the sun while the sunburn heals.

DIET—No special diet. Increase fluid intake.

CALL YOUR DOCTOR IF

The following occur after sunburn:
- Oral temperature rises to 101°F (38.3°C).
- Vomiting, chills, tiredness, weakness occurs.
- Pain and fever persist longer than 48 hours.

THORACIC OUTLET OBSTRUCTION SYNDROME (Cervical Rib Syndrome; Serratus Anticus Syndrome)

GENERAL INFORMATION

DEFINITION—Pain and weakness from compression of nerves in the neck. These nerves affect the shoulders, arms and hands.

SIGNS & SYMPTOMS—One or more of the following:
• Pain, numbness and tingling in the neck, shoulders, arms and hands.
• Weakness in the arms and fingers.
• Headache; cold intolerance.

CAUSES & RISK FACTORS—The nerves and blood vessels that supply the shoulder, arms and hands start in the neck and pass as a bundle near the cervical ribs and collarbone. Pressure on this bundle creates symptoms. Pressure may be caused by:
• An extra rib in the lower neck (cervical rib).
• Overdevelopment of the neck muscles, as may be required with some contact sports or may result from intense weightlifting programs.
• Prolonged period with the arm or neck in an abnormal position, as can occur during surgery, when unsonscious for any reason, or while sleeping with a too-firm object under the neck.
• Injury from overextending the arm or shoulder.
• Tumor that has spread to the head and neck area from another part of the body.
• Muscle weakness and drooping in the shoulder.

HOW TO PREVENT
• Avoid shoulder and neck injury whenever possible. Wear seatbelts and use padded headrests in cars. Use shoulder pads or other protective equipment appropriate for your sport.
• Women with large breasts should wear a bra that provides good support.
• Change sleeping positions. Try sleeping on one side, or sleep without a firm pillow.
• If symptoms are caused by overdeveloped muscles in the neck, reduce exercises that affect these muscles.

WHAT TO EXPECT

DIAGNOSTIC MEASURES
• Your own observation of symptoms.
• Medical history and exam by a doctor.
• X-rays of the neck and shoulder area to look for an extra cervical rib or a tumor.

SURGERY—Sometimes necessary if a cervical rib is causing pressure on nerves and blood vessels.

NORMAL COURSE OF DISORDER
• If caused by overdevelopment of neck muscles, the disorder is usually curable with physical therapy and decreased exercises that affect these muscles.
• If caused by injury while unconscious or asleep, the disorder is usually curable with new sleeping habits and physical therapy.
• If caused by a cervical rib, the disorder is usually curable with surgery.
• If caused by a tumor, treatment may be unsuccessful.

POSSIBLE COMPLICATIONS
• Permanent numbness or loss of arm or hand strength if thoracic outlet obstruction syndrome is not treated.
• Postsurgical complications (rare).

HOW TO TREAT

NOTE—Follow your doctor's instructions. These instructions are supplemental.

MEDICAL TREATMENT
• Doctor's treatment.
• Surgery to relieve pressure on the nerves and blood vessels if a cervical rib is the underlying cause.
• Physical therapy.

HOME TREATMENT—Use heat to relieve pain. Use a heating pad, heat lamp, hot showers or warm compresses.

MEDICATION—You may use nonprescription drugs, such as acetaminophen or aspirin, to relieve pain. Your doctor may prescribe a muscle relaxant. Medication cannot correct the underlying condition.

ACTIVITY—Your doctor may prescribe physical therapy and exercises less likely to cause neck muscle overdevelopment.

DIET—No special diet.

CALL YOUR DOCTOR IF

• You have symptoms of thoracic outlet obstruction syndrome.
• Symptoms don't improve in 2 weeks, despite treatment.

TOENAIL, INGROWN

GENERAL INFORMATION

DEFINITION—A common condition in which one or both edges of a nail grows into the flesh of a toe, usually the great (big) toe. This can lead to infection and inflammation. Until treated, this problem may markedly hamper athletic performance.

SIGNS & SYMPTOMS—Pain, tenderness, redness, swelling and heat in the toe where the sharp nail edge pierces the surrounding fold of tissue. Once tissue surrounding the nail becomes inflamed, infection often develops.

CAUSES & RISK FACTORS—An ingrown toenail is likely to occur with one of the following conditions:
• The nail is more curved than normal.
• The toenail is clipped back too far, allowing tissue to grow up over it.
• Shoes fit poorly, forcing the toe of the shoe against the nail and surrounding tissue.
• Injury to the nail or infection of the nail.
• You participate in activities that requires sudden stops ("toe jamming").

HOW TO PREVENT
• Wear roomy, well-fitting shoes and socks.
• Carefully cut toenails straight across and not too short.
• If you have diabetes mellitus or circulatory disease or other disorder that causes poor healing, be very careful in trimming your toenails. Foot injury is dangerous with these disorders because of impaired blood circulation to the feet.
• If you frequently handle heavy objects in your work, consider wearing work shoes with steel toe boxes.
• Keep feet clean and dry.

WHAT TO EXPECT

DIAGNOSTIC MEASURES
• Your own observation of symptoms.
• Medical history and physical exam by a doctor if needed.

SURGERY—Sometimes necessary. The type of surgery will depend on how severe the condition is. It may involve just removing overgrown skin tissue or removing a portion of the toenail or complete removal of the toenail.

NORMAL COURSE OF DISORDER—Curable with treatment. If there is an infection, medicine usually relieve symptoms within 1 week. If an ingrown toenail occurs repeatedly despite preventive measures, then surgery is usually recommended.

POSSIBLE COMPLICATIONS—An ingrown toenail may become very painful, red and swollen with pus if treatment for infection is delayed too long. Sometimes a bloody growth called proud flesh builds up on the side of the nail.

HOW TO TREAT

NOTE—Follow your doctor's instructions if provided. These instructions are supplemental.

MEDICAL TREATMENT—May be necessary for diagnosis, non-surgical care and surgery. After surgery, your doctor will provide instructions for care of the wound.

HOME TREATMENT
The following home treatment may help prevent the need for surgery:
• Soak the toe for 20 minutes twice a day in a gallon of warm water. You may add either 2 tablespoons of epsom salts or 2 tablespoons of a mild detergent.
• Lift the nail corners gently, and wedge a very small piece of cotton under the ingrown nail edges. This will lift the nail slightly so it can grow past the skin tissue it is digging into. Replace the cotton daily. Do not cut a V in the middle of the nail. This is not helpful.

MEDICATION
• Your doctor may prescribe antibiotics to fight infection.
• There are nonprescription products that may soften the nail and the skin around it, which can help relieve the pain. Follow directions carefully. These products should not be used if you have diabetes mellitus or a blood circulation problem.

ACTIVITY
• Resume your normal activities as soon as symptoms improve. You may need to wear sandals or a shoe with the toe cut out until the toe heals.
• If you have surgery, your doctor will instruct you about aftercare, such as keeping the foot propped up as much as possible.

DIET—Eat a well-balanced diet.

CALL YOUR DOCTOR IF

• You have symptoms of an ingrown toenail that persist despite self-treatment.
• The following occur during treatment or after surgery:
  Fever.
  Increased pain.
  Signs of infection (pain, redness, tenderness, swelling or heat) in the toe.

WARTS
(Verruca Vulgaris)

GENERAL INFORMATION

DEFINITION—Benign tumors caused by a virus in the outer skin layer. Warts are not cancerous. They are contagious from person to person and from one area to another on the same person. They appear most often on the fingers, hands and arms. They are common in athletes who share locker room facilities and have close personal contact with each other.

SIGNS & SYMPTOMS—A small, raised bump on the skin with the following description:
• Warts begin very small (1 mm to 3 mm) and grow larger.
• Warts have a rough surface and clearly defined borders.
• They are usually the same color as the skin, but sometimes darker.
• Warts often appear in clusters around a "mother wart."
• If you cut into the wart's surface, it contains small black dots or bleeding points.
• Warts are painless and don't itch.

CAUSES & RISK FACTORS—Invasion of the outer skin layer (epidermis) by the *papilloma* virus. The virus makes some cells to grow more rapidly than normal. Warts are very common. By adulthood, 90% of all people have antibodies to the virus, indicating a history of at least one wart infection.

HOW TO PREVENT—To keep from spreading warts, don't scratch them. Warts spread readily to small cuts and scratches.

WHAT TO EXPECT

DIAGNOSTIC MEASURES
• Your own observation of symptoms.
• Medical history and physical exam by a doctor if needed.

SURGERY—Electrosurgery or cryotherapy is sometimes used.

NORMAL COURSE OF DISORDER—There is no one specific treatment for warts that works for everybody. Some warts go away on their own, others are cured with nonprescription drugs, while other may require a doctor's care that could include surgery. There are also many "home remedies" that may work for some people. Nonsurgical treatment for warts may take some time, so be patient.

POSSIBLE COMPLICATIONS
• Spread to other body parts.
• Secondary infection of a wart.

• Warts recur after treatment.
• Minor scars left by surgery.

HOW TO TREAT

NOTE—Follow your doctor's instructions if provided. These instructions are supplemental.

MEDICAL TREATMENT
• Cryotherapy (freezing cells to destroy them). This is a doctor's office procedure that doesn't require anesthesia or cause bleeding. Freezing stings or hurts slightly while being done, and pain may increase a bit after thawing. Treatments may be necessary 3 to 5 times a week to destroy the wart.
• Electrosurgery (using heat to destroy cells). This treatment can usually be completed in one office visit, but healing takes longer, and secondary bacterial infections and scarring are more common.

HOME TREATMENT
• Often no treatment is needed.
• There are many home (or folk) remedies for warts. Family members or friends may recommend trying different treatments. Since warts often disappear on their own, it is hard to know if the treatment worked or the warts just cleared up on their own.
• In one medical study, common duct tape was used to treat warts. The cure rate compared to other forms of treatment. For details on this method, do an internet search.

MEDICATION
• There are nonprescription drugs for treatment of warts. Most are applied to skin daily for several weeks. Also available is a freezing aerosol product. Follow the instructions provided with any product that you purchase.
• Your doctor may prescribe stronger drugs or injections for removing the warts.

ACTIVITY—No restrictions.

DIET—No special diet.

CALL YOUR DOCTOR IF

• You have warts and you want them removed.
• After removal by cryosurgery or electrocautery, signs of infection (fever, swelling, redness, pain or pus) appear at the treatment site.
• Warts don't disappear completely after treatment.
• Other warts appear after treatment.

WARTS, PLANTAR

 GENERAL INFORMATION

DEFINITION—Warts on the soles of the feet. Plantar warts seem to grow inward ("into the skin"). They are sometimes mistaken for calluses or corns, but the little dark spots in plantar warts help distinguish them from other skin problems.

SIGNS & SYMPTOMS
- Pinhead-sized bump that grows to 2 mm or 3 mm. Shaving off the top reveals small black dots, pinpoint bleeding and an underlying translucent core.
- Pain on walking. The wart compresses underlying tender tissue.
- Plantar warts may occur singly or in adjacent clusters.

CAUSES & RISK FACTORS—Infection with the human *papilloma* virus, which passes from person to person by direct contact. The virus invades the skin, making Infected cells reproduce faster than normal cells. Plantar warts are contagious and are most common In association with the following:
- Repeated injury to the skin due to puncture wounds, excessive perspiration, increased heat or friction of foot covering and protective gear.
- Fall and spring seasons.
- Having other warts.

HOW TO PREVENT
- Don't touch warts on other people. Don't wear another person's shoes.
- Change shoes frequently (the wart virus breeds in moist places), and allow shoes to dry out before putting them on again.
- Wear thong sandals in locker rooms, showers, health clubs or swimming pools.

 WHAT TO EXPECT

DIAGNOSTIC MEASURES
- Your own observation of symptoms.
- Medical history and physical exam by a doctor if needed.

SURGERY—Sometimes performed in a doctor's office to remove painful, nonhealing plantar warts.

NORMAL COURSE OF DISORDER—Usually curable in 6 to 12 weeks with treatment or they disappear. Some cases are slow to heal or are resistant to treatment. Recurrence is common.

POSSIBLE COMPLICATIONS—Inflammation and arthritic changes in other parts of the body due to abnormal gait and posture caused by painful plantar warts.

 HOW TO TREAT

NOTE—Follow your doctor's instructions if provided. These Instructions are supplemental.

MEDICAL TREATMENT—Your doctor may pare away the overlying callused skin and apply chemical cauterants, such as trichloracetic acid, 20% salicylic acid or 20% formalin. Sometimes plantar warts are removed using other methods, such as lasers.

HOME TREATMENT
- Insert pads or cushions in your shoes to make walking more comfortable.
- Soak feet in 1/2 gallon of warm water with 2 tablespoons of mild detergent.
- Apply the sticky side of medicated plaster directly onto the wart. Push it down, and keep it dry and in place for 2 days.
- After 2 days, remove bandage and plaster. If skin tears as you remove the tape, loosen the tape with nail polish remover on a cotton-tip applicator inserted between the skin and the tape. (Wart will look whitish.) Wash 2 times daily for 2 days with soap and water, and scrub with a brush or toothbrush. Expose the wart to air.
- Scrape gray wart tissue with the point of a sterilized nail file after a bath or shower,
- Repeat entire process for 2 weeks. If wart becomes sore, skip treatment for 2 or 5 days.
- Wear a pad cut from adhesive foam. Cut a hole for the wart, and attach the pad to prevent pressure directly on the wart.
- If the wart is close to the base of a toe, have a shoe repairman sew a metatarsal bar on the bottom of the shoe.

MEDICATION
- For minor discomfort, you may use non-prescription drugs such as acetaminophen.
- Your doctor may prescribe chemically treated plaster for you to apply. Follow Instructions carefully.

ACTIVITY—No restrictions. Because walking aggravates the wart, find the most comfortable way to walk without putting weight on the wart.

DIET—No special diet.

 CALL YOUR DOCTOR IF

- You have a plantar wart that does not respond to self-treatment.
- The treated area becomes infected, with redness, heat, increased pain and tenderness.

YIPS

GENERAL INFORMATION

DEFINITION—A definition of yips is—a state of nervous tension affecting an athlete (such as a golfer) in the performance of a crucial action. Yips affects the performance of many amateur and professional golfers, both male and female. Similar nervous and anxiety-like conditions can affect other athletes, as well as musicians, health care workers (such as dentists) and others.

SIGNS & SYMPTOMS
• There is a wide range of yips symptoms from slight spasms to total body involvement.
• Motions that are not controlled (such as sudden tremors, jerking, spasm or freezing) of the hand or wrist that can make putting all but impossible. Terms such as twitches, staggers, jitters and jerks are used to describe the movements.
• Yips may begin with missing short golf putts. A player may progress to fear of missing and the fear of putting.
• The condition comes and goes, occurring more frequently during tournaments and competitive play.

CAUSES & RISK FACTORS
• The exact cause of the yips is yet to be determined. It may be a problem of nerves (focal dystonia), performance anxiety, or a combination of the two. Focal dystonia is a nerve problem that results in sudden, contractions of a muscle or group of muscles, resulting in twisting or turning. In the case of the yips, the muscles involved are usually those of the lower arm or hand. Anxiety and stress may make this symptom worse.
• One study found that those who experience the yips also appear to have faster than average heart rates, increased muscle activity in the wrists and tend to grip the putter with greater force.
• Golfers who have played for approximately 25 years or more appear to be most prone to the condition.
• The yips most often affects men in their 40s and 50s who have played a lot of tournament golf.

HOW TO PREVENT
• There are no known preventive methods for yips.
• Some physical and mental techniques may help. Practice different strokes during your warm-up sessions to avoid using the same muscles repeatedly. Stretch before and after your game to reduce anxiety levels and loosen your muscles.

WHAT TO EXPECT

DIAGNOSTIC MEASURES
• Your own observations of symptoms. There are no clinical methods or medical tests for diagnosing yips.
• Medical history and physical exam by a doctor if needed.

SURGERY—Not necessary or useful for this disorder.

NORMAL COURSE OF DISORDER—Yips symptoms differ for different people. There is no specific therapy and most attempts at a cure are usually a trial and error process.

POSSIBLE COMPLICATIONS—There are no medical complications from yips. The symptoms may cause some golfers to give up the game.

HOW TO TREAT

NOTE—Follow your doctor's instructions if provided. These instructions are supplemental.

MEDICAL TREATMENT—Usually not necessary.

HOME TREATMENT
• There is no proven cure for the yips. To date, no medical treatments, medications or supplements are effective in curing the problem. Research is ongoing.
• There are numerous products and suggestions for cures listed on the internet. Golf books, and anecdotes from family or friends suggest many ways to treat yips.
• Try changing golfing techniques. Some golfers have found relief from the yips by using an alternative grip or putter, which may ease the strain.
• Mental therapy is not proven, but may help some golfers. Mental training techniques, include relaxation, imaging, goal setting, hypnosis or positive thinking. These techniques may help lower anxiety and increase concentration.

MEDICATION—Medicine is usually not necessary for this disorder.

ACTIVITY—Maintain your normal activity levels.

DIET—No special diet.

CALL YOUR DOCTOR IF

You have symptoms of yips that are painful.

REHABILITATION

Rehabilitation is a process of restoring full function to the musculoskeletal system. Rehabilitation consists of patient education regarding proper posture and body mechanics and the appropriate exercises. Exercises include stretching to restore muscle and joint flexibility, and strengthening exercises to improve muscle strength and motor control. A complete program will also include balance activities and a gradual return to functional activities.

Because an injury results in weakness, muscle incoordination, and loss of joint function, the initial exercises performed following injury must be gentle and safe. Proper progression of the rehabilitation program will ensure the most effective recovery of an injury and return to optimal function. For this reason, many doctors will recommend that you see a professional physical therapist or athletic trainer to guide you through your rehabilitation.

How to Use the Exercises That Follow

This section includes exercises to help you in rehabilitation of any area of the body following injury. These exercises are arranged by area of the body and have been organized in a progression from easy to more difficult. Turn to the exercise for the area of the body that has been injured and begin with the exercises to restore range of motion (ROM). This will provide a gentle warm-up as you increase your muscle and joint mobility. Perform the exercises slowly while being aware of any pain. Once completed, progress to the next exercise under ROM and onto those under strength.

We recommend that you get clearance from your doctor before performing these exercises.

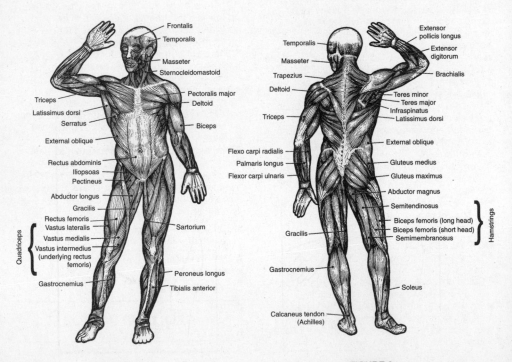

FIGURE 1

FIGURE 2

These exercises have been designed for the rehabilitation and reconditioning of an athlete following injury. They have not been designed for the conditioning of a person beginning a sport or an exercise program. Rehabilitation of an injured athlete restores full flexibility, strength, endurance and balance to restore optimal function. While the exercises described here can be useful to the beginning athlete, exercises specifically designed for conditioning would be better. Many good resources are available that detail conditioning programs for those who are beginning a sport or an exercise program.

Muscles and Muscle Groups Affected by the Exercises

For each exercise in this section we have listed the tissues affected. Many of these tissues are individual muscles or muscle groups. For individual muscles, see Figures 1 and 2 on page 483. Some of the muscles affected by the exercises are not visible on these drawings because they underlie other muscles. For those muscles, we will tell you where they are located in relation to the visible muscles.

Often groups of muscles rather than individual muscles are affected by an exercise. Some of these groups have specific names, such as the hamstrings and the quadriceps, which are labeled on Figures 1 and 2. Others are defined by function. These functions are illustrated in Figures 3-6 and described in the figure captions.

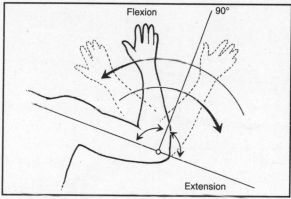

FIGURE 3

Extension (Figure 3) is the act of straightening a limb or joint.

Flexion (Figure 3) is the act of bending a limb at a joint.

Abduction (Figure 4) is the act of moving a limb away from the midline of the body (represented by the spine).

Adduction (Figure 5) is the act of moving a limb toward the midline of the body (represented by the spine).

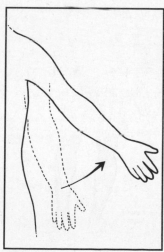

FIGURE 4

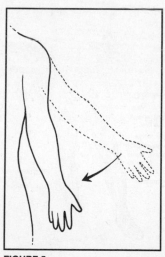

FIGURE 5

Pronation Figure 6) is the act of rotating the forearm while the elbow is flexed to 90° so that the palm of the hand is turned downward toward the floor or while the elbow is fully extended and the forearm rotated so the palm of the hand faces toward the back. With reference to the entire body, pronation is the act of lying face downward (on one's stomach).

Supination (Figure 6) is the act of rotating the forearm while the elbow is flexed to 90° so that the palm of the hand is turned upward toward the ceiling or while the elbow is fully extended and the forearm rotated so the palm of the hand faces forward.

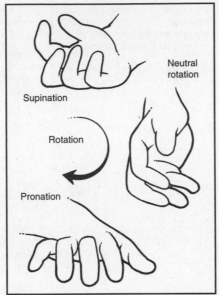

FIGURE 6

Other Terms Used

A few other terms are used in describing the tissues affected by these exercises. Their definitions are as follows:

Medial—Toward the midline of the body (represented by the spine).

Lateral—Away from the midline of the body (represented by the spine); pertaining to a side.

Anterior—In front. This definition assumes that the palms of the hands are facing forward.

Posterior—In back. This definition assumes that the palms of the hands are facing backward.

Dorsal—Same as posterior.

NECK EXERCISES

If you experience any neck pain or injury, you should be examined by a doctor. If at any time during these exercises you experience pain, numbness or tingling in your hands, or dizziness, consult with your doctor, physical therapist or athletic trainer. Perform all exercises gently and slowly, respecting your pain. All exercises should be done while sitting or standing with proper posture.

RANGE OF MOTION

CHIN TUCKS
Affected tissues: Muscles and joints of the neck.
Position: Sitting or standing with good posture.
Action: Always look forward. Place two fingers on your chin, and gently move your chin and face back until you feel a stretch at your hairline (see Figure 7).
Repetitions: Hold each stretch for 10 seconds and repeat 10 times.

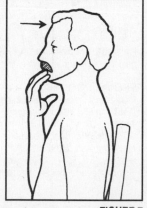

FIGURE 7

NECK FLEXION
Affected tissues: Muscles and joints of the neck.
Position: Sitting or standing with good posture.
Action: Slowly bend head forward while allowing your chin to move toward your chest.
Repetitions: Hold each motion for 3-5 seconds, and repeat 5-10 times.

NECK EXTENSION
Affected tissues: Muscles and joints of the neck.
Position: Sitting or standing with good posture.
Action: Bend elbows and place hands between neck and shoulders to stabilize your neck. Slowly look up to the ceiling. Gently try to increase the range with every motion.
Repetitions: Hold each motion for 3-5 seconds, and repeat 3-5 times.

HEAD ROTATIONS, RIGHT & LEFT
Affected tissues: Muscles and joints of the neck.
Position: Sitting or standing with good posture.
Action: Slowly turn and look as far as possible to the right. Do the same thing to the left.
Repetitions: Hold 3-5 seconds. Return to starting position. Repeat 5-10 times.

SIDEBENDING, RIGHT & LEFT
Affected tissues: Muscles and joints of the neck.
Position: Sitting or standing with good posture. Keep eyes and nose facing forward as you move your head.
Action: Slowly bend your head and neck to one side toward the shoulder, and try to place your ear over the shoulder. If the stretch causes no pain or other symptoms in the neck or arm, reach toward the floor with your opposite arm.
Repetitions: Hold stretch for 10 seconds, and repeat 5 to 10 times. Then stretch your neck to the other side.

NECK EXERCISES (continued)

STRENGTH

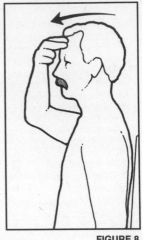

ISOMETRIC (performing muscle contraction without movement)
FLEXION, EXTENSION, SIDEBENDING
Muscles: All muscles of the neck.
Position: Sitting.
Action: Hold your head still, and use your hands to gently press on your forehead, then the back of your head, and then the right and left sides of your head (see Figure 8).
Repetitions: Hold pressure in each position for 2 seconds, and perform each action 5 to 10 times.

SHOULDER ROLLS
Muscles: Trapezius and other muscles of the neck.
Position: Sitting or standing.
Action: Slowly shrug your shoulders up toward your ears, then pull your shoulders back and squeeze the shoulder blades together. Lower your shoulders to the starting position. Do this in a slow continuous motion.
Repetitions: Repeat this routine 10 to 15 times.

FIGURE 8

UPPER BACK EXERCISES

The upper back refers to the region of the thoracic spine and the area around the scapula and ribs. There are many conditions and injuries of the upper back that require restoration of mobility and strength.

RANGE OF MOTION

CORNER STRETCH
Affected tissues: Pectoralis muscles and shoulder capsule.
Position: Stand close to a corner of a room and face it. Hold your arms out straight to the sides, then bend them up at the elbows to make 90-degree angles. Your upper arms will be parallel to the floor, your lower arms reaching straight up. Place them on the wall. Put one foot and knee toward the corner.
Action: Keeping your foot and knee in the corner and your arms against the walls, lean your body into the corner. You should feel a stretch across your chest and front shoulder area. Keep your chin tucked in. Return to starting position.
Repetitions: Hold for 30 seconds, and repeat 2 to 3 times.

TOWEL STRETCH, VERTICAL & HORIZONTAL
Affected tissues: Pectoralis muscles, ligaments and muscles between the vertebrae.
Position: Roll up a small bath towel tightly, and wrap some tape around it. The diameter should be abut 2-4 inches. Sit down on the floor, and place the towel vertically between your shoulder blades. Lie down on the towel, allowing your shoulders to fall toward the floor. Support your head with a small pillow. Repeat stretch. This time placing the towel horizontally under your back. Let your spine bend backward over the towel.
Action: Breathe deeply, and with each deep breath allow your shoulders to sink toward the floor.
Repetitions: Hold for at least 2-3 minutes, and repeat 2 to 3 times.

UPPER BACK EXERCISES (continued)

STRENGTH

SUPERMAN SQUEEZE (scapular retraction)
Muscles: Shoulder retractors (the trapezius and the rhomboid, which underlies the trapezius), posterior deltoid and external rotator.
Position: Lie on the floor face down with your arms at your sides or standing with good posture.
Action: Squeeze your shoulder blades together, and reach toward your feet with your hands. Increase the difficulty by lifting your hands off the ground, palms facing downward. If you do not have neck symptoms, raise your head off the floor (continue to look at the floor).
Repetitions: Hold for a count of five, and repeat 10 times, which completes one set. Progress to 3 sets of 10.

TRUNK EXTENSIONS
Muscles: Paraspinals (the muscles parallel to the spine).
Position: Lie face down on the floor with your feet under an immovable object. Place your arms at your sides.
Action: Slowly lift your head, shoulders and upper back off of the floor. Return to starting position. To increase the difficulty, fold your hands behind your neck, and lift up (be careful that you do not pull on your neck).
Repetitions: Repeat 10 to 15 times.

SHOULDER EXERCISES

RANGE OF MOTION

PENDULUM EXERCISE
Affected tissues: Shoulder muscles and shoulder capsule.
Position: Stand and bend forward with the uninvolved arm supporting the upper body on a table or the back of a chair. Holding a 1-pound weight (such as a can of soup) in the involved hand, allow the arm to hang toward the floor.
Action: With the arm hanging freely toward the floor, shift your body weight from one foot to the other, allowing the involved arm to swing gradually like a pendulum.
Repetitions: Perform the exercise for 1 to 2 minutes as needed and before and after shoulder strengthening exercises.

CANE EXERCISES
Affected tissues: Shoulder muscles and shoulder capsule.
Position: Lie on the floor on your back with knees bent and both arms straight up toward the ceiling holding a cane, long stick or broom handle.
Action: (1) Keeping your arms straight, slowly lower the cane over your head toward the floor. Return to starting position. (2) Keeping your arms straight, slowly lower the cane to one side and then the other.
Repetitions: Hold each stretch as tolerated, and repeat 10 to 15 times.

KNEELING REACH STRETCH
Affected tissues: Shoulder muscles and shoulder capsule.
Position: Begin on the floor on your hands and knees.
Action: Keeping your hands stationary, slowly sit back onto your heels. To increase the stretch, begin with your hands farther from your knees, and slowly sit back onto your heels.
Repetitions: Hold each stretch for 15 to 20 seconds, and repeat 5 to 10 times.

SHOULDER EXERCISES (continued)

INTERNAL AND EXTERNAL ROTATION
Affected tissues: Pectoralis muscles and shoulder capsule.
Position: Standing, holding a towel behind your back with one hand behind your neck and the other hand behind your waist.
Action: Gently move the towel up and down, as if you were drying off your back,
Repetitions: Repeat 8-10 times, pause, then do the same thing, reversing your hand positions.

CORNER STRETCH (more advanced)
Affected tissues: Pectoralis muscles and shoulder capsule.
Position: Stand close to a corner of a room and face it. Hold your arms out straight to the sides, then bend them up at the elbows to make 90-degree angles (your upper arms will be parallel to the floor, your lower arms reaching straight up) and place them on the wall. Put one foot and knee in the corner.
Action: Keeping your foot and knee in the corner and your arms against the walls, push your chest into the corner. Keep your chin tucked in, and breathe deeply. Return to starting position.
Repetitions: Hold for 30 seconds, and repeat 3-5 times.

STRENGTH

SUPERMAN SQUEEZE (scapular retraction)
Muscles: Shoulder retractors (the trapezius and the rhomboid, which underlies the trapezius), posterior deltoid and external rotator.
Position: Lie on the floor face down with your arms at your sides or standing with good posture.
Action: Squeeze your shoulder blades together, and reach toward your feet with your hands. Increase the difficulty by lifting your hands off the ground, palms facing downward. If you do not have neck symptoms, raise your head off the floor (continue to look at the floor).
Repetitions: Hold for a count of five, and repeat 10 times, which completes one set. Progress to 3 sets of 10.

WALL PUSH-UPS
Muscles: Shoulder protractors (pectoralis muscles and serratus).
Position: Stand, facing the wall with feet about two feet from the wall.
Action: Place both hands flat on the wall, with straight arms shoulder-width apart at shoulder height. Bend your elbows and lower body toward the wall until chest is a few inches from the wall. Squeeze chest muscles as you push back to starting position.
Repetitions: Repeat 10 times, which completes one set. Progress to 3 sets of 10.

FLEXION AND ABDUCTION
Muscles: Rotator cuff and deltoid.
Position: Stand with the involved arm at your side holding little to no weight, letting pain be your guide.
Action: (1) Slowly raise the arm in front of you to 90 degrees, then slowly return. (2) Slowly raise the arm out to your side to 90 degrees, then slowly return. With both movements, keep the shoulder blade from rising up toward your ear. You can perform this exercise with both arms at the same time.
Repetitions: Repeat 8 to 10 times, which completes one set. Progress to 3 sets of 10.

ROTATOR CUFF EXERCISES

The rotator cuff is a group of four muscles that provide the shoulder with dynamic stability and keep the shoulder girdle (bony arch formed by the collarbones and shoulder blades) depressed. Rotator cuff strengthening is critical to rehabilitation of any shoulder injury and will also help prevent reinjury.

STRENGTH

SCAPTION
Muscles: Supraspinatus.
Position: Stand with no weight or a 1-pound weight in the hand of each arm.
Action: Slowly raise the arms 45 degrees from the front. Keep your shoulder blade depressed, and raise the arm no higher than 90 degrees. Keep thumbs pointed downward, leading with pinky fingers.
Repetitions: Repeat 10 times, which completes one set. Begin with one set, progressing to 3 sets, with brief pauses between each set.

EXTERNAL ROTATOR
Muscles: Infraspinatus and teres minor.
Position: Lie on the uninvolved side on the floor with a towel between the involved elbow and your body. Elbow should be bent to 90 degrees flexion.
Action: Holding no weight or a 1- to 2-pound weight, slowly raise your hand toward the ceiling while keeping the elbow at your side on the towel (see Figure 9). Slowly return to starting position.
Repetitions: Repeat 10 times, which completes one set. Begin with one set, progressing to 3 sets, with brief pauses between each set.

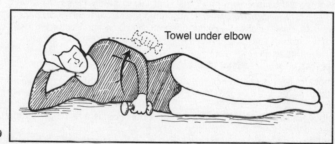

Towel under elbow

FIGURE 9

INTERNAL ROTATION
Muscles: Subscapularis.
Position: Lie on the floor on your back with the involved elbow bent to 90 degrees. Place a towel between your elbow and body to keep the shoulder in proper position.
Action: Holding no weight or a 1- to 2-pound weight, keep your elbow bent. Slowly lower your hand toward the floor, then bring hand in toward stomach.
Repetitions: Repeat 10 times, which completes one set. Begin with one set, progressing to 3 sets, with brief pauses between each set.

ELBOW EXERCISES

Restoring motion to an injured elbow should be done cautiously. It is important to progress with minimal pain and perform active motion.

RANGE OF MOTION

ELBOW FLEXION
Affected tissues: Triceps muscles and elbow capsule (posterior).
Position: Stand or sit with the involved arm at your side.
Action: Slowly bend the elbow, gently assisting with the other hand.
Repetitions: Hold each flex for at least 20 seconds, and repeat 3-5 times.

EXTENSION
Affected tissues: Biceps muscles and front of elbow joint capsule.
Position: Sit on a chair, and lean forward so that the upper part of the involved arm is flat on a table. Flex the lower arm upward at a right angle to the table.
Action: Slowly attempt to straighten the elbow using the triceps muscles and gravity (see Figure 10). Use the other arm to support arm while straightening.
Repetitions: Hold each stretch for at least 30 seconds, and repeat 3-5 times.

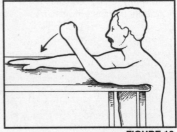

FIGURE 10

SUPINATION
Affected tissues: Wrist pronators.
Position: Sit on a chair with the involved arm at your side and the elbow bent to 90 degrees. Support arm with a pillow.
Action: Attempt to turn your palm toward the ceiling, gently assisting with the other hand (see Figure 11).
Repetitions: Hold each stretch for at least 30 seconds, and repeat 3-5 times.

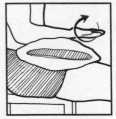

PRONATION
Affected tissues: Wrist supinators.
Position: Sit on a chair with the involved arm at your side and the elbow bent to 90 degrees. Support arm with a pillow.
Action: Attempt to turn your palm toward the floor, gently assisting with the other hand.
Repetitions: Hold each stretch for at least 30 seconds, and repeat 3-5 times.

FIGURE 11

STRENGTH

FIGURE 12

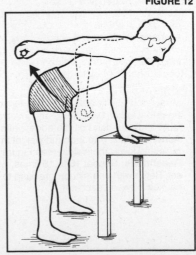

BICEPS CURLS
Muscles: Biceps.
Position: Stand and hold a weight (1 to 2 pounds to start) at your side in the hand of the involved arm with your palm facing forward.
Action: Slowly bend the elbow, bringing the weight toward your shoulder, then slowly return to starting position.
Repetitions: Repeat 10 times, which completes one set. Progress to 3 sets of 10 with a short pauses between sets.

TRICEPS EXTENSIONS
Muscles: Triceps.
Position: Stand with knees slightly bent, and bend forward with the involved arm extended back, horizontal to the ground. Hold a weight (1 to 2 pounds to start).
Action: Slowly bend the elbow and then straighten it (see Figure 12).
Repetitions: Repeat 10 times, which completes one set. Progress to 3 sets of 10 with a short pauses between sets.

WRIST AND HAND EXERCISES

RANGE OF MOTION

WRIST FLEXION AND EXTENSION
Affected tissues: Ligaments and tendons of the wrist.
Position: Sit on a chair with the forearm of the involved arm resting on a table so that your hand is off the edge.
Action: Allow your wrist to fully flex and extend using your muscles. Gently assist with the other hand.
Repetitions: Hold each stretch for at least 20 to 30 seconds, then repeat 2-5 times.

ULNAR AND RADIAL DEVIATIONS
Affected tissues: Ligaments and tendons of the wrist.
Position: Sit on a chair with the forearm and hand of the involved arm flat on a table, palm down.
Action: Keeping the hand flat and assisting with the other hand. 1) Move the hand inward toward the thumb. 2) Move hand outward toward the pinky finger.
Repetitions: Hold each stretch for at least 20 to 30 seconds, then repeat 2-5 times.

PRONATION
Affected tissues: Wrist supinators.
Position: Sit on a chair with the involved arm at your side and your elbow bent to 90 degrees.
Action: Turn your palm toward the floor, gently assisting with the other hand, just above the wrist.
Repetitions: Hold each stretch for at least 30 seconds, and repeat 2 to 5 times.

SUPINATION
Affected tissues: Wrist pronators.
Position: Sit on a chair with the involved arm at your side and the elbow bent to 90 degrees.
Action: Attempt to turn your palm toward the ceiling, gently assisting with the other hand, just above the wrist.
Repetitions: Hold each stretch for at least 30 seconds, and repeat 2 to 5 times.

ACTIVE FIST
Affected tissues: Ligaments and tendons of the fist and hand.
Position: Sitting or standing.
Action: Attempt to make a clenched fist with the involved hand. If necessary, use the other hand to gently assist any finger joints that cannot fully flex actively.
Repetitions: Hold each stretch for 20 to 30 seconds, then repeat.

COMPLETE OPENING
Affected tissues: Ligaments and tendons of the hands and fingers.
Position: Sitting or standing.
Action: Attempt to fully open the hand. With your other hand, gently assist any finger joints that cannot fully open.
Repetitions: Hold each stretch for at least 30 seconds, and repeat 2 to 5 times.

STRENGTH

WRIST FLEXION
Muscles: Wrist flexors and the extensors of the forearm.
Position: Sit on a chair with the involved arm resting on a table and your hand off the edge, palm up.
Action: Hold a 1- to 2-pound weight in the hand, and slowly raise and lower the weight (see Figure 13).
Repetitions: Repeat 10 to 15 times, which completes one set. Begin with one set, progressing to 3 sets, with brief pauses between each set.

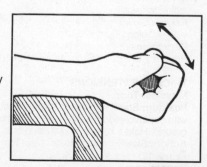

FIGURE 13

WRIST AND HAND EXERCISES (continued)

WRIST EXTENSION
Muscles: Wrist flexors and the extensors of the forearm.
Position: Sit on a chair with the involved arm resting on a table and your hand off the edge, palm down.
Action: Hold a 1- to 2-pound weight in the hand, and slowly raise and lower the weight.
Repetitions: Repeat 10 times, which completes one set. Begin with one set, progressing to 3 sets, with brief pauses between each set.

GRIPPING EXERCISES
Muscles: Wrist and finger flexors.
Position: While sitting or standing, hold a tennis ball, or any small squeezable sphere in the involved hand.
Action: Grip and squeeze the object.
Repetitions: Hold for a count of five, and repeat 10 to 15 times, which completes one set. Progress to 3 sets with short pauses in between.

WRIST PRONATION AND SUPINATION
Muscles: Pronators and supinators of the forearm.
Position: Sit with the involved forearm resting on a table and your hand at the table edge.
Action: While holding a 1- to 2-pound weight fixed at the end of a bar or stick, slowly turn the palm up toward the ceiling and then down toward the floor.
Repetitions: Repeat 10 times, which completes one set. Progress to 3 sets with short pauses in between.

LOW BACK EXERCISES

RANGE OF MOTION

FLEXION EXERCISES, SINGLE LEG (Williams Flexion Exercises)
Affected tissues: Muscles and joints of the low back.
Position: Lie on a firm surface on your back with your legs flat on the floor.
Action: With your hands and arms, pull one knee toward your chest. Then return the leg to its starting position. Be sure to continue normal breathing.
Repetitions: Hold approximately 30 seconds, and repeat 3 times with each leg.

FLEXION EXERCISES, DOUBLE LEG (Williams Flexion Exercises)
Affected tissues: Muscles and joints of the low back.
Position: Lie on a firm surface on your back with your legs flat on the floor.
Action: With your hands and arms, pull both knees toward your chest. Then release, allowing your arms to straighten, but still holding on to your legs. Do not hold your breath; continue normal breathing.
Repetitions: Hold approximately 30 seconds, and repeat 3 times.

CAT EXERCISES
Affected tissues: Muscles and joints of the back.
Position: Begin on a firm surface on your hands and knees with your back flat.
Action: Keeping your arms straight, allow your low back to sink (like a sway-back horse). Return to flat back position, and raise your back (like an angry cat). Return to flat back position.
Repetitions: Repeat each step 10 times.

LOW BACK EXERCISES (continued)

EXTENSION EXERCISES (McKenzie Extension)
Affected tissues: Muscles and joints of the low back.
Position: Lie on a firm surface on your stomach. Place your hands, palms down, next to your shoulders.
Action: Slowly press up, keeping your pelvis on the floor (see Figure 14). This should create an arch in your lower back. Be sure to respect your pain. As you progress, you can extend your lower back more fully by pressing up until your elbows are extended. Keep your hips on the floor.
Repetitions: Repeat each step 3 to 6 times.

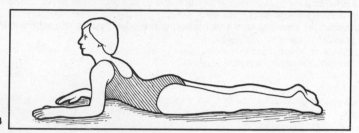

FIGURE 14

SUPINE TWISTS
Affected tissues: Muscles and ligaments of the low back.
Position: Lie on your back on a firm surface with your arms extended out to the sides at 90 degrees to your body and your legs extended flat on the floor.
Action: Reach one leg toward the opposite hand, twisting through the lower back (see Figure 15). Return to starting position.
Repetitions: Hold each stretch for 20 to 30 seconds, and repeat 2 to 3 times on each side.

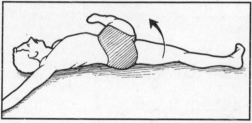

FIGURE 15

STRENGTH

PELVIC TILTS
Muscles: Abdominals and gluteals.
Position: Lie on the floor on your back with your knees bent and your feet flat on the floor.
Action: Press your lower back to the floor as you tighten your buttock muscles.
Repetitions: Hold this position for a count of 10. Count out loud to ensure you are not holding your breath. Repeat 10 times.

CRUNCHES
Muscles: Abdominals.
Position: Lie on the floor on your back with your feet under a chair or sofa.
Action: With arms extended, reaching toward knees, curl up, completely lifting shoulder blades off the floor. Hold one second and lower slowly. A progression of this exercise would be to fold arms across the chest and perform the same movement. Further progression would be to place hands behind your head and perform the same movement.
Repetitions: Repeat 10 times. Do 1-3 sets.

TRUNK EXTENSIONS
Muscles: Paraspinals (the muscles parallel to the spine).
Position: Lie on the floor face down with your feet under an immovable object. Place your arms at your sides.
Action: Slowly lift your head, shoulders and upper back off the floor. Return to starting position. To increase the difficulty, fold your hands behind your neck and lift up (don't pull on your neck).
Repetitions: Repeat 10 times.

POSTURE & BODY MECHANICS

POSTURE
Proper sitting posture and the use of good body mechanics are essential components of a spinal rehabilitation program. Poor sitting posture will frequently perpetuate or delay the recovery from a spinal injury. Alternatively, good sitting posture, as well as the use of good body mechanics, will enhance and expedite the recovery process.

SITTING POSTURE
• A good sitting posture maintains the spinal curves normally present in the erect standing position. This is usually your "neutral spine" position and it is your most comfortable position.
• To find your neutral spine position, sit on a chair and fully flex your spine (slouch), now completely straighten and extend your lumbar spine. Now, relax off the fully extended position by about 10%, finding your most comfortable position. This is your neutral spine position. Your spinal curves should be similar to your erect standing position now.
• When you sit in a chair, you want to maintain this neutral spine position. Always try to sit all the way back in the chair with both feet flat on the floor.

BODY MECHANICS
• Proper body mechanics refers to the technique used while lifting, bending, moving, reaching, etc. When you perform any of the activities, you should try to maintain the neutral spine position.
• When you move from a sitting position to standing, be sure to scoot to the edge of the chair, and then stand up, while maintaining your neutral spine. When you move from standing to sitting, it is just the reverse. You do not want to lean forward at the trunk when you move in and out of the chair.
• When moving from sitting to a sidelying position, start at the edge of the bed, come down on your elbow as you simultaneously lift both legs up onto the bed. If you sleep on your side, you may be more comfortable with a standard pillow between your knees and thighs. Moving from lying down to sitting would be the reverse.
• Frequent bending and lifting should be avoided with acute back pain. When you do need to move to a lower position, keep your neutral spine position and squat down by bending your knees, not your low back. You should use this technique for all bending, whether you are leaning forward using a low sink or picking something up from the floor.
• If you lift something, keep the item at about hip level and close to your body. When reaching overhead for something, use a step stool so you can reach at shoulder height or lower. Again, be sure to keep your neutral spine position while doing these activities.
• When moving a heavy object, it is easier to maintain a neutral spine position if you push the object, rather than pull it. So, if you have a choice, always push an object rather than pull.

HIP & PELVIS EXERCISES

RANGE OF MOTION

HAMSTRING STRETCHES, SEATED
Affected tissues: Muscles and tendons of the posterior thigh (hamstrings).
Position: Sit on the floor with one leg stretched out in front and the other leg bent with the heel close to your groin.
Action: While keeping the knee of the extended leg straight and your back straight, lean slowly forward, until you feel a mild stretch in the back of your thigh. Repeat with other leg.
Repetitions: Hold for 20-30 seconds for each leg. Progress to 3 sets with short pauses in between.

HIP & PELVIS EXERCISES (continued)

HAMSTRING STRETCHES, SUPINE
Affected tissues: Muscles and tendons of the posterior thigh (hamstrings).
Position: Lie on the floor on your back with your legs stretched out.
Action: Grasp one thigh with both hands, and straighten the knee actively using the quadriceps muscle (see Figure 16). Return to starting position, and repeat with the other leg.
Repetitions: Hold for 20-30 seconds for each leg. Progress to 3 sets with short pauses in between.

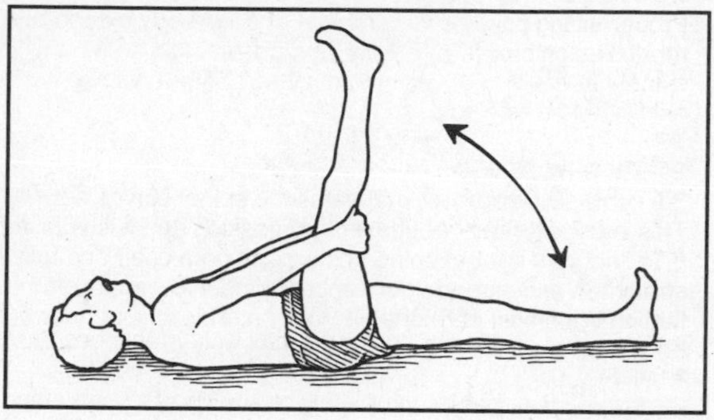

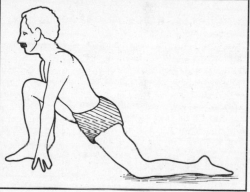

FIGURE 16

WALL GROIN STRETCHES
Affected tissues: Groin muscles.
Position: Lie on the floor on your back, with your buttocks close to the wall.
Action: Straighten your legs so they extend up the wall (your buttocks should be about 6 inches away from the wall). Allow your legs to slowly fall away (from each other) until you feel a mild stretch on your inner thighs. Keep your heels resting against the wall. You can place your hands on the outside of your legs to prevent them from spreading too wide and to allow full relaxation while stretching.
Repetitions: Hold for 20-30 seconds. Progress to 3 sets with short pauses in between.

HIP FLEXOR STRETCHES
Muscles: Rectus femoris and iliopsoas.
Position: Begin on the floor on your hands and knees.
Action: Step forward with the foot on the uninvolved side until the knee of the opposite leg is nearly straight. Lean over the extended leg, leaving the knee on the floor (see Figure 17). Contract the muscles in the buttocks of the trailing leg, and extend your pelvis toward the floor. To stretch your quadriceps muscles, reach back and pull the ankle of the trailing leg toward the buttock.
Repetitions: Hold for 30 seconds and repeat 2-3 times.

FIGURE 17

QUAD STRETCHES
Muscles: Quadriceps.
Position: Stand on the uninvolved leg and use the hand on that side to balance yourself against a wall or counter.
Action: Bend the knee of the involved leg and use your hand to assist bringing your heel toward your buttocks, until you feel a mild stretch on the front thigh. Be sure to keep you thigh parallel with your standing leg.
Repetitions: Hold for at least 20-30 seconds. Then perform stretch with the opposite leg. Repeat 3-5 times.

PIRIFORMIS AND GLUTE STRETCHES
Muscles: Gluteals and piriformis (a muscle underlying the gluteus maximus).
Position: Sit on the floor with your left leg straight. Cross the right foot over the left knee onto the floor. Place your right hand on the floor behind your right hip area.
Action: Pull your right knee toward your left shoulder with your left hand.
Repetitions: Hold for at least 20-30 seconds. Then perform stretch with the opposite leg. Repeat 3-5 times.

HIPS & PELVIS EXERCISES (continued)

STRENGTH

GLUTE SETS
Muscles: Gluteals.
Position: Standing or lying supine.
Action: Squeeze your buttocks together.
Repetitions: Hold each squeeze for 5 seconds. Repeat this action 10 to 15 times, which completes one set. Perform a total of 3 sets, with short pauses between sets.

BRIDGES
Muscles: Gluteals and hamstrings.
Position: Lie on the floor on your back with your knees bent to about 90 degrees and your feet flat on the floor.
Action: Lift your pelvis completely off the floor, straightening your hips. Hold for 5 seconds and then slowly lower.
Repetitions: Repeat this action 10 to 15 times slowly, which completes one set. Perform a total of 3 sets, with short pauses between sets.

STRAIGHT LEG RAISES FOR HIP ABDUCTION
Muscles: Gluteus maximus and gluteus medius.
Position: Lie on the floor on the uninvolved side with your legs straight.
Action: Raise the top leg about 6 to 8 inches, and then lower it. Lead with your heel, toes pointing down.
Repetitions: Repeat this action 10 to 15 times, which completes one set. Perform a total of 3 sets, with short pauses between sets.

STRAIGHT LEG RAISES FOR HIP ADDUCTION
Muscles: Adductors.
Position: Lie on the floor on the uninvolved side with the top knee bent and the foot flat on the floor in front of the knee of the bottom leg (see Figure 18).
Action: Raise the extended bottom leg about 6 to 8 inches off the floor, and then lower it.
Repetitions: Repeat this action 10 to 15 times, which completes one set. Perform a total of 3 sets, with short pauses between sets.

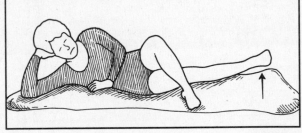

FIGURE 18

HIP EXTENSION IN STANDING
Muscles: Gluteals and hamstrings.
Position: Stand on the uninvolved leg and use hand on wall for balance support. Comfortably bend involved knee.
Action: With the knee bent, gently push foot and thigh back, contracting your gluteal muscles. Slowly lift and lower back to starting position. Keep pelvis and low back stable while moving the thigh back.
Repetitions: Repeat this action 10 to 15 times, which is one set. Perform 1-3 sets with short pauses between sets.

KNEE EXERCISES

RANGE OF MOTION

HEEL SLIDES
Affected tissues: Soft tissue structures at front of knee, quadriceps.
Position: Lying supine or sitting on floor or bed with legs out as straight as possible.
Action: Bend and straighten knee by sliding your heel up toward your buttocks and then back to your starting position.
Repetitions: Perform 10 times, trying to bend knee further with each repetition. Do 1-3 sets.

WALL SLIDES
Affected tissues: Soft tissue structures at front of knee, quadriceps.
Position: Lie on the floor on your back with your feet against a wall (see Figure 19).
Action: Slowly slide the foot of the involved leg down the wall until the desired degree of stretch is felt in the knee. Use the other foot to help remove the involved leg from the stretch.
Repetitions: Hold each stretch for at least 20-30 seconds, and repeat 5 times.

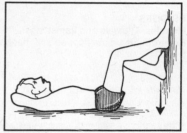

FIGURE 19

SEATED SCOOTS
Affected tissues: Soft tissue structures at front of knee, quadriceps.
Position: Sit in a chair with your feet flat on the floor.
Action: Scoot forward in the chair while attempting to keep your feet firmly on the floor. You should feel a stretch along the front of your knee. Then return to starting position.
Repetitions: Hold for at least 20-30 seconds, and repeat 5 times.

STRENGTH

QUAD SETS
Muscles: Quadriceps.
Position: Sit or lie on the floor on your back with your knees straight (see Figure 20).
Action: Tighten the quadriceps muscles by pushing the back of your knees into the floor. The quadriceps muscles should tighten. Do both legs at the same time.
Repetitions: Hold for at least 5 seconds, and repeat 10 times, which completes one set. Perform a total of 3 sets, with short pauses between sets.

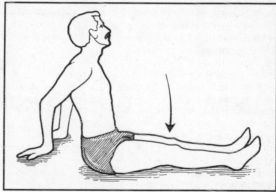

FIGURE 20

HAMSTRING SETS
Muscles: Hamstrings.
Position: Lie on the floor on your back with a small rolled towel under your knees.
Action: Dig heel into floor, tightening your hamstrings.
Repetitions: Hold for at least 5 seconds, and repeat 10-15 times, which completes one set. Perform a total of 3 sets, with short pauses between sets.

STRAIGHT LEG RAISES
Muscles: Quadriceps and hip flexors.
Position: Lie on the floor on your back with your involved knee straight. Bend your uninvolved knee.
Action: Tighten the quadriceps muscles of the involved leg as if pressing the back of the knee to the floor. Raise the leg 6 to 8 inches off of the floor, and then lower it without allowing the foot to touch the floor. Raise and lower 10 times. As an option, you may place an ankle weight on the ankle or knee to increase the difficulty.
Repetitions: Repeat 10 times, which completes one set. Perform a total of 3 sets, with short pauses between sets.

KNEE EXERCISES (continued)

KNEE EXTENSIONS
Muscles: Quadriceps.
Position: Sit on a chair or the edge of a bed with your knees bent.
Action: Slowly straighten the knee of the involved leg to the count of two, and return to the bent position on a count of four. As an option, place an ankle weight on the ankle to increase the difficulty.
Repetitions: Repeat 10 times, which completes one set. Perform a total of 3 sets, with short pauses between sets.

HAMSTRING CURLS
Muscles: Hamstrings.
Position: Stand on the uninvolved leg, and hold onto the back of a chair or a wall.
Action: Keep the knee of the involved leg pointed toward the ground, and bend the knee by pulling the heel toward the buttocks. As an option, you may place an ankle weight on the ankle to increase the difficulty.
Repetitions: Repeat 10 to 15 times, which completes one set. Perform a total of 3 sets, with short pauses between sets.

WALL SLIDES
Muscles: Quadriceps, hip extensors, hamstrings.
Position: Standing with back against a wall, feet shoulder-width apart, 1 1/2 to 2 feet away from wall.
Action: Slowly slide down wall, knees bending as you move. Do not allow knees to go past your toes while bending. Return to starting position. Keep back against wall during entire exercise.
Repetitions: Repeat 10 times, which completes one set. Progress to 3 sets of 10, with short pauses between sets.

STEP-UPS
Muscles: Lower extremity muscles.
Position: Stand in front of step 8 to 15 inches high.
Action: Place your involved leg/foot on the step and slowly push up, keeping the knee aligned over the foot. Then slowly lower. As an option, you may progress to higher steps.
Repetitions: Repeat 10 times, which completes one set. Progress to 3 sets of 10, with short pauses between sets.

ANKLE AND FOOT EXERCISES

RANGE OF MOTION

ANKLE CIRCLES
Affected tissues: Ligaments, muscles and tendons around the ankle.
Position: Sit in a chair or on the floor.
Action: Move the involved foot and ankle slowly in a circular motion.
Repetitions: Make 10 circles in each direction.

STANDING DORSIFLEXION STRETCHES
Affected tissues: Leg muscles (gastrocnemius and soleus) and ankle joint.
Position: Stand in front of a wall, with the involved ankle behind the uninvolved leg. Toes are pointed straight, not to the side, and heels are down. You should feel a stretch in your calf.
Action: Lean toward the wall while keeping the heel of the involved foot on the floor.
Repetitions: Hold for 20-30 seconds. Repeat 5 times throughout the day.

ANKLE AND FOOT EXERCISES (continued)

STRENGTH

HEEL RAISES
Muscles: Calf, gastrocnemius and soleus muscles.
Position: Standing next to counter on involved leg. Put two fingers on counter to assist with balance.
Action: Raise your heel off of the floor and slowly lower.
Repetitions: Repeat 10 times, which completes one set. Progress to 3 sets, with short pauses in between sets.

STRUT WALKING
Muscles: Mostly the calf muscles.
Position: Walking.
Action: Step forward on the involved leg, and land on the heel of the foot, then overemphasize the push-off to appear as if you are strutting.
Repetitions: Perform 15 to 20 steps at various times throughout the day.

TOE TAPPERS
Muscles: Muscles of the front of the leg, anterior tibialis.
Position: Sitting.
Action: Keeping your heels on the floor, lift the front of the foot up off the ground.
Repetitions: Repeat 10 to 20 times, which completes one set. Perform a total of 3 sets, with short pauses between sets.

TOWEL SCRUNCHES
Muscles: All muscles of the foot.
Position: Sit in a chair with the involved foot on a towel.
Action: Keeping your heels on the floor, use your toes to scrunch up the towel.
Repetitions: Perform until fatigued twice during an exercise session.

BALANCE ACTIVITIES

1. Standing balance: Stand on the involved foot next to a chair. Balance on the involved foot. To progress,, do the same thing while moving your arms up and down. Further progression would be to do the same thing with your eyes closed.

2. Heel to toe walking in a straight line: Try to walk on a straight line, placing your heel just ahead of your toes on the previous step. Do this forward and backwards 5 times.

3. Side stepping: Keeping toes pointed forward, step to the right with the right foot, and then step with your left foot to your right foot. As you progress, move more quickly, as in sidestepping quickly in a game of tennis. Do this to the left as well.

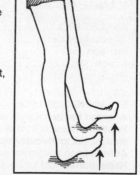

4. Cariocas: This is a grapevine step. Step to the right with your right foot, now cross in front of your right foot with your left. Step to the right again with your right foot, now cross behind your right foot with your left. Continue repeating crossing in front, then behind. Do this down a long hall. Repeat going to the left. As you progress, increase your speed.

5. Heel walking: Walk on your heels for 15-20 steps (see figure 21).

6. Toe walking: Walk on the balls of your feet for 15-20 steps.

FIGURE 21

As you progress, it is ideal to address balance activities and movements that are more "sport specific". These are movements that you will be required to perform once returning to your sport activities. For example, in basketball, you would need to progress to running, jumping, cutting, and rapid start and stop movements, before safely returning to a competitive game of basketball. If you need assistance with these higher level balance activities, consult you health care provider, physical therapist or trainer.

APPENDIX 1

R.I.C.E. (Rest, Ice, Compression, Elevation)

R.I.C.E. is an acronym (a word coined from first letters) for the most important elements—*rest, ice, compression* and *elevation*—in first aid for many injuries. This acronym appears repeatedly throughout this book—and in medical literature in general—in reference to athletic injuries. Use the word *R.I.C.E.* to jog your memory when you are faced with such injuries as contusions, sprains, strains, dislocations or uncomplicated fractures.

REST

Stop using the injured part, and rest it as soon as you realize an injury has taken place. Continued exercise or other activity could cause further injury, delay healing, increase pain and stimulate bleeding. Use crutches to avoid bearing weight on injuries of the foot, ankle, knee or leg. Use splints for injuries of the hand, wrist, elbow or arm. After medical treatment, the injured part may require immobilization with splints or a cast to keep the area at rest until it heals.

ICE

Ice helps stop internal bleeding from injured blood vessels and capillaries. Sudden cold causes small blood vessels to contract. This contraction of blood vessels decreases the amount of blood that can collect around the wound. The more blood that collects, the longer the healing time. Ice can be safely applied in several ways using the following instructions:

- For injury to a small area, such as a finger, toe, foot or wrist, immerse the injured area in a bucket of ice water. Use ice cubes to keep the water cold, as ice dissolves.
- For injury to a larger area, use ice packs. Avoid placing ice directly on the skin. Before applying the ice, place a towel, cloth, or one or two layers of an elasticized compression bandage (Ace bandage) on the skin to be iced. To make the ice pack, put ice chips or ice cubes in a plastic bag, or wrap them in a thin towel. Place the ice pack over the cloth. The pack may sit directly on the injured part, or it may be wrapped in place.
- Ice the injured area for about 30 minutes (no matter what form of ice treatment you are using).
- Remove the ice to allow the skin to warm for 15 minutes.
- Reapply the ice.
- Repeat the icing and warming cycles for 3 hours while following the instructions below for compression and elevation. If pain and swelling persist after 3 hours, consult your doctor (if you have not already done so). Your doctor may change the icing schedule after the first 3 hours. Regular ice treatment is often discontinued after 72 hours. At that point, heat is often more comfortable. Or you might try contrast baths of the injured area—alternating 5 minutes of hot weather with 5 minutes of ice water.

COMPRESSION

Compression decreases swelling by slowing bleeding and limiting the accumulation of blood and plasma near the injured site. Without compression, fluid from adjacent normal tissues seeps into the injury area. The more blood and fluid that accumulate around an injury, the slower the healing. Following are instructions for safely applying compression to an injury:

- Use an elasticized bandage (Ace bandage) for compression, if possible. If you do not have one available, any kind of cloth will suffice for a short time. Wrap the injured part firmly, wrapping over the ice also. Begin wrapping below the injury site, and extend above the injury site.
- Be careful not to compress the area so tightly that the blood supply is impaired. Signs of blood supply deprivation include pain, numbness, cramping and blue or dusky-colored nails. Remove the compression bandage immediately if any of these symptoms appears. Leave the bandage off until all signs of impaired circulation disappear. Then rewrap the area—less tightly this time.

ELEVATION

Elevating the injured part above the level of the heart is another way to decrease swelling and pain at the injury site. Elevate the iced, compressed area in whatever way is most convenient. Prop an injured leg on solid objects or pillows. Elevate an injured arm by lying down and placing pillows under the arm or placing them on the chest with the arm folded across. The whole upper part of the body may be elevated gently with pillows or a reclining chair or by raising the head of the bed on blocks.

APPENDIX 2

Care of Casts

A cast immobilizes a part of the body that has been injured. Casts are used most commonly after bone fractures. A cast is usually applied by placing a splint along the injured part and wrapping it with gauze saturated with plaster of Paris. Before the injury heals, it may be necessary to change the cast one or more times. The time needed for healing determines how long a cast remains in place. Some casts are needed for only 2 weeks. Others are necessary for several months. X-rays through a cast reveal whether bone alignment is satisfactory. They are also used in later stages to check for signs of healing.

AFTER YOU LEAVE THE DOCTOR'S OFFICE

• Don't allow pressure on any part of the cast—no matter what type of casting material was used—until it is completely dry. Any depression that develops will create pressure on the skin underneath, making ulcer formation likely. Drying time varies depending on the type of material used, thickness of the cast, temperature and humidity. Drying can require 24 hours or longer.
• Keep the cast dry, especially at first. If the cast accidentally gets wet and a soft area appears, return to the doctor's office, emergency room or outpatient surgical facility for repairs.
• Whenever possible, elevate the body part enclosed in the cast. This decreases the chance of tissue swelling inside the cast. Prop a leg in a cast on a pillow when in bed or on a footstool or chair when sitting. Prop an arm in a cast on a pillow placed on the chest. Elevate the foot of the bed at night for any injury requiring a cast below the abdomen.

SWELLING INSIDE A CAST

No matter how carefully the injured tissues are handled and no matter how expertly a cast is applied, swelling sometimes occurs inside a cast. Swelling should be reported immediately to the doctor. The following are common symptoms and signs of swelling:

• Severe, persistent pain.
• Change in color of tissues beyond the cast, such as a change to blue or gray under the fingernails or toenails.
• Coldness of the tissues beyond the cast, even though the rest of the body is warm.
• Numbness or complete loss of feeling in the skin beyond the cast.
• Feeling of tightness under the cast after it dries.
• With a leg cast, inability to raise or curl the big toe.

INFECTION INSIDE A CAST

Sometimes the injured area becomes infected during healing. Detecting the infection in its early stages may be difficult if the infected area is covered by a cast. Infection should be reported immediately to the doctor. Following are common signs and symptoms of infection:

• Leakage of fluid through the cast.
• Increasing pain or soreness of the skin under the cast.
• Fever accompanied by a general ill feeling.

ITCHING INSIDE A CAST

Itching can be a maddening problem for a person with a cast—especially during hot weather. Even if you can reach the itch, don't scratch the skin inside the cast. Because the skin is in a hot, moist environment, it is very vulnerable to damage, Scratching is more likely to injure the skin than under normal circumstances. If no incision was made in the skin enclosed by the cast, you may sprinkle cornstarch into the cast to relieve itching. If an incision was made, consult your doctor for pain medication. Itching is a form of mild pain.

Although slow to relieve itching, applying an ice bag over the cast or heating it with a hair dryer may help.

BATHING WITH A CAST

You may find bathing difficult when wearing a cast. The cast must be kept dry at all times, so do not take showers. If the cast is on a limb, such as your arm or leg, you may take tub baths. Position a chair or other support by the tub so you can prop the injured part out of the water while bathing. If the cast is on the trunk of the body, you should take sponge baths until the cast is removed.

Alternately, a "rubber dam" cast cover can be used over a cast on an extremity to allow you to shower. Ask your doctor or a pharmacy or medical supply store for this.

APPENDIX 3

Safe Use of Crutches

Crutches are often a necessary aid to walking when a person has injured a foot, ankle, leg or hip. Proper use of crutches can allow safe, satisfactory mobility. Improper use can cause further accidents.

BEFORE YOU USE CRUTCHES
• Practice using crutches under supervision before trying them out on your own.
• Reread these instructions frequently while getting used to crutches until using the crutches becomes automatic.
• Use a backpack to carry necessary belongings while using crutches. Never try to carry anything in your hands or arms.

FITTING CRUTCHES
You will be fitted for your crutches at the place where you rent or buy them—usually a medical supply store. The following points are important in ensuring a proper fit:

1. Stand straight.
2. Adjust the length of the crutches so 2 or 3 fingers can fit between the top of the crutch and the armpit (about 2 inches).
3. Adjust the hand grip so your elbow bends about 25 degrees, as shown in Figure 1.
   Warning: Don't bear any weight in the armpits. This can cause permanent damage to the nerves of the arm and hand.

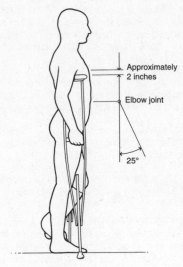

Approximately 2 inches

Elbow joint

25°

Figure 1

MOVING ON CRUTCHES
There are 4 major gaits used by people who need crutches:
Swing-Through Gait—Fastest and most difficult.
Swing-To Gait—Slower and easier and good to use until you become skillful with crutches and can advance to a faster gait.
Shuffle Gait—Slowest of all, and most appropriate for older people.
Three-Point Gait—Can be used only when a slight amount of weight can be borne on the weak side.
The last three gaits are described here. When you are ready to progress to a faster gait, such as the swing-through gait, you will need instructions and supervision from your trainer, nurse or doctor. Also described are instructions on ascending and descending stairs and curbs. These are general suggestions that apply to everyone on crutches.

APPENDIX 3 (continued)

SWING-TO GAIT
This is a good gait for beginners.
1. Place both crutches forward simultaneously, 12 inches in front of your feet, 6 to 8 inches wider than your toes on both sides (see Figure 2).
2. Push your hands down against the handles, and shift your weight forward.
3. Swing your body to a point directly between the crutches. Let the heel on the healthy side land first.
   Note: The swing-through gait is the same as the swing-to gait except that the body swings through and lands in front of the crutches (see Figure 3).

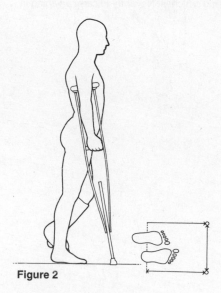

Figure 2

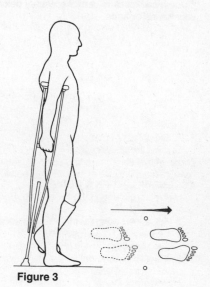

Figure 3

SHUFFLE GAIT
This gait should be used when the swing-to gait is too difficult:
1. Place both crutches forward simultaneously, 12 inches in front of your feet, 6 to 8 inches wider than your toes on both sides (see Figure 4).
2. Push your hands down against the handles as you shift your body weight forward.
3. Slide the strong leg forward a few inches to a point between the crutches.
4. Follow with the weak leg, ending with the legs together.

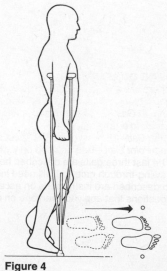

Figure 4

APPENDIX 3 (continued)

THREE-POINT GAIT

Use this gait only when you are able to bear slight, increasing weight on the weak leg (see Figure 5).

1. Place both crutches and the weak foot forward simultaneously, with the weak foot between the crutches. The weight is borne on the strong foot.
2. Push against the handles, and shift your weight forward.
3. Swing your body forward with weight on your hands, and bear a slight amount of weight on the weak foot.
4. End with the strong foot ahead of the crutches.

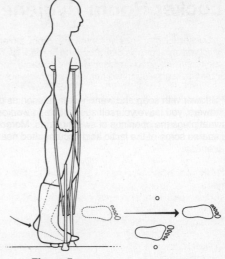

Figure 5

ASCENDING STEPS & CURBS

1. Keep crutches on the lower step. Body weight is on the hands.
2. Raise the strong foot to the step above, trailing the weak leg (see Figure 6).
3. Straighten the strong leg, and advance the crutches to the next step.

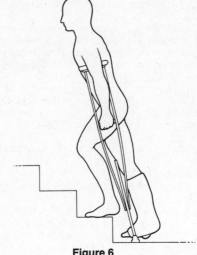

Figure 6

DESCENDING STEPS & CURBS

1. Place crutches on the lower step, and extend the weak leg forward. Body weight is on the hands (see Figure 7).
2. Bend the strong leg, and slowly lower the body.
3. Quickly move the strong leg to the lower step.

Reminder for ascending and descending steps with crutches: "The good goes up, the bad goes down."

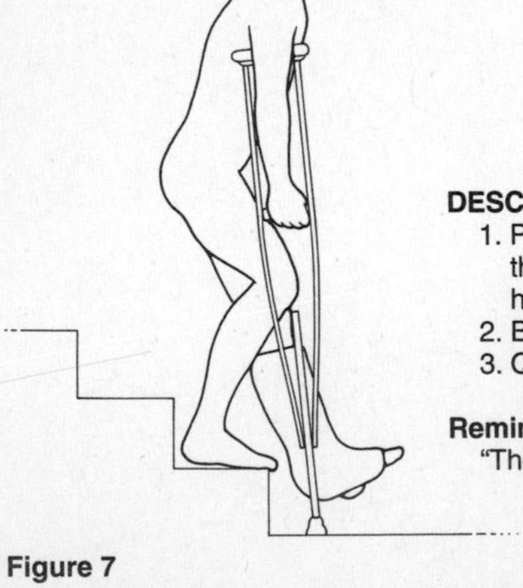

Figure 7

APPENDIX 4

Locker Room Hygiene

Locker rooms, shower rooms and other athletic club facilities can provide an ideal environment in which harmful germs can grow and spread. Many bacteria and fungi thrive in dark, moist environments such as these, and crowded facilities enable germs to spread easily from person to person. Following are some suggestions to help you minimize your risk of illness.

• Shower with soap and warm water as soon as possible after each workout. If you avoid or delay showers, you leave yourself susceptible to *workout breakout*—a skin condition that develops when dry sweat plugs the openings of sweat glands. Moreover, warm showers make you feel better and disperse some of the lactic acid accumulated near muscles, which sometimes causes muscle soreness.

• After each shower, use a clean towel that has been laundered with very hot water and detergent in a home or commercial laundry. Never share someone's towel. Unhygienic towels can spread disease such as pink eye, skin eruptions, virus infections or fungus infections.

• Bring your own stool to sit on, if possible. Store your stool in your locker when not in use. Avoid sitting on benches used by others. A damp bench can harbor bacterial, viral and fungal infections, spreading them easily from one person to another. If you must sit on a bench, dry off first and put your clothes on before doing so.

• Wear shoes whenever possible in the locker room. After showering, dry your feet last. Make sure you dry carefully between the toes, and dust your feet with nonprescription antifungal powder to help prevent athlete's foot. Use shower sandals to help prevent the spread of athlete's foot.

• Avoid touching team members or other persons who share the athletic facilities, especially during outbreaks of colds or the flu. When you can't avoid touching others, wash your hands with soap and warm water before putting your fingers or food touched by your fingers into your mouth. Colds, flu and other viruses are more likely to be spread by hand-to-mouth contact than by breathing air contaminated with sneezes and coughs.

• Lockers must be well ventilated to reduce odors and to enable athletic clothing and equipment to dry. Locker rooms should have automatic temperature and ventilation controls. Spray your locker with an antiseptic spray at least once a week.

• Insist that shower rooms and floors of locker rooms be periodically treated with antiseptic solutions.

APPENDIX 5

Nutrition for Athletes

Nutrition is the foundation of any athlete's training program. It is essential to maintain good nutrition at all times for optimal athletic performance, even if competition is only seasonal. Poor dietary intake can diminish any gains made in performance, even if the athlete is participating in a well-designed training program. A diet with sufficient macronutrient content (protein, carbohydrates and fat) will allow the athlete to take advantage of the physiological and hormonal effects of these nutrients.

One problem in determining optimal dietary intake is that there is no one ideal diet that will fit every individual athlete. Another problem is that the nutrient demands of different sports vary widely. Current research reveals a wide range of recommendations regarding the makeup of an optimal diet for athletes. The following information is intended to provide a starting point for athletes in evaluating their dietary intake. These guidelines may be modified as time passes and ongoing research provides additional information regarding nutrition and athletic performance.

Present Dietary Guidelines

One tool that has recently been designed to help all individuals achieve a healthy diet is the Food Guide Pyramid developed by the U.S. Department of Agriculture (USDA). This pyramid provides a visual guideline as to the types of foods and how much of each a person should consume every day. The USDA recommends that we eat more of the foods at the bottom of the pyramid and less of the foods at the top.

At the base of pyramid is the bread, cereal, rice and pasta group, from which it is recommended that we eat 6 to 11 servings a day. (One serving = 1 slice of bread, 1/2 bagel, 1 small muffin, 1 4-inch pancake or waffle, 1/2 to 3/4 cup cooked cereal, 1/2 cup rice or pasta, 1 ounce or 1 cup ready-to-eat cereal or 1/2 potato).

On the next level of the pyramid are the vegetable group and the fruit group. It is recommended that we eat 3 to 5 servings of vegetables and 2 to 4 servings of fruit a day. (One serving = 1/2 cup of vegetables, 1 medium fruit or 1 cup of salad. Note that potatoes and corn are starchy vegetables and are considered part of the bread and cereal group).

On the next level of the pyramid are the milk, yogurt and cheese group and the meat, poultry, fish, dry beans, eggs and nuts group. It is recommended that we eat 2 to 3 servings a day from each of these groups. (One serving of the former = 1 cup of milk or yogurt, 1 ounce of cheese or 1/2 cup of ice cream. One serving of the latter = 3 ounces of meat, 1.5 cups of beans, 2/3 cup of cottage cheese and 4 tablespoons of peanut butter. Note that cottage cheese is high in protein and is considered part of the meat and poultry group.)

At the top of the pyramid is the fats, oils and sweets group. The USDA recommends that we eat foods from this group sparingly.

Although these basic guidelines apply to athletes, they were originally designed with the general population in mind. Therefore, some guidelines may need to be adjusted to meet the nutritional needs of athletes engaged in sport. Following are guidelines for athletes.

Caloric Intake

Athletes involved in regular training and competition will probably need an increased number of total calories in their diets to offset the energy demands and increased metabolic rate accompanying such activity levels. One current recommendation suggests multiplying the weight of the athlete in kilograms (kg) by a range of 35 to 50 to produce an estimate of the number of calories required daily to maintain weight and fuel performance. (To determine your weight in kilograms, multiply your weight in pounds by .454.) For an athlete weighing 100 kg (220 pounds), the recommendation would be 100 x 35 to 50 = 3,500-5,000 calories per day.

Carbohydrates

Carbohydrates are the main source of energy for activity. Carbohydrates are stored in the liver and muscles as glycogen and converted to glucose for use during activity. The current recommendations for carbohydrate intake for athletes range from 40 to 70 percent of total caloric intake. Typically, athletes will require anywhere from 5 to 10 grams of carbohydrates per kilogram of body weight per day (g/kg/day) to maintain their weight and fuel performance.

Carbohydrates are classified as simple or complex. Simple carbohydrates contain mostly sugar. Complex carbohydrates should make up the majority of the carbohydrates consumed daily. Examples of complex carbohydrates are potatoes, rice, dried beans, fresh fruits and vegetables, and whole-grain breads and cereals. These foods also provide dietary fiber, an important element in regulating bowel function.

Protein
The current recommendations for protein intake for athletes range from 15 to 30 percent of total caloric intake. Typically athletes will require anywhere from 1.2 to 2.0 g/kg/day to maintain their lean body mass. Athletes attempting to increase their percentage of lean body mass might benefit from a range of 1.5 to 2.0 g/kg/day.

Fat
The current recommendations for fat intake for athletes range from 20 to 40 percent of total caloric intake.

Fluids
Dehydration has an acute and detrimental impact on athletic performance. Even a slight degree of dehydration significantly decreases the ability of the body to dissipate heat. This, in turn, has a significant adverse effect on performance. Water remains the fluid of choice for hydration purposes. Water is absorbed most rapidly if it is cooler than room temperature, but not ice cold. Fluids containing caffeine are not recommended.

Recommendations for a typical person are to drink at least eight 8-ounce glasses of water daily. Clearly those involved in regular training will need to increase this amount. It is currently recommended that athletes drink 1 to 1.5 milliliters (ml) of fluid per kilocalorie of energy expended. (To convert from ounces to milliliters, multiply the number of ounces by 29.5).

There is evidence to support the use of fluids containing glucose during periods of extended exercise. During exercise lasting longer than 60 minutes, athletes will typically begin to deplete stores of muscle glycogen. Athletes may benefit from drinking 600 to 1000 ml of fluid per hour containing up to 6 percent carbohydrates. If fluid contains more than 6 percent carbohydrates, the carbohydrate content may interfere with and slow absorption of the fluid.

Additional Recommendations for Female Athletes
Some supplements may be necessary for female athletes. Calcium supplements may be recommended for women who exercise so strenuously that their regular menstrual periods cease. These women are at higher risk of developing osteoporosis (a condition that involves loss of bone mass and density) at an early age.

Iron supplements may also be recommended for some women. Normally iron stores are not directly diminished by exercise. However, if iron-deficiency anemia develops as a result of other causes, such as excessive menstruation, an iron supplement is essential to ensure optimal physical performance.

Eating Schedules for Athletes

Before Competition or Exercise
There is little consensus as to the timing or makeup of meals eaten before competition or vigorous exercise. Current recommendations contain a wide range of information. A meal should be consumed anywhere from two to five hours prior to the start of competition or exercise. This will allow ample time for the meal to be digested and energy to be stored before exercise begins. Foods should be selected based on prior knowledge of palatability and ease of digestion.

A meal consumed before competition or exercise should contain higher amounts of complex carbohydrates than usual and smaller amounts of protein and fat. Digestion of complex carbohydrates will allow for a slow, steady release of glucose into the bloodstream. Plenty of fluids should also be consumed as part of this meal. It is especially important to avoid fluids containing caffeine prior to competition or exercise.

After Competition or Exercise
During strenuous exercise, stores of muscle and liver glycogen are depleted. Research has shown that glycogen is more readily stored during the first four hours following competition or exercise. Ingesting a meal that is high in carbohydrates within this time period will allow glycogen stores to be more rapidly replenished, thus enabling the athlete to resume high-intensity training sooner following competition or vigorous exercise. Rehydration is another important aspect of meals eaten after competition or exercise.

(continued on next page)

APPENDIX 5 (continued)

Other Considerations

Any athlete who trains regularly should be aware that vigorous exercise may transform some body fat into lean mass (muscle). As a result, while the overall body weight of the athlete may not change, the percentage of body fat may decrease, while the ratio of lean body weight to overall body weight may increase. Athletes who discontinue training for any reason may need to decrease their caloric intake. Without the regular vigorous activity that burns calories for fuel, extra calories may be stored as body fat, rapidly increasing both the percentage of body weight and the overall body weight of the athlete.

While there has been a significant amount of research into the effects of supplementing the diet with micronutrients (vitamins and minerals), very little of this research has shown a positive effect on performance enhancement. Most research shows that the micronutrient needs of athletes are met without supplementation. However, obviously supplementation is beneficial for those with deficiencies of specific micronutrients.

Sports nutrition has become a very controversial and lucrative business. While there are some products being marketed that genuinely improve performance, athletes should always beware of any products or information that make extraordinary claims. Many of these products and diet plans are marketed on the basis of unproven anecdotal results that have not been supported by sound research. There are many quality resources detailing nutritional needs and planning for athletes that are readily available to anyone desiring more information.

APPENDIX 6

Common Injuries Associated with Various Sports

Almost any of the injuries and medical problems described in this book could occur during participation in any sport or vigorous physical activity. The most likely ones associated with popular sports are listed below, sport by sport.

Aerobic Dance: Muscle, ligament or tendon sprain or strain in any area of the shoulder, arm, abdominal wall, pelvis, leg, ankle or foot; "runner's knee"; shin splints; hamstring injury; foot or leg exostosis or stress fracture.

Archery: Epicondylitis ("tennis elbow"); finger sprain or strain; strain of upper arm muscles, especially biceps; pneumothorax; puncture wounds (from off-target arrows).

Baseball: Epicondylitis ("tennis elbow" or "pitcher's elbow"); strain of upper arm muscles; olecranon elbow fracture; radiohumeral elbow joint sprain; shoulder dislocation; acromioclavicular strain; shoulder bursitis; shin splints; finger fracture or dislocation; laceration; contusion; abrasion; puncture wound (from cleats); hematoma under fingernail or toenail.

Basketball: Finger dislocation or fracture; thumb sprain; ankle sprain; groin muscle sprain; "runner's knee"; shin splints; shoulder dislocation; acromioclavicular strain; shoulder bursitis; hematoma under toenail; contusion; abrasion; laceration.

Boating (Includes Sailing, Canoeing, Kayaking): Cold injury (hypothermia); heat illness; wrist sprain or strain; shoulder tendinitis or bursitis; epicondylitis ("tennis elbow"); knee contusion or abrasion (from kneeling).

Bowling: Epicondylitis ("tennis elbow"); toe contusion; back, shoulder or arm sprain or strain.

Boxing: Facial laceration, especially around the eyes; jaw fracture; head injury, including concussion, epidural hematoma, subdural hematoma or cauliflower ear; neck sprain or dislocation; internal abdominal injury to spleen, liver or kidney; hematoma under fingernail or toenail; contusion; abrasion.

Cycling: Contusion or pressure injury to the perineum (area between the scrotum and anus in males, between the vagina and anus in females), causing numbness in genitals and upper legs; boils on buttocks due to heat and moisture; carpal tunnel syndrome; "runner's knee"; sprain or strain of pelvic, upper leg or lower leg muscles, tendons or ligaments; ankle sprain; contusion; abrasion; laceration.

Diving: Hand, thumb, wrist or shoulder sprain or strain; head and neck injury; back strain; Osgood-Schlatter's disease.

Fencing: Hematoma under toenail; contusion; abrasion; laceration; puncture wound; back, shoulder or arm sprain or strain.

Football: Every injury listed in this book. The most common ones include those to the head, neck, knee, ankle and pelvic and leg muscles.

Golf: Epicondylitis ("golf elbow"); shoulder bursitis and tendinitis; upper back sprain; contusion or head injury from flying ball.

Gymnastics: Neck or back strain; radius (bone in forearm) stress fracture; shoulder, elbow, wrist, knee, ankle or foot sprain or strain; Osgood-Schlatter's disease; shin splints; hematoma under nailbed; contusion; abrasion; laceration.

Handball: Finger dislocation or fracture; thumb sprain; ankle sprain; groin muscle sprain; "runner's knee"; shin splints; shoulder dislocation; acromioclavicular strain; shoulder bursitis; hematoma under fingernail or toenail; contusion; abrasion; laceration.

Hiking & Backpacking: Muscle, ligament or tendon strain or sprain in any area of the shoulder, arm, abdominal wall, pelvis, leg, ankle or foot; "runner's knee"; shin splints; hamstring pull; foot or leg exostosis; stress fracture; hematoma under toenail; contusion; abrasion; laceration; puncture wound; snakebite.

Hockey: Every injury listed in this book. The most common ones include those to the head, neck, knee, ankle and pelvic or leg muscles.

Jogging: Muscle, ligament or tendon sprain or strain in any area of the shoulders, arms, abdominal wall, pelvis, legs, ankles or feet; "runner's knee"; shin splints; hamstring injury; foot or leg exostosis or stress fracture; contusion; abrasion; laceration; puncture wound; snakebite.

Mountain Climbing: Abrasion; contusion; laceration; shin splints; dislocation, fracture, sprain or strain of any muscle group or joint; snakebite; head injury; internal chest or abdomen injury; altitude sickness; dehydration; cold injury (hypothermia or frostbite).

(continued on next page)

Racquetball: Eye injury; hematoma under toenail; contusion; abrasion; laceration; shoulder-area bursitis; sprain or strain of the shoulder, neck, back, arm, wrist, hip, upper leg, knee, lower leg or ankle; shin splints; epicondylitis ("tennis elbow").

Scuba Diving: Decompression illness; contact dermatitis (skin rash) if hypersensitive to wet suit material.

Skating (Ice Skating, Roller Skating): Coccyx (tailbone) fracture or contusion from falling; cold injury (ice skating only); foot stress fracture; "runner's knee"; shin splints; Osgood-Schlatter's disease; sprain or strain in the upper leg, knee, lower leg, ankle or foot; hematoma under toenail; contusion; abrasion; laceration.

Skiing (Downhill Skiing, Slalom Skiing, Cross-Country Skiing): Osgood-Schlatter's disease; shin splints; hematoma under toenail; contusion; abrasion; laceration; sprain or strain of ligaments, muscles or tendons of the back, neck, shoulder, chest, abdominal wall, arm, wrist, pelvis, leg, knee, ankle or foot; knee cartilage injury; tendinitis and bursitis of the shoulder, knee or hip; epicondylitis ("tennis elbow"); dehydration; altitude sickness; cold injury (hypothermia); sunburn; injury to the retina of the eye from sun glare.

Soccer: Every injury listed in this book. The most common ones are those to the hip, pelvis and lower extremities.

Softball: Epicondylitis ("tennis elbow" or "pitcher's elbow"); strain of upper arm muscles; olecranon elbow fracture; radiohumeral elbow joint sprain; shoulder dislocation; acromioclavicular strain; shoulder bursitis; shin splints; finger fracture or dislocation; laceration; contusion; abrasion; puncture wound (from cleats); hematoma under fingernail or toenail.

Squash: Eye injury; hematoma under toenail; contusion; abrasion; laceration; shoulder-area bursitis; sprain or strain of the shoulder, neck, back, arm, wrist, hip, upper leg, knee, lower leg or ankle; shin splints; epicondylitis ("tennis elbow").

Surfing: Head injury; sprain or strain of the shoulder, lower back, hip or knee; shin splints; cold injury (hypothermia); sunburn; contact dermatitis from wax on surfboard and sensitivity to wet suits; contusion; abrasion; laceration.

Swimming: Eye injury (from pool chemicals); verruca (warts) from damp poolside areas; sprain or strain of the shoulder, lower back, hip or knee areas; cold injury (hypothermia); sunburn.

Tennis: Epicondylitis ("tennis elbow"); shoulder-area bursitis; eye injury; shin splints; hematoma under toenail; contusion; abrasion; laceration; sprain or strain of the shoulder, neck, back, arm, wrist, hip, upper leg, knee, lower leg or ankle.

Track & Field Events (Sprints, Relays, High Jump, Discus, Long Jump, Hurdles, Javelin Throw, Pole Vault, Shot Put): Muscle, ligament or tendon sprain or strain of any area of the shoulder, arm, abdominal wall, pelvis, leg, ankle or foot; "runner's knee"; shin splints; hamstring injury; foot or leg exostosis or stress fracture; hematoma under toenail; contusion; abrasion; laceration; puncture wound.

Trampoline: Sprain or strain of the hand, thumb, wrist or shoulder; head and neck injury; back strain; Osgood-Schlatter's disease.

Volleyball: Finger dislocation or fracture; thumb sprain; ankle sprain; shin splints; groin muscle sprain; "runner's knee"; shoulder dislocation; acromioclavicular strain; shoulder bursitis; hematoma under fingernail or toenail; contusion; abrasion; laceration.

Walking: Injuries are unlikely, but possibilities include muscle, ligament or tendon strain or sprain in any area of the shoulder, arm, abdominal wall, pelvis, leg, ankle or foot; "runner's knee"; hamstring pull; foot or leg exostosis; stress fracture; contusion; abrasion; laceration; snakebite.

Water Polo: Eye injury (from pool chemicals); verruca (warts) from damp poolside areas; sprain or strain of the shoulder, lower back, hip or knee; cold injury (hypothermia); sunburn; contusion; abrasion; laceration.

Water Skiing: Head injury; epicondylitis ("tennis elbow"); contusion; abrasion; laceration; sprain or strain of the back, neck, shoulder, chest, abdominal wall, arm, wrist, pelvis, leg, knee, ankle or foot; shin splints; knee cartilage injury; tendinitis and bursitis of the shoulder, knee or hip; cold injury (hypothermia); sunburn; injury to the retina of the eye from sun glare.

Weightlifting: Strain or sprain of the muscles, tendons or ligaments of the neck, shoulder, arm, wrist, finger, abdominal wall, hip, pelvis, leg (especially quadriceps), knee, ankle, foot or toe; elbow dislocation; dehydration from fluid loss due to sweating.

Wrestling: Laceration of areas around the eye; head injury, including concussion, epidural hematoma, subdural hematoma or cauliflower ear; neck sprain or dislocation; internal abdominal injury to the spleen, liver or kidney; hematoma under fingernail or toenail; contusion; abrasion; shoulder dislocation, Osgood-Schlatter's disease. Almost any other injury is possible, but because this sport is usually well supervised, injuries are minimal.

APPENDIX 7

Medical Conditions That Disqualify an Individual for Sports Participation

NONCOLLISION, NONCONTACT SPORTS (see next page for collision and contact sports)
(Competitive running of marathons; track and field; tennis; racket sports; competitive swimming; bowling; golf; archery).

Temporary Disqualifications
• Active infection, including:
Respiratory infection.
Kidney infection.
Infectious mononucleosis.
Hepatitis.
Acute rheumatic fever.
Active tuberculosis.
• Joint inflammation resulting from infection or recent injury.

Permanent Disqualifications
• Chronic diseases, including:
Those that involve serious bleeding tendencies, such as hemophilia.
Inadequately controlled diabetes.
Severe chronic obstructive pulmonary disease.
Valvular heart disease (mitral stenosis, aortic stenosis).
Previous heart surgery (sometimes).
High blood pressure with a known cause, such as chronic kidney disease, coarctation (constriction of a small segment of the aorta), adrenal tumors or congenital arteriosclerosis. This disqualification does not include essential hypertension or high blood pressure due to an unknown cause that is under control with medications. Vigorous exercise after adequate training is recommended for persons with this condition.

Exceptions
Persons with mild forms of the preceding conditions may benefit from noncontact, noncollision exercise programs if they have medical supervision and frequent monitoring of their conditions. Consult your doctor for guidance if you have any of the following:
• High blood pressure.
• Asthma.
• Early obstructive pulmonary disease.
• Well-controlled diabetes.
• Convulsive disorders controlled by medication.
• Absence of one kidney.
• Absence of one testicle or undescended testicles.
• Previous heart attack.
• Previous heart surgery.

APPENDIX 7 (continued)

COLLISION AND CONTACT SPORTS
(Football; hockey; rugby; lacrosse; baseball; basketball; soccer; wrestling; boxing).

Temporary Disqualifications
- Active infection, including:
  Respiratory infection.
  Kidney infection.
  Infectious mononucleosis.
  Hepatitis.
  Acute rheumatic fever.
  Active tuberculosis.
- Joint inflammation resulting from infection or recent injury.
- Skin disease in an active phase (boils, impetigo, herpes).
- Fractures and dislocations.

Permanent Disqualifications
- Physical immaturity in comparison with others competing in the same group.
- Chronic diseases, including:
  Those that involve serious bleeding tendencies, such as hemophilia.
  Inadequately controlled diabetes.
  Severe chronic obstructive pulmonary disease.
  Valvular heart disease (mitral stenosis, aortic stenosis).
  Previous heart surgery (sometimes).
  High blood pressure with a known cause, such as chronic kidney disease, coarctation (constriction of a small segment of the aorta), adrenal tumors or congenital arteriosclerosis. This disqualification does not include essential hypertension or high blood pressure due to an unknown cause that is under control with medications. Vigorous exercise after adequate training is recommended for persons with this condition.
- Hernia (no disqualification after successful surgical repair).
- Congenital musculoskeletal abnormalities that prevent competitive function, such as clubfoot or osteogenesis imperfecta.
- Loss of one eye or blindness in one eye.
- Repeated head injuries or repeated concussions accompanied by unconsciousness.
- Epilepsy or other convulsive disorder not controlled with medication.
- Previous head or brain surgery.
- Absence of one kidney.
- Absence of one testicle.

APPENDIX 8

Stress & Psychosomatic Illness in Athletics

Competitive sports—by their nature—cause stress. Vigorous exercise programs can also cause stress if one takes a program seriously or tries to keep up with friends or others. To a certain degree, stress can have positive effects and push us to greater achievement. But how much stress one can easily handle varies from person to person.

Stress, particularly that due to competitive excitement, fear or anger, causes the body to liberate chemicals that stimulate the adrenal glands. These glands release adrenaline (sometimes called epinephrine). Adrenaline has the following effects on the body:
* Rapid heartbeat.
* Increased blood pressure.
* Tremor.
* Headache.
* Excessive sweating.
* Body hair "standing on end."
* Dry mouth and throat.

Under ordinary circumstances, vigorous exercise "burns off" the breakdown products (catecholamines) of adrenalin. If all the chemicals produced by stress are not burned off, the positive effects of exercise may become negative and self-defeating. Common stress-related disorders are:
* Insomnia.
* Mental and emotional upheavals.
* Skin eruptions, such as eczema and neurodermatitis.
* Digestive system problems, including peptic ulcers, colitis and irritable colon.
* Endocrine disorders, including overactive thyroid, adrenal gland or pituitary gland overactivity or underactivity, changes in menstrual patterns, impotence or premature ejaculation in men or orgasmic dysfunction in women.
* Lung disorders associated with spasm of the bronchial tubes, such as asthma.
* Pain syndromes, such as chronic or recurrent disabling headaches or back pain.

Other causes of stress that can occur in anyone, athlete or not, include:
* Regular conflict with others.
* Recent death of a loved one—spouse, child or friend.
* Loss of anything valuable.
* Injury or severe illness.
* Being fired or changing jobs.
* Recent move to a new home.
* Sexual difficulties.
* Business, academic or financial reverses or taking on a large debt.
* Constant fatigue.

Many doctors believe that stress has a role in almost any disorder. Few doubt that stress can complicate an illness or delay healing from an injury or surgery by preventing normal recovery, prolonging pain and sustaining disability.

SELF-HELP TIPS FOR COPING WITH STRESS

Here are some tips that may help you reduce stress:
* Learn a meditation technique and practice it regularly—daily if possible. There are many methods available. Most of them include "tuning in to" and giving complete attention to a word, sound, sentence or concept that you silently repeat to yourself. Don't try to banish other thoughts that enter your mind during your period of concentration, but don't focus on them enough to stop you from meditating. The purpose of meditation is to empty your mind of all disturbing thoughts for a given period of time to encourage mental relaxation. Mental relaxation, in turn, will help reduce stress.

The transcendental meditation program is a different technique that has been shown through extensive physiological research to be effective in reducing stress. It is taught in most communities in individualized instruction sessions through the International Meditation Society.

(continued on next page)

APPENDIX 8 (continued)

• Take a short period of time away from any stressful situation you encounter during a day. Practice a muscle-tensing and muscle-relaxing technique. Close your eyes and take a series of deep breaths. Then start with the muscle groups in your face. Consciously tense them and hold the contraction for a few seconds. Then consciously relax them. Continue through all major muscle groups in the body—neck, shoulders, hands, abdomen, back and legs. When you become skillful, you can use this technique to relax quickly any time you need to in almost any environment.

• Avoid taking your problems to bed with you. At the end of the day, spend a few minutes reviewing your entire day's experiences, event by event, as if you're replaying a tape. Release all negative emotions you have harbored (anger, feelings of insecurity or anxiety). Relish all good energy or emotion (loving thoughts, praise, feeling good about your work or yourself). Reach a decision about unfinished events, and release mental or muscular tension. Then you're ready for a relaxing and emotionally healing sleep.

PSYCHOSOMATIC ILLNESS

Psychosomatic illness is a term used to describe an illness in which factors other than physical ones dominate. These factors may also play an important part in complications. Such illnesses are real—not imagined, as many people think. We can't separate our body from our mind or our spirit. Most illnesses have some connection with these elements, even if the links between mind, spirit and body are poorly defined at times.

Although medical researchers are beginning to understand the basic mechanisms, we still have much to learn about psychosomatic illness. One group of researchers believes that mental, emotional or spiritual stress can trigger almost any illness in a person genetically predisposed to that illness. Such illnesses include asthma, cancer, digestive disturbances and heart disease. All these and others are more common in certain families. Yet not all people in these families succumb to the same illnesses.

SUGGESTIONS FOR IMPROVING, PREVENTING OR COPING WITH PSYCHOSOMATIC ILLNESS

• Define and resolve all personal conflicts, if possible. Confront areas of personal conflict in your spiritual, emotional, occupational, civic or recreational involvements. If you can't resolve these conflicts alone, seek help from family, friends or competent counselors.

• Seek a balanced life of work, intellectual and physical challenges, recreation, intimacy, reflection and rest. Be moderate in all your activities.

• Maintain a positive attitude whenever possible.

• Allow yourself to give and receive love.

• Be a friend. Considerate, respectful and loving attitudes toward yourself and others are powerful allies.

APPENDIX 9

Aging & Exercise

People of all ages benefit from regular exercise. Many persons aged 65 and older exercise regularly and stay as physically fit as their general health allows. These persons grow older with a style and vigor far surpassing those of their sedentary contemporaries. Following are some specific ways in which exercise and fitness are beneficial in aging:
● More people reach age 65 and older who are physically fit than those who are not. Those who remain physically active continue to have more stamina than their inactive counterparts.
● Although exercise probably does not retard the aging process, it reduces the likelihood of untimely death from medical problems that are caused in part by a sedentary lifestyle. These include coronary artery disease, high blood pressure, stroke, kidney disease, chronic lung disease and depression.

THE BENEFITS OF AEROBIC EXERCISE
Aerobic exercise is the most effective way to achieve physical and psychological benefits. An exercise is aerobic if it provides:
● Sustained physical activity that uses major muscle groups of the body.
● Regulated-intensity, long-duration exercise for 20 minutes or more.
Proper aerobic benefit is based on sufficient exercise to accelerate the heart rate to a prescribed level and keep it there a certain length of time. Three to five aerobic exercise sessions a week are necessary for maximum benefit. The best forms of aerobic exercise include brisk walking, swimming, bike riding, jogging, rope jumping and rowing, Sports such as bowling, tennis and golf have good recreational effects, but they do not require enough effort to allow one to reach sustained aerobic levels.
Persons over 65 receive the same benefits from aerobic exercise as do younger persons—even if they choose the less strenuous forms of exercise. Following is an explanation of the effects of aerobic exercise on the body.

EXERCISE & THE CARDIOVASCULAR SYSTEM
Older persons are most at risk of cardiovascular problems. Exercise benefits the cardiovascular system in the following ways:
● Increases the number of circulating red blood cells (thus providing more oxygen and better nourishment to all body cells).
● Increases the blood flow during exercise.
● Increases production of the enzymes necessary for changing glucose into usable energy by body cells.
● Increases the amount of high-density lipoproteins in the circulating blood. These protect against hardening of the arteries, which is responsible for heart attacks, strokes and chronic kidney failure.

EXERCISE & CIRCULATION TO THE BRAIN AND OTHER BODY PARTS
Exercise in a healthy person produces an increase in an enzyme that helps prevent the deposit of fibrin (a clotting factor in the blood) in the blood vessels to the brain and other body parts. Fibrin deposits on the lining of the blood vessels narrow the arteries and decrease the blood supply to the cells supplied by the affected blood vessels. Narrowed arteries and decreased blood flow can result in stroke, heart attack and lack of sufficient blood supply to the kidneys and legs, causing kidney failure.

EXERCISE & THE LUNGS
Regular exercise can increase one's maximum breathing capacity, improving or preventing chronic lung disease.

EXERCISE & THE MUSCULOSKELETAL SYSTEM
Regular, adequate exercise helps maintain the normal size and contour of muscles and bones. The combination of exercise and adequate calcium intake is an important factor in preventing osteoporosis (softening of the bones), a common disorder in women past menopause. (In addition to exercise and calcium, bone-building drugs may also be necessary to prevent osteoporosis.) Exercise promotes healthy new bone formation in all age groups. This new bone protects against bone fractures that commonly occur in older people of both sexes.

(continued on next page)

APPENDIX 9 (continued)

EXERCISE & THE MIND
Exercise helps rid the body of ("burn off") undesirable levels of catecholamines (breakdown products of adrenaline, which is released by the body as a reaction to physical or mental stress). The following results have been documented in many studies:
● Regular exercise has a positive influence on one's sense of well-being and self-esteem.
● An exercise program can be very beneficial in relieving depression—it is now commonly prescribed as part of therapy.

EXERCISE & SEXUALITY
Exercise has the following beneficial effects on sexuality:
● Men who remain physically active maintain a higher level of testosterone than their sedentary contemporaries.
● People who exercise regularly are generally healthier emotionally, have a better self-image and enjoy increased muscular strength. These factors are all important in meaningful sexual relationships.
● People who are fit—no matter what their age—are more sexually attractive to others.

CONCLUSIONS
Regular exercise has proved to be of great benefit in minimizing the negative effects of aging. If you are an older person who has not remained physically fit, discuss a fitness program with your doctor. Follow his or her suggestions about what exercise you can safely perform.

APPENDIX 10

Chronic Disease & Exercise

Some persons suffer from serious disease that can last many years. Each case must be evaluated on an individual basis, but many of these persons can benefit from regular exercise. It can play a vital role in improving their sense of well-being. In a few instances, it may help retard progress of the disease. Three of the most serious and common forms of chronic disease—heart disease, chronic obstructive pulmonary (lung) disease and diabetes—are discussed in this section.

HEART DISEASE & EXERCISE

The most common types of heart disease are coronary artery disease and hardening of the arteries (atherosclerosis or arteriosclerosis). Three important risk factors for developing heart disease are hypertension (high blood pressure), obesity and a sedentary lifestyle. Exercise plays an important role in controlling hypertension and obesity, making it significant in the treatment of heart disease. The known benefits of cardiovascular fitness include:
- Increased blood supply to the heart.
- Decreased oxygen demand.
- Increased blood flow through the coronary arteries.
- Increased efficiency of heart muscle function.
- Indirect evidence of decreased electrical irritability of the heart, lessening the chance that abnormal or life-threatening heartbeat irregularities will occur.
- Indirect evidence of delayed development of hardening of the arteries. These benefits are possible for men and women in all age groups, but the most positive evidence of benefit is in men over 40.

After Heart Disease is Diagnosed—Many medical centers throughout the world have developed rehabilitation centers for patients who have had heart attacks. The American College of Sports Medicine has established guidelines and certification programs for exercise leaders trained in cardiac rehabilitation techniques. These centers prescribe exercise after a thorough evaluation and supervise the exercise carefully with monitors. Following a heart attack a cardiac patient can frequently benefit from enrolling in one of these programs in a YMCA, college or university physical education department or cardiac rehabilitation center. It is unsafe for a recent cardiac patient to try to develop an exercise program at home. A specialized facility, under the supervision of trained professionals, can offer monitoring of your responses to individually designed exercise programs. Repeated studies have shown that such careful programs have brought quicker recovery, earlier return to work, an enhanced feeling of well-being, and less likelihood of developing a subsequent heart attack. Ask your doctor for a referral.

CHRONIC OBSTRUCTIVE PULMONARY DISEASE & EXERCISE

COPD (chronic obstructive pulmonary disease) is any long-term lung disorder characterized by gradually increasing breathing difficulty. Some underlying diseases that produce COPD include chronic bronchitis, bronchiectasis, emphysema, asthma and other disorders associated with spasm of the bronchial tubes. For a full description of each of these diseases, see *Complete Guide to Symptoms, Illness & Surgery* by H. Winter Griffith, M.D., published by Perigee Books.

Exercise Programs—Supervised exercise and activity can enhance breathing function and improve the patient's sense of well-being. However, exercise programs for people with this disorder must be individualized. A physical therapist or doctor can teach the patient how to increase his or her breathing skill and capacity. Breathing retraining begins with exercises using forced expiration against pursed lips and other techniques to use the diaphragm and accessory muscles of the chest wall. When breathing rehabilitation reaches an acceptable level, a program of walking can increase breathing capacity and general health. See your doctor for detailed instructions.

(continued on next page)

APPENDIX 10 (continued)

DIABETES & EXERCISE

Diabetes is a disease of metabolism characterized by the body's inability to produce enough insulin to process carbohydrates, fat and protein efficiently. Non-insulin-dependent diabetes can often be controlled with a treatment program that includes diet, exercise, weight loss and oral medication (sometimes). Insulin-dependent diabetes can usually be controlled with regular injections of insulin in addition to the diet and exercise program. Therefore, diabetic patients, whether insulin-dependent or non-insulin-dependent, benefit from exercise—even though the role of exercise in treatment is still not well understood. However, people with diabetes should be medically evaluated and educated before beginning an exercise or athletic program.

Benefits
- Exercise helps control appetite in diabetic persons who need to lose weight. Exercise by itself does not necessarily lead to weight loss, but it does affect the "appetite control center" in the hypothalamus, decreasing appetite. In some persons with non-insulin-dependent diabetes, weight loss alone reduces blood sugar levels.
- Exercise helps improve glucose (sugar) tolerance in some diabetic persons. This allows a reduction of insulin (for insulin-dependent individuals) or oral medication (for non-insulin-dependent individuals).
- Exercise appears to reduce the likelihood of cardiovascular disease (heart attack, stroke, kidney failure, hypertension). These conditions are more likely to occur in people with diabetes, so exercise becomes an aid in prevention. To sustain the protective effect, exercise must be performed regularly throughout one's lifetime.

Risks
- Prolonged or overly vigorous exercise may increase the effect of insulin or oral antidiabetic medicines, causing them to lower blood sugar too much. This could produce symptoms of hypoglycemia (low blood sugar), including confusion, weakness, sweating, paleness or loss of consciousness. Treatment includes drinking a high-sugar drink, such as orange juice with added sugar, and notifying your doctor as soon as possible.
- Complications of diabetes (diabetic retinopathy, peripheral neuropathy, decreased kidney function) may worsen with overly enthusiastic training or activity, depending on the activity chosen. See recommendations below, and consult your doctor for more information.

Recommendations
- Don't start or return to an intensive exercise program until your diabetes is under control. Then consult your doctor about the suitability of the exercise program you have chosen.
- Under medical guidance, learn to balance your insulin dosage with exercise and diet. For instance, prior to heavy exercise, you may need to reduce the insulin dose and increase food intake.
- If you use insulin, inject it into a nonexercising part—such as the abdomen—rather than the arm or leg.
- If you have diabetic retinopathy, don't jog, lift weights or attempt any exercise that jars the head or increases pressure in the eye.
- Because diabetes increases the risk of developing cardiovascular problems, all persons with diabetes (particularly those over 40) should have medical clearance before beginning any strenuous exercise program or sports activity.
- Special precautions are necessary for individuals with diabetes who drink alcohol or must take other medications, such as aspirin, beta-adrenergic blockers and nonsteroidal anti-inflammatory medicines. Each of these can cause hypoglycemia during exercise. If you take these drugs, you must reduce your exercise level to compensate for resulting blood sugar changes.

APPENDIX 11

Mental Retardation, Sports & Exercise

Athletic activity and recreation are important for everyone, regardless of mental capacity. Sports and athletic activities can make a positive difference in problems experienced by persons who are mentally retarded. These problems include poor physical fitness, obesity, restlessness, boredom, hyperactivity and social immaturity. Most health professionals and social workers believe that children and adults who are mildly to moderately retarded can and should participate safely in athletic activities, as long as they are supervised adequately. This section presents guidelines to parents or guardians of mentally retarded children and adults who are considering an exercise program or athletic competition for them.

RECOMMENDATIONS

• Encourage and stress activities that require gross motor (large muscle) coordination rather than fine motor coordination.

• Stress the right kinds of activities. Children and adults who are mentally retarded find more satisfaction and success in participating in dual and individual sports rather than in team sports. Children who are retarded may benefit from noncompetitive sports with normal children.

• Teach and encourage games, which are more interesting than exercises. The following sports and activities are recommended: tennis, folk dancing, shooting baskets, running races, playing catch, boating, bicycling and hiking. Less suitable activities that are not recommended include basketball, football and baseball.

• Match competitors evenly so each person has a chance to win sometimes. Have children participate with each other according to their developmental ages rather than their chronological ages. Otherwise, some individuals may fail repeatedly, damaging their self-esteem and turning a positive situation into a negative one.

• Keep records of improvement, and share them with the person who is retarded.

• Support development of athletic opportunities at the community level. For more information about programs for persons who are mentally retarded, contact either of the following:

The Special Olympics, Inc.
1325 G St., N.W.
Suite 500
Washington, D.C. 20005
202-628-3630
www.specialolympics.org

Arc of the United States
1010 Wayne Ave., Suite 650
Silver Spring, MD 20910
301-565-3842
www.thearc.org

APPENDIX 12

Sexual Activity & Contraception in Athletes

Several medical studies and reports conclude that men and women who are well conditioned and vigorously engaged in sports and competition have more frequent sexual intercourse—and enjoy it more—than their sedentary counterparts. The energy drain that results from sexual intercourse is negligible among athletes, who are physically fit. The amount of energy expended is estimated to be equal to running a 100-yard dash.

CONTRACEPTIVE CONSIDERATIONS

Athletes use the same contraceptive measures as others, but some forms of birth control may require special considerations for athletes. The use of diaphragms, cervical caps or rubber condoms obviously has no effect on sports ability or performance. However, the following forms of contraception for women merit examination:

• Contraceptive creams and jellies sometimes cause vaginal and vulva irritation that can interfere with athletic performance. These side effects usually disappear readily once the cream or jelly is discontinued. Occasionally, local treatment with topical steroid creams is necessary.

• Oral contraceptive pills cause significant physiological changes. At present, we do not know enough to encourage or discourage their use in women athletes. Some women retain excess fluid while on the pill, and this may decrease performance. On the other hand, the pill increases the body's blood volume. Exercise enhances the body's ability to deal with the body's blood volume because the heart functions more efficiently and circulation is better. Both of these factors can enhance endurance and other aspects of performance. The physiological changes experienced with oral contraceptives vary from woman to woman, so the decision to use the pill should be based on factors other than physical activity.

• Injections of long-acting progesterone can cause fluid retention and irregular periods. Fluid retention may decrease athletic performance.

• Intrauterine devices (IUDs) have significant negative effects on women athletes and should not be used. Following are some of the reported problems associated with using IUDs:

(1) Higher percentage of pelvic infections in athletes than in sedentary women using IUDs.

(2) Higher degree of unpredictable intervals between menstrual periods in athletes than in sedentary women using IUDs.

(3) Much higher frequency of heavy, prolonged bleeding. Some medical studies have reported that 60% to 75% of IUD users experience excessive flow. This significant increase in bleeding can lead to anemia and decreased oxygen-carrying capacity of the blood, eventually affecting athletic performance.

APPENDIX 13

Pregnancy, Sports & Vigorous Exercise

Fitness and continued recreational activities during pregnancy are important for mother and unborn child. Increased oxygenation provided by exercise helps nourish the fetus. Continuing exercise and recreation at the prepregnancy level (within the limitations described below) are feasible and recommended for the first several months of pregnancy. However, starting a new vigorous fitness program during pregnancy is not wise. Pregnancy affects posture and center of gravity and balance. Changes occur in the respiratory system, the cardiovascular system, total body weight and the body's ability to dissipate heat.

RECOMMENDATIONS DURING PREGNANCY
• If you are planning to become pregnant, start a fitness program and attain as high a level of physical fitness as possible prior to conception. This maximizes your chances of a healthy pregnancy.
• If you continue to exercise after conception, you should increase your caloric nutritional intake to allow for a 23- to 27-pound weight gain during pregnancy. Carefully follow your doctor's nutritional recommendations regarding vitamins, folic acid, iron and other supplements.
• After conception, continue to exercise at your prepregnancy level, but don't increase the frequency or vigor of your program. During the first 3 or 4 months, avoid repeated prolonged exercise. Reduce activity by the 5th month. Toward the end of your pregnancy, your body will let you know you should decrease your activity. The signals for this include increased weight, decreased breathing capacity, increased clumsiness and change in your center of gravity. Pay attention to your body's signals—don't push beyond your capacity. By the 7th month and until 4 weeks after delivery, confine exercise to the limited amount prescribed by your doctor.
• Avoid activities in hot weather that increase your body temperature. If you are not sure what your temperature is, take it rectally after an average workout under average conditions. If your body temperature is higher than 101°F, take steps to prevent temperature elevation. Consider these measures:
  Select a cooler time of day for exercise.
  Wear loose, light clothing.
  Increase water intake to prevent dehydration.
  Temporarily decrease the vigor or duration of your exercise program.
• Avoid saunas, hot tubs, whirlpools and steam rooms during pregnancy. Any of these may cause harmful increases in body temperature.
• Don't train at high altitudes, because oxygen levels are lower.
• Avoid scuba diving while pregnant. Increased pressure can have adverse effects on the fetus.
• Avoid contact or collision sports, which can lead to harmful abdominal injuries. It is probably better to avoid or restrict fast running, cross-country skiing, aerobic dance exercises (except for special prenatal classes) or speed sports of any sort.
• During the later months of pregnancy, avoid downhill skiing. Your center of gravity will have changed, making spills much more likely—even if you are a skilled athlete.
• Stop all exercise and report to your doctor immediately if any of the following occurs:
  Abdominal pain.
  Bleeding from the vagina.
  Rupture of the fetal membranes—signaled by a gush of water from the vagina.
  Cessation of fetal movement.

RECOMMENDATIONS FOLLOWING DELIVERY
• Resume your training program and full vigorous exercise and competition as soon as all pain in the genitals and abdomen has disappeared. If you had an episiotomy (an incision that enlarges the vaginal opening), the recovery time will be a little longer. You should be able to gradually resume your regular activities within 3 to 4 weeks after delivery.
• Avoid inserting anything into the vagina (such as tampons or douching chemicals) for 3 to 4 weeks following delivery. Until that time, the dilated cervix that allowed delivery of your baby forms a fertile entry for germs into the reproductive organs, making you susceptible to infection. Use sanitary napkins for continued bleeding. Talk to your doctor about resuming sexual relations. The usual recommendation is to avoid vaginal intercourse for a few weeks following delivery, whether or not there has been an episiotomy.
• If you wish to breast-feed your baby, it should cause no major problems that would interfere with your exercise program. Be careful to use adequate breast support and to increase your fluid intake during exercise to prevent dehydration.

APPENDIX 14

Drugs in Sports

The use of drugs by amateur and professional athletes has received much publicity in recent years. Many athletes believe that drugs are essential for optimum performance. The issue of whether drugs can enhance physical performance remains controversial and unresolved. However, the physiological effects that drugs have on the body can be documented. This section is devoted to examining the most common drugs used by athletes. Questions of legality or ethics are best answered by the prevailing view in sports medicine: The use of drugs is generally considered unethical—in some cases illegal—and such use is usually forbidden by organizations that govern competitive athletics.

ANABOLIC STEROID HORMONES
Some athletes take synthetic male hormones (anabolic steroids) in the hope of increasing strength or muscle mass. The most common synthetic male hormones taken by athletes include testosterone, methandrostenolone and nandrolone.

Effects in Women—Muscle mass increases when the hormone is taken for a sufficiently long period of time. However, side effects and adverse reactions include the following:
* Growth of hair on the face and other body parts.
* Enlargement of the clitoris.
* Deepening of the voice.
* Acne.
* Baldness.
* Change in sex drive (usually increased).
* Irregular menstrual periods.
* Depression.

Effects in Men—Strength and body weight sometimes increase. However, many side effects and adverse reactions are possible. These include:
* Decreased levels of FSH (follicle-stimulating hormone) and leutenizing hormone. These in turn cause decreased male hormone production, decreased sperm production and testicular atrophy.
* A decrease in high-density lipoprotein, which may increase the likelihood of hardening of the arteries, stroke and kidney disease.
* Increased incidence of liver tumors.
* Increased aggressiveness.
* Acne.
* Depression.
* Change in sex drive (sometimes lessened, sometimes increased).
* Increased risk of soft tissue injuries such as tendon ruptures and muscle strains.

The consensus among medical experts is that the use of anabolic steroid hormones by both men and women poses greater risk and danger from adverse effects than is justified by any possible benefit. Physicians uniformly advise against using them. Their use is condemned by the Medical Commission of the International Olympics Committee.

AMPHETAMINES
These drugs are central nervous system stimulants. Athletes take them believing they will help their performance in competition. Studies show that performance is actually diminished, despite the feeling on the part of the athlete that his or her performance is outstanding, The toxic effects of amphetamines are:
* Tremor.
* Confusion.
* Restlessness.
* Loss of appetite.
* Delusions and hallucinations.
* High blood pressure.
* Heartbeat irregularities.

Amphetamines are particularly dangerous if taken with other stimulants such as cocaine, appetite suppressants and caffeine.

APPENDIX 14 (continued)

CAFFEINE

Caffeine is also a central nervous system stimulant. When taken in small, infrequent doses, caffeine seems to have few if any long-lasting ill effects. However, new evidence suggests a correlation between consumption of any coffee—including decaffeinated coffee—and an increase in low-density lipoproteins. High levels of these fatty elements in the blood are known to increase the likelihood that atherosclerosis (hardening of the arteries), heart disease, kidney disease and stroke will develop. This effect is noted with the consumption of as little as 2 cups of coffee per day.

The immediate effects of caffeine consumption vary from person to person, depending on individual factors. Most people can tolerate 2 cups a day. However, too much caffeine will produce the following:
- Nervousness, irritability and rapid heartbeat.
- Insomnia.
- Increased urine output.
- Symptoms of low blood sugar (hypoglycemia), including tremor, weakness and increased irritability.

Some people believe caffeine consumption relieves fatigue, but this is an artificial effect. Use of caffeine does not result in increased athletic performance.

COCAINE

This central nervous system stimulant has similar effects to those of amphetamines and caffeine—but stronger. Cocaine is illegal and addicting. Its use can lead to delusions, psychosocial problems, tremor, restlessness and damage to nasal tissues (if "snorted"). An overdose of cocaine can be fatal. Its damaging effects on the central nervous system increase greatly when it is taken with other stimulants such as amphetamines, appetite suppressants or caffeine. Medical experts have documented no benefits from the use of cocaine among athletes.

NICOTINE

This is the addicting factor in tobacco smoke that makes smoking cessation so difficult for many persons. Nicotine causes constriction of the peripheral blood vessels. It also causes an increase in heart rate that does not result in increased cardiac output. The results of these two effects are increased fatigue and diminished athletic performance.

PRESCRIPTION & NONPRESCRIPTION DRUGS

All effective medications have potential side effects for at least some individuals. Do not expect to be able to perform at your accustomed level if you are taking any medication.

Safety precautions for athletes are similar to those for the general population. The most important additional precaution for athletes relates to fluid loss that accompanies heavy sweating. Drugs most likely to become dangerous under these conditions are:
- Digitalis (a heart medicine).
- Diuretics (medicine to treat high blood pressure and heart problems).
- Steroid hormones.

All the above can cause excessive loss of sodium and potassium from the body. The effects of these drugs may be accelerated by fluid loss, as in heavy sweating, diarrhea and vomiting, particularly in hot weather. Excessive sweating due to any cause may require a dose modification of digitalis, diuretics or hormones. Let your doctor know if you exercise vigorously. If you take these or any other medication that affects sodium and potassium metabolism in the body, see Sodium Imbalance and Potassium Imbalance in the Sports Medicine section of this book.

APPENDIX 15

Physical Therapy Methods & Techniques

Rehabilitation, when applied to athletic injuries, means restoration to health. Traditionally this has meant exercising muscles to restore strength, endurance and normal range of motion. A broader interpretation includes other methods and techniques that facilitate the healing process.

Physical agents such as heat, cold, and massage can be used in conjunction with exercise programs—and sometimes medications—to hasten rehabilitation. These can often be used at home under the supervision of a doctor, physical therapist or trainer. These trained professionals can oversee progress, shifting from one type of exercise to another when advisable. The different methods are explained in greater detail below.

COLD (CRYOTHERAPY)

During the past several years, cold treatment has been used increasingly in first aid and in rehabilitation of athletic injuries. Localized cold treatments provide these important benefits:
- Reduction and control of swelling (edema).
- Facilitation of active or passive joint motion, allowing a return to exercise sooner than is possible without cryotherapy. Ice is applied before exercise during the healing phase.
- Reduction of pain and muscle spasm. Because ice can be applied prior to exercise, reducing pain and muscle spasm, muscle and joint movements can start sooner without interfering with the healing process. A thin margin of safety regarding when exercise should start and continue makes clinical supervision necessary during rehabilitation.

Ice can be applied in the form of ice packs, ice compresses or ice massage. Ice massage is particularly helpful for sore muscles or muscles in spasm. The techniques of ice massage are as follows:
- Fill a large styrofoam cup with water and freeze.
- Tear a small amount of foam from the top so ice protrudes.
- Massage firmly over the injured area in a circle about the size of a softball.
- Do this for 7 to 10 minutes at a time 3 or 4 times a day, and also before workouts or competition.

HEAT

When heat is applied to an injury, it dilates (enlarges) small blood vessels in the area, increasing blood flow. The increased blood supply nourishes the tissues and hastens healing. Heat also reduces pain in an injured area and reduces muscle spasm. But heat increases the chance that small capillaries will leak blood and plasma into soft tissues around the injury. While dilation of the blood vessels and increased blood flow are desirable in healing, capillary leakage is undesirable. It leads to greater fluid accumulation and swelling, which retards the healing process. To be beneficial, heat should not be applied until the capillaries have had a chance to seal and stop leaking. This usually requires 24 to 48 hours following injury—if ice, compression and elevation were used immediately.

Depending on the type of injury, heat can be applied in several ways: hot compresses, hydrocollator packs (see Glossary), heat lamps, heating pads, whirlpool baths or hot tubs, ultrasound, or diathermy (seldom used now—see Glossary).

Your doctor or therapist must prescribe the best program for you and provide supervision and guidance throughout your rehabilitation program. You will need instructions about when to start, how long to apply heat during each treatment and how long to continue with heat treatments. These factors are determined by many variables, such as type and extent of injury, previous medical history and healing rate.

MASSAGE

Gentle massage is useful for treating sore muscles. It consists of gentle or firm stroking of the injured area. Strokes should be directed toward the heart. The appropriate amount of pressure and the length of the massage should be determined by the person receiving the massage. Massage that increases pain is too hard. When properly administered, massage can reduce fluid accumulation and swelling around an injury. It will stimulate circulation through the veins and lymphatic vessels. However, *overzealous* massage can aggravate an injury and increase bleeding.

APPENDIX 16

Exercise & Air Pollution

Exercising while breathing polluted air not only decreases performance—it may be hazardous to your health. Polluted air can take either of two forms: it can be polluted by tobacco smoke as you inhale it into your lungs, or it can be polluted by chemicals in the general environment around you.

TOBACCO SMOKE

Tobacco smoke contains up to 4% by volume of carbon monoxide, which greatly reduces the blood's capacity to transport oxygen efficiently to all cells in the body. It may take 24 hours for the blood to return to its normal oxygen-carrying capacity after inhaling the smoke of one cigarette. In addition, smoking tobacco increases airway resistance, preventing the inhaled oxygen from reaching the alveoli (air sacs in the lungs), where oxygen filters into the bloodstream. These effects have a profound effect on athletic performance. An athlete cannot reach peak fitness levels and smoke cigarettes.

ENVIRONMENTAL AIR POLLUTION

Environmental air pollutants can have similar—if not so dramatic—effects on an athlete. However, breathing polluted air may be somewhat inescapable in some urban areas. Environmental pollutants include hydrocarbons, oxidants, carbon monoxide, sulfur oxides, peroxyacetyl nitrates and others. Any or all of these can cause bronchial irritation, excessive mucus production, decreased efficiency of the bronchial cilia (hairlike structures that move and filter mucus), and decreased resistance to respiratory tract infections. Exercising in highly polluted areas, such as along expressways, may adversely affect performance and health. When you exercise, try to do it in an area with the cleanest air possible.

APPENDIX 17

Common Types of Bone Fractures

AVULSION
A small portion of bone, with ligament or tendon attached, is pulled away from the main bone segment.

COMMINUTED
The bone is fractured into three or more segments. This type of fracture usually must be immobilized with surgical screws or pins for healing.

COMPLETE
The fractured bone fragments are completely separated. A clean break usually heals relatively quickly.

COMPOUND (OPEN)
At least one bone fragment penetrates the skin or a skin wound overlying the fracture, allowing bone to be exposed (be visible). When the injury area is open to the outside, the risk of complicating infections increases.

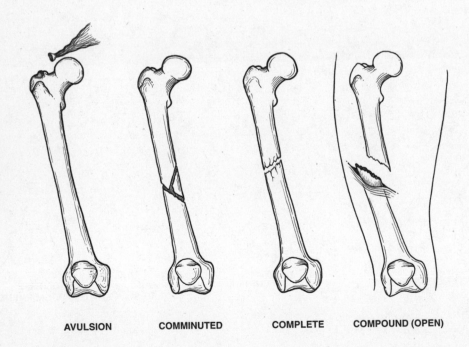

| AVULSION | COMMINUTED | COMPLETE | COMPOUND (OPEN) |

APPENDIX 17 (continued)

COMPRESSION
This type of fracture occurs when the mass of bone is compressed, usually by forces in opposite directions. Compression fractures are most common in the spinal vertebrae.

FATIGUE
This is a complete or incomplete hairline fracture that develops after repeated stress to the bone rather than as the result of a single significant stress.

GREENSTICK
This is an incomplete fracture, with bone fragments joined by at least some bone. Greenstick fractures heal more quickly than other fractures.

SPIRAL
Shearing forces cause the fractured segments to separate in a spiral fashion.

STRESS (SEE FATIGUE)

TRANSVERSE (WITH DISPLACEMENT)
The complete fractured bone segments are displaced in relation to each other. These fractures require strength and skill to return the bone fragments to a functional position for healing.

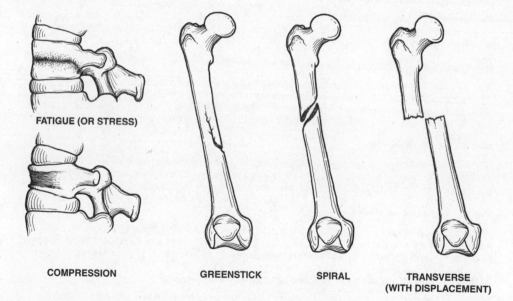

FATIGUE (OR STRESS)

COMPRESSION GREENSTICK SPIRAL TRANSVERSE (WITH DISPLACEMENT)

APPENDIX 18

Using the Web for Health Information

People who look for health and medical information have many choices on the World Wide Web. It is important to know the source and if it is reliable. Look at the web page address. These types of addresses often have excellent websites:

- Addresses that end in .gov are hosted by the U.S. government.

- Addresses that end in .org are hosted by nonprofit organizations, such as the American Heart Association.

- Addresses ending in .edu are provided by universities.

Websites which advertise products (.com) can be good sources for medical information also, but should be read with some caution. It is often helpful to compare several different web resources on the same topic.

Information obtained from the web is not a substitute for your health care provider's instructions and advice. Words on the computer screen can not replace the knowledge and experience that your health care provider can share with you.

Selected Websites

This is a selected list of websites that provide medical information. In addition to these sites, there are many others (sponsored by different types of organizations) that are useful for valid and quality medical information, patient education materials, and helpful ideas for managing your health.

Family Doctor familydoctor.org

The American Academy of Family Physicians provides information for general educational purposes for the whole family. All of the information has been written and reviewed by physicians and patient education professionals.

Healthfinder www.healthfinder.gov/

The U.S. Department of Health & Human services along with other federal agencies designed this web site as a gateway to consumer health information. It provides access to selected online publications, clearinghouses, databases, web sites, and support and self-help groups. It also links to government agencies and not-for-profit organizations that produce reliable information for the public.

Medem www.medem.com

Medem is a web site project of several organizations — including the American Medical Association, the American Academy of Pediatrics, and the American College of Obstetricians and Gynecologists. It is a comprehensive and trusted source of healthcare content on the internet.

Medlineplus www.medlineplus.gov

A web site established by the National Library of Medicine, the world's largest biomedical library and creator of the medline database. An alphabetical list of medical and health topics consists of hundreds of specific diseases, conditions and wellness issues. Health information in spanish is also included.

National Health Information Center www.health.gov/nhic

This site is run by the U.S. department of Health and Human Services. It provides links to many organizations that have information about specific medical topics.

American Orthopaedic Society for Sports Medicine www.sportsmed.org

This site provides information for patients about prevention, treatment and rehabilitation of common sports injuries. It also helps you find a doctor in your location.

APPENDIX 19

Exercise for Good Health

Exercise is a part of a healthy lifestyle at any age. It helps you feel and look better, aids in weight loss, and can lower the risk for many common diseases. Exercise can be fun—even though it may not seem fun at first. Talk to your health care provider about exercising. People who have not been active, have health problems, are pregnant, or elderly may need special advice.

REASONS OR EXCUSES PEOPLE GIVE FOR NOT EXERCISING
People have many reasons for not exercising. Look for ways to overcome the ones that affect you personally.
* *Not enough time or exercising is inconvenient:* Find available time slots. Take exercise breaks at work. Walk for 10-15 minutes at a time.
* *Lack of energy:* Plan exercise time during the day or week when you do feel more energetic. Convince yourself that exercise will actually boost your energy level.
* *It is not enjoyable or it is boring:* Watch television while you exercise. Do gardening or mow the lawn. Exercise with a friend. Join an exercise class.
* *Fear of injury or have had a recent injury:* Learn how to warm up and cool down. Wear proper shoes for the activity. Pick activities that have little risk.
* Lack of confidence in being able to exercise: Exercise with friends who have the same skill level. Take a class to learn a new skill. Walking is the easiest exercise.
* *Not able to maintain an exercise routine due to travel for work or other conflicting schedules:* Walk in hotel halls and take stairs instead of elevators. Pack stretch bands and jump rope and use them in your room. Pick places to stay with pools or fitness rooms.
* *Family or friends are not supportive or encouraging:* Ask your family for support. Invite family or friends to exercise with you. Join a fitness class or hiking club.
* *No place to walk nearby such as a park or sidewalks or weather is bad:* Always have activities that you can do indoors. Exercise to a video tape. Walk in the mall. Ride an exercise bike.
* *Family obligations take too much time:* Exercise with the kids, such as walking or swimming. Plan on exercising when kids are at school, playing or sleeping.

WHAT TO DO TO GET STARTED
* Plan on making exercise or physical activity a part of your everyday life. Do things you enjoy. Many people are getting their exercise doing things such as biking, skiing and tennis. Others prefer less active recreation such as walking, gardening or golf.
* Children and adults should try to get at least 30-60 minutes of exercise a day. You can break this into shorter periods of 10 or 15 minutes during the day.

PARTS OF AN EXERCISE PLAN
* Endurance: Find an activity that makes you breathe harder, on most or all days of the week. That's called "endurance activity," because it builds your stamina.
* Muscle strength: Lack of use lets muscles waste away. Start lifting weights and increase the weight slowly.
* Balance: Do things to help your balance. Stand on one foot, then the other, without holding onto anything for support. Walk heel-to-toe (the toes of the foot in back should almost touch the heel of the foot in front when you walk this way).
* Stretch: Stretching won't build your endurance or muscles, but it can help keep you limber and flexible.

SUGGESTIONS FOR BEING ACTIVE
* Walk, cycle, jog, or skate to work, school, stores, etc. Walk during breaks at work. Keep a comfortable pair of shoes handy in your office or car.
* Park the car farther away from where you want to go.
* Take the stairs instead of the elevator.
* Play actively with children or pets.
* Garden at home, or do home repair work.
* Exercise while watching television. Ride an exercise bike, walk in place, lift weights or stretch.

APPENDIX 19 (continued)

CAUTIONS
- Don't overdo the activity. Listen to your body. A few muscle aches are to be expected, but not pain.
- Start off a new routine at an easy pace. Then increase your time and effort. If you can talk without any trouble at all, your activity is probably too easy. If you can't talk at all, it's too hard.
- Use the correct equipment, especially shoes.
- Take 3-5 minutes to warm up. For example, start off a walk at a slow pace and then increase to a brisk pace.
- Be aware of any warning signs of heart problems: Severe sweating, chest and arm pain, and dizziness.
- Drink plenty of water to replace any lost fluids.

GLOSSARY

A

Abduction—Moving or pushing an arm or leg away from the median line of the body.

Acute—Symptoms that are severe and/or brief in duration.

Adduction—Moving or pulling an arm or leg toward the median line of the body.

Amenorrhea—Abnormal absence of menstrual periods.

Angiography—An x-ray study of blood vessels. The blood vessels to be studied are injected with a chemical that is opaque to x-rays, so abnormalities can be easily detected on the x-ray film.

Angulation—Deviation from a straight line, as in a badly set bone.

Anterior—The front part.

Anterior Cruciate Ligament Injury—A frequent injury to one of the important ligaments in the knee. Sometimes the extent of injury can be diagnosed simply. At other times, arthroscopic surgery is necessary for diagnosis. Most injuries to the anterior cruciate ligament can be repaired surgically with good results. Rehabilitation is as important in recovery as is precise surgical repair.

Antihypertensives—Medications used to treat high blood pressure (hypertension).

Arteriography—An x-ray procedure to study arteries. The arteries to be studied are injected with a chemical that is opaque to x rays, so abnormalities can be easily detected on the x-ray film.

Arthrogram—A diagnostic technique for examining the interior of an injured joint. The joints to be studied are injected with a chemical that is opaque to x-rays, so abnormalities can be easily detected on the x-ray film.

Arthroscopy—A procedure carried out with an arthroscope. An arthroscope is an instrument with a system of lenses and lights that enables a surgeon to view the inside of a joint. It is used most often to study the knee joint. Arthroscopy reveals abnormalities inside the joint. Some surgical procedures can also be accomplished with it. The opening into the joint is minimal, and healing is usually more rapid after arthroscopic surgery than after traditional surgery to repair an injured joint.

Aspiration—A surgical procedure to remove accumulated blood or fluid by suctioning through a needle and syringe.

Athlete's Heart—A normal, healthy, efficient heart in a well-conditioned athlete, but larger than the heart of someone of the same age, height and weight who is not well conditioned. An athlete's heart usually returns to "normal" size when conditioning ceases.

Atrophy—Wasting away of any part, organ, tissue or cell.

Audiometry—A test of the sense of hearing. Audiometry is usually done in a special soundproof room with sensitive devices that record the intensity of tone heard by the one being tested.

Aura—Unusual or bizarre sensations of sight, hearing, smell or taste that precede a seizure or migraine headache.

Avulsion—Forceful tearing away of any part of a structure.

B

Back Board—An inflexible board made of wood or plastic to keep an injured person's back from bending while being transported to an emergency room or hospital.

Beta-Adrenergic Blockers—A class or family of drugs that blocks the effects of adrenaline at selected sites in the sympathetic nervous system. There are many brands available in the United States by prescription. "Beta blockers" are used to reduce angina attacks, lower blood pressure, stabilize irregular heartbeat and reduce the frequency of migraine headaches. They are very useful and important drugs, but they must be taken under a doctor's supervision.

GLOSSARY

Biofeedback—A training process of providing visual or auditory evidence of the status of the musculoskeletal system, cardiovascular system, skin surface temperature and autonomic nervous system. Biofeedback practitioners work with patients to teach them to manage a number of problems, including reduction of stress levels, lowering of blood pressure, treatment of headaches and reduction of muscle spasm and pain. The instruments used in biofeedback training are very sensitive galvanometers that record minute changes in body function with great sensitivity.

Biopsy—Removal by surgery or aspiration of a small amount of tissue or fluid for laboratory examination and diagnosis. Biopsy is most often used to differentiate between cancerous and noncancerous tissue.

Blocker's Disease—An overgrowth of bone in the middle third of the arm (approximately where the deltoid muscle attaches to the humerus). It is caused by repeated injury at that site. This overgrowth may be termed an *exostosis or a myositis ossificans* if the bony part infiltrates a muscle.

Bone Scan—Nuclear medicine diagnostic test to identify areas of rapid turnover in bone (such as stress fractures, tumors, infections). Also known as a technetium bone scan or Tc 99 bone scan.

Bronchi (Bronchial Tubes)—Hollow air passages that branch from the largest segment (the windpipe or trachea) into the lungs. Oxygen-containing air passes into the lungs through the bronchial tubes, and waste gases (mostly carbon dioxide) pass out of the lungs through them.

Bronchioles—Tiny air passages (too small to be seen except through a microscope) that serve the same purpose as the bronchi.

Bronchoscopy—A surgical procedure using a bronchoscope, an instrument with lenses and lights that is inserted through the throat past the vocal cords and into the bronchial tubes.

After administering anesthesia, a surgeon passes the bronchoscope into the trachea and the largest branching segments of the bronchi. Foreign bodies that may have been inhaled accidentally can be removed. In addition, fluid may be removed or tissues may be biopsied and examined to detect tumors or infections.

Buerger's Disease (Thromboangiitis Obliterans)—A serious disease of unknown cause that leads to blockage of the small and medium arteries—usually in the legs and feet. Smoking, exposure to cold and any form of physical or emotional stress are important factors that make Buerger's disease more likely to occur.

C

Calcium Deposit—Abnormal hardening of soft tissue, usually from repeated injury.

Capillaries—The smallest (microscopic) blood vessels in the body. Capillaries form a network throughout the body through which substances can be exchanged between cells and the circulating blood. The substances exchanged include fluids, nourishment, waste materials, electrolytes, oxygen and carbon dioxide.

Carbohydrates, Complex—Starches and fiber found in food (mostly whole grains, fresh fruits and vegetables). Carbohydrates are essential for human nutrition, and complex carbohydrates are healthier than simple carbohydrates (sugars).

Carbohydrates, Simple—Sugars found in foods. Many high-carbohydrate foods are refined and depleted of their fiber and starch. Simple sugars are not as nutritious to human bodies as complex carbohydrates. "Junk foods" are frequently very high in simple carbohydrates. They cause a quick rise in blood sugar, followed by a sudden drop in blood sugar.

Carbonic Anhydrase Inhibitors—A class or family of drugs that inhibits the action of carbonic anhydrase, an enzyme. These medicines force the kidneys to excrete increased amounts of sodium and water, reducing excess body fluid.

Cardiovascular—Relating to the heart and blood vessels.

Cartilage—Rubbery, fibrous, dense connective tissue—harder than ligaments, softer than bone. Cartilage usually is found between bones and permits smooth movement of joints. It also helps shape flexible parts of the nose and external ear. The most frequent and significant cartilage injury associated with athletics is damage to the crescent-shaped cartilage in the knee (meniscus).

Cast—A stiff dressing or casing made of dressings impregnated with plaster of Paris or other hardening material such as plastic. Casts are used to immobilize various parts of the body in cases of fractures, dislocations and moderate or severe sprains.

CAT (Computerized Axial Tomography) Scan—See CT scan.

Caudad—Directed toward the tail; opposite of *cephalad*.

Cauterization—A surgical procedure to destroy tissue using a hot instrument, an electric current or a chemical substance.

Cephalad—Directed toward the head; opposite of *caudad*.

Cerebrospinal Fluid—Fluid that bathes the brain and the spinal cord.

Chondral—Pertaining to cartilage.

Chronic—The opposite of acute. Chronic means prolonged or slow to heal.

Circulatory System—The system that provides blood to the body. Parts of the system include the heart, arteries, arterioles, capillaries, venules, veins, blood, plasma and lymphatic vessels and fluid.

Circumduction Exercises—Active or passive circular exercise movements of any part of the body.

Colicky—Intermittent or fluctuating. Colicky pain usually refers to abdominal pain caused by spasms of the urinary tract or intestinal tract. The pain corresponds to strong contractions of surrounding involuntary muscles.

Compartment Syndrome—(1) Acute traumatically induced excess pressure in a muscle compartment. This may lead to pain, pressure, numbness, weakness or paralysis. If untreated, it may result in the permanent death of muscle bellies (the fleshy, contractile parts of muscles) and contracture of joints. (2) Chronic or exercise-induced periodic excess pressure in a muscle compartment (usually of the leg) associated with pain and decreased level of performance and relieved by rest.

Congestive Heart Failure—A complication of many serious diseases in which the heart loses its full pumping capacity. Blood backs up into other organs, especially the lungs, producing shortness of breath. Blood also backs up into the liver, causing production of fluid that distends the abdomen or accumulates in the feet, ankles and legs.

Connective Tissue—The body's supporting framework of tissue, consisting of strands of collagen, elastic fibers between muscles and around muscle groups and blood vessels, and simple cells.

Contracture—Shortening or distortion of a tissue, usually a muscle. Contractures may be temporary or may be permanent if caused by scar tissue.

Contusion—A bruising injury that does not break the skin. The brain can also be contused through the skull, usually leading to temporary unconsciousness.

COPD (Chronic Obstructive Pulmonary Disease)—A disease that results from any of several lung diseases—usually incurable—that lead to increasing breathing difficulty. The chronic diseases that lead to COPD include emphysema, asthma, chronic bronchitis, tuberculosis, fungus infections of the lung and bronchiectasis.

Corticosteroids—Synthetic medications similar in structure and function to natural hormones produced by the core of the adrenal glands. Cortisone, hydrocortisone, dexamethasone and others belong to the family of corticosteroid drugs.

Costochondral—Relating to the rib and its attached cartilage. *Costa* means rib. *Chondral* means cartilage.

Cotton Mouth—Dry mouth from dehydration or anxiety. People with "cotton mouth" spit whitish sputum that looks like cotton.

Crazy Bone—See Funny Bone.

Crepitation—The sensation that small balloons or pockets of air beneath the skin are breaking when the skin is pressed with the fingers. Crepitation also refers to the grating feeling produced when two joint surfaces rub against each other.

Cryokinetics—The use of cold for physical therapy.

Cryosurgery—A simple surgical procedure in which tissue is destroyed by below-freezing temperatures. Liquid nitrogen is frequently used as the freezing chemical agent in cryosurgery.

CT (Computerized Tomography) Scan—Previously called CAT scan. A computerized x-ray procedure that provides exceptionally clear images of parts of the body. CT scans aid in the diagnosis of disorders that may not be diagnosed by less sophisticated x-ray studies.

Culture—The growth of microscopic organisms (viruses, bacteria or fungi) or cells in a special environment that supports them so they can be examined.

Cutaneous—Relating to the skin.

Cystoscopy—Examination of the inside of the lower urinary tract using a cystoscope. A cystoscope has a special system of lenses and lights. It is passed from the urethra into the bladder. The cystoscope is used for examination of the bladder and ureters, some surgical procedures on the prostate gland and biopsies of tissue inside the bladder.

D

Delirium—A brief, reversible mental disturbance characterized by delusions, hallucinations, emotional excitement, physical restlessness and incoherence. Delirium can be caused by infections, head injuries, decreased blood supply to the brain, medications and psychotic disorders.

Diathermy—Heating deep within body tissues that is done with a special machine. Tissues can be heated without damaging the skin. Diathermy was once popular in physical therapy, but other treatments are now more common.

Displacement—Removal from the normal position or place.

Distal—Distant from a midline or other point of reference. The opposite of *distal* is *proximal.*

Diuretics—A class or family of drugs used to force the kidney to excrete more sodium than usual. Increased sodium excretion causes increased water excretion, so urine volume increases. The increased sodium excretion is desirable and therapeutic in disorders causing abnormal fluid retention (edema) due to heart failure, liver failure or kidney failure. Unfortunately, some diuretics increase excretion of potassium, which must be replaced—usually with potassium supplements—to avoid serious adverse effects.

Dorsal Spine—The vertebral bodies below the neck and above the lumbar spine. Also known as the thoracic spine. Dorsal spine vertebrae have ribs attached.

Dorsiflexion—Backward bending, especially of the hand or foot.

E

Ear, Nose & Throat (ENT) Specialist—A physician with special postgraduate training in diagnosing and treating disorders and diseases of the ear, nose and throat.

Ecchymosis—A small area of bleeding under the skin or mucous membrane forming a non-elevated, rounded or irregular blue or purplish patch.

ECG (Electrocardiogram)—A graphic representation of the electrical current generated by the electrical system that controls heart muscle cells. The ECG is a useful tool in diagnosing the presence and severity of many forms of heart disease. However, the heart may be severely impaired and still show no typical or characteristic ECG changes, so the ECG is only one of the tools used to detect and monitor heart disorders.

Edema—Accumulation of abnormal quantities of fluid in spaces between the cells of the body. Edema can occur in almost any location in the body. The most common sites include the feet and ankles, skin, abdomen, liver and brain.

EEG (Electroencephalogram)—A recording of electrical activity in the brain. An EEG is done with a galvanometer connected to electrodes attached to the skull. The EEG is useful in detecting brain damage and in diagnosing seizure and sleep disorders.

Electrolytes—Chemicals dissolved in the blood and inside body cells. Electrolytes play an essential role in all body functions and must be maintained within narrow limits to preserve health. The major electrolytes include sodium, potassium, chloride, calcium, phosphorus, magnesium and carbon dioxide. They are ingested through food. The kidneys and lungs regulate the rate at which they are excreted. Levels that are too high or too low in body cells can lead to serious illnesses, including heart rhythm disturbances, fluid accumulation, dehydration and dangerously low blood pressure. In the worst cases, electrolyte disturbances can be life-threatening.

Electromyogram—A recording of the electrical activity of nerve and muscle cells, measured with an extremely sensitive galvanometer. The electromyogram is used to help detect and diagnose a variety of disorders of the peripheral nerves and muscles.

Erythema—Redness and warmth of the skin caused by congestion of the capillaries. Erythema may be caused by many factors, including infection, sunburn, inflammation or direct injury.

Erythema Multiforme—A disease characterized by a vivid red skin eruption that appears suddenly on the face, neck, forearms, legs, feet and hands. This disorder results from hypersensitivity to some drugs and also sometimes appears spontaneously—probably as a result of a defect in the immune system.

Etiology—The cause of a disease or injury.

Eversion—An outward turning.

F

Fatigue Fracture—Also known as a stress fracture. A bony fracture produced by repetitive low-level forces rather than a single large trauma. Fatigue fractures may not be initially apparent in x-rays.

Fibrosis—The formation of fibrous tissue. Fibrosis is caused by many factors, including injury, inflammation and infection.

Fibrositis—An inflammatory condition affecting connective tissues and muscles, joints, ligaments and tendons. Fibrositis has many causes, including repeated injury, infections or overuse of a part. The disease usually resolves itself without treatment, but recurrence is frequent.

Flank—The area of the body that extends from the bottom of the ribs to the upper edge of the hip on either side of the body.

Flatulence—Intestinal gaseousness caused by failure of the intestines to completely process some complex carbohydrates, such as those found in beans, onions and bran. Exercise may increase flatulence, because it hastens the passage of food through the

GLOSSARY

intestinal tract, sometimes not allowing enough time for complete digestion.

Fracture—A break in a bone, cartilage, tooth or other rigid body tissue.

Fungus—A microorganism that causes infection of the skin; mucous membranes of the mouth, vagina or rectum; or other organs (particularly the lungs).

Funny Bone (Crazy Bone)—Where the ulnar nerve passes through a groove on the inner side of the elbow joint. When injured, it produces a disabling, temporary burning and numbness along the inner side of the forearm and hand.

G

Gastrointestinal (GI) Tract—The digestive tract, beginning with the mouth, continuing through the esophagus, stomach, duodenum, small intestine and large intestine, and ending in the rectum. The GI tract is about 26 feet long.

H

Heartburn—A burning sensation in the chest perceived as arising from the region of the heart. Heartburn is not related to heart disease. It is caused by stomach acid or stomach contents that spill into the lower esophagus, irritating the sensitive membrane lining it.

Hemarthrosis—Collection of blood in a joint from broken capillaries or larger blood vessels.

Hematocrit—A blood test to detect anemia and other blood disorders. The test shows what percentage of whole blood is occupied by red blood cells. The normal hematocrit range is 35% to 45%. The remainder of the blood is made up of white blood cells, platelets, serum, plasma and electrolytes. The hematocrit range varies with age and sex.

Hematoma—A dome-shaped collection of blood—usually clotted—under the skin, the scalp or inside the abdomen. The hematoma is formed by bleeding from a broken blood vessel.

Hemoglobin—A chemical component of red blood cells that carries oxygen from air breathed in to all cells in the body. The blood test for hemoglobin is used to detect anemia and other blood disorders. The normal hemoglobin range is 12 to 18 grams per 100 cubic centimeters.

Hernia—Protrusion of an organ or tissue through an abnormal opening.

Hip Pointer—A bruise or contusion of the top part of the ilium, one of the bones of the pelvis.

Hyaluronidase—An enzyme that neutralizes the adverse effects of hyaluronic acid, the cement substance of tissues.

Hyper—A prefix meaning above, beyond or excessive. For example, *hyperextended* means bent beyond normal limits; *hyperventilation* means excessive breathing.

Hypo—A prefix meaning below or deficient. For example, *hypogastric* means below the stomach; *hypoglycemia* means too little sugar in the blood.

I

Id Reaction—A rash associated with, but located remotely from, the main lesions of a disease. The cause is probably an allergic or hypersensitive reaction to the germ causing the original disease. A common example is an itchy rash with blisters that appears on the hands and forearms of people who have athlete's foot.

Iliotibial Band Syndrome—Pain in the knee region (common in runners). The pain is caused by injury to the iliotibial tract—a fibrous band that forms a ligament that helps support and stabilize the knee. Treatment consists of rest, physical therapy, rehabilitation and occasionally surgery.

Incision—A cut made with a sharp instrument through the skin or other tissue.

Inflammation—A protective tissue response to injury or destruction of tissues. Signs of inflammation include pain, warmth, redness, swelling and loss of function. While inflammation is a part of the normal healing process, it may become self-sustaining and thus require treatment.

Insulin—A hormone manufactured in the pancreas that facilitates the metabolism of glucose (sugar) by the body's cells. A deficiency in the production of insulin results in the disease *diabetes mellitus* (sugar diabetes).

Intravenous—Inside a vein. Medications, electrolyte solutions (such as saline or potassium) and blood transfusions are given intravenously through a needle inserted into a vein.

Inversion—To turn inward.

Ipsilateral—The same side of the body.

J

Joint Capsule—The thin, cartilaginous, fatty, fibrous, membranous structure that envelopes a joint. Fluid inside the joint capsule lubricates the area, allowing bones to glide smoothly against each other.

K

Knee, Internal Derangement of—Injury to any of the internal structures of the knee joint, including the meniscus (articular cartilage), ligaments, tendons, fat pad under the patella (kneecap) and the uppermost part of the tibia (the major bone in the lower leg).

L

Laryngoscope—An instrument used to inspect and treat the muscular structures in the larynx and vocal cords.

Lateral—Toward the outside or away from a midline.

Lesion—A wound, injury or abnormal skin growth.

Ligament—A band of fibrous tissue that connects bone to bone or cartilage to bone, supporting and strengthening a joint.

Lumbar Spine—The vertebral bodies below the dorsal spine and above the sacrum. These are mobile vertebrae without attached ribs.

Lupus Erythematosus—An inflammatory disease of the connective tissues, believed to be caused by a defect in the body's immune system, in which the body attacks its own normal tissues.

Luxation—Dislocation of bones in a joint so that they are no longer in the correct functional positions relative to each other. *Subluxation* means an incomplete or partial dislocation.

M

Massage—Therapeutic kneading and stroking of skin and muscles.

Medial—Toward the midline or closer to a midline than any other structure. For example, the breastbone (sternum) is medial to the right rib cage.

Mind-Altering Drugs—Drugs or medications that interfere with normal function of the brain. This group includes narcotics such as heroin, morphine, Demerol and codeine; major tranquilizers; hallucinogenic agents such as LSD; marijuana; cocaine; amphetamines; and barbiturates and other sedatives.

Moleskin—A heavy, downy cotton twill material used to wrap around joints for support or to protect the skin under bandages, splints or casts. It is also used to reduce friction over tender skin.

MRI (Magnetic Resonance Imaging)—A special radiological study that allows visualization of scarred or damaged areas of the brain. The MRI is useful in diagnosing epilepsy and other disorders of the brain and central nervous system.

Muscle—An organ that produces movement by contractions. There are two major kinds of muscles: voluntary (striated) and involuntary

GLOSSARY

(nonstriated). Striated muscles are under voluntary control and include most of the muscles in the body. Involuntary muscles form the largest mass of the heart and surround blood vessels, lymphatic vessels, the urinary tract and the intestinal tract.

N

Necrosis—Death. Tissue death (avascular necrosis) results from deprivation of blood supply.

Neuritis—Any inflammatory condition of a nerve. Neuritis may have many causes, including injury. Treatment is difficult and recurrence frequent.

Nonsteroidal Anti-Inflammatory Drugs (NSAIDs)—Oral and injectable medications that interrupt the inflammation cascade and thereby eliminate symptoms. (While steroids can fight inflammation, they are classified differently.).

O

Oligomenorrhea—Abnormally infrequent or irregular menstruation.

Ophthalmologist—A medical doctor who specializes in medical or surgical disorders of the eye.

Oral Surgeon—A dentist who specializes in tooth extractions and surgery on the gums and other structures in the mouth.

Osteomalacia—A condition characterized by softening of the bones. Symptoms include pain, tenderness, muscle weakness and weight loss. The cause is a deficiency in vitamin D and calcium.

Osteomyelitis—Infection of the bone and bone marrow, frequently associated with open (compound) fractures of bones. The broken skin accompanying such fractures allows bacteria to enter the injured area and infect injured tissues. Bone has relatively poor resistance to infection because of its sparse blood supply.

Overtraining Syndrome—A group of symptoms caused by overwork of muscles and other tissues during vigorous athletic activity. The outstanding symptom is pain in muscles, bones or joints. The first symptoms include dull aching of the joints after a hard workout. If training continues at the same level of intensity, pain will occur during and after workouts. The only successful treatment is to decrease the level of activity until the symptoms disappear. Training can then be resumed as long as symptoms don't reappear.

P

Pain—A sensation of discomfort, hurt, stress or agony resulting from stimulation of specialized nerve endings. Pain means something is wrong, and it should not be ignored. The saying "No pain, no gain" is outmoded.

Periodic Paralysis—A rare disease characterized by a rapidly progressive form of paralysis associated with abnormal serum potassium levels. This is an inherited disease. Attacks may be triggered by vigorous exercise. They are more likely to occur on the day following a workout rather than during the workout.

PET (Positron Emission Tomography)—A sophisticated, expensive radiological procedure that allows visualization of various parts of the body not observable by more traditional x-ray studies.

Phonophoresis—The use of ultrasound to enhance the delivery of topically applied drugs. The procedure enables the drugs to penetrate through the skin more effectively and reach an injured area of muscle, tendon or other tissue.

Plantar Fasciitis—A partial or complete tear in the fascia (fibrous connective tissue) on the bottom of the foot. It is characterized by pain just under the heel bone. Causes include inadequate arch supports, poorly fitting shoes or shoes with soles that are too stiff, sudden turns or stops and weak ankles. Rest is the only successful treatment.

Plantar Flexion—Bending or pointing of the toes toward the floor.

Plastic Surgeon—A medical doctor who specializes in surgery concerned with the restoration, reconstruction, correction or improvement in the shape and appearance of body structures that are defective or misshapen by injury, disease or growth and development.

Platelets—Blood cells (smaller than red or white blood cells) that assist in the blood-clotting process.

Podiatrist—A doctor who specializes in the diagnosis and treatment of medical and surgical problems of the feet.

Polycythemia—An abnormal increase in the red blood cells of the body. The disease has 3 forms: (1) Polycythemia vera, which involves overproduction of red blood cells, white blood cells and platelets.
(2) Secondary polycythemia, a complication of diseases or factors other than blood cell disorders. (3) Stress polycythemia, which is associated with decreased blood plasma. Stress polycythemia can occur in athletes who become dehydrated during competition or heavy workouts in very hot weather. Secondary polycythemia and stress polycythemia are curable by correcting the underlying cause.

Popliteal Space—The space behind the knee joint. The space is bounded by ligaments and contains soft tissues including nerves, fat, membranes and blood vessels.

Porphyria—A serious inherited disease of the metabolism characterized by excretion of porphyrins. Attacks can be triggered by pregnancy, excessive exposure to sunlight and use of barbiturates or birth control pills.

Posterior—The rear part.

Postural Drainage—A physical therapy procedure for treating chronic lung diseases such as bronchiectasis or lung abscess. The patient is placed so that the part of the lung involved is higher than the trachea and the head. Forced coughing in this position helps clear the lungs and bronchial tubes of harmful accumulated secretions.

Prodrome—An early warning symptom of illness. For example, a migraine headache may be preceded by a pins-and-needles sensation in an extremity or by an aura that is composed of visual symptoms.

Prognosis—Prediction of the course of an injury or disease, including its end result.

Progressive Resistance Exercise (PRE)—Exercise that forces muscles into bearing heavier and heavier loads.

Pronation—Rotation of a body part (usually the hand or foot) backward, inward or downward. The muscles in the forearm can produce pronation of the hand; the muscles in the lower leg can produce pronation of the foot.

Proteinuria—Passing of protein in the urine. This is sometimes associated with kidney disease, but it may occur normally following many forms of strenuous exercise such as rowing, football, track, long-distance running, swimming and calisthenics. There is no evidence that exercise-induced proteinuria increases the risk of developing chronic kidney disease.

Proximal—Nearest to a point of reference. The opposite of *proximal* is *distal*.

Pulmonary—Pertaining to all parts of the lung.

Pyelogram—A special x-ray study of the urinary tract in which dye is injected into a vein and x-rays are done repeatedly to follow the dye's progress through the urinary tract.

R

Radioactive Technetium Study—See Bone Scan.

Radioactive Uptake Studies—Special x-ray studies showing concentration of injected radioactive materials in various tissues and organs of the body.

GLOSSARY

Retina—One of the three major segments of the eye. The retina is located in the back of the eyeball, and it has many layers. The layers of the retina contain blood vessels, nerve endings and the specialized rods and cones that make it possible for us to distinguish shapes and colors.

Rotator Cuff—A structure around the shoulder joint capsule composed of intermingled muscle and tendon fibers. The rotator cuff provides stability and strength to the shoulder joint.

Rupture—Forcible tearing or disruption of a tissue.

S

Secondary Infection—An infection that follows and sometimes complicates a primary infection. A secondary infection is usually caused by a different germ than the one that caused the first infection. For example, a secondary bacterial skin infection on the feet can occur over a preexisting fungus infection on the feet.

Sedatives—Drugs to lessen anxiety or excitement. Most effective sedatives are habit-forming.

Soft Tissues—All tissues of the body except bone.

Sonogram—A diagnostic test in which high-frequency sound waves are transmitted into the body. Their reflections or echoes create images of body organs or the outline of a fetus.

Spearing—An aggressive move in which a person butts his or her helmeted head into the chest or midsection of an opponent. This is a hazardous maneuver that may cause neck injury to the aggressor and severe direct injury to the opponent.

Spine Board—An inflexible board (also called a back board) made of wood or plastic that immobilizes the spine while an injured person is transported to an emergency facility.

Splint—A rigid support made from metal, plaster or plastic and used to immobilize an injured or inflamed part of the body.

Spondylolisthesis—Spondylolysis with displacement of one of the vertebral bones forward of the one below.

Spondylolysis—A congenital defect in which a small area of bone in the spine does not fuse completely. This causes weakness in the spine and makes it subject to more frequent and more serious injury. People with spondylolysis should probably not engage in heavy lifting or in contact sports.

Stitch in the Side—Pain, usually in the upper abdomen, accompanying vigorous physical activity. This is probably caused by spasm of the diaphragm, the big muscle that separates the chest from the abdomen and that moves with breathing. Treatment is to stop exercise until the pain disappears.

Stress Fracture—See Fatigue Fracture.

Subacute—An intermediate stage in the progress of an injury or disease that is between acute and chronic, closer in nature to the acute stage than the chronic.

Subcutaneous—Below the skin.

Subluxation—Incomplete or partial dislocation of bones in a joint, usually associated with an injury to the attached ligaments.

Supination—Rotation of a hand or foot outward on its long axis. The movement is done with the muscles of the forearm or lower leg.

Syncope—Fainting—a mild form of shock with a short period of unconsciousness and usually a rapid recovery.

Synovium—A thin layer of connective tissue with a free smooth surface that lines the capsule of a joint. Synovial fluid lubricates and facilitates movements of the joint.

T

Technetium Scan—See Bone Scan.

Tenderness—Discomfort produced when any injured area is touched or pressed.

Tendon—A fibrous cord by which a muscle is attached to a bone.

Thoracic Spine—See Dorsal Spine.

Tinnitus—Ringing in the ears caused by a disorder of the eighth cranial nerve. Disorders can be caused by virus infections, occasionally by blood clots to the brain and commonly by taking medications such as aspirin.

Traction—A form of physical therapy in which a pulling force is exerted on a muscle or joint.

Tranquilizers—A class or family of drugs used to lessen anxiety or nervousness. Most major tranquilizers are habit-forming.

Trauma—A direct wound or injury.

Triad, Unhappy—A classic football injury that results from being hit on the lateral side of the knee with the foot on the ground. The blow causes sprains of the medial collateral ligament and the anterior cruciate ligament and tears the meniscus (knee cartilage). This injury usually requires surgery to repair.

U

Ultrasound—A form of physical therapy in which deep heat is applied to an injured area using sound waves that are outside the normal range of human hearing. Ultrasound treatments require special equipment and professional supervision.

Ultrasound, Diagnostic—Use of sound waves to examine the structures of the body. It is especially significant for tendon and muscle injuries in sports medicine, but is also utilized to view the kidneys and the uterus or a developing fetus.

Ultrasound, Therapeutic—A form of physical therapy in which deep heat is applied to an injured area using ultrasound waves that are outside the normal range of human hearing. Ultrasound treatments require special equipment and professional supervision.

V

Vesicle—A fluid-containing, blisterlike skin eruption. For example, the lesions of chickenpox are vesicles.

Vitiligo—A loss of pigment in scattered areas of the skin.

W

Whiplash—A nonmedical popular term meaning an injury to the neck caused by hyperextension and/or hyperflexion.

Whirlpool—Equipment that provides turbulent water and is used to treat many athletic injuries.

X

X-rays—Diagnostic procedures to study internal structures not visible to the naked eye.

Y

Yeast—A general term applied to single-budding microscopic fungus cells. Yeast infections can occur on the skin, mucous membranes and organs of the body, such as the lungs.

INDEX

INDEX

INDEX

INDEX

INDEX

INDEX

INDEX

EMERGENCY FIRST AID

ANAPHYLAXIS (Severe Allergic Reaction)

Symptoms

Itching, rash, hives, runny nose, wheezing, shortness of breath, paleness, cold sweats, low blood pressure, coma, cardiac arrest.

Treatment

If Victim Is Unconscious, Not Breathing:

1. Yell for help. Don't leave the victim.
2. Have someone dial 911 (emergency) for an ambulance or medical help.
3. Begin mouth-to-mouth breathing immediately.
4. If there is no heartbeat, give external cardiac massage.
5. Don't stop cardiopulmonary resuscitation (CPR) until help arrives.

If Victim Is Unconscious and Breathing:

1. Dial 911 (emergency) for an ambulance or emergency medical help. Have the person lie down with feet elevated.
2. If you can't get help immediately, take patient to nearest emergency facility.

BLEEDING

Symptoms

Bright red blood pumping from an injured artery or darker blood if a large vein has been injured. Bleeding caused by any serious injury should be treated in an emergency facility.

Treatment

1. Dial 911 (emergency) for an ambulance or emergency medical help.
2. If you can't get help immediately, take patient to nearest emergency facility.
3. Cover entire injured area using a thick sterile pad or clean cloth, towel, or similar material or hands. Place the pad directly over the entire wound, and press firmly with the heel of your hand. If the wound is in a limb (and no bone injury), elevate it above the heart. This helps reduce blood flow.
4. Apply strong pressure directly to injured area for 10 minutes or more while awaiting ambulance or while transporting victim to emergency facility.
5. If bleeding continues, apply indirect pressure. Press the artery at the next pressure point (pressure points are difficult and sometimes dangerous to use, and should only be used by someone trained in first aid).
6. Cover and/or dress the wound as soon as possible.

CONVULSIONS

Symptoms

Unconsciousness; jerking or twitching of the arms, legs or face; loss of bowel or bladder control (sometimes). After consciousness is regained, memory loss.

Treatment

1. When the victim begins to fall, soften the fall by catching his body, laying it down gently and turning the head to one side.
2. Don't restrain the person. Clear the area of any objects so the victim won't be injured.
3. Don't try to separate the teeth or insert objects to keep the patient from biting his tongue. Doing so can cause injury.
4. Don't throw ice water on the patient.
5. Don't attempt to force water or any fluid until the patient is fully conscious and asks for fluids.
6. Call for medical help, and stay with any patient who has a convulsion immediately after the first convulsion. Also stay with any pregnant woman who has a convulsion.

FRACTURES, DISLOCATIONS OR SEVERE SPRAINS

Symptoms

Extreme pain and tenderness in the injured area; change in appearance of injured part, such as swelling, protruding bone or blood under skin. An extremity, such as a finger, arm or leg, may be bent out of normal alignment.

Treatment

1. Dial 911 (emergency) for an ambulance or emergency medical help.
2. Control any bleeding (see page 557).
3. Treat all fractures in the position found if possible. Gently support the injured part by hand, place the victim in a comfortable position, and support with rolled up blankets.
4. If emergency help is delayed, immobilize the injured part by securing it to not injured part of the body with padding and bandages, arm to body, leg to leg.
5. If leg, back or neck is severely injured and possibly fractured or dislocated, keep patient warm and immobilized until the ambulance arrives. Don't move the victim.
6. Watch for signs of shock (see page 560).

HEAD, NECK OR BACK INJURY

Symptoms

Head injury: Drowsiness or confusion; vomiting and nausea; blurred vision; pupils of different sizes; loss of consciousness—either temporarily or for long periods; amnesia or memory lapses; irritability; headache; bleeding of the scalp if the skin is broken.

Neck or back injury: Pain in the neck or back; paralysis or difficulty moving; loss of sensation in the extremities.

Treatment

1. Assume that all injuries to the head (including the face), neck or back—whether the patient is conscious or unconscious—may also involve damage to the spinal cord.
2. Call 911 (emergency) for an ambulance or medical help.
3. Avoid moving the patient if at all possible.
4. If the injured person is unconscious and lying face down so he or she cannot breathe, obtain assistance from several people to carefully support the entire body, and roll it to one side. Use a rolled-up blanket, pillows or other such objects to stabilize the victim's head to keep it from moving.
5. Give mouth-to-mouth breathing if the victim is not breathing but has a heartbeat.
6. If there is no heartbeat, give external cardiac massage.
7. Don't stop cardiopulmonary resuscitation (CPR) until help arrives.

HEART ATTACK

Symptoms

Chest pain that lasts more than 2 minutes and radiates into the jaw or arm; unexplained heavy sweating; weakness; nausea; pale skin; irregular pulse.

Treatment

If Victim Is Unconscious, Not Breathing:

1. Yell for help. Don't leave the victim.
2. Have someone dial 911 (emergency) for an ambulance or medical help.
3. Begin mouth-to-mouth breathing immediately.
4. If there is no heartbeat, give external cardiac massage.
5. Don't stop cardiopulmonary resuscitation (CPR) until help arrives.

If Victim Is Unconscious and Breathing:

1. Dial 911 (emergency) for an ambulance or emergency medical help.
2. If you can't get help immediately, take patient to nearest emergency facility.

SHOCK

Symptoms

Moist, cold, pale skin; fast, weak pulse; rapid breathing; disorientation or confusion; anxiety with feelings of impending doom; low blood pressure (sometimes so low that it cannot be read); unconsciousness (sometimes).

Treatment

1. Loosen tight clothing. Then, cover the person with a coat or blanket to prevent heat loss. You can lie down next to and hug the person to share your body heat until help arrives. Place insulation between the person and the ground. Do not use hot-water bottles or electric blankets to try to warm the person.
2. Check for breathing and pulse every so often.
3. Do not give any food or liquids. If the person asks for water, moisten the lips, but do not allow him or her to drink any fluids.
4. If the person vomits, roll him or her on the side so the vomit does not back up into the windpipe and lungs.

Conversion to Metric Measures

When You Know	Symbol	Multiply By	To Find	Symbol
VOLUME				
teaspoons	tsp.	4.93	milliliters	ml
tablespoons	tbsp.	14.79	milliliters	ml
fluid ounces	fl. oz.	29.57	milliliters	ml
cups	c.	0.24	liters	l
pints	pt.	0.47	liters	l
quarts	qt.	0.95	liters	l
gallons	gal.	3.79	liters	l
LENGTH				
inches	in.	25.4	millimeters	mm
inches	in.	2.54	centimeters	cm
feet	ft.	30.48	centimeters	cm
yards	yd.	0.91	meters	m
TEMPERATURE				
Fahrenheit	F	0.56 (after subtracting 32)	Celsius	C